Autism and Child Psychopathology Series

Series Editor

Johnny L. Matson, Department of Psychology,
Louisiana State University, Baton Rouge, LA, USA

Brief Overview

The purpose of this series is to advance knowledge in the broad multidisciplinary fields of autism and various forms of psychopathology (e.g., anxiety and depression). Volumes synthesize research on a range of rapidly expanding topics on assessment, treatment, and etiology.

Description

The **Autism and Child Psychopathology Series** explores a wide range of research and professional methods, procedures, and theories used to enhance positive development and outcomes across the lifespan. Developments in education, medicine, psychology, and applied behavior analysis as well as child and adolescent development across home, school, hospital, and community settings are the focus of this series. Series volumes are both authored and edited, and they provide critical reviews of evidence-based methods. As such, these books serve as a critical reference source for researchers and professionals who deal with developmental disorders and disabilities, most notably autism, intellectual disabilities, challenging behaviors, anxiety, depression, ADHD, developmental coordination disorder, communication disorders, and other common childhood problems. The series addresses important mental health and development difficulties that children and youth, their caregivers, and the professionals who treat them must face. Each volume in the series provides an analysis of methods and procedures that may assist in effectively treating these developmental problems.

More information about this series at http://www.springer.com/series/8665

Johnny L. Matson
Editor

Functional Assessment for Challenging Behaviors and Mental Health Disorders

Second Edition

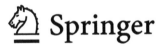 Springer

Editor
Johnny L. Matson
Department of Psychology
Louisiana State University
Baton Rouge, LA, USA

ISSN 2192-922X   ISSN 2192-9238   (electronic)
Autism and Child Psychopathology Series
ISBN 978-3-030-66269-1   ISBN 978-3-030-66270-7   (eBook)
https://doi.org/10.1007/978-3-030-66270-7

This Springer imprint is published by the registered company Springer Nature Switzerland AG
The registered company address is: Gewerbestrasse 11, 6330 Cham, Switzerland

Describe the Book and Its Content

This book is an update and expansion of a successful book published by the proposed editor in 2012 entitled *Functional Assessment for Challenging Behaviors* (Springer). In addition to updating existing chapters, new chapters have been added, including a chapter on definitions and rationale, a general overview, research on mental health disorders, report writing, the role of treatment planning, and treatment associated with mental health disorders.

The book is organized into parts. The topic of the first part is foundations and consists of four chapters that define the field of functional assessment while also providing a rational for the approach along with historical background information. The second part consists of 10 chapters that cover various aspects of assessment, which constitutes the core of functional assessment. There are various techniques such as tests, observational methods, and experimental functional assessment. The chapters describe specific techniques and the research that has emerged to support them. Finally, five chapters are included in a part on treatment. Topics covered include how functional assessment helps guide what treatments are selected and also report on the studies that have emerged. Also, due to the nature of the vulnerable population (i.e., autism, intellectual disabilities, mental health, and children), a chapter on informed consent and ethical issues is also included.

Targeted Market Segments

The focus of the volume is graduate students and professionals in psychology, special education, psychiatry, school psychology, and rehabilitation psychology. Special emphasis is on Board Certified Behavior Analysts (BCBA), BCBA's in training, and departments of applied behavior analysis.

Keywords

Functional assessment; Experimental functional analysis; Questions about behavior function; Applied behavior analysis; Anxiety; Challenging behaviors; Assessment; Autism; Intellectual disabilities

Contents

About the Editor

Johnny L. Matson, Ph.D. is professor and distinguished research master in the Department of Psychology at LSU. He has served as major professor for 71 Ph.D.s over a 42-year career and has over 850 publications including 48 books. He is founding editor of the *Review Journal of Autism and Developmental Disorders*.

Part I
Foundations

Chapter 1
Definition and Rationale for Functional Assessment

Jeff Sigafoos, Russell Lang, and Mandy Rispoli

Introduction

Assessment is widely acknowledged to be a necessary and fundamental component of any therapeutic, rehabilitation, behavioral, or education intervention (Goldstein, Allen, & Deluca, 2019; Pierangelo & Giuliani, 2017; Strauser, Tansey, & Chan, 2020). Kramer, Bernstein, and Phares (2019), for example, view assessment as a critical, if not dominant, part of clinical psychology practice. They further argue that assessment is essential for understanding the problems that precipitate intervention referral. Strauser and Greco (2020) explain that assessment has long been viewed as a critical service within the broad rehabilitation field—a field that includes mental health counseling. In behaviorally based treatment programs, assessment underpins several indispensable steps of the intervention process. For example, various types of assessment protocols are implemented to assist clinicians in (a) identifying, defining, and prioritizing target behaviors, (b) recording focal dimensions of target behaviors (e.g., frequency, latency, and duration), and (c) scrutinizing a range of variables to ascertain their influence, if any, on the expression of target behaviors (O'Brien, Oemig, & Northern, 2010). Shute, Leighton, Jang, and Chu (2016) reviewed the long history of educational assessment and called for its expansion to achieve "rigorous and ubiquitous measurement of the whole student learning

J. Sigafoos (✉)
School of Education, Victoria University of Wellington, Wellington, New Zealand
e-mail: jeff.sigafoos@vuw.ac.nz

R. Lang
Department of Curriculum and Instruction, Texas State University, San Marcos, TX, USA
e-mail: rl30@txstate.edu

M. Rispoli
Department of Special Education, Purdue University, West Lafayette, IN, USA
e-mail: mrispoli@purdue.edu

© Springer Nature Switzerland AG 2021
J. L. Matson (ed.), *Functional Assessment for Challenging Behaviors and Mental Health Disorders*, Autism and Child Psychopathology Series,
https://doi.org/10.1007/978-3-030-66270-7_1

experience" (p. 34). These examples illustrate the general consensus regarding the need for assessment and its intrinsic link into the overall intervention process. This is true of many fields including clinical and educational psychology, rehabilitation, general and special education, speech-language pathology, social work, and occupational therapy (Brown, Stoffel, & Muñoz, 2019; Chan et al., 2020; Frey, 2019; Groth-Marnat & Wright, 2016; Jordan & Franklin, 2015; Matson, 2007; Shipley & McAfee, 2016).

The need for, and value of, assessment is particularly clear when it comes to the treatment of challenging behavior and mental health disorders (Callaghan, 2019; Matson, 2007, 2012; Matson & Williams, 2014). Challenging behaviors, such as verbal and physical aggression, disruptive behavior, destruction of property, irritability, self-injury, stereotyped movements, and tantrums, are prevalent among children and adults with various types of disability (Bowring, Totsika, Hastings, Toogood, & Griffith, 2017; Simó-Pinatella, Mumbardó-Adam, Alomar-Kurz, Sugai, & Simonsen, 2019). Challenging behavior is also frequently seen in persons with dementia (Stokes, 2000), and among individuals who have experienced traumatic brain injury resulting in loss of behavioral inhibition (McNett, Sarver, & Wilczewski, 2012). Mental health disorders (e.g., anxiety, obsessive-compulsive disorder, conduct disorder, emotional and behavioral disorders, hallucinations, delusions, disordered speech, and depression) are also found in such populations, as well as in the general population (Alderman, 2003; Downs et al., 2018; Einfeld, Ellis, & Emerson, 2011; Fodstad, 2019; Froján-Parga, de Prado-Gordillo, Álvarez-Iglesias, & Alonso-Vega, 2019; Scholten et al., 2016; Whitney & Peterson, 2019).

It is well established that challenging behavior and mental health disorders can—depending on their topography, frequency, and severity—result in serious negative consequences both in the short term and in the long term (Pilgrim, 2020). Self-injurious behavior and aggression directed toward others, for example, can lead to serious physical injury to the person's self and others, respectively (Huisman et al., 2018; Tremblay, 2002). Additional negative impacts can arise across a host of cognitive, developmental, and adaptive functioning domains. Adverse effects may be seen in the areas of learning, academic achievement, emotional and social development, physical health, participation (e.g., community, educational, and vocational participation), peer acceptance, and overall quality of life (Bruffaerts et al., 2018; Evans, Banerjee, Leese, & Huxley, 2007; Gur, 2017; Matson, Sipes, Fodstad, & Fitzgerald, 2011).

In light of these potential adverse outcomes, provision of effective intervention is essential. Intervention specifically aimed at preventing and reducing challenging behavior and promoting mental health should be major priorities for individuals with or at risk for exhibiting challenging behavior or developing mental health disorders. Assessment has a critical role in the development of preventative and treatment programs for challenging behavior and mental health disorders. Designing and implementing effective intervention will depend, to a large extent, on obtaining reliable and valid assessment data. Along these lines, certain types of assessment data, specifically data obtained from one or more functional assessment methods, are increasingly being recognized as key elements in the design of effective therapeutic supports for individuals with, or at risk of developing, challenging behavior (Dixon, Vogel, & Tarbox, 2012) and/or mental health disorders (Daffern & Howells, 2002; Davies et al., 2019).

The present chapter aims to define and contextualize the broad class of functional assessment methods that have been used to inform treatments for challenging behavior and mental health disorders. Matson and Williams (2014) pointed out that functional assessment is "a foundational strategy" that underpins contemporary [behavioral] interventions aimed at reducing challenging behavior (p. 58). Indeed, developing interventions for challenging behaviors based on the results of a prior functional assessment is considered best practice (Dixon et al., 2012). The relevance of functional assessment strategies for supporting people with mental health disorders is also being increasingly recognized (Davies et al., 2019; Froján-Parga et al., 2019). Daffern and Howells (2002), for example, concluded that functional assessment data is of considerable value to the development of effective psychological interventions for reducing aggression among psychiatric inpatients.

In light of the widely acknowledged relevance and foundational nature of functional assessment methods for the treatment of challenging behavior and mental health disorders, this chapter will first review how various researchers define this group of methods in the literature. Following this, we consider the theoretical and applied rationale for the use of functional assessment methods for informing interventions to address challenging behavior and mental health disorders. Rationale and indications for using common functional assessment methods will then be considered. In considering the utility of different functional assessment methods, a number of factors will be explored, such as (a) the nature of the challenging behavior, (b) population studied, (c) who does the assessment, and (c) where the assessment occurs. Various studies will be described to exemplify the varying types, applications, and rationale for the use of different functional assessment methods.

Defining and Contextualizing Functional Assessment

Assessment can be broadly defined as a systematic/structured process for gathering information (Goldstein et al., 2019; Pierangelo & Giuliani, 2017; Strauser et al., 2020). Various assessment methods and tools have been developed to capture the wide range of information that may be useful when designing interventions. In terms of the specific types of information sought in therapeutic, rehabilitation, or behavioral/education endeavors, Strauser and Greco (2020) noted that assessment is often directed at gathering information related to "the client's aptitudes, achievement, intelligence, personality, interests, and behavior" (p. 1). Cognitive, emotional, physiological, and motor responses are also common assessment targets (O'Brien et al., 2010).

Functional assessment fits within this broader definition. It is also a process for gathering information. Smith, Vollmer, and St. Peter Pipkin (2007), for example, defined functional assessment as "any procedure or set of procedures designed to produce information" (p. 192). However, unlike the broader definition of assessment articulated by Strauser and Greco (2020), Smith et al. (2007) further explained that functional assessment methods seek a specific type of information, namely, "information about the events that precede or follow problem behavior" (p. 192). In a paper focusing on forensic mental health services, Davies et al. (2019) defined functional assessment as a systematic process for discerning the "specific circumstances under which behaviours that challenge occur and what they achieve for the person" (n.p.). In a definition emphasizing its application for specific mental health disorders (i.e., delusions, hallucinations, and disordered speech), Froján-Parga et al. (2019) described functional assessment as a "pretreatment ideographic set of assessments which aim to identify variables associated with the occurrence of a specific behavior, in order to develop an idiosyncratic intervention aimed at promoting behavioral changes" (p. 1). Echoing these sentiments while focusing on the assessment of challenging behaviors among children with developmental disabilities, Newcomb and Hagopian (2018) defined functional assessment as "a client-driven process that often involves multiple methods aimed at determining the specific environmental variables (i.e., reinforcers) that maintain or exacerbate problem behavior and the conditions under which it is more likely to occur" (p. 101). In the context of searching for studies on the quality of functional assessments included in school-based behavior intervention plans, Pennington, Simacek, McComas, McMasters, and Elmquist (2019) defined functional assessment as "any assessment designed to identify the function maintaining the target behavior" (p. 29).

As the above sample of definitions illustrate, functional assessment methods focus on gathering information related to the variables that control (i.e., trigger/evoke and reinforce/maintain) specified target behaviors. Information of this type is used to formulate hypotheses regarding the function or purpose of the targeted behaviors. To these ends, and in line with the above definitions, Steege, Pratt, Wickerd, Guare, and Steuart Watson (2019) delineated a number of features that should be evident in the functional assessment of challenging behavior. First, they noted that functional assessment should be undertaken in a systematic and formal manner. Second, the functional assessment process should be aimed at identifying the operant functions or purposes of the behavior. Third, various types of functional assessment methods should be used so as to effectively and comprehensively answer two basic questions: Why is the behavior occurring and what interventions are indicated? Similar criteria would seem applicable for the functional assessment of mental health disorders.

In a functional assessment, the emphasis is on understanding the purpose of the behavior, rather than attempting to ascertain meaning from the form of the behavior (Daffern & Howells, 2002). That is, the emphasis is on why the person is engaging in the behavior rather than what specific form of behavior (e.g., aggression versus self-injury, hallucinations versus disordered speech) is occurring. Moreover, functional assessment focuses on understanding or explaining specific behaviors (e.g., disruption, off-task behavior, swearing), rather than formulating a diagnosis (e.g., attention-deficit/hyperactivity disorder) to account for the person's behaviors

(Fabiano & Pyle, 2019). In addition to this more specific focus on function over form, functional assessment methods are defined and distinguished by their underlying theoretical and applied rationale.

Theoretical and Applied Rationale

In terms of its defining theoretical underpinnings, functional assessment is most closely associated with operant theory and with research and practice in the field of applied behavior analysis (ABA; Smith et al., 2007). In the operant paradigm, the causes of behavior are to be found through a careful examination (or assessment) of the environmental events that surround occurrences and non-occurrences of precisely defined behaviors (Skinner, 1981). Two kinds of environmental events are specifically sought in this type of operant or contingency analysis of behavior. These are (a) the antecedent stimuli that trigger, evoke, or set the occasion for behavior, and (b) the consequences which reliably follow behavior and function to reinforce and maintain behavior at strength. The events that proceed challenging behavior (i.e., antecedents) are important to identify because antecedent events will often come to trigger—or more technically evoke—the challenging behavior. The events that reliably follow occurrences of challenging behavior (i.e., consequences) are equally important to identify because certain consequent events might function as effective types of reinforcing stimuli and thus could be maintaining a challenging behavior. Generally, functional assessment methods are designed to look for controlling variables (antecedents and consequences) by carefully examining the external environment, including interactions that occur with others in the environment. Arguably, however, events or stimulations that occur inside the body (e.g., pain or dysfunctional thought patterns) might also influence behavior (Overskeid, 2018; Skinner, 1963). Consequently, functional assessment methods might need to include attempts to assess the internal (i.e., inside the body) environment. In such cases, the aim is to identify any internal events or private behaviors (e.g., internal speech) that might be influencing a person's propensity to engage in challenging behavior or which might be exacerbating symptoms (e.g., expressions of a delusionary nature) of a mental health disorder.

In operant theory, challenging behavior is viewed as learned behavior sensitive to environmental variables and is considered in terms of its controlling environmental variables (i.e., antecedents and maintaining consequences/reinforcers). Ostensibly, from an operant paradigm, when one has identified the controlling antecedents and consequences of a targeted challenging behavior, one has in fact identified its causes. Functional assessment might thus be loosely defined as the systematic search for the causes of behavior. In this vein, functional assessment seeks to answer questions such as "What variables control this behavior" and what environmental factors "contribute to the occurrence of the behavior" (Smith et al., 2007, p. 189). In practice, identification of controlling variables is intended to generate hypotheses regarding the function or purpose of behavior.

In considering the value of functional assessment methods for addressing mental health concerns, Davies et al. (2019) articulated a position consistent with operant theory by stating that all behavior is functional. The intended meaning here is that all behavior, including challenging behavior, serves a function or purpose for the individual. In line with this, functional assessment could also be broadly defined as the search for the functions or purposes of behavior. In behavior analytic accounts, challenging behavior is conceptualized as learned/operant behavior. Furthermore, it is behavior that can be explained by referencing its controlling antecedents and consequences and interpreted in terms of its function or purpose. This general conceptualization constitutes the overarching theoretical rationale for the use of functional assessment in the understanding and treatment of challenging behavior and, increasingly, mental health disorders.

The applied rationale for functional assessment follows directly from the overarching theoretical rationale. In sum, the emphasis is on "why" a behavior occurs as opposed to "what" the behavior looks like (i.e., the focus is on function over form) and the results are then used to inform intervention selection and implementation procedures. Specifically, if challenging behaviors are learned (i.e., operant behaviors) and are predominantly controlled by environmental variables, then they might be effectively reduced by altering environments to replace stimuli and contingencies that support challenging behavior with those that support more appropriate behaviors.

The idea of changing environments in order to change behavior is not a recent development (Davison, 2019); nor is the application of that approach at an individual level via in depth assessment of a single case (Shapiro, 1957). However, Hoffman and Hayes (2019) point out that functional assessment represents a notable departure from the nearly ubiquitous and long-standing psychiatric/medical model wherein disorders are defined in a somewhat homogenous way based primarily on the appearance (form) of the behavioral symptoms associated with a given condition. The use of the *Diagnostic and Statistical Manual* (American Psychiatric Association, 2013) to identify a disorder and then using the diagnosis to guide the selection of a treatment package illustrates this general psychiatric/medical model.

In contrast to the above-noted psychiatric/medical model, the functional assessment process focuses on identifying the purpose (function) of an operationally defined challenging behavior for a specific individual within a given environment. Intervention is then aligned with the functional properties of the target behavior and is further tailored for acceptability and/or sustainability in the individual's typical environments. Specifically, intervention components are selected and modified such that the reinforcement contingencies maintaining challenging behavior are disrupted and the same reinforcers are then made contingent on appropriate behavior, such as appropriate communicative and social behaviors.

The tight alignment between functional assessment and function-based intervention underlies the mechanism of behavior change. This function-matched intervention approach should be individualized for a specific person, their specific goals, obstacles, and environments. Gordon Paul (1969) is often cited for summarizing this in a single question, "What treatment, by whom, is most effective for this individual with that specific problem, under which set of circumstances, and how does it come about?" (p. 44; Hoffman & Hayes, 2019). A proper and thorough functional assessment answers those questions or, at least generates hypotheses that can be evaluated through a person's response to individually tailored intervention components.

As noted earlier, functional assessment is intended to reveal the contingent changes that occur in the environment immediately before and immediately after the targeted behavior. For example, a functional assessment may indicate that a person's challenging behavior occurs when a task demand is presented and that the behavior appears to be maintained (negatively reinforced) by the resulting removal of that task demand. In this scenario, the presentation of the task demand prior to the occurrence of any challenging behavior would be conceptualized as the antecedent and the subsequent removal of the task demand when challenging behavior occurs would be viewed as the controlling/reinforcing consequence.

In most cases, functional assessment results are conceptualized in terms of positive (i.e., obtaining preferred stimuli) and negative reinforcement (i.e., escaping from or avoiding unwanted or aversive stimuli). The identified reinforcement contingencies then become the basis of the intervention logic by informing the selection of specific intervention components and guiding procedures for implementation. For example, Table 1.1 displays various ways in which the function of challenging behavior would inform procedures used to implement a differential reinforcement intervention package. Differential reinforcement involves selecting an appropriate behavior to be reinforced and placing the challenging behavior on extinction (EXT) (i.e., withholding of reinforcement following challenging behavior). The specific

Table 1.1 Examples of how the results of a functional assessment might inform the application of extinction and reinforcement procedures

Challenging behavior	Function identified via functional assessment	Corresponding extinction and reinforcement procedures
Self-injury	Obtain attention	Extinction: Attention is withheld and the challenging behavior is ignored Reinforcement: Hand raising is reinforced by teacher attention
Self-injury	Avoid social interaction	Extinction: Attention is given (i.e., avoidance/escape is blocked) Reinforcement: Activating a speech-generating device that says "I need time alone now" is reinforced with a break from social interaction
Self-injury	Obtain preferred tangible item	Extinction: The preferred item is withheld Reinforcement: Handing communication partner a picture of the preferred item is reinforced by access to the preferred item.
Self-injury	Avoid undesirable task demands	Extinction: The task demand is maintained Reinforcement: A verbal request for a break from work is reinforced by providing a break from work.

behavior selected for reinforcement, the reinforcer used, and the procedures used in EXT all depend on the results from a functional assessment.

The application of procedures and technologies derived from the operant paradigm in an effort to achieve socially valid outcomes (e.g., to reduce challenging behavior in people with developmental disabilities) is the defining characteristic of ABA (Baer, Wolf, & Risley, 1968). The functional assessment process has become a hallmark of ABA due to the effectiveness and efficiency of function-based interventions across a wide array of environments, diagnoses, and types of challenging behaviors (Saini, Fisher, Retzlaff & Keevy, 2020). For example, functional assessment procedures have been implemented with success in school environments in the USA (Lloyd, Weaver, & Staubitz, 2016) where evidence-based practice is required by law and efficiency is often cited as a primary concern. Further, functional assessment has been used to address challenging behavior across the life span, including during early childhood (e.g., Arndorfer & Miltenberger, 1993). It has also been used with people having varying diagnoses including developmental disability, emotional disorders, behavioral disorders, and various mental health conditions, such as anxiety, depression, and obsessive-compulsive disorder (Gage, Lewis, & Stichter, 2012). Given the wide range of use, it is not surprising that a number of functional assessment methods have been developed and evaluated.

Rationale for Different Functional Assessment Methods

Under the umbrella of functional assessment, Smith et al. (2007) defined two specific types or classes of assessment methods. Specifically, they defined functional analysis as a functional assessment method that requires the direct manipulation of various antecedent and consequent conditions with the aim of experimentally isolating the effects, if any, of such manipulations on a person's propensity to engage in pre-defined challenging behaviors. They also defined the term 'functional behavioral assessment' as a broader and more generic process of gathering information surrounding a person's challenging behavior. For example, as part of the process of undertaking a functional behavioral assessment, information might be sought not only on the antecedents that evoke the behavior and the consequences that maintain the defined challenging behavior (i.e., the triggers and reinforcers), but also on additional relevant circumstances, such as the person's preferences, cultural and linguistic background, inter-personal relationships, and social support network (Crone, Hawkins, & Horner, 2015; Davies et al., 2019). Along with data on controlling antecedents and consequences, this latter type of information can also be useful for intervention planning.

Functional assessment methods have also been classified as involving primarily indirect versus more direct, observation-based protocols (Froján-Parga et al., 2019). Indirect methods include interviewing informants using a structured interview protocol or administration of one or more of several validated informant-based rating scales. Direct assessment methods include conducting observations of behavior either in the natural environment or during structured sessions in which antecedent and consequent variables are controlled and manipulated to directly assess for different functions. With these two broad classes there are a number of more specific methods, tactics, or protocols that have been developed to assess the variables controlling challenging behavior. Rojahn, Whittaker, Hoch, and González (2007) provided a comprehensive overview of a number of the main indirect and direct functional assessment methods.

Indirect and direct assessment methods are not mutually exclusive and there appears to be no particular reason why these two classes of functional assessment methods could not be combined into a comprehensive assessment package. Indeed, information from indirect and direct functional assessment methods could be seen as complementary. However, each of these specific methods has indications and contraindications that need to be considered when selecting the specific type of functional assessment protocol to be used and how it will be applied. Different functional assessment methods will often have differing rationale indicating differing indications for use. The method or methods used, and the manner in which these are applied, will often need to vary in line with a number of factors, such as (a) the nature of the challenging behavior, (b) the unique characteristics of the individual, (c) who does the assessment, and (c) where the assessment needs to occur.

Indirect Functional Assessment

The purpose of indirect assessment is to gather qualitative and/or quantitative data regarding a specific target behavior from other respondents who know the focus individual well. Such respondents may be family members, caregivers, teachers, direct support personnel, and/or other service providers with deep knowledge of the focus learner and their challenging behavior. This is called an indirect assessment because the information about the person's challenging behavior comes about indirectly via reports from others. Thus the information obtained represents others' perspectives about the person's challenging behavior, which may have been gained by interacting with the person for a considerable period of time and across a range of settings and contexts. Indirect assessments are often conducted early in the functional assessment process as a means of gathering initial data and incorporating multiple stakeholder views and knowledge into the process.

There are three primary categories of indirect assessments: interviews, rating scales, and checklists. The intent of interviews is to gather as much relevant information as possible to inform the next steps in the functional assessment process and to begin to consider behavior intervention components that might be pursued or which are contraindicated. Due to the often open-ended response format of many such interview protocols, this approach could be seen as offering opportunities for the interviewer to explore both the breadth and depth of stakeholders' knowledge of the target behavior and the circumstances of the focus learner. Interviews may be highly structured and follow a specific sequence of questioning, or they might be less structured, enabling some flexibility in the questions asked and the opportunity for follow-up questions. Interview questions may involve describing the history of target behaviors, identifying potential biological factors that may affect the target behavior (such as medications, sleep, health conditions, or diet) and describing events that are likely to evoke or set the occasion for the target behavior. In some interviews, questions about previous interventions attempted and their results may also be sought.

Though respondents need not have knowledge and background in behavior analysis or functional assessment, interviews can begin to help the respondent identify potentially relevant antecedents, reinforcers, and contextual variables. For example, the Functional Assessment Interview (O'Neil et al., 2015) is a structured interview that addresses the history of the target behavior, potential motivating factors (i.e., establishing operations, antecedents, and reinforcers). In one section, the Functional Assessment Interview prompts the respondent to consider the communicative properties of the individual's behaviors. Respondents are asked to consider specific functions of communication such as requesting access to an object, requesting help, or protesting and map those to a variety of behavioral topographies such as pointing, crying, or tantrums. As such, interviews can be quite helpful in the initial stages of forming a hypothesis of behavioral function, as a way to make meaningful data collection accessible to respondents from a variety of backgrounds and roles.

Interview protocols have also been developed that are designed to be conducted with the focus individual. The Student-Assisted Functional Assessment Interview (Kern, Dunlap, Clarke, & Elfner, 1994) and the Student Guided Functional Assessment interview (Reed, Thomas, Sprague, & Horner, 1997) are both intended to be used with students who are able to reflect on their own behavior, articulate what may be causing or motivating their behaviors, and communicate their preferences for intervention components (Kern et al., 1994). Results from such student interviews may be of considerable value for informing the selection and application of additional functional assessment components and to inform the design of acceptable and potentially effective behavioral interventions.

Overall, interviews are considered to be a beneficial starting point in the functional assessment process. They allow for rich data collection from a variety of stakeholders. However, interviews can often require a substantial amount of time to complete (e.g., 90 minutes for the Functional Assessment Interview), which may not be feasible for some stakeholders. Additionally, due to the narrative nature of responses, combing through the results and pulling out relevant information to inform the rest of the assessment or intervention can be challenging. It is also often unclear if an informants' information provided during an interview is reliable and valid. For example, informants' perceptions might be biased due to holding inaccurate beliefs regarding the causes of challenging behavior.

Unlike interviews, rating scales are designed to quantify respondent views of environmental conditions that they perceive to be influencing a person's challenging behavior. For example, respondents may be asked to estimate the likelihood of a certain behavior occurring given specific conditions. One such rating scale is the Questions About Behavioral Function (Matson & Vollmer, 1995). This scale consists of 25 items that are rated on a Likert scale. Each item is mapped to a potential reinforcer for challenging behavior, that is attention, escape, physical tangible, or nonsocial reinforcers. The scores of each item are then summed and the condition(s) with the highest scores are hypothesized to be the function of the target behavior.

There are a number of functional assessment tools that combine brief interviews with rating scales. For example the Function Analysis Screen Tool (FAST, Iwata & DeLeon, 2005) begins with questions regarding the history and contexts surrounding the target behavior followed by a 16-item rating scale. Each of these items is linked to a specific function, social attention, social escape, sensory stimulation, or pain attenuation. The intent of the FAST protocol is to provide information that will inform subsequent and more direct functional assessment processes.

There are several potential advantages to the use of rating scales as a form of indirect functional assessment. Generally such scales are fairly quick and easy to administer, and can offer meaningful participation in the functional assessment process for multiple stakeholders. Some rating scales that are paired with interviews also enable access to data on the history of behavior and information about past intervention efforts, including those that worked and those that were not successful. However, as with interview information, the accuracy and reliability of data from rating scale results is often unknown and in some cases that information may be highly unreliable (Dracobly, Dozier, Briggs, & Juanico, 2018). This is likely due to varying perspectives, different experiences with the focus individual and the target behavior, and possible attitude biases. In light of these limitations, indirect assessments might be recommended as a starting point from which to design a more direct functional assessment package.

Direct Naturalistic Observations

One method of gathering objective data is to conduct direct observations of the target behavior in the natural context in which the person is expected to engage and where the behavior has been known to occur or is likely to occur. A well-designed direct observational method offers the opportunity to directly gather objective descriptive data on environmental factors that are evoking the target behavior (i.e., antecedents) and the consequences that maintain the target behavior (i.e., reinforcement). Direct observation allows the examiner to observe the challenging behavior first hand without depending on others' perspectives. Direct observation data, sometimes called descriptive data or antecedent-behavior-consequence (ABC) data, is recorded in a continuous manner by an observer. Direct observation data should be collected across multiple days and for sufficient durations to enable identification of patterns of antecedents and consequences (O'Neill, Albin, Storey, Horner, & Sprague, 2015).

There are two primary methods of collecting direct observational data. One is to use open-ended recording in which the observer writes a summary of what occurred prior to and immediately following any instances of challenging behavior. The potential benefits of this approach are the ability to record detailed and often highly individualized antecedents and consequences. Challenges with open-ended direct observation data pertain to the feasibility of recording observations while continuing to observe the individual. Often challenging behaviors may occur in a rapid sequence. The need to divert attention from the individual being observed in order to write a narrative description may cause the assessor to miss additional instances of the behavior that were evoked by different antecedents and which produced different consequences. Additionally, open-ended data can also be difficult to interpret and summarize and thus might lead to only very tentative hypotheses regarding the function of the person's challenging behavior (O'Neill et al., 2015).

To reduce time spent recording antecedents and consequences and to aid in summarizing data, observers may opt to use a selection-based direct observational approach. Selection-based direct observation data systems include pre-entered antecedents and pre-filled consequences. The observer simply checks off which antecedents and consequences were observed for each occurrence of challenging behavior. Selection-based direct observation systems are often more efficient to complete than open-ended observations. However, because of the pre-filled options, some individualized antecedents or consequences may not be included. In such situations, the observer might supplement a selection-based data system with open-ended recording as needed.

There are several potential advantages of undertaking direct observation as part of a functional assessment. First, direct observations may help place the target behavior in context and reveal consistent patterns of antecedents and consequences, which can in turn point to specific hypotheses as to the function of the challenging behavior. Due to the observational nature of the data, direct observation may also enable the assessor to collect useful data in an unobtrusive manner, that is, without disrupting the individual's typical routines or activities.

It is important to note that there are potential limitations to the conclusiveness of data gathered from direct observation. In addition, conducting direct observations accurately will often require explicit training of the observers. For example, observers need to be trained to record only those events in the environment that are directly seen or heard and refrain from making inferences as to the person's motivation. This can be challenging because there may be a tendency for observers to infer certain emotions or intentions (e.g., "The child became angry." "The child was trying to make the teacher angry").

Because environmental variables are not being directly manipulated by the observer, the data about antecedent-behavior-consequence relations that are ascertained via more naturalistic observations are correlational in nature. This can lead to potential false positives of hypothesized behavior function. For example, when conducting direct observations in a classroom setting, the observer might record that each instance of challenging behavior is followed by teacher attention in the form of a verbal reprimand. The observer might therefore hypothesize that the challenging behavior is maintained by positive reinforcement, in the form of the teacher's attention. Indeed, teachers often provide large amounts of verbal attention for student behaviors throughout the day, but this does not mean that the child's challenging behavior occurs to get the teacher's attention. Because the teacher always provided a reprimand, the observer cannot assess whether the target behavior would continue to occur in the absence of this consequence being provided by the teacher. Related to this, when antecedents and consequences are only recorded based on the presence of challenging behavior, it is unknown if those same antecedents and consequences events may be present when challenging behavior is absent. In other words, direct observations under naturalistic conditions do not demonstrate whether there is, in fact, a functional relation between any specific antecedents and consequences and increased occurrences of the challenging behavior (Sasso et al., 1992). Thus relying solely on direct observation data to determine the function of challenging behaviors may be problematic as there is the possibility of falling into the error that correlation implies causation (Lerman & Iwata, 1993).

Experimental-Functional Analysis

One approach to moving beyond correlational data is to systematically manipulate environmental variables by undertaking an experimental-functional analysis of the person's challenging behavior. An experimental-functional analysis allows for the demonstration of a cause/effect (or functional) relation between antecedents, behavior, and consequences. With respect to challenging behavior, an experimental-functional analysis would seem to provide the best empirical test regarding that function or purpose of behavior.

In an experimental-functional analysis, the individual participates in different activities/social conditions to determine whether certain specific classes of stimuli either do or do not evoke and reinforce the person's challenging behavior. Within each condition, various dimensions (e.g., frequency, latency, or magnitude) of the target behavior could be measured (Beavers, Iwata, & Lerman, 2013). Experimental-functional analyses typically comprise three test conditions: social positive reinforcement (e.g., access to attention, objects, or activities), social negative reinforcement (e.g., escape from task demands), and a control condition (e.g., play or ignore). Within each condition, antecedents or establishing operations are arranged to determine if they evoke challenging behavior. For example, if the hypothesized function of the behavior is to access attention, then the attention condition may begin with the removal or withdrawal of attention. This would then establish the opportunity for the individual to engage in attention-seeking behavior if attention is a reinforcer for the target behavior. As part of this assessment, if problem behavior occurred in response to the antecedent condition, then the presumed reinforcer (e.g., attention) would be provided to determine if this contingency was maintaining the person's problem behavior. This systematic structure allows the examiner to experimentally test for the hypothesized function(s) in a controlled assessment context.

There are a number of different experimental-functional analysis methods that have been developed for assessing the function of challenging behavior. Though the structure of each varies, each method involves the systematic manipulation of antecedent and/or consequence stimuli. The gold-standard method involves the experimental-functional analysis protocol developed by Iwata, Dorsey, Slifer, Bauman, and Richman (1982/1994). This method involves arranging and repeating various tasks and social conditions across a number of 10- to 15-min sessions. The conditions arranged (e.g., prompting task engagement, verbally reprimanding instances of challenging behavior) are meant to be analogues of the contingencies that have shaped the behavior (e.g., enabling escape from task demands, recruiting attention from adults). The rationale is that certain conditions may evoke more challenging behavior and thus indicate the function of that behavior.

Implementing the analogue functional analysis approach requires considerable competence because assessors need to be mindful of the potential problems that may arise by repeatedly exposing the person to conditions that might reinforce and strengthen challenging behavior. There also needs to be attention given to the potential safety risks to individuals who engage in dangerous behaviors (Kahng et al., 2015). Time requirements (LaRue et al., 2010) and issues of efficiency also need to be considered (Saini et al., 2020). Still, the approach developed by Iwata and colleagues has certainly stood the test of time and proven to be a highly effective approach for identifying the operant function of a wide range of challenging behavior across a wide range of populations.

The impressive utility of Iwata, Dorsey, et al. (1982/1994) experimental-functional analysis methodology has spawned a number of variations on this gold-standard protocol. For example, the pairwise functional analysis model (Iwata, Duncan, Zarcone, Lerman, & Shore, 1994) evaluates two conditions in an alternating format. Such an arrangement is of value when comparing a single hypothesized function to a control condition. Another variation is the brief functional analysis approach described by Cooper, Wacker, Sasso, Reimers, and Donn (1990), which was designed to enable examiners to assess the relation between antecedent and response patterns as well as antecedent-response-consequence patterns in a single 90-min session (Badgett & Falcomata, 2015). Some brief functional analysis models also include a contingency reversal condition (Northup et al., 1991), which can serve as a pilot for behavioral intervention components. Due to the relatively brief nature of conditions, low-frequency behaviors may not be readily captured in an analogue functional analysis model. For behaviors that are low frequency but high intensity, a latency functional analysis (Neidert, Iwata, Dempsey, & Thomason-Sassi, 2013) may be considered. In a latency functional analysis the behavior is measured by the time between the presentation of the antecedent and the occurrence of the target behavior. Research has also led to a trial-based functional analysis method (Sigafoos & Saggers, 1995). For example, brief (1-min) trials are distributed into naturally occurring routines. When selecting an experimental-functional analysis method practitioners should consider the resources and time available to conduct the functional analysis, the setting in which the functional analysis will be conducted, and the nature of the target behavior with respect to frequency and intensity (Rispoli et al., 2015).

While some researchers advocate for modifying functional analysis conditions based on ambiguous or inconclusive data (Fisher, Greer, Romani, Zangrillo, & Owen, 2016), others recommend designing functional analysis with idiosyncratic and individualized variables at the outset (Roscoe, Schlichenmeyer, & Dube, 2015). Advances in functional analysis research have highlighted the importance of designing functional analysis conditions based on the results of indirect and descriptive assessments (Tiger, Hanley, & Bessette, 2006). For example, if indirect assessment and direct observation results indicate the target behavior occurs to access ritualistic activities (e.g., Rispoli, Camargo, Machalicek, Lang, & Sigafoos, 2014), then an experimental condition in which challenging behavior is followed by access to rituals should be designed and conducted.

Functional analysis individualization may also involve altering the structure of reinforcement contingencies. In most functional analysis research, the putative reinforcer is designed to be delivered in isolation within that specific condition. For example, to assess whether challenging behavior is maintained by negative reinforcement, the escape condition would include removal of task demands contingent upon challenging behavior. Recently, however, researchers have begun to explore combining multiple reinforcers into a single condition in a synthesized contingency format (Hanley, Jin, Vanselow, & Hanratty, 2014). That is, if an individual's target behavior appears to be maintained by access to attention and escape from task demands, then the functional analysis should provide simulations and contingent access to both attention and escape. The utility of synthesized functional analysis contingencies is the subject of much debate and mixed results from this method have been reported (Fisher et al., 2016). As such, the implications for synthesized contingencies in practice will depend on the results of additional research. What is promising, however, is that researchers continue to adapt and refine functional analysis approaches to improve the efficient and feasible identification of functions of behavior.

Summary and Conclusion

In light of its fundamental importance, the skills required to conduct assessments represent key areas of competence for practitioners involved in providing therapy, rehabilitation, behavioral interventions, and/or educational services. Practitioners in many fields (e.g., applied behavior analysis, clinical psychology, school psychology, teaching, rehabilitation counseling, and speech-language pathology) therefore need to understand the indications for various broad assessment approaches. They also need to gain competence in the selection and implementation of numerous specific evidence-based assessment tools and protocols. Competencies with respect to interpreting and using assessment data to inform and evaluate interventions are also crucial for optimizing intervention outcomes. This is particularly true for the understanding and treatment of challenging behavior and/or mental health concerns (Matson, 2012) as well as for the broader range of services that may be indicated for individuals who present with challenging behavior and mental health concerns. A thorough understanding of a person's challenging behavior and/or mental health concerns will most likely require a comprehensive assessment that includes implementing a number of different functional assessment methods. To this end, the present chapter has defined functional assessment and reviewed the underlying rationale and indications for use of various functional assessment methods.

Most research into functional assessment has focused on its use for identifying the operant function of challenging behaviors, such as self-injury and aggression, in persons with developmental disabilities. For this purpose, functional assessment has proven remarkably useful and highly adaptable to meet individuals' unique circumstances. There is also growing recognition regarding the utility of functional assessment for understanding mental health issues. Froján-Parga et al. (2019), for example, conducted an important meta-analytic study into the use of functional assessment and function-based treatments for reducing hallucinatory speech, delusional speech, and disorganized speech in adults. They synthesized the results of 23 studies involving 24 adults. In these studies, an experimental analysis based on the Iwata, Dorsey, et al. (1982/1994) protocol was the most frequently used functional assessment method (used in 41% of the cases). However, interview-based indirect assessments (25%) and direct, naturalistic observations (12.5%) were also used. And in 20.8% of the cases, multiple functional assessment methods were employed (e.g., interviews plus experimental analyses or interviews plus naturalistic observations). Froján-Parga et al.'s analyses showed that all of these functional assessment methods and the subsequently implemented (function-based) interventions were "proven to be effective" (p. 6). In the absence of any significant differences in outcomes across the different assessment methods and interventions applied, they concluded that the range of functional assessment methods employed across these studies all seemed to be "precise enough to establish the environmental contingencies of these problem behaviors" (p. 8). The authors further note that atypical vocalizations, rather than being merely bizarre, may serve important functions or purposes that need to be identified and considered when planning interventions to reduce such behaviors. To this end, functional assessment (whether indirect, descriptive, and/or experimentally based) represents "a key therapeutic tool to enhance the therapeutic power of our intervention" (p. 7).

In line with Froján-Parga et al.'s (2019) conclusions, the different functional assessment methods canvassed in this chapter (e.g., interview protocols, rating scales, direct naturalistic observations, and experimental-functional analysis methods) are all ultimately aimed at discovering the function or purpose of behavior. The primary reason for doing so stems from the fact that knowledge of behavioral function has proven to be critical to the development of effective interventions. Functional assessment is indeed a key therapeutic tool. Functional assessment is based on overarching, compelling rationale; that all behavior is functional and that behavioral function is revealed when its controlling antecedents and consequences are identified.

References

Alderman, N. (2003). Contemporary approaches to the management of irritability and aggression following traumatic brain injury. *Neuropsychological Rehabilitation, 13*, 211–240. https://doi.org/10.1080/09602010244000327

American Psychiatric Association. (2013). *Diagnostic and statistical manual of mental disorders* (5th ed.). Washington, DC: American Psychiatric Association.

Arndorfer, R. E., & Miltenberger, R. G. (1993). Functional assessment and treatment of challenging behavior: A review with implications for early childhood. *Topics in Early Childhood Special Education, 13*, 82–105.

Badgett, N., & Falcomata, T. S. (2015). A comparison of methodologies of brief functional analysis. *Developmental Neurorehabilitation, 18*, 224–233. https://doi.org/10.3109/17518423.2013.792298

Baer, D. M., Wolf, M. M., & Risley, T. R. (1968). Some current dimensions of applied behavior analysis. *Journal of Applied Behavior Analysis, 1*, 91–97. https://doi.org/10.1901/jaba.1968.1-91

Beavers, G. A., Iwata, B. A., & Lerman, D. C. (2013). Thirty years of research on the functional analysis of problem behavior. *Journal of Applied Behavior Analysis, 46*, 1–21.

Bowring, D. L., Totsika, V., Hastings, R. P., Toogood, S., & Griffith, G. M. (2017). Challenging behaviours in adults with intellectual disability: A total population study and exploration of risk indices. *British Journal of Clinical Psychology, 56*, 16–32. https://doi.org/10.1111/bjc.12118

Brown, C., Stoffel, V. C., & Muñoz, J. P. (2019). *Occupational therapy in mental health: A vision for participation* (2nd ed.). Philadelphia, PA: F. A. Davis.

Bruffaerts, R., Mortier, P., Kiekens, G., Auerbach, R. P., Cuijpers, P., Demyttenaere, K., … Kessler, R. C. (2018). Mental health problems in college freshman: Prevalence and academic functioning. *Journal of Affective Disorders, 225*, 97–103. https://doi.org/10.1016/j.jad.2017.07.044

Callaghan, P. (2019). Mental health assessment. In C. L. Cox, R. Turner, & R. Blackwood (Eds.), *Physical assessment for nurses and healthcare professionals* (pp. 267–285). Hoboken, NJ: Wiley.

Chan, F., Yaghmaian, R., Chen, X., Wu, J.-R., Lee, B., Iwanaga, K., & Tao, J. (2020). The World Health Organization International Classification of Functioning, Disability, and Health as a framework for rehabilitation assessment. In D. R. Strauser, T. N. Tansey, & F. Chan (Eds.), *Assessment in rehabilitation and mental health counseling* (pp. 12–34). New York, NY: Springer. https://doi.org/10.1891/9780826162434

Cooper, L. J., Wacker, D. P., Sasso, G. M., Reimers, T. M., & Donn, L. K. (1990). Using parents as therapists to evaluate appropriate behavior of their children: Application to a tertiary diagnostic clinic. *Journal of Applied Behavior Analysis, 23*, 285–296.

Crone, D. A., Hawkins, L. S., & Horner, R. H. (2015). *Building positive behavior support systems in schools, 2nd edition: Functional behavioral assessment*. New York, NY: Guilford Press.

Daffern, M., & Howells, K. (2002). Psychiatric inpatient aggression: A review of structural and functional assessment approaches. *Aggression and Violent Behavior, 7*, 477–497.

Davies, B., Lowe, K., Morgan, S., John-Evans, H., Griffiths, J., Tarmey, L., & Fitoussi, J. (2019). Development of a behavioural assessment tool for use in forensic mental health services. *Mental Health Practice, 22*(5). https://doi.org/10.7748/mhp.2019.e1350

Davison, G. C. (2019). A return to functional analysis, the search for mechanisms of change, and the nomothetic idiographic issue in psychosocial interventions. *Clinical Psychological Science, 7*, 51–53. https://doi.org/10.1177/2167702618794924

Dixon, D. R., Vogel, T., & Tarbox, J. (2012). A brief history of functional analysis and applied behavior analysis. In J. L. Matson (Ed.), *Functional assessment for challenging behaviors* (pp. 3–24). New York, NY: Springer. https://doi.org/10.1007/978-1-4614-3037-7_2

Downs, J., Blackmore, A. M., Epstein, A., Skoss, R., Langdon, K., Jacoby, P., … Glasson, E. J. (2018). The prevalence of mental health disorders and symptoms in children and adolescents with cerebral palsy: A systematic review and meta-analysis. *Developmental Medicine and Child Neurology, 60*, 30–38. https://doi.org/10.1111/dmcn.13555

Dracobly, J. D., Dozier, C. L., Briggs, A. M., & Juanico, J. F. (2018). Reliability and validity of indirect assessment outcomes: Experts versus caregivers. *Learning and Motivation, 62*, 77–90. https://doi.org/10.1016/j.lmot.2017.02.007

Einfeld, S. L., Ellis, L. A., & Emerson, E. (2011). Comorbidity of intellectual disability and mental disorder in children and adolescents: A systematic review. *Journal of Intellectual and Developmental Disability, 36*, 137–143. https://doi.org/10.1080/13668250.2011.572548

Evans, S., Banerjee, S., Leese, M., & Huxley, P. (2007). The impact of mental illness on quality of life: A comparison of severe mental illness, common mental disorder and healthy population samples. *Quality of Life Research, 16*, 17–29. https://doi.org/10.1007/s11136-006-9002-6

Fabiano, G. A., & Pyle, K. (2019). Best practices in school mental health for attention-deficit/hyperactivity disorder: A framework for intervention. *School Mental Health: A Multidisciplinary Research and Practice Journal, 11*(1), 72–91. https://doi.org/10.1007/s12310-018-9267-2

Fisher, W. W., Greer, B. D., Romani, P. W., Zangrillo, A. N., & Owen, T. M. (2016). Comparisons of synthesized and individual reinforcement contingencies during functional analysis. *Journal of Applied Behavior Analysis, 49*, 596–616. https://doi.org/10.1002/jaba.314

Fodstad, J. C. (2019). Editorial: Special issue on mental health issues in autism spectrum disorder. *Review Journal of Autism and Developmental Disorders, 6*, 243–245. https://doi.org/10.1007/s40489-019-00178-7

Frey, J. R. (2019). Assessment for special education: Diagnosis and placement. *The Annals of the American Academy of Political and Social Science, 683*, 149–161. https://doi.org/10.1177/0002716219841352

Froján-Parga, M. X., de Prado-Gordillo, M. N., Álvarez-Iglesias, A., & Alonso-Vega, J. (2019). Functional behavioral assessment-based interventions on adults' delusions, hallucinations and disorganized speech: A single case meta-analysis. *Behaviour Research and Therapy, 120*, 1–10. https://doi.org/10.1016/j.brat.2019.103444

Gage, N. A., Lewis, T. J., & Stichter, J. P. (2012). Functional behavioral assessment-based interventions for students with or at risk for emotional and/or behavioral disorder in school: A hierarchical linear modeling meta-analysis. *Behavioral Disorders, 37*, 55–77.

Goldstein, G., Allen, D., & Deluca, J. (Eds.). (2019). *Handbook of psychological assessment* (4th ed.). London: Academic Press. https://doi.org/10.1016/B978-0-12-802203-0.00022-5

Groth-Marnat, G., & Wright, A. J. (Eds.). (2016). *Handbook of psychological assessment* (6th ed.). Hoboken, NJ: Wiley.

Gur, A. (2017). Challenging behavior, functioning difficulties, and quality of life of adults with intellectual disabilities. *International Journal of Developmental Disabilities, 64*, 45–52. https://doi.org/10.1080/20473869.2016.1221233

Hanley, G. P., Jin, C. S., Vanselow, N. R., & Hanratty, L. A. (2014). Producing meaningful improvements in problem behavior of children with autism via synthesized analyses and treatments. *Journal of Applied Behavior Analysis, 47*, 16–36. https://doi.org/10.1002/jaba.106

Hoffman, S. G., & Hayes, S. C. (2019). The future of intervention science: Process-based therapy. *Clinical Psychological Science, 7*, 37–50. https://doi.org/10.1177/2167702618772296

Huisman, S., Mulder, P., Kuijk, J., Kers, tholt, M., van Eeghen, A., Leenders, A., … Hennekam, R. (2018). Self-injurious behavior. *Neuroscience and Biobehavioral Reviews, 84*, 483–491. https://doi.org/10.1016/j.neubiorev.2017.02.027

Iwata, B., & DeLeon, I. (2005). *The functional analysis screening tool*. Gainesville, FL: The Florida Center on Self-Injury, University of Florida.

Iwata, B. A., Dorsey, M. F., Slifer, K. J., Bauman, K. E., & Richman, G. S. (1994). Toward a functional analysis of self-injury. *Journal of Applied Behavior Analysis, 27*, 197–209. https://doi.org/10.1901/jaba.1994.27-197. (Reprinted from *Analysis and Intervention in Developmental Disabilities, 2*, 3–20, 1982).

Iwata, B. A., Duncan, B. A., Zarcone, J. R., Lerman, D. C., & Shore, B. A. (1994). A sequential, test-control methodology for conducting functional analyses of self-injurious behavior. *Behavior Modification, 18*, 289–306. https://doi.org/10.1177/01454455940183003

Jordan, C., & Franklin, C. (Eds.). (2015). *Clinical assessment for social workers: Qualitative and quantitative methods* (4th ed.). New York, NY: Oxford University Press.

Kahng, S., Hausman, N. L., Fisher, A. B., Donaldson, J. M., Cox, J. R., Logo, M., & Wiskow, K. M. (2015). The safety of functional analysis of self-injurious behavior. *Journal of Applied Behavior Analysis, 48*, 107–114. https://doi.org/10.1002/jaba.168

Kern, L., Dunlap, G., Clarke, S., & Elfner, K. (1994). Student-assisted functional assessment interview. *Assessment for Effective Intervention, 19*, 29–39. https://doi.org/10.1177/073724779401900203

Kramer, G. P., Bernstein, D. A., & Phares, V. (2019). *Introduction to clinical psychology* (8th ed.). Cambridge, UK: Cambridge University Press. https://doi.org/10.1017/9781108593823

LaRue, R. H., Lenard, K., Weiss, M. J., Bamond, M., Palmieri, M., & Kelley, M. E. (2010). Comparison of traditional and trial-based methodologies for conducting functional analyses. *Research in Developmental Disabilities, 31*, 480–487.

Lerman, D. C., & Iwata, B. A. (1993). Descriptive and experimental analyses of variables maintaining self-injurious behavior. *Journal of Applied Behavior Analysis, 26*, 293–319.

Lloyd, B. P., Weaver, E. S., & Staubitz, J. L. (2016). A review of functional analysis methods conducted in public school classroom settings. *Journal of Behavioral Education, 25*, 324–356. https://doi.org/10.1007/s10864-015-9243-y

Matson, J. L. (Ed.). (2007). *Handbook of assessment for persons with intellectual disability.* Boston: Academic Press.

Matson, J. L. (Ed.). (2012). *Functional assessment for challenging behaviors.* New York, NY: Springer. https://doi.org/10.1007/978-1-4614-3037-7

Matson, J. L., Sipes, M., Fodstad, J. C., & Fitzgerald, M. E. (2011). Issues in the management of challenging behaviours of adults with autism spectrum disorder. *CNS Drugs, 7*, 597–606. https://doi.org/10.2165/11591700-000000000-00000

Matson, J. L., & Vollmer, T. R. (1995). *User's guide: Questions about behavioral function (QABF).* Baton Rouge, LA: Scientific Publishers.

Matson, J. L., & Williams, L. W. (2014). Functional assessment of challenging behavior. *Current Developmental Disorders Reports, 1*, 56–66. https://doi.org/10.1007/s40474-013-0006-y

McNett, M., Sarver, W., & Wilczewski, P. (2012). The prevalence, treatment and outcomes of agitation among patients with brain injury admitted to acute care units. *Brain Injury, 26*, 1155–1162. https://doi.org/10.3109/02699052.2012.667587

Neidert, P. L., Iwata, B. A., Dempsey, C. M., & Thomason-Sassi, J. L. (2013). Latency of response during the functional analysis of elopement. *Journal of Applied Behavior Analysis, 46*, 312–316. https://doi.org/10.1002/jaba.11

Newcomb, E. T., & Hagopian, L. P. (2018). Treatment of severe problem behaviour in children with autism spectrum disorder and intellectual disabilities. *International Review of Psychiatry, 30*, 96–109. https://doi.org/10.1080/09540261.2018.1435513

Northup, J., Wacker, D., Sasso, G., Steege, M., Cigrand, K., Cook, J., & DeRaad, A. (1991). A brief analysis of aggressive and alternative behavior in an outclinic setting. *Journal of Applied Behavior Analysis, 24*, 509–522.

O'Brien, W. H., Oemig, C. K., & Northern, J. J. (2010). Behavioral assessment with adults. In J. Thomas & M. Hersen (Eds.), *Handbook of clinical psychology competencies* (pp. 283–307). New York, NY: Springer. https://doi.org/10.1007/978-0-387-09757-2_11

O'Neill, R. E., Albin, R. W., Storey, K., Horner, R. H., & Sprague, J. R. (2015). *Functional assessment and program development for problem behavior: A practical handbook.* Stamford, CT: Cenage Learning.

Overskeid, G. (2018). Do we need the environment to explain operant behavior? *Frontiers in Psychology, 9*, 373. https://doi.org/10.3389/fpsyg.2018.00373

Paul, G. (1969). Behavior modification research: Design and tactics. In C. M. Franks (Ed.), *Behaviour therapy: Appraisal and status* (pp. 29–62). New York, NY: McGraw-Hill.

Pennington, B., Simacek, J., McComas, J., McMaster, K., & Elmquist, M. (2019). Maintenance and generalisation in functional behavioral assessment and behavior intervention plan literature. *Journal of Behavioral Education, 28*(1), 27–53. https://doi.org/10.1007/s10864-018-9299-6

Pierangelo, R. A., & Giuliani, G. A. (2017). *Assessment in special education: A practical approach* (5th ed.). New York, NY: Pearson.

Pilgrim, D. (2020). *Key concepts in mental health* (5th ed.). London: Sage.

Reed, H., Thomas, E., Sprague, J. R., & Horner, R. H. (1997). The student guided functional assessment interview: An analysis of student and teacher agreement. *Journal of Behavioral Education, 7*, 33–49. https://doi.org/10.1023/A:1022837319739

Rispoli, M., Camargo, S., Machalicek, W., Lang, R., & Sigafoos, J. (2014). Functional communication training in the treatment of problem behavior maintained by access to rituals. *Journal of Applied Behavior Analysis, 47*, 580–593. https://doi.org/10.1002/jaba.130

Rispoli, M., Burke, M. D., Hatton, H., Ninci, J., Zaini, S., & Sanchez, L. (2015). Training head start teachers to conduct trial-based functional analysis of challenging behavior. *Journal of Positive Behavior Interventions, 17*, 235–244.

Rojahn, J., Whittaker, K., Hoch, T. A., & González, M. L. (2007). Assessment of self-injurious and aggressive behavior. In J. L. Matson (Ed.), *Handbook of assessment in persons with intellectual disabilities* (pp. 281–319). Boston: Academic Press.

Roscoe, E. M., Schlichenmeyer, K. J., & Dube, W. V. (2015). Functional analysis of problem behavior: A systematic approach for identifying idiosyncratic variables. *Journal of Applied Behavior Analysis, 48*, 289–314. https://doi.org/10.1002/jaba.201

Saini, V., Fisher, W. W., Retzlaff, B. J., & Keevy, M. (2020). Efficiency in functional analysis of problem behavior: A quantitative and qualitative review. *Journal of Applied Behavior Analysis, 53*, 44–66. https://doi.org/10.1002/jaba.583

Sasso, G. M., Reimers, T. M., Cooper, L. J., Wacker, D., Berg, W., Steege, M., et al. (1992). Use of descriptive and experimental analyses to identify the functional properties of aberrant behavior in school settings. *Journal of Applied Behavior Analysis, 25*, 809–821.

Scholten, A. C., Haagsma, J. A., Crossen, M. C., Olff, M., Van Beeck, E. F., & Polinder, S. (2016). Prevalence of and risk factors for anxiety and depressive disorders after traumatic brain injury: A systematic review. *Journal of Neurotrauma, 33*, 1969–1994. https://doi.org/10.1089/neu.2015.4252

Shapiro, M. B. (1957). Experimental method in the psychological description of the individual psychiatric patient. *International Journal of Social Psychiatry, 3*, 89–102.

Shipley, K. G., & McAfee, J. G. (2016). *Assessment in speech-language pathology: A resource manual* (5th ed.). Boston: Cengage Learning.

Shute, V. J., Leighton, J. P., Jang, E. E., & Chu, M.-W. (2016). Advances in the science of assessment. *Educational Assessment, 21*, 34–59. https://doi.org/10.1080/10627197.2015.1127752

Sigafoos, J., & Saggers, E. (1995). A discrete-trial approach to the functional analysis of aggressive behaviour in two boys with autism. *Australia & New Zealand Journal of Developmental Disabilities, 20*, 287–297.

Simó-Pinatella, D., Mumbardó-Adam, C., Alomar-Kurz, E., Sugai, G., & Simonsen, B. (2019). Prevalence of challenging behaviors exhibited by children with disabilities: Mapping the literature. *Journal of Behavioral Education, 28*, 323–343. https://doi.org/10.1007/s10864-019-09326-9

Skinner, B. F. (1963). Behaviorism at fifty. *Science, 140*, 951–958. https://doi.org/10.1126/science.140.3570.951

Skinner, B. F. (1981). Selection by consequences. *Science, 213*, 501–504. https://doi.org/10.1126/science.7244649

Smith, R. G., Vollmer, T. R., & St. Peter Pipkin, C. (2007). Functional approaches to assessment and treatment of problem behavior in persons with autism and related disabilities. In P. Sturmey & A. Fitzer (Eds.), *Autism spectrum disorders: Applied behavior analysis, evidence, and practice* (pp. 187–234). Austin, TX: Pro-Ed.

Steege, M. W., Pratt, J. L., Wickerd, G., Guare, R., & Steuart Watson, T. (2019). *Conducting school-based functional behavioral assessments: A practitioner's guide* (3rd ed.). New York, NY: Guilford Press.

Stokes, G. (2000). *Challenging behaviour in dementia: A person-centred approach*. London: Routledge.

Strauser, D. R., & Greco, C. E. (2020). Introduction to assessment in rehabilitation. In D. R. Strauser, T. N. Tansey, & F. Chan (Eds.), *Assessment in rehabilitation and mental health counseling* (pp. 1–11). New York, NY: Springer. https://doi.org/10.1891/9780826162434

Strauser, D. R., Tansey, T. N., & Chan, F. (Eds.). (2020). *Assessment in rehabilitation and mental health counseling*. New York, NY: Springer. https://doi.org/10.1891/9780826162434

Tiger, J. H., Hanley, G. P., & Bessette, K. K. (2006). Incorporating descriptive assessment results into the design of a functional analysis: A case example involving a preschooler's hand mouthing. *Education and Treatment of Children, 29*, 107–124.

Tremblay, R. E. (2002). Prevention if injury by early socialization of aggressive behavior. *Injury Prevention, 8*(Suppl IV), iv17–iv21. https://doi.org/10.1136/ip.8.suppl_4.iv17

Whitney, D. G., & Peterson, M. D. (2019). US national and state-level prevalence of mental health disorders and disparities of mental health care use in children. *Journal of American Medical Association: Pediatrics, 173*, 389–391. https://doi.org/10.1001/jamapediatrics.2018.5399

Chapter 2
A Brief History of Functional Analysis: An Update

Karen Nohelty, Claire Burns, and Dennis Dixon

Introduction

This chapter serves as an update to a previously published chapter on the "Brief History of Functional Analysis" (Dixon, Vogel, & Tarbox, 2012). This chapter will briefly outline the history of behaviorism and applied behavior analysis (ABA) as well as the development of behavioral functional analysis (FA). As ABA has developed as a discipline, so too has the field's understanding of using functional assessments to develop comprehensive interventions to increase adaptive and decrease maladaptive behaviors.

Key people and early studies will be discussed, including the evolution from Watson's stimulus-response theory to Skinner's experimental analysis of behavior to Baer, Wolf, and Risley's definition of ABA and the first publication of the *Journal of Applied Behavior Analysis (JABA)*. This chapter will then review the first published experimental functional analysis (EFA) by Iwata and colleagues (Iwata, Dorsey, Slifer, Bauman, & Richman, 1994).

After a synopsis of the emergence of the field and the procedures for FA, more recent adaptations of FA from its origins to expansion across methodology, populations, behaviors, and settings (e.g., school, home, telehealth) will be discussed. The implementation of analysis in developing FA procedures to address idiosyncratic variables will be reviewed. Considerations for conducting full EFAs versus abbreviated or targeted EFAs is touched upon, with an emphasis on best practices in analysis and modifications beyond the standard structure to best utilize FAs to get useful information for treatment planning. A review of methodologies in interpreting EFA results will be shared, as well as nonexperimental methods for conducting an FA. Finally, this chapter will review commonly cited barriers to FAs as well as

K. Nohelty · C. Burns · D. Dixon (✉)
Center for Autism and Related Disorders, Woodland Hills, CA, USA
e-mail: D.Dixon@centerforautism.com

© Springer Nature Switzerland AG 2021
J. L. Matson (ed.), *Functional Assessment for Challenging Behaviors and Mental Health Disorders*, Autism and Child Psychopathology Series,
https://doi.org/10.1007/978-3-030-66270-7_2

trends in the more recent literature and potential future directions. Readers are directed to subsequent chapters for specific details on methodology, reporting, populations, topography, ethical consideration, informed consent, and treatment planning. Regarding terminology, the terms "functional analysis" (FA) and "experimental functional analysis" (EFA) will be used throughout the chapter for consistency, but it should be noted that different disciplines may use other terms to describe the same procedures; for examples, in school settings, the term Functional Behavior Assessment (FBA) is common.

Historical Roots of Behavior Analysis

Prior to the advent of behaviorism, the field of psychology was primarily focused on mental processes. John B. Watson is widely credited with bringing behaviorism to the forefront of the field. He argued that the construct that should be studied in psychology was observable behavior. Watson introduced stimulus-response (S-R) theory, which suggests that that the understanding of behavior should be based on the relationship between the environmental stimulus (S) and the observable response (Watson, 1913). This theory laid the groundwork for the three-term contingency, or the relations between the stimulus, response, and consequence (Catania, 1984).

B. F. Skinner expanded the field of behaviorism by identifying and describing operant behavior, in addition to the definition of respondent behavior based on Watson and Ivan Pavlov's work (Skinner, 1938). Principles of operant behavior better explain those behaviors that could not be adequately explained by Watson's S-R theory by acknowledging the role of consequences that are resultant of the behavior itself. Skinner's stimulus-response-stimulus (S-R-S), or what now is more commonly referred to as antecedent-behavior-consequence (ABC), three-term contingency model of behavior describes the environmental variables that increase or decrease the likelihood that a behavior will occur (Moxley, 1996). This model gave rise to the term "functional analysis," which is the study of external variables that allows us to predict and change behavior based on an assumption of cause and effect between the environment and behavior (Skinner, 1953). Skinner then expanded this to the methodology of "experimental analysis of behavior," which included using a highly controlled experimental setting to observe emitted behavior. This experimental manipulation of aspects of the environment could demonstrate a clear relationship between these manipulations and the behavior of interest (Cooper, Heron, & Heward, 2014).

Some behavioral theories include structuralism, methodological behaviorism, and radical behaviorism. Structuralism focuses only on observable and describable behaviors and does not include experimental manipulations or attempt to draw causal claims regarding behavior. Methodological behaviorism also focuses only on operationally defined behavior and avoids private events but, unlike structuralism, investigates functional relationships through experimentation. Skinner's radical behaviorism also acknowledged that private events such as emotions and thoughts can also be considered behavior. He also noted that these private events are related to environmental events in the same way as observable behavior (Skinner, 1974). Skinner provided operational definitions for radical behaviorism and discussed private events and the psychological constructs of consciousness, will, and feeling, which he conceptualized as verbal behavior (Skinner, 1945).

Development of Applied Behavior Analysis

Early research on behavior analysis focused on animals such as pigeons and rats. For example, Skinner's operant chambers, or the "Skinner box," created arbitrary contingencies to study the relation between simple responses by animals and stimuli such as lights and sounds as well as primary reinforcers such as food and water (Catania, 1984). In the 1950s and 1960s, the focus of research on the experimental analysis of behavior shifted to investigate how these principles applied to humans. Early studies focused on individuals with intellectual and developmental disabilities or severe mental health concerns (e.g., schizophrenia) and were typically conducted in highly controlled settings such as laboratories, hospitals, or residential facilities (Fuller, 1949; Lindsley, 1956; Orlando & Bijou, 1960).

Both the subject matter[1] of applying behavioral principles to human participants as well as the emergence of single-subject data analysis, which indicated a shift from traditional large *n* studies, made funding and publication challenging for this field (Cooper et al., 2014). However, as more research emerged to support the evidence for behavioral approaches, the field of ABA began to take shape, including training programs through universities in the 1960s–70s as well as the advent of publication of the *Journal of Applied Behavior Analysis (JABA)* in 1968. The same year that JABA began publication, Baer, Wolf, and Risley (1968) published an article outlining best practices in research and practice in the field. These seminal events spurred the advancement of the field of ABA. Since that time, the field has expanded and has many applications across populations, settings, and fields. Based on current research and best practice, Cooper et al. (2014) provided the most widely used definition of ABA as "the science in which tactics derived from the principles of behavior are applied systematically to improve socially significant behavior and experimentation is used to identify the variables responsible for behavior change."

Origin of Procedures to Determine the Function of Behaviors

The early understanding of behavior modification included a focus on punishment and reinforcement of behavior, without much attention given to the reinforcement histories of behaviors, which lent itself to the use of more extreme contingencies

---

[1] For additional information on single-subject design, see Cooper et al. (2014).

(Mace, 1994). However, the field then began to shift to have a greater emphasis on procedures to determine the maintaining variables of the behavior. Carr's (1977) review on hypotheses of self-injurious behavior (SIB) set that stage for developing and testing hypotheses as to the function of behaviors to inform the intervention techniques. Carr's (1977) review identified positive reinforcement and negative reinforcement as well as sensory or automatic contingencies.

The focus on *consequences* of behavior within the three-term contingency generated some general principles, including that consequences can only impact subsequent behavior, they influence response classes, and the immediacy of the consequence influences that magnitude of the effect. The consequences impact whether the future frequency of the behavior will increase or decrease, and the operations are currently described as positive reinforcement, negative reinforcement, positive punishment, or negative punishment. The antecedent is also an important component of functional analyses as the environmental conditions that impact the occurrence of the behavior are considered to be the discriminative stimulus (Cooper et al., 2014).

Understanding the antecedents and consequences of behaviors enable researchers and clinicians to reliably and validly demonstrate behavior change. One of the early publications on this topic, "Some Current Dimensions of Applied Behavior Analysis" by Baer et al. (1968), described the reversal and multiple baseline techniques used to demonstrate reliable control over behavior. The reversal design involves establishing a baseline of the behavior then beginning the experimental condition to determine whether there is a subsequent change in the behavior. If so, then the experimental condition is discontinued to re-establish a baseline and then applied again to determine whether it can again establish behavior change. If a reversal design is not feasible or the behavior change is not reversible (i.e., acquired skills), a multiple baseline technique may be more appropriate, which involves considering multiple behaviors so as to compare the experimental condition across behaviors rather than removing the experimental condition from one to re-establish a baseline. A multielement design (also called an alternating treatments design) involves the concurrent implementation of multiple treatments (alternating treatments across sessions) to determine which treatment is most effective (Cooper et al., 2014). An experimental design, such as those listed above, can be used to examine the effects of different variables (e.g., social positive, social negative, and intrinsic reinforcement) on the occurrence of SIB to test hypotheses for the function of that behavior (Carr, 1977). Previous research on SIB focused on intervention strategies, with varied results (Carr, 1977). However, reviews in the late 1970s proposed that SIB, across individuals, could be maintained by multiple variables and understanding the variables surrounding SIB could lead to better interventions (Carr, 1977). While the idea was present that SIB could be controlled by multiple variables, a systematic method of assessing those variables had not yet been demonstrated in the literature.

The First Comprehensive Experimental Functional Analysis

In 1982, Iwata and colleagues addressed this area of need by publishing the ground-breaking article "Toward a Functional Analysis of Self-Injury", which remains to this day the model for implementation of EFAs (republished in 1994). Iwata and colleagues developed an assessment protocol using analogue conditions in which environmental events were manipulated in order to provide information about the function of a given challenging behavior. Assessments were conducted in an inpatient setting with nine individuals with developmental delay. Participants were each exposed to controlled conditions (eight participants were assessed with four different conditions and one participant was assessed with three conditions) using a multielement design (Iwata et al., 1994).

The social disapproval condition (often referred to as the attention condition) consisted of a room in which a variety of toys were accessible. At the start of the condition, the experimenter directed the participant to "play with the toys" and proceeded to engage in the outward behavior of reading a book or a magazine. If the participant engaged in SIB, the experimenter provided "statements of concern and disapproval" and brief physical contact (e.g., putting a hand on the participant's shoulder). Otherwise, the experimenter ignored all responses from the participant. This condition was designed to assess if social disapproval maintained engagement in the behavior of SIB (Iwata et al., 1994).

In the academic demand condition (often referred to as the escape or demand condition), participant-specific educational activities were presented by the experimenter at a table. A three-prompt procedure was used to present the demands. After providing the instruction and waiting 5 seconds, if the correct response was not exhibited, the instruction was repeated with a model prompt. After an additional 5 seconds, if the correct response was not exhibited, the instruction was repeated with a physical prompt. If the participant engaged in SIB, the experimenter immediately ended the trial and looked away for 30 seconds. This condition was designed to assess if escape from demands was a maintaining variable in the engagement of SIB (Iwata et al., 1994).

In the unstructured play condition (usually referred to as the play condition), a variety of toys were available, but there were no educational activities. Without presenting demands, the experimenter remained close to the participant and provided toys to the participant intermittently. The experimenter ignored occurrences of SIB and instead provided social praise and brief physical contact for the absence of SIB (at minimum every 30 seconds). This condition was designed to be the control, with attention and items freely available in the absence of demands. It was expected that minimal SIB would occur during this condition due to the availability of social attention and physical items (Iwata et al., 1994). However, research since Iwata's landmark study has indicated that there are situations when the rate of the behavior is higher in the play condition; specifically, the behavior may be maintained by automatic variables if a pattern of high, relatively stable occurrences of the behavior is observed across all conditions, including play (Hagopian et al., 1997).

In the alone condition, the room was devoid of toys or other items that might provide engagement. The participant remained in the room by themselves. This condition was designed to assess if there was an automatic function to the individual's SIB by providing an environment without external stimulation (Iwata et al., 1994).

One condition was presented each session and sessions were 15 minutes in length. Alternating conditions were randomly presented in a successive sequence. Presentation of conditions continued until one of three conditions were met: (1) visual analysis indicated stability in level of SIB, (2) unstable levels of SIB were observed for 5 days, (3) 12 days passed (Iwata et al., 1994).

This study indicated that an individual's learning history impacted his/her presentation of challenging behavior. In six out of nine participants, SIB consistently occurred at higher levels in one condition. However, this condition was not the same across participants. Providing empirical support for the idea that one topography of behavior may have a different function across individuals, this study demonstrated that experimental analysis of the contingencies surrounding a behavior could yield powerful information. Additionally, this landmark study demonstrated a protocol that could successfully be used to identify the function of an individual's SIB (Iwata et al., 1994).

Expansion of Functional Analyses

Iwata's work was groundbreaking in that he coalesced previous research into a methodology to analyze the contingencies surrounding a challenging behavior to determine the variables maintaining that behavior (i.e., the function). Analysis was part of ABA history from its inception; Iwata identified a more precise way of identifying the function to lead to the use of more effective interventions and reinforcers. The long-term value of Iwata's work lies in the framework for how this analysis could be conducted, allowing it to be applied in a multitude of situations. While his work was a major advancement for our field, it was just a stepping-stone for further refinement in the procedures of EFA. Ensuring that analysis was the focus, researchers who followed applied the principles from Iwata's 1982 study to numerous other situations.

Summarizing the strides taken since Iwata's original study, in 2003, Hanley and colleagues conducted a review of EFA literature through the year 2000, encompassing a total of 277 studies, to provide information across various dimensions of EFAs included in research (e.g., population characteristics, setting characteristics, response topographies, condition types; Hanley, Iwata, & McCord, 2003). Beavers and colleagues replicated this review in 2013, including 158 EFA studies from January 2001 through May 2012, providing a picture of how EFAs changed in the field in the ensuing decade. In the following sections regarding expansion of EFAs, comparison of results between these two reviews will be included to provide information regarding trends in the research regarding how EFAs are conducted (Beavers, Iwata, & Lerman, 2013).

The methodology developed by Iwata and colleagues has been replicated numerous times with each major variable expanded and generalized. The resulting body of work has demonstrated the remarkable range of utility of EFA procedures. In the sections that follow, expansions and modifications to the original Iwata EFA are described, including expansions across methodology, populations, behaviors, and settings/individuals.

Expansion Across Methodology

Iwata's EFA study described several conditions that were consistent with the current understanding within the field of the functions of behavior (i.e., attention, escape/demand, play, alone). However, a function that was not directly addressed in Iwata's study was tangible reinforcement (where access to items/activities is the maintaining variable). The tangible condition is similar to the attention condition, except access to toys/items/activities were provided in the absence of social attention and was first described by Mace and West (1986). However, their analysis was complicated by a dual function of escape from demands and tangible. It was first investigated as a discrete function in a study by Day, Rea, Schussler, Larsen, and Johnson (1988). Since these initial developments of the tangible conditions, it has been included in EFAs more commonly. In 2003, Hanley and colleagues noted that 38.3% of studies incorporating EFAs included a tangible condition; this number increased to 54% in 2013 (Beavers et al., 2013). However, a recommendation made by Hanley et al. (2003) and continued by Beavers et al. (2013) in their review was to only include a tangible condition when initial data (e.g., observations, interview) suggest that tangible items may be a maintaining variable; the tangible condition has been shown to be more prone to a false-positive outcome and its increasing use may have contributed to the increase in multiple controlled outcomes observed in the 2013 review.

Iwata's original study involved the use of a multielement design (Iwata et al., 1994); however, this is not the only experimental design that could be used to gather information on the variables maintaining a behavior. A review by Hanley et al. (2003) found that the multielement design was most widely used (81.2% of EFA studies), followed by the reversal design (15.5% of EFA studies). Ten years later, these rates varied only slightly (multielement 79.1% and reversal 12%; Beavers et al., 2013). The pairwise design is also used in EFA, but less commonly; it is often used when multielement designs do not yield clear outcomes (Hanley et al., 2003).

In contrast to Iwata's original study which involved the manipulation of antecedents and consequences, another EFA methodology includes manipulation only of the antecedent of the behavior. Carr and Durand (1985) first established this methodology by manipulating only the antecedents of challenging behaviors such as aggression, tantrums, and self-injurious behavior by teaching functional communication as a replacement behavior and using differential reinforcement. These same authors then demonstrated maintenance and generalization of these results in a subsequent study (Durand & Carr, 1991). A 2003 review by Hanley and colleagues indicated that antecedent-only methodology was widely published in the research literature, included in 20.2% of EFA studies (Hanley et al., 2003); however, by 2013, the use of this methodology had decreased, to 12% (Beavers et al., 2013). This decrease suggests that the benefits of programming both antecedent and consequences outweigh the potential extra effort in implementation of consequences (Beavers et al., 2013).

Expansion Across Populations

Early in its development, EFAs were primarily conducted with individuals with intellectual and/or developmental disabilities (Beavers et al., 2013). While still the primary population for this method of assessment, the procedures have been demonstrated with individuals with other diagnoses, including attention deficit hyperactivity disorder, conduct disorder, dementia, Tourette syndrome, schizophrenia, and traumatic brain injury (Beavers et al., 2013; DuPaul & Ervin, 1996). The procedures have been increasingly used with individuals without disabilities as well. From 2003 to 2013, the percentage of EFAs conducted with individuals without disabilities increased from 9.0% to 21.5% (Beavers et al., 2013; Hanley et al., 2003). At the same time, studies incorporating EFAs with individuals with autism spectrum disorder (ASD) also increased 20.9–37.3% (Beavers et al., 2013, Hanley et al., 2003). Various reasons could explain the increase, including an increase in prevalence of ASD within the population, increased public awareness of ASD, and increased focus on research with individuals with ASD among behavior analysts.

EFAs have also been conducted with individuals of varying ages. While the majority of studies have been, and continue to be, conducted with children, adults make up a sizeable proportion of the individuals studied (24.7% in studies from 2001–2012, Beavers et al., 2013). While initially studies were conducted with school age children, Kurtz et al. (2003) implemented the techniques with very young children (10 months to 4 years 11 months of age) who engaged in SIB.

Expansion Across Behaviors

Since 1982 when Iwata and colleagues introduced functional analysis for SIB, the procedure has been applied to a multitude of topographies. In 2003, Hanley found that SIB (64.6% of EFAs) was the most commonly assessed behavior; by 2013, Beaver and colleagues found that aggression (47.5% of EFAs) was most commonly assessed. Additional topographies include vocalizations, property destruction, disruption, elopement, noncompliance, stereotypy, tantrums, and pica. From 2003 to 2013 a general trend was observed in expanding EFA procedures to different topographies, including licking/ mouthing/sniffing objects, rumination, expelling/packing food, disrobing, inappropriate sexual behavior, and nail biting. Additionally, in the past 10 years, an increase in assessing multiple topographies in one EFA was observed, from 27.8% to 75.9% of studies (Beavers et al., 2013, Hanley et al., 2003). Recently, an emphasis has also been placed on conducting EFAs for inappropriate behaviors that occur during mealtime. In 2019, Saini and colleagues conducted a systematic review of literature on EFAs conducted for this topography. Their findings supported the notion that EFAs could be effectively conducted on mealtime behaviors. While they found escape was identified as the reinforcer in the vast majority of cases (92%), the identification of multiple functions for one topography and individual was also prevalent.

One concern when conducting EFAs is the potential risk of injury to the individual, due to setting up contingencies that are designed to elicit the challenging behavior (Fritz, Iwata, Hammond, & Bloom, 2013). In order for the results of an EFA to be interpretable, observation of the challenging behavior needs to occur; however, when assessing contingencies surrounding severe challenging behavior that is unsafe to the individual (e.g., SIB) or others (e.g., aggression), a standard EFA may not be possible (Fritz et al., 2013). In 2002, Smith and Churchill identified a potential method to reduce this risk by focusing on precursor behaviors, which precede the target behavior (i.e., severe challenging behavior that is unsafe). If the precursor behavior and target behavior are members of the same response class, analysis of the precursor behavior will enable identification of the function without eliciting the target behavior. In their study, Smith and Churchill identified precursor behaviors that reliably preceded challenging behaviors and demonstrated that there was correspondence in function identified from an EFA for the precursor behavior and the challenging behavior (Smith & Churchill, 2002). In 2013, Fritz and colleagues took this concept further by identifying precursor behaviors using a checklist, identifying the function of precursor and severe challenging behavior via an EFA and then implementing an intervention based on the analysis of the precursor behavior. They found that rates of precursor and challenging behaviors decreased following this intervention (Fritz et al., 2013). In 2018, Hoffmann and colleagues replicated these results with preschool children; an intervention implemented based on the results of the precursor analysis alone (without an EFA completed on the challenging behavior) resulted in reduction of both precursor and severe challenging behavior (Hoffmann, Sellers, Halversen, & Bloom, 2018).

Challenging behaviors that occur at low rates may lead to an EFA with inconclusive results as the behavior may occur infrequently or not all during the assessment process. To address this challenge, Kahng, Abt, and Schonbachler (2001) conducted extended functional analyses, lasting an eight-hour day, with conditions varying across days. Using these procedures, they were able to identify the function and developed a successful intervention to reduce the challenging behavior. The authors noted concerns with this procedure, including the potential difficulty in staffing this extended assessment as well as ethical concerns over exposing the individual to the assessment for this extended duration. In 2004, Tarbox and colleagues identified an alternative procedure, involving starting the assessment when the challenging behavior occurred, that also resulted in identification of function and implementation of an effective treatment for two participants. Another approach that can aid in addressing safety concerns is a latency-based FA, which uses latency to the target behavior as the dependent variable (Davis et al., 2013; Falcomata, Muething, Roberts, Hamrick, & Shpall, 2016; Heath & Smith, 2019; Iwata & Dozier, 2008).

Expansion Across Settings and Individuals

The high degree of environmental control required to conduct an EFA may create a barrier for many clients, as it may not be possible to carry out an EFA in a clinical setting. Additionally, the more well controlled the conditions, the less potential for ecological validity. The assessment setting is often different from the one in which the behavior most often occurs in the natural environment or is at least altered (Hanley et al., 2003), and the EFA setting has been shown to sometimes be related to differences in the EFA results (Lang et al., 2008). One recommendation to address the differences in circumstances is to include people in the assessment who the client has a previous learning history with, such as parent or caregiver, teachers, or peers (Hanley et al., 2003).There was a shift in the research in the late twentieth and early twenty-first centuries to investigate the utility and accuracy of EFAs in other settings, particularly home and school (Iwata & Dozier, 2008). Although there may be some loss in environmental control, there is also value in conducting EFAs in the context in which challenging behaviors most often occur.

Schools

Based on a review by Anderson, Rodriguez, and Campbell (2015), the first research study was published on FA in the school setting in 1981 (Weeks & Gaylord-Ross, 1981). The number of yearly studies on school-based FAs has increased since that time, indicating more widespread interest in applying FAs to address challenging behavior in schools. Since 1997, schools have been mandated to use FAs to develop Behavior Intervention Plans (BIPs) by the Individuals with Disabilities Education Act (Allday, Nelson, & Russel, 2011). Anderson et al.'s (2015) review indicated that many studies reported using more than one form of FA, with over 60% using experimental analysis. Nearly half of the studies used non-experimental methods. Although EFAs are recommended in schools, there are several barriers to conducting thorough EFAs in this setting.

As research on FAs in schools gained traction in the early 2000s, several issues were identified, including lack of inclusion of low-rate challenging behaviors, students with disabilities as participants, and academic behaviors as the target outcome (Ervin et al., 2001). Scott, Liaupsin, Nelson, and McIntyre (2005) conducted a descriptive analysis of barriers to team-based FAs based on feedback from FA teams in schools. Of the 13 teams interviewed, 11 indicated that a referral for an FA was due to a crisis behavior. The other two teams indicated that the referral was made for challenging behaviors that were not at a crisis level that had been occurring for more than 6 months. No proactive strategies were reportedly tried prior to the referral for all 13 teams, and one team noted that no interventions had been attempted in the past while the other 12 reported that only punitive strategies had been implemented. The authors advocated the need for sufficient systems to support FA teams in schools. Proactive use of FAs is recommended but based on these results is not being utilized adequately in schools. This and other studies continue to indicate that although there is significant research to indicate the effectiveness of interventions based on FAs in schools, these techniques are not being applied consistently or successfully in schools due to a variety of barriers (Allday et al., 2011). Similarly, in a statewide survey of practitioners working with individuals with ASD either in schools, private programs, or who had a Board Certified Behavior Analyst (BCBA) certification, two-third of participants endorsed a belief that FA is the best assessment tool for informing treatment, but only one-third routinely used FA for this purpose (Roscoe, Phillips, Kelly, Farber, & Dube, 2015).

The question of who is qualified to conduct a functional analysis of behavior has been addressed frequently in the literature. Some have emphasized the limitations and potential harm of attempting to conduct an FA without proper training and have strongly recommended that only those with a BCBA or a certain level of training in behavior analysis conduct FAs for severe challenging behaviors (Hanley, 2012). Anderson et al.'s (2015) review pointed out that in published studies on school-based FAs, although teachers conducted data collection, a researcher always directed how the FA was conducted. They also noted that teachers were more likely to be involved in data collection for descriptive assessments, but researchers were more likely to conduct experimental designs, which is consistent with two earlier reviews, one by Solnick and Ardoin (2010) which found that teachers rarely participated in data collection and another by Allday et al. (2011) which reported that teachers often completed interview or rating scales but rarely were involved in active data collection. This review highlighted the consideration that the school-based FA research literature may not represent current clinical practice in schools. However, there is a substantial amount of literature indicating that teachers effectively implement EFAs when there is adequate training and consultation (Erbas, Tekin-Iftar, & Yucesoy, 2006; McKenney, Waldron, & Conroy, 2013; Rispoli et al., 2015). Erbas et al. (2006) also found that teachers rated functional analysis more positively following training.

Home and Residences

Another setting where challenging behaviors frequently occur is the home or residence of the individual. Arndorfer, Miltenberger, Woster, Rortvedt, and Gaffaney (1994) conducted descriptive and experimental FAs in the home setting, with parents included as active participants. This study included the use of the functional assessment interview (FAI), ABC data, and motivation assessment scale (MAS). The authors noted that brief EFA, which is discussed later in this chapter in greater detail, may be more appropriate in this setting than standard EFA. They found that data obtained from parental interview and ABC assessment was sufficient to determine the functions of the behavior and were consistent with an EFA. Additionally, parents were able to complete the EFA with instruction from the researcher. This study emphasized the importance of future research on feasibility and validity of FAs conducted by parents and teachers in naturalistic settings. Similarly, Thomason-Sassi, Iwata, & Fritz (2013) found that FAs conducted by caregivers who had received training or in the home setting were sufficiently consistent with FAs conducted by trained staff in clinic settings. However, they noted that this study did not directly investigate procedural integrity, so this variable should be evaluated in the future.

Emphasis in the parent training literature involves education on the functions of behavior and development of behavior plans to address challenging behaviors in children. Many manualized interventions emphasize the use of behavioral principles for parents to understand their child's behavior, including the Research Units Behavioral Intervention (RUBI; Bearss et al., 2018), Parent Child Interaction Therapy (PCIT), Managing the Defiant Child (Barkley, 1997), Defiant Teens (Barkley & Robin, 2013), the Incredible Years (Webster-Stratton, 2001), and Positive Parenting Program (Triple P; Sanders, 2003), among many others. Therefore, having parents participate in and understand FAs and how they inform treatment approaches would likely be beneficial to fidelity of intervention implementation by caregivers.

Technology and Telehealth

Another area that holds significant implications for behavioral assessment and intervention is the use of technology, such as mobile-based applications and use of telehealth for assessment, intervention, and training. For example, several mobile-based applications have been developed to collect behavioral data. ABA providers have been using programs designed specifically to allow behavior technicians to collect fast and reliable data and enable supervisors to review clients' progress for years. More recently, apps have been developed for other professionals, such as teachers, as well as parents or caregivers. Apps include programs to prompt and reward appropriate behaviors as well as track ABC data (7 Apps for Applied Behavior Analysis Therapy, 2017). Many research studies have focused on the effect of app-based interventions on improvement in functional communication. For example, one study by Law, Neihart, and Dutt (2018) found that training in parent implementation of the Map4speech app resulted in high levels of procedural integrity by parents and an increase in functional communication in children. However, few have evaluated the use of an app to conduct an FA of behavior. This may be an area of future research to incorporate technology-based systems within the context of parent training.

Telehealth services have been used to train caregivers, teachers, and direct care staff to successfully implement assessment and treatment based on ABA (Boisvert, Lang, Andrianopoulos, & Boscardin, 2010; Ferguson, Craig, & Dounavi, 2019; Tomlinson, Gore, & McGill, 2018). The use of telehealth by professionals also has implications for barriers to FAs such as lack of resources in certain areas. One study investigated the use of telehealth by behavior consultants to conduct FAs with children with ASD who lived significant distances from medical facilities that offer these types of services (Wacker et al., 2013). FAs were conducted by parents in local clinics during weekly telehealth meetings with behavior consultants who were located in a Teleconsultation Center. For EFAs, functions of challenging behaviors were identified with high interrater agreement for 18 out of 20 cases. These results support the use of telehealth to conduct FAs remotely (Wacker et al., 2013). Similar results were reported by another study that evaluated the use of telehealth to train parents to conduct an FA and provide behavioral intervention to address challenging behaviors and increase functional communication (Machalicek et al., 2016).

Idiosyncratic Variables

Standard test conditions for EFAs include attention, escape, tangible, play, and alone. However, there are situations in which elements not contained within those conditions impact the occurrence or non-occurrence of a target behavior that have been examined more frequently in recent years. Idiosyncratic variables are those that are particular to a given individual or situation and impact rate of the target behavior. Failure to identify idiosyncratic variables can result in identification of the incorrect function of the behavior, leading to an unsuccessful intervention. Carr et al. (1997) conducted EFAs with three individuals, demonstrating that idiosyncratic stimuli impacted the outcomes of the EFAs. For one of the individuals, slightly higher frequency of challenging behaviors were observed in the demand condition over the attention condition, which indicated an escape function of the behavior. However, subsequent analysis indicated that the behavior occurred more often in situations where small objects that could be manipulated (e.g., small balls, wristband) were absent. Additionally, Carr et al. (1997) identified guidelines to aid in identifying if idiosyncratic variables are present, thus requiring further analysis. A review conducted by Schlichenmeyer, Roscoe, Rooker, Wheeler, and Dube (2013) identified over 30 idiosyncratic variables that impacted outcomes in EFAs. Additionally, they identified strategies utilized by researchers to identify idiosyncratic variables (i.e., informal observation, anecdotal report, descriptive assessments, manipulation and observation, indirect assessments). Overall, they noted an increase in the rigor used in analyzing idiosyncratic variables.

Taking the process of identifying idiosyncratic variables further, Roscoe et al. (2015) delineated a systematic approach for identifying idiosyncratic variables.

Following inconclusive standard EFA results, the researchers were able to identify a function for the challenging behavior for five out of six participants using an indirect assessment questionnaire and/or a descriptive analysis.

In conducting EFAs, it is important to analyze the situation for the specific patient and not rely on standard EFA conditions. The goal of an EFA is to identify the variable(s) maintaining the challenging behavior. At times, this may involve using the standard EFA conditions; however, they may be insufficient to determine the maintaining variables. Before conducting an EFA, it is critical to gather information about the patient and their environment to enable design of conditions that will more likely identify the maintaining variables surrounding their challenging behavior. The standard EFA conditions should be used as a tool and should not replace analysis on the part of the behavior analyst. The procedures used to analyze function of behavior will continue to evolve as more research is gathered on idiosyncratic variables.

Functional Analysis Duration

One potential barrier to conducting an EFA is the time required to complete the procedure. Full EFAs include at least three observations across a minimum of two conditions, while a brief EFA includes two or fewer observations in each condition (Hanley et al., 2003). The brief EFA has gained popularity and is designed to be conducted within 90 minutes (Northup et al., 1991). Wallace and Iwata (1999) investigated the reliability of data when the 15-minute conditions were retrospectively shortened by deleting data from the last 5 or 10 minutes of the session. Their results suggested that duration of each session could be shortened while still yielding informative and accurate data.

In addition to brief EFAs, another way to conduct an EFA in a limited amount of time is to test one function through a repeated-measures analysis, which includes a single test condition compared to a control. This is most often used when indirect measures such as caregiver report or rating scales support one hypothesized function, and if the EFA indicates that this condition is related to the behavior it has implications for more immediate treatment; however, if a clear function is not established, then a more traditional EFA that evaluates several test conditions is warranted (Iwata & Dozier, 2008). This may expedite the EFA process and lead to faster implementation of intervention; however, if the hypothesized function is not clearly determined then follow-up EFAs may be required.

Another variation of EFAs are alone series, which are employed when there is strong evidence that the behavior is automatically maintained and so a series of alone conditions are repeated to test this hypothesis (Iwata & Dozier, 2008). Situations where it is not possible to employ rigorous methodological control and integration into the natural context is beneficial often call for trial-based EFAs (Larkin, Hawkins, & Collins, 2016; Rispoli, Ninci, Neely, & Zaini, 2014; Ruiz, 2017). Trial-based EFAs involve embedding short trials (e.g., 1–3 minutes) into the natural context/environment where antecedents and consequences are manipulated during the course of the shortened trial. They are therefore a useful alternative when there are limited resources or other limitations to conduct a traditional EFA (Bloom, Iwata, Fritz, Roscoe, & Carreau, 2011).

Interpretation of Functional Analyses

Visual inspection or visual analysis is the standard method of interpreting data in single subject design research; this is the primary method of interpreting EFA results as well (Kazdin, 2011). Following the collection and graphing of data from an EFA, the graphs are viewed to identify "patterns of responding within and across conditions to determine, which, if any, of the variables may be responsible for behavioral maintenance" (Hagopian et al., 1997). Elements analyzed include "number of data points within a specific condition or phase, variability of data points, level of data, and the direction and degree of trends" (Roane, Fisher, Kelley, Mevers, & Bouxsein, 2013). Following visual analysis of the graphed data, the results are categorized. Hagopian et al. (1997) identified 12 categories of results, corresponding to the variable(s) maintaining the challenging behavior: (1) undifferentiated; (2) attention; (3) escape from demands; (4) tangible; (5) automatic; (6) attention and escape; (7) attention and tangible; (8) tangible and escape; (9) automatic and escape; (10) automatic and attention; (11) automatic and tangible; and (12) attention, tangible, and escape. However, there are potential downsides to the use of visual analysis, including the subjective nature of the analysis, the lack of specified procedures, low interrater agreement, and the challenge in interpreting data that is highly variable or includes minimal differences in level (Danov & Symons, 2008, Hagopian et al., 1997). Interrater agreement of at least 70% is considered necessary, at least 80% is considered adequate, and of at least 90% is considered good (House, House, & Campbell, 1981). In a survey conducted by Danov and Symons (2008) in which graphs were mailed to faculty and graduate student trainees without a specific visual inspection criterion, overall mean interrater agreement was 0.63. Experts had only slightly higher mean (0.65 compared with 0.63) and no rater reached the standard of good (over 90%). Categories accounting for multiple functions and undifferentiated results received lower agreement. Single social functions resulted in the highest interrater agreement. In 2015, Ninci et al. conducted a meta-analysis of interrater agreement on visual inspection results (19 articles were identified for inclusion, not necessarily functional analysis graphs) and found an overall weighted score of 0.76 (Ninci, Vannest, Willson, & Zhang, 2015).

Accurate interpretation of the function is critical to implementing an appropriate, function-based intervention (Roane et al., 2013). Over the past several decades, procedures have been developed to improve this method. Hagopian et al. (1997) developed structured criteria for interpreting EFA data that included a list of steps to follow. Without using the criteria, the interrater agreement of predoctoral interns was low (0.46); after training (didactic instruction, modeling, practice with feedback) on the criteria, interrater agreement significantly improved (0.81). While this criterion should not replace visual inspection or be applied rigidly (as it does not encapsulate all potential situations), the researchers demonstrated that decision making rules could be operationalized and individuals could be trained in the use of these procedures to increase interrater agreement. In 2013, Roane and colleagues extended these results, applying a modified criterion, allowing the criteria to be applied to a greater range of EFAs (i.e., not requiring a specific number of data points per condition, so allowing for varied lengths of EFAs to be interpreted with this criteria). Additionally, they used training similar to that of Hagopian et al. (1997) to train master's-level students and postbaccalaureate behavior therapists. During pretraining, when they were provided with the written criteria only, they achieved 0.73 and 0.80 interrater agreement, respectively. After the training, they received 0.98 and 0.95, respectively, indicating that the procedures can be used to train non-experts in visual inspection.

However, results of visual inspection are not always conclusive. When variability in the data lead to an undifferentiated function, the results need to be clarified. A recent review of published research indicated that differentiated results lead to the identification of a function in 94% of cases; while this is a high percentage, it is likely that publication bias resulted in a percentage that is higher than is what is seen in general clinical settings (Beavers et al., 2013). In recent years, procedures have been developed to aid in clarifying inconclusive results to aid in identifying effective function-based interventions; the literature supports the use of a combination of various approaches to identify a function in these situations (Saini, Greer, & Fisher, 2015). In a summary of 176 cases, Hagopian, Rooker, Jessel, and DeLeon (2013) found that a function was identified following the implementation of a standard EFA only in 47% of cases. They then implemented initial modifications to the EFA that they classified into one of three categories (or a combination): antecedent modifications (e.g., using more challenging demand condition tasks), changes to consequences (e.g., providing varied forms of attention), or design modifications (e.g., using a reversal instead of a multielement design) and were able to obtain differentiated results in 84% of total cases. Following secondary modifications, a function was identified for a total of 93% of cases. The most effective initial modification was change to the EFA design. When an EFA resulted in inclusive results for aggression, Saini et al. (2015) used multiple strategies to determine the function, including graphing topographies separately, conducting an EFA for one topography only, modifying the EFA procedures to aid in discrimination between conditions, and evaluating treatments matched to a proposed function.

Recently, research has been conducted on training staff to analyze undifferentiated EFA results. Chok, Shlesinger, Studer, and Bird (2012) implemented a training program (including instruction, modeling, practice, and feedback) for BCBAs that involved teaching four component skills in conducting an EFA: accurately implementing the EFA conditions, interpreting EFA graphs, identifying next steps for undifferentiated graphs, and determining function-based interventions to implement based on EFA results. All three participants demonstrated a significant increase over baseline in all four areas. Schnell, Sidener, DeBar, Vladescu, and Kahng (2018) trained graduate students in making appropriate decisions when presented with undifferentiated EFA data. Computer-based training was used to teach the students that included multi-media modes of presentation, interaction, and quizzes. For 19 out of 20 students, identification of the function (or lack of differentiation) and the next step (i.e., brief EFA, multielement EFA, extended alone condition, pairwise analysis, refer client to treatment) improved over baseline following treatment and maintained 2 weeks following treatment. However, for both of the articles discussed above, training was conducted with prepared graphs as opposed to with graphs that resulted from an EFA with a client.

Nonexperimental Methods for Functional Analysis

Although EFAs have numerous advantages over nonexperimental methods of functional analysis, due to a variety of limitations it is often not possible to conduct an EFA. Nonexperimental methods most often consist of direct observation or descriptive analysis or indirect assessments through interviews and rating scales (Healy & Brett, 2014). Direct or descriptive assessments often consist of identifying relevant information or recording of data such as frequency, duration, and ABC. These methods do not include experimental modification of variables that may be related to the behavior (Herzinger & Campbell, 2007). Indirect assessments include interviews, and questionnaires or scales such as the Questions About Behavior Function (QABF; Paclawskyj, Matson, Rush, Smalls, & Vollmer, 2000), the Motivation Assessment Scale (MAS; Durand, 1989) and the Motivation Analysis Rating Scale (MARS; Wiesler, Hanzel, Chamberlain, & Thompson, 1985). The Functional Assessment Interview (FAI), which is adapted from O'Neill et al. (1997), is also widely used to gather information.

One study compared types of functional assessments (i.e., indirect, descriptive, and experimental) and found that descriptive assessments typically did not yield conclusive information, while indirect and experimental assessments provided what were considered conclusive findings. The authors noted that "current results suggest that indirect and experimental functional assessment procedures may be the most cost-effective and reliable options" (Tarbox et al., 2009). Additionally, Fee, Schieber, Noble, and Valdovinos (2016) compared indirect and direct assessments. Indirect assessments investigated were the QABF, the MAS, and FAI. These measures were compared to brief EFAs (Northup et al., 1991). There were inconsistencies in results across measures, and the authors suggested that using them in conjunction with one another to increase the accuracy of the results. They also noted that information gained from indirect assessments can be beneficial in understanding parent or caregiver's perception of the functions of behaviors, even if these are not the primary functions identified through direct assessment. This understanding of parent or caregiver perception has implications for treatment, as it may inform parent training following identification of the primary function (Fee et al., 2016).

Future Directions

Several barriers to FAs and limitations of current practice have been identified in the present chapter. Some of the most commonly cited obstacles include issues measuring low-rate behaviors, time commitment, risk of harm, changing reinforcers over time, multiple topographies and functions, and lack of investment from stakeholders (Hanley, 2012). The last several decades have yielded research to address some of the primary initial limitations of the initial FA procedures; however, there continue to be barriers to conducting FAs in real-world settings that are not always reflected in research studies. Ecological validity continues to be a primary concern within the field. It is important moving forward that clinicians and researchers continue to attempt to expand the procedures for FAs to better fit the real-world needs of clients and continue to critically think about the analysis component of FAs (Dixon et al., 2012). Subsequent chapters in this volume are aimed at addressing considerations for practical application of the FAs that expand the methodologies described in the present chapter.

References

7 Apps for Applied Behavior Analysis Therapy. (2017, February 23). Retrieved from: https://online.sju.edu/graduate/masters-special-education/resources/articles/7-apps-for-applied-behavior-analysis-therapy

Allday, R. A., Nelson, J. R., & Russel, C. S. (2011). Classroom-based functional behavioral assessment: Does the literature support high Fidelity implementation? *Journal of Disability Policy Studies, 22*(3), 140–149. https://doi.org/10.1177/1044207311399380

Anderson, C. M., Rodriguez, B. J., & Campbell, A. (2015). Functional behavior assessment in schools: Current status and future directions. *Journal of Behavioral Education, 24*(3), 338–371. https://doi.org/10.1007/s10864-015-9226-z

Arndorfer, R. E., Miltenberger, R. G., Woster, S. H., Rortvedt, A. K., & Gaffaney, T. (1994). Home-based descriptive and experimental analysis of problem behaviors in children. *Topics in Early Childhood Special Education, 14*(1), 64–87. https://doi.org/10.1177/027112149401400108

Baer, D. M., Wolf, M. M., & Risley, T. R. (1968). Some current dimensions of applied behavior analysis. *Journal of Applied Behavior Analysis, 1*(1), 91–97. https://doi.org/10.1901/jaba.1968.1-91

Barkley, R., & Robin, A. L. (2013). *The defiant teen: 10 steps to resolve conflict and build your relationships.* New York, NY: Guilford Press.

Barkley, R. A. (1997). *Managing the defiant child: A guide to parent training.* Guilford Publications.

Bearss, K., Johnson, C. R., Handen, B. L., Butter, E., Lecavalier, L., Smith, T., & Scahill, L. (2018). *Parent training for disruptive behavior: The RUBI Autism Network, clinician manual.* New York, NY: Oxford University Press.

Beavers, G. A., Iwata, B. A., & Lerman, D. C. (2013). Thirty years of research on the functional analysis of problem behavior: Thirty years of functional analysis. *Journal of Applied Behavior Analysis, 46*(1), 1–21. https://doi.org/10.1002/jaba.30

Bloom, S. E., Iwata, B. A., Fritz, J. N., Roscoe, E. M., & Carreau, A. B. (2011). Classroom application of a trial-based functional analysis. *Journal of Applied Behavior Analysis, 44*(1), 19–31. https://doi.org/10.1901/jaba.2011.44-19

Boisvert, M., Lang, R., Andrianopoulos, M., & Boscardin, M. L. (2010). Telepractice in the assessment and treatment of individuals with autism spectrum disorders: A systematic review. *Developmental Neurorehabilitation, 13*(6), 423–432. https://doi.org/10.3109/17518423.2010. 499889

Carr, E. G. (1977). The motivation of self-injurious behavior: A review of some hypotheses. *Psychological Bulletin, 84*(4), 800–816.

Carr, E. G., & Durand, V. M. (1985). Reducing behavior problems through functional communication training. *Journal of Applied Behavior Analysis, 18*(2), 111–126. https://doi.org/10.1901/jaba.1985.18-111

Carr, E. G., Yarbrough, S. C., & Langdon, N. A. (1997). Effects of idiosyncratic stimulus variables on functional analysis outcomes. *Journal of Applied Behavior Analysis, 30*(4), 673–686. https://doi.org/10.1901/jaba.1997.30-673

Catania, A. C. (1984). The operant behaviorism of B. F. Skinner. *Behavioral and Brain Sciences, 7*(4), 473–475. https://doi.org/10.1017/S0140525X00026728

Chok, J. T., Shlesinger, A., Studer, L., & Bird, F. L. (2012). Description of a practitioner training program on functional analysis and treatment development. *Behavior Analysis in Practice, 5*(2), 25–36. https://doi.org/10.1007/BF03391821

Cooper, J. O., Heron, T. E., & Heward, W. L. (2014). *Applied behavior analysis* (2nd ed.). Harlow, UK: Pearson Education Limited.

Danov, S. E., & Symons, F. J. (2008). A survey evaluation of the reliability of visual inspection and functional analysis graphs. *Behavior Modification, 32*(6), 828–839. https://doi.org/10.1177/0145445508318606

Davis, T. N., Durand, S., Bankhead, J., Strickland, E., Blenden, K., Dacus, S., … Machalicek, W. (2013). Brief report: Latency functional analysis of elopement. *Behavioral Interventions, 28*(3), 251–259. https://doi.org/10.1002/bin.1363

Day, R. M., Rea, J. A., Schussler, N. G., Larsen, S. E., & Johnson, W. L. (1988). A functionally based approach to the treatment of self-injurious behavior. *Behavior Modification, 12*(4), 565–589.

Dixon, D. R., Vogel, T., & Tarbox, J. (2012). A brief history of functional analysis and applied behavior analysis. In J. L. Matson (Ed.), *Functional assessment for challenging behaviors.* New York, NY: Springer Science + Business Media.

DuPaul, G. J., & Ervin, R. A. (1996). Functional assessment of behaviors related to attention-deficit/hyperactivity disorder: Linking assessment to intervention design. *Behavior Therapy, 27*(4), 601–622. https://doi.org/10.1016/S0005-7894(96)80046-3

Durand, V. M. (1989). *The motivation assessment scale.* New York, NY: Pergamon Press.

Durand, V. M., & Carr, E. G. (1991). Functional communication training to reduce challenging behavior: Maintenance and application in new settings. *Journal of Applied Behavior Analysis, 24*(2), 251–264. https://doi.org/10.1901/jaba.1991.24-251

Erbas, D., Tekin-Iftar, E., & Yucesoy, S. (2006). Teaching special education teachers how to conduct functional analysis in natural settings. *Education and Training in Developmental Disabilities, 41*(1), 28–36. JSTOR.

Ervin, R. A., Radford, P. M., Bertsch, K., Piper, A. L., Ehrhardt, K. E., & Poling, A. (2001). A descriptive analysis and critique of the empirical literature on school-based functional assessment. *School Psychology Review, 30*(2), 193–210. https://doi.org/10.1080/02796015.2001.12086109

Falcomata, T. S., Muething, C. S., Roberts, G. J., Hamrick, J., & Shpall, C. (2016). Further evaluation of latency-based brief functional analysis methods: An evaluation of treatment utility. *Developmental Neurorehabilitation, 19*(2), 88–94. https://doi.org/10.3109/17518423.2014.910281

Fee, A., Schieber, E., Noble, N., & Valdovinos, M. G. (2016). Agreement between questions about behavior function, the motivation assessment scale, functional assessment interview, and brief functional analysis of children's challenging behaviors. *Behavior Analysis: Research and Practice, 16*(2), 94–102. https://doi.org/10.1037/bar0000040

Ferguson, J., Craig, E. A., & Dounavi, K. (2019). Telehealth as a model for providing behaviour analytic interventions to individuals with autism spectrum disorder: A systematic review. *Journal of Autism and Developmental Disorders, 49*(2), 582–616. https://doi.org/10.1007/s10803-018-3724-5

Fritz, J. N., Iwata, B. A., Hammond, J. L., & Bloom, S. E. (2013). Experimental analysis of precursors to severe problem behavior: Analysis of precursors. *Journal of Applied Behavior Analysis, 46*(1), 101–129. https://doi.org/10.1002/jaba.27

Fuller, P. R. (1949). Operant conditioning of a vegetative human organism. *The American Journal of Psychology, 62*, 587–590. https://doi.org/10.2307/1418565

Hagopian, L. P., Fisher, W. W., Thompson, R. H., Owen-DeSchryver, J., Iwata, B. A., & Wacker, D. P. (1997). Toward the development of structured criteria for interpretation of functional analysis data. *Journal of Applied Behavior Analysis, 30*(2), 313–326. https://doi.org/10.1901/jaba.1997.30-313

Hagopian, L. P., Rooker, G. W., Jessel, J., & DeLeon, I. G. (2013). Initial functional analysis outcomes and modifications in pursuit of differentiation: A summary of 175 inpatient cases: FA modifications. *Journal of Applied Behavior Analysis, 46*(1), 88–100. https://doi.org/10.1002/jaba.25

Hanley, G. P. (2012). Functional assessment of problem behavior: Dispelling myths, overcoming implementation obstacles, and developing new lore. *Behavior Analysis in Practice, 5*(1), 54–72. https://doi.org/10.1007/BF03391818

Hanley, G. P., Iwata, B. A., & McCord, B. E. (2003). Functional analysis of problem behavior: A review. *Journal of Applied Behavior Analysis, 36*(2), 147–185. https://doi.org/10.1901/jaba.2003.36-147

Healy, O., & Brett, D. (2014). Functional behavior assessments for challenging behavior in autism. In V. B. Patel, V. R. Preedy, & C. R. Martin (Eds.), *Comprehensive guide to Autism* (pp. 2881–2901). New York, NY: Springer. https://doi.org/10.1007/978-1-4614-4788-7_191

Heath, H., & Smith, R. G. (2019). Precursor behavior and functional analysis: A brief review. *Journal of Applied Behavior Analysis, 52*(3), 804–810. https://doi.org/10.1002/jaba.571

Herzinger, C. V., & Campbell, J. M. (2007). Comparing functional assessment methodologies: A quantitative synthesis. *Journal of Autism and Developmental Disorders, 37*(8), 1430–1445. https://doi.org/10.1007/s10803-006-0219-6

Hoffmann, A. N., Sellers, T. P., Halversen, H., & Bloom, S. E. (2018). Implementation of interventions informed by precursor functional analyses with young children: A replication. *Journal of Applied Behavior Analysis, 51*(4), 879–889. https://doi.org/10.1002/jaba.502

House, A. E., House, B. J., & Campbell, M. B. (1981). Measures of interobserver agreement: Calculation formulas and distribution effects. *Journal of Behavioral Assessment, 3*(1), 37–57.

Iwata, B. A., Dorsey, M. F., Slifer, K. J., Bauman, K. E., & Richman, G. S. (1994). Toward a functional analysis of self-injury. *Journal of Applied Behavior Analysis, 27*(2), 197–209.

Iwata, B. A., & Dozier, C. L. (2008). Clinical application of functional analysis methodology. *Behavior Analysis in Practice, 1*(1), 3–9.

Kahng, S., Abt, K. A., & Schonbachler, H. E. (2001). Assessment and treatment of low-rate high-intensity problem behavior. *Journal of Applied Behavior Analysis, 34*(2), 225–228. https://doi.org/10.1901/jaba.2001.34-225

Kazdin, A. E. (2011). *Single-case research designs: Methods for clinical and applied settings* (2nd ed.). New York, NY: Oxford University Press.

Kurtz, P. F., Chin, M. D., Huete, J. M., Tarbox, R. S. F., O'Connor, J. T., Paclawskyj, T. R., & Rush, K. S. (2003). Functional analysis and treatment of self-injurious behavior in young children: A summary of 30 cases. *Journal of Applied Behavior Analysis, 36*(2), 205–219. https://doi.org/10.1901/jaba.2003.36-205

Lang, R., O'Reilly, M., Machalicek, W., Lancioni, G., Rispoli, M., & Chan, J. M. (2008). A preliminary comparison of functional analysis results when conducted in contrived versus natural settings. *Journal of Applied Behavior Analysis, 41*(3), 441–445. https://doi.org/10.1901/jaba.2008.41-441

Larkin, W., Hawkins, R. O., & Collins, T. (2016). Using trial-based functional analysis to design effective interventions for students diagnosed with autism spectrum disorder. *School Psychology Quarterly, 31*(4), 534–547. https://doi.org/10.1037/spq0000158

Law, G. C., Neihart, M., & Dutt, A. (2018). The use of behavior modeling training in a mobile app parent training program to improve functional communication of young children with autism spectrum disorder. *Autism, 22*(4), 424–439. https://doi.org/10.1177/1362361316683887

Lindsley, O. R. (1956). Operant conditioning methods applied to research in chronic schizophrenia. *Psychiatric Research Reports, 5*, 118–139.

Mace, F. C. (1994). The significance and future of functional analysis methodologies. *Journal of Applied Behavior Analysis, 27*(2), 385–392. https://doi.org/10.1901/jaba.1994.27-385

Mace, F. C., & West, B. J. (1986). Analysis of demand conditions associated with reluctant speech. *Journal of Behavior Therapy and Experimental Psychiatry, 17*(4), 285–294.

Machalicek, W., Lequia, J., Pinkelman, S., Knowles, C., Raulston, T., Davis, T., & Alresheed, F. (2016). Behavioral telehealth consultation with families of children with autism spectrum disorder. *Behavioral Interventions, 31*(3), 223–250. https://doi.org/10.1002/bin.1450

McKenney, E. L. W., Waldron, N., & Conroy, M. (2013). The effects of training and performance feedback during behavioral consultation on general education middle school teachers' integrity to functional analysis procedures. *Journal of Educational and Psychological Consultation, 23*(1), 63–85. https://doi.org/10.1080/10474412.2013.757152

Moxley, R. A. (1996). The import of Skinner's three-term contingency. *Behavior and Philosophy, 24*(2), 145–167. JSTOR.

Ninci, J., Vannest, K. J., Willson, V., & Zhang, N. (2015). Interrater agreement between visual analysts of single-case data: A meta-analysis. *Behavior Modification, 39*(4), 510–541. https://doi.org/10.1177/0145445515581327

Northup, J., Wacker, D., Sasso, G., Steege, M., Cigrand, K., Cook, J., & DeRaad, A. (1991). A brief functional analysis of aggressive and alternative behavior in an outclinic setting. *Journal of Applied Behavior Analysis, 24*(3), 509–522. https://doi.org/10.1901/jaba.1991.24-509

O'Neill, R. E., Horner, R. H., Albin, R. W., Sprague, J. R., Storey, K., & Newton, J. S. (1997). *Functional assessment and program development for problem behavior*. Pacific Grove, CA: Cole Publishing.

Orlando, R., & Bijou, S. W. (1960). Single and multiple schedules of reinforcement in developmentally retarded children. *Journal of the Experimental Analysis of Behavior, 3*(4), 339–348. https://doi.org/10.1901/jeab.1960.3-339

Paclawskyj, T. R., Matson, J. L., Rush, K. S., Smalls, Y., & Vollmer, T. R. (2000). Questions about behavioral function (QABF): A behavioral checklist for functional assessment of aberrant behavior. *Research in Developmental Disabilities, 21*(3), 223–229. https://doi.org/10.1016/S0891-4222(00)00036-6

Rispoli, M., Burke, M. D., Hatton, H., Ninci, J., Zaini, S., & Sanchez, L. (2015). Training head start teachers to conduct trial-based functional analysis of challenging behavior. *Journal of Positive Behavior Interventions, 17*(4), 235–244. https://doi.org/10.1177/1098300715577428

Rispoli, M., Ninci, J., Neely, L., & Zaini, S. (2014). A systematic review of trial-based functional analysis of challenging behavior. *Journal of Developmental and Physical Disabilities, 26*(3), 271–283. https://doi.org/10.1007/s10882-013-9363-z

Roane, H. S., Fisher, W. W., Kelley, M. E., Mevers, J. L., & Bouxsein, K. J. (2013). Using modified visual-inspection criteria to interpret functional analysis outcomes: Functional analysis interpretation. *Journal of Applied Behavior Analysis, 46*(1), 130–146. https://doi.org/10.1002/jaba.13

Roscoe, E. M., Phillips, K. M., Kelly, M. A., Farber, R., & Dube, W. V. (2015). A statewide survey assessing practitioners' use and perceived utility of functional assessment. *Journal of Applied Behavior Analysis, 48*(4), 830–844. https://doi.org/10.1002/jaba.259

Ruiz, S. (2017). Impact of trial-based functional analysis on challenging behavior and training: A review of the literature. *Behavior Analysis: Research and Practice, 17*(4), 347–356. https://doi.org/10.1037/bar0000079

Saini, V., Greer, B. D., & Fisher, W. W. (2015). Clarifying inconclusive functional analysis results: Assessment and treatment of automatically reinforced aggression. *Journal of Applied Behavior Analysis, 48*(2), 315–330. https://doi.org/10.1002/jaba.203

Sanders, M. R. (2003). Triple P – Positive parenting program: A population approach to promoting competent parenting. *Australian E-Journal for the Advancement of Mental Health, 2*(3), 127–143. https://doi.org/10.5172/jamh.2.3.127

Schlichenmeyer, K. J., Roscoe, E. M., Rooker, G. W., Wheeler, E. E., & Dube, W. V. (2013). Idiosyncratic variables that affect functional analysis outcomes: A review (2001–2010): Idiosyncratic variables. *Journal of Applied Behavior Analysis, 46*(1), 339–348. https://doi.org/10.1002/jaba.12

Schnell, L. K., Sidener, T. M., DeBar, R. M., Vladescu, J. C., & Kahng, S. (2018). Effects of computer-based training on procedural modifications to standard functional analyses. *Journal of Applied Behavior Analysis, 51*(1), 87–98. https://doi.org/10.1002/jaba.423

Scott, T. M., Liaupsin, C., Nelson, C. M., & McIntyre, J. (2005). Team-based functional behavior assessment as a proactive public school process: A descriptive analysis of current barriers. *Journal of Behavioral Education, 14*(1), 57–71. https://doi.org/10.1007/s10864-005-0961-4

Skinner, B. F. (1938). *The behavior of organisms.* New York, NY: Appleton-Century-Crofts.

Skinner, B. F. (1945). The operational analysis of psychological terms. *Psychological Review, 52*(5), 270–277. https://doi.org/10.1037/h0062535

Skinner, B. F. (1953). *Science and human behavior.* New York, NY: Simon and Schuster.

Skinner, B. F. (1974). *About behaviorism.* New York, NY: Knopf.

Smith, R. G., & Churchill, R. M. (2002). Identification of environmental determinants of behavior disorders through functional analysis of precursor behaviors. *Journal of Applied Behavior Analysis, 35*(2), 125–136. https://doi.org/10.1901/jaba.2002.35-125

Solnick, M. D., & Ardoin, S. P. (2010). A quantitative review of functional analysis procedures in public school settings. *Education and Treatment of Children, 33*(1), 153–175. https://doi.org/10.1353/etc.0.0083

Tarbox, J., Wilke, A. E., Najdowski, A. C., Findel-Pyles, R. S., Balasanyan, S., Caveney, A. C., … Tia, B. (2009). Comparing indirect, descriptive, and experimental functional assessments of challenging behavior in children with autism. *Journal of Developmental and Physical Disabilities, 21*(6), 493. https://doi.org/10.1007/s10882-009-9154-8

Thomason-Sassi, J. L., Iwata, B. A., & Fritz, J. N. (2013). Therapist and setting influences on functional analysis outcomes. *Journal of Applied Behavior Analysis, 46*(1), 79–87. https://doi.org/10.1002/jaba.28

Tomlinson, S. R. L., Gore, N., & McGill, P. (2018). Training individuals to implement applied behavior analytic procedures via telehealth: A systematic review of the literature. *Journal of Behavioral Education, 27*(2), 172–222. https://doi.org/10.1007/s10864-018-9292-0

Wacker, D. P., Lee, J. F., Dalmau, Y. C. P., Kopelman, T. G., Lindgren, S. D., Kuhle, J., … Waldron, D. B. (2013). Conducting functional analyses of problem behavior via TELehealth. *Journal of Applied Behavior Analysis, 46*(1), 31–46. https://doi.org/10.1002/jaba.29

Wallace, M. D., & Iwata, B. A. (1999). Effects of session duration on functional analysis outcomes. *Journal of Applied Behavior Analysis, 32*(2), 175–183. https://doi.org/10.1901/jaba.1999.32-175

Watson, J. B. (1913). Psychology as the behaviorist views it. *Psychological Review, 20,* 158–177.

Webster-Stratton, C. (2001). The incredible years: Parents, teachers, and children training series. *Residential Treatment for Children & Youth, 18*(3), 31–45. https://doi.org/10.1300/J007v18n03_04

Weeks, M., & Gaylord-Ross, R. (1981). Task difficulty and aberrant behavior in severely handicapped students. *Journal of Applied Behavior Analysis, 14*(4), 449–463. https://doi.org/10.1901/jaba.1981.14-449

Wiesler, N. A., Hanzel, T. E., Chamberlain, T. P., & Thompson, T. (1985). Functional taxonomy of stereotypic and self-injurious behavior. *Mental Retardation, 23,* 230–234.

Chapter 3
How Maintaining Variables Are Defined and Established in Functional Assessment

William E. Sullivan, Emily L. Baxter, Andrew R. Craig, Nicole M. Derosa, and Henry S. Roane

How Maintaining Variables Are Defined and Established in Functional Assessment

Historically, psychiatric conditions have been assessed and classified by identifying correlations among samples of behavior that are considered to be symptomatic of a particular disorder. For example, autism spectrum disorder can be classified by observing social-communication deficits and restricted patterns of behavior that covary within an individual (APA, 2013). Although this structural approach is helpful in classifying individuals who display similar patterns of behavior, it provides little to no information about the causal factors that contribute to the development and maintenance of those behaviors that comprise the disorder. An alternative approach involves examination of an individual's behavior and the enviornmental context in which the behavior occurs, thereby viewing the maintenance of those behaviors as an interaction between individual-level factors and the environment. Through such a functional approach, behavior is classified based on the purpose that it serves for the individual.

In *The Behavior of Organisms*, B. F. Skinner (1953) offered a comprehensive description of the processes that govern operant behavior. In parallel with natural selection, wherein specific traits are selected because individuals who possess those traits are more likely survive and re-produce, specific behaviors within a given context are selected because of the consequences they produce through a process termed *operant selection*. That is, when a specific behavior produces a favorable outcome for the organism, the principle of reinforcement states that the future probability of that behavior will increase under similar situations. Based on this notion, early

W. E. Sullivan (✉) · E. L. Baxter · A. R. Craig · N. M. Derosa · H. S. Roane
Department of Pediatrics, SUNY Upstate Medical University, Syracuse, NY, USA
e-mail: sullivaw@upstate.edu

© Springer Nature Switzerland AG 2021

J. L. Matson (ed.), *Functional Assessment for Challenging Behaviors and Mental Health Disorders*, Autism and Child Psychopathology Series,
https://doi.org/10.1007/978-3-030-66270-7_3

research suggested that even severe forms of challenging behavior (e.g., aggression and self-injurious behavior; SIB) may be learned and selected under certain circumstances because of the consequences they produce (Carr, 1977; Carr, Newsom, & Binkoff, 1976; Iwata, Dorsey, Slifer, Bauman, & Richman, 1982/1994; Lovaas & Simmons, 1969). Thus, when conceptualizing challenging behavior within a functional approach, the specific environmental variables that precede (antecedents) and follow (consequences) challenging behavior are key. This functional relation between behavior and the environment is particularly important because once identified, those reinforcement contingencies can be leveraged in treatment.

In this chapter, we describe the ways in which functions of challenging behavior are defined and established during the functional assessment process. We begin by providing a brief synopsis of the various functional-assessment strategies that have been employed in the literature. A comprehensive review of these procedures is beyond the scope of this chapter, but will be briefly described to provide readers with sufficient context to understand how functions of challenging behavior are generally assessed. From there, common functions of challenging behavior that have been reported in the literature will be reviewed. Each of these functions generally falls into one of three broad categories of reinforcement (i.e., social-positive, social-negative, and automatic reinforcement) and will be presented accordingly. Finally, we will discuss the implications of categorizing behavior by function in terms of treatment utility.

Functional-Assessment Strategies

Generally speaking, functional assessment refers to a set of procedures that assess those environmental variables that surround the occurrence of challenging behavior. These procedures operate under a number of key assumptions (Erchul & Martens, 2010; Martens & Ardoin, 2010; Martens, Witt, Daly, & Vollmer, 1999): (a) challenging behavior is the focus of the assessment and is not merely considered a sign indicating an underlying disorder, (b) challenging behavior is learned and varies systematically across environmental situations, (c) challenging behavior occurs in a predictable pattern that may be identified through repeated measurement, and (d) the maintaining contingencies identified through functional assessment can be modified during treatment.

The extant literature suggests that social-positive, social-negative, and automatic reinforcement are primary categories into which the functions of challenging behavior may be divided (Carr, 1977; Cataldo et al., 2012; Fisher, Greer, Romani, Zangrillo, & Owen, 2016; Hanley, Iwata, & McCord, 2003). Following the occurrence of challenging behavior, social-positive reinforcement involves the *addition* of a reinforcing event or stimulus (e.g., delivering attention or preferred tangibles). Social-negative reinforcement refers to the *removal* of an aversive event or stimulus (e.g., escape difficult academic tasks) contingent on challenging behavior. Both of these forms of reinforcement are socially mediated, meaning that these reinforcement contingencies are controlled by others in the environment (e.g., others reactions to challenging behavior). Alternatively, the term "automatic reinforcement" applies to reinforcement that occurs independent of others' responses and results from the internal consequences that challenging behavior produces (e.g., sensory induction or reduction; Cataldo et al., 2012; Derby et al., 1994). These categories of reinforcement will be explored more fully throughout this chapter. At this point, it is important to recognize that hypotheses regarding behavioral function are based largely on one or more of these categories.

As one conducts a functional assessment, information is gathered regarding the behavior, the conditions under which it occurs, and its relation to the aforementioned categories of reinforcement. The strategies for obtaining such information have generally fallen into three categories (Roane, Sullivan, Martens, & Kelley, 2019): (1) indirect assessment, (2) descriptive assessment, and (3) functional analysis. In the following sections we will briefly describe these procedures in order to clarify how functions of challenging behavior are defined and established during functional assessment.

Indirect Assessment

Indirect assessment describes an assortment of procedures that are designed to efficiently assesses the function of challenging behavior, outside of the time and place in which it occurs. These procedures include interviews (e.g., Functional Assessment Interview [FAI], O'Neill et al., 1997) and rating scales (e.g., Motivation Assessment Scale [MAS], Durand & Crimmins, 1988; Questions About Behavioral Function [QABF], Matson & Vollmer, 1995; Functional Analysis Screening Tool [FAST], Iwata, DeLeon, & Roscoe, 2013) that rely on reports from informants who are familiar with the individual's challenging behavior, such as parents, teachers, or caregivers. For example, the FAI is a structured interview that gathers information about the topography of challenging behavior, the events that lead to its occurrence, responses to challenging behavior, the individual's communicative ability, potential reinforcing stimuli, and their treatment history. The entire interview lasts between 45 and 90 min and aids the assessor in developing functional hypotheses regarding challenging behavior.

Similarly, the MAS, QABF, and FAST ask informants to report on challenging behavior and the environmental variables suspected to influence its occurrence. However, unlike the FAI, MAS, QABF, and FAST utilize Likert scales (e.g., QABF ranges 0 [Never] to 3 [Always]) and have informants rate how often challenging behavior occurs across environmental situations. Item ratings are then summed across domains, and the domain(s) with the highest rating is suggestive of the potential function(s) of challenging behavior.

Common to each of the indirect assessment strategies is that potential functions are hypothesized based on the environmental events that were reported by others to occasion challenging behavior in the natural environment (e.g., school or home). Although these procedures are practical and efficient, the outcomes are based on the *perceptions* of the informants rather than actual sampling of behavior through direct observation of its occurrence. Because these strategies rely on the informant's recall of past events, errors and bias in reporting may occur leading to erroneous functional hypotheses (Iwata et al., 2013; Kazdin, 1977, 2011). An alternative, more direct, functional assessment method is to observe challenging behavior in the time and place in which it actually occurs and collect data on the events that surround its occurrence using descriptive-assessment methodology.

Descriptive Assessment

Descriptive assessment involves the direct observation of challenging behavior across a variety of naturalistic contexts, with little to no direct manipulation of the contingencies that might impact challenging behavior (e.g., Castillo et al., 2018; Lerman & Iwata, 1993; Mace & Lalli, 1991; Martens, DiGennaro, Reed, Szczech, & Rosenthal, 2008). Typically, descriptive assessments begin with an observation of challenging behavior across different settings (e.g., home, school, or community activities; Erchul & Martens, 2010), sometimes in the form of *scatterplot recording* (Touchette, MacDonald, & Langer, 1985). Scatterplot recording is designed to determine what settings are associated with challenging behavior, such that more focused observations can be conducted to assess the specific environmental events that occur during those times (Eckert, Martens, & DiGennaro, 2005).

During these more focused observations, data are collected on challenging behavior and the sequence of events the precede and follow its occurrence. That is, the environmental variables that are suspected to be functionally related to challenging behavior are assessed. For example, data may be collected through Antecedent-Behavior-Consequence (A-B-C) recording (Bijou, Peterson, & Ault, 1968; Mace & Lalli, 1991; O'Neil, Horner, Albin, Storey, & Sprague, 1990). This type of data collection involves recording the conditions that immediately precede challenging behavior (antecedents), the challenging behavior itself (behavior), and the consequence(s) that follow behavior. Data are collected in this manner until a clear sequence of events emerge such that a function(s) of challenging behavior can be hypothesized.

Another way of examining the relationship between challenging behavior and its consequences during descriptive assessments, such that functional hypotheses can be made, is to engage in sequential recording. This data-collection strategy involves recording challenging behavior and its consequences (i.e., attention and tangible [social-positive], escape [social-negative], no consequence [automatic]) in brief intervals (e.g., 10 s) as they occur in sequence across an observation period (Martens et al., 2008). Data are then analyzed by examining the probability of a consequence given the occurrence of challenging behavior (i.e., conditional probabilities; see McComas et al., 2009, for a review of these calculations). From there, the consequence(s) that has(have) the highest probability of following challenging behavior is hypothesized to be a likely function (Martens et al., 2008). For example, if attention had a high probability of following the occurrence of challenging behavior, and was rarely delivered in the absence of challenging behavior, then an attention (social-positive) function would be hypothesized.

Descriptive assessments offer advantages relative to indirect assessments in that they involve direct observation of the individual in their natural environment while permitting an analysis of the associations between the targeted form of challenging behavior and potential environment events that might maintain that behavior. This direct observation of an individual's challenging behavior is not without limits, however. That is, descriptive assessments typically do not involve direct manipulation of environmental variables to assess their impact on challenging behavior and allow hypothesis testing about the role of those variables on the maintenance of challenging behavior, as is the case in a functional analysis (Miltenberger, 2012).

Functional Analysis

Functional analysis (FA; Iwata et al., 1982/1994) measures challenging behavior while systematically manipulating environmental variables that putatively occasion challenging behavior. Iwata et al. (1982/1994) developed brief (i.e., 10 min) test and control conditions to identify function(s) of challenging behavior (i.e., SIB). Each test condition was designed to mimic naturally occurring contingencies that were suspected to maintain challenging behavior and consisted of three components: (1) a discriminative stimulus that signaled the availability of a specific type of reinforcement, (2) a motivational component that increased the momentary value of the reinforcer being tested, and (3) delivery of the specific reinforcer contingent on challenging behavior. The test conditions were designed to test for various forms of social-positive (i.e., attention), social-negative (i.e., escape), and automatic (i.e., sensory stimulation or reduction) reinforcement. To do so, each form of reinforcement suspected to influence challenging behavior was isolated and delivered contingent on challenging behavior. The control condition, to which levels of challenging behavior in the test conditions were compared, consisted of access to reinforcement independent of behavior. That is, preferred tangible items and attention were freely available in the absence of demands. The test condition(s) associated with the elevated levels of challenging behavior, relative to the control condition, suggested that challenging behavior was maintained by that type of reinforcement in the natural environment.

Contemporary functional-analysis methodology borrows heavily from the methods used by Iwata et al. (1982/1994). For a comprehensive review of this methodology, please refer to Chap. 11 of the current volume. The key aspect of functional analysis that is pertinent to the current chapter is that the environmental variables suspected to occasion challenging behavior are systematically manipulated such that causal inferences can be drawn regarding behavioral function. Furthermore, it is important to recognize that each of the test conditions is specifically designed to determine if challenging behavior is a function of one or more of the categories of reinforcement reviewed above (i.e., social-positive, social-negative, and/or automatic). In the following sections, we will further examine each category of reinforcement for which challenging behavior has been shown to be a function and provide a selective review of the literature documenting these findings.

Categories of Reinforcement

As described previously, challenging behavior can be learned through the process of operant selection. When challenging behavior produces a desirable stimulus change, challenging behavior may be reinforced and more likely to occur again in the future under similar situations. Through functional assessment methodology, the reinforcing stimuli purported to maintain challenging behavior are assessed. Accordingly, the reinforcement contingencies identified as maintaining challenging behavior are classified into functions that corresponds with the broad categories of reinforcement (i.e., social-positive, social-negative, and automatic) described previously.

Social-Positive Reinforcement

Social-positive reinforcement describes the process of increasing the future likelihood of a behavior by presenting a stimulus (a "positive reinforcer") contingent on its occurrence (Cooper, Heron, & Heward, 2007). For example, an individual may engage in challenging behavior because it produces access to tangible items or attention that are mediated by others in their environment. Based on collective reviews of 981 published functional analyses by Hanley et al. (2003) and Beavers, Iwata, and Lerman (2013), challenging behavior was found to be maintained by social-positive reinforcement in 32.7% of the published functional analyses. Of those cases, 21.7% were maintained by access to *attention* and 11% by *tangible* reinforcers. Additionally, challenging behavior can be maintained by access to control over social situations, a function which has been termed *mand compliance* or *social control* (e.g., Bowman, Fisher, Thompson, & Piazza, 1997; Owen et al., 2020). In the sections below, we will review the literature on challenging behavior maintained by these three forms of social-positive reinforcement.

Attention Challenging behavior can be maintained by contingent access to attention. For example, when a student tells an inappropriate joke in the classroom and her/his peers laugh at the joke, that student may be more likely to tell those jokes again in the future (provided that peer laughter is a desirable consequence for the student). Likewise in the home setting, if a child engages in challenging behavior while their parent's attention is diverted toward another activity (e.g., working on the computer) and the child is reprimanded following its occurrence, the child may learn to engage in challenging behavior to gain their parent's attention under similar situations. Comparable to the examples noted above, numerous studies have confirmed a functional relation between challenging behavior and access to attention (e.g., Berg et al., 2000; Bloom, Iwata, Fritz, Roscoe, & Carreau, 2011; Dolezal &

Kurtz, 2010; Fahmie, Iwata, Harper, & Querim, 2013; Greer et al., 2013; Ndoro, Hanley, Tiger, & Heal, 2006).

When examining the role of attention in functional assessment with the goal of identifying the contingency maintaining challenging behavior in the natural environment, it is important to consider the topography and quality of attention that is being delivered. Different topographies (e.g., verbal or physical) and quality (e.g., enthusiastic or apathetic) of attention can affect behavior differently, and preference for different varieties or quality of attention is idiosyncratic to the individual (Gardner, Wacker, & Boelter, 2009; Kodak, Northup, & Kelley, 2007; Lang et al., 2014). For example, to some individuals, rich descriptive praise (e.g., "Wow, Delilah! I love how you said 'Excuse me' when you walked past me! Great job!") may be a desired form of attention, whereas negative statements or reprimands (e.g., "I don't like it when you push past me. Stop shoving!") may not be a desired form of attention. Other individuals, however, may be more likely to engage in challenging behavior to gain access to reprimands and less likely to engage in a behavior to access praise. Recognizing the impact of individual differences in preferred types of attention is important when examining the role of attention as a reinforcer for challenging behavior.

Given that the topography and quality of attention delivered contingent on challenging behavior may vary across persons (e.g., *verbal attention*—praise, neutral conversation, reprimands, or instructions; *physical attention*—hugs, high fives, or a pat on the back; *non-verbal attention*—eye contact, crossing arms, or facial expressions), a clinician would want to confirm the type of attention of which challenging behavior is a function. This goal may be accomplished via interviews (i.e., indirect assessments) with key stakeholders who are familiar with the individual's challenging behavior and/or direct observation of the behavior and the attention that is delivered in the natural environment (i.e., descriptive assessment). For example, Hanley, Jin, Vanselow, and Hanratty (2014) describe the use of a structured open-ended interview in combination with brief observations to help identify the type of attention that is typically delivered contingent on challenging behavior. Furthermore, Morris and Vollmer (2019) developed a method for assessing preference for different topographies of attention and social interactions (the social interaction preference assessment) in which participants chose which social interaction they would like to engage in briefly with the therapist across 5-trials sessions. Gathering this information may help one to better understand the type of attention that may function as a reinforcer for a given individual's challenging behavior.

Tangible Challenging behavior can also be maintained by contingent access to tangible items or activities. For example, a child may engage in aggression to gain access to a toy with which their sibling is playing. That is, the child may learn that aggression will result in their sibling handing them the toy. As a second example, a child with autism spectrum disorder may engage in high-pitched screaming whenever the battery on their tablet dies, and their parent quickly comes in their room to plug in the tablet for them. Thus, the child may be more likely to scream in the future when their tablet runs out of batteries because doing so allows them continued access to their tablet. Such relations have been identified repeatedly in the existing literature (e.g., Gabor, Fritz, Roath, Rothe, & Gourley, 2016; Holehan et al., 2020; Sullivan et al., 2020).

In functional assessment, it is important to identify the items or activities for which the individual is motivated to engage in challenging behavior to obtain. When considering access to which items or activities may maintain challenging behavior, it is important to first determine the items that are delivered contingent on the behavior in the natural environment. Similar to the methods described above for identifying the specific forms of attention that may maintain challenging behavior, the clinician may conduct indirect preference assessments to collect these data (e.g., Hanley et al., 2014).

An important initial step in completing a preference assessment is to determine an array of preferred items/activities for an individual. Tools such as the Reinforcer Assessment for Individuals with Severe Disabilities (Fisher, Piazza, Bowman, & Amari, 1996) questionnaire have been developed to accomplish this task. This assessment requires respondents to provide several examples of preferred items in a wide range of different categories such as preferred edible items (e.g., chips, carrots, chocolate chips), toys, sounds (e.g., music or white noise), or physical activities (e.g., running or jumping on a trampoline). After an array of items have been identified

There are several preference-assessment methodologies that have been examined in the existing literature (e.g., DeLeon & Iwata, 1996; Fisher et al., 1992; Pace, Ivancic, Edwards, Iwata, & Page, 1985; Roane, Vollmer, Ringdahl, & Marcus, 1998). Each of these methods can be employed to help determine potential tangible items that are likely to serve as reinforcers for challenging behavior. While these methods have a variety of procedural differences, they share common elements which include: (a) presentation of an array of potentially preferred items, (b) direct measurement of an item engagement/selection response, and (c) a ranking of items based on engagement/selection responses. Generally speaking, items associated with more selections (or more engagement) in a preference assessment tend to be more effective positive reinforcers (e.g., Fisher et al., 1992).

Mand compliance An individual's motivation to obtain various reinforcers may fluctuate rapidly (Bowman et al., 1997), making it difficult to identify the exact reinforcement contingency for which challenging behavior is a function at any given moment. As such, the individual may ask or request (herein referred to as a *mand*) for various reinforcers and engage in challenging behavior if those mands go unreinforced. Under these situations, the terminal reinforcer may differ from moment to moment. If the initial mand (e.g., "I want a cookie," "I want you to play with me," "I want you to be quiet") goes unreinforced but the resulting challenging behavior produces the reinforcer, the individual may learn to engage in challenging behavior to get others in their environment to comply with their mands. Thus, challenging behavior can be viewed as a precurrent response that increases the probability of others complying with the individual's mands (Fisher, 2001).

Bowman et al. (1997) were among the first to document that challenging behavior can be a function of increasing caregiver compliance with mands. Two participants who engaged in self-injurious behaviors, aggression, and property destruction were included in the study. A standard functional analysis was completed with both participants, but the analyses produced undifferentiated results (i.e., no clear function was identified). Next, Bowman and colleagues conducted a *mand analysis*. In the mand analysis, a therapist initially complied with all mands for 2 min, which served as a control condition. Once the control condition was completed, the therapist then altered what they were doing (i.e., deviated from the last mand), and contingent on challenging behavior, the therapist complied with what the participant manded for (i.e., test condition). For example, if the participant manded for a toy the therapist complied with this request only following the occurrence of challenging behavior. For both participants, challenging behavior occurred at consistently higher rates in the test condition relative to the control condition, suggesting that the participants' challenging behavior was a function of increasing the therapist's compliance with their mands.

More recently, Owen et al. (2020) conducted a follow-up study on challenging behavior maintained by increased mand compliance across a large cohort of individuals (i.e., 16 participants from two different treatment centers). First, a standard functional analysis was completed for all participants, with 14 of the 16 participants showing undifferentiated or multiply controlled patterns of responding. Following the functional analyses, mand analyses were completed for all participants using similar procedures to those of Bowman et al.'s (1997) test and control conditions described above. With the exception of one participant, challenging behavior occurred at elevated rates during the test condition relative to the control. Thus, Owen and colleagues were able to establish that participants' challenging behavior was a function of increasing caregiver compliance with their mands and in turn developed function-matched treatments that effectively suppressed challenging behavior.

Social-Negative Reinforcement

Negative reinforcement is the process by which the future probability of a behavior is increased by removing a stimulus (a "negative reinforcer") from the environment contingent on the behavior. In 1953, Skinner pointed out that removal of events that are subjectively aversive ["for example, a loud noise, a very bright light, extreme cold or heat, or electric shock" (p. 73)] tends to serve as a negative reinforcer. *Social-negative* reinforcement is a more specific process in which the negatively reinforcing operation is mediated by another person (see, e.g., Cooper et al., 2007). That is, someone other than the individual whose behavior is being reinforced removes the subjectively aversive stimulus whenever the behavior of interest occurs.

Two types of social-negative reinforcement contingencies exist. If, on the one hand, an individual's behavior leads to the *removal* of an aversive stimulus, and *escape* contingency is said to be present. On the other hand, if engaging in a specific behavior *prevents* the presentation of an aversive stimulus, an *avoidance* contingency is said to be present.

Escape In functional analyses (Iwata et al., 1982/1994), the condition designed to test for an escape function typically involves the presentation of some aversive task or stimulus (e.g., school demands). Contingent on challenging behavior, the aversive task or stimulus is briefly removed. These types of escape contingencies represent a particularly prevalent function of challenging behavior (for review, see Geiger, Carr, & LeBlanc, 2010), though prevalence estimates for escape-maintained challenging behavior vary. For example, in a sample of 32 children diagnosed with ASD, Love, Carr, and LeBlanc (2009) found that roughly half engaged in some form of challenging behavior to escape from demands. More comprehensive analysis of extent data, however, suggest the prevalence of escape-maintained challenging behavior may be lower. Specifically, Hanley et al. (2003) and Beavers et al. (2013) found that 32.2% of cases ($n = 297$) demonstrated escape-maintained challenging behavior.

In the context of behavior that is maintained by escape from demands, however, not all demands are equally aversive (similar to individual preferences for different types of attention of preferred items/activities). That is, for a given individual, presentation of a specific type of demand (e.g., math problems) might evoke substantially more or less challenging behavior than presentation of other types of demands (e.g., cleaning up a messy area). If the therapist were to deliver demands that are not particularly evocative in the escape condition of a functional analysis, the analysis outcomes might suggest that escape is a less pressing function of challenging behavior than it is in reality. In the worst-case scenario, the demands used may not evoke any challenging behavior at all, thus leading to the erroneous conclusion that escape is not a clinically significant function of challenging behavior. Thus, when an individual presents with behavior that it suspected to be maintained by escape from demands, an important initial question is which specific demands to use in assessment and treatment procedures.

There are several different means for determining the types of demands to deliver in functional analyses. For example, demands may be identified through indirect assessment such as interviews with caregivers, teachers, or other stakeholders in the care of the individual (see, e.g., Cooper et al., 1992). By contrast, direct demand-assessment methodologies have also been developed to determine the specific demands to be used in behavioral assessment and treatment procedures while circumventing the issues with indirect measures. For example, Roscoe, Rooker, Pence, and Longworth (2009) assessed the effects of different demand types on the rates of challenging behavior emitted by four individuals with developmental disabilities during the escape condition of a functional analysis. These researchers first identified 12 tasks for each participant that were similar to the tasks included in their individualized education plans. Therapists then presented each participant with one task per session of the pre-functional-analysis demand assessment. If the participant complied with the demand, brief praise was delivered. If, however, the participant engaged in challenging behavior, she or he earned a brief break from instructions. Based on the outcomes from this assessment, Roscoe and colleagues identified demands that occasioned high rates of challenging behavior and low levels of compliance and those that occasioned low rates of challenging behavior and high levels of compliance.

Though less-often reported in the literature than escape from demands (see Beavers et al., 2013; Hanley et al., 2003), challenging behavior may also occur to produce escape from other putatively aversive and socially mediated antecedent stimuli. For example, Harper, Iwata, and Camp (2013) identified four participants whose challenging behavior occurred in the control and escape conditions of a functional analysis. The authors hypothesized that the participants engaged in challenging behavior to escape from social interaction with therapists, which was provided in both of these conditions (i.e., control and escape). In a subsequent assessment, all participants engaged in challenging behavior to terminate therapist-provided social interaction. In light of these outcomes, it is important to be sensitive to potential indicators that an individuals' behavior may be maintained by escape from situations that may not appear to be aversive from the assessor's perspective (e.g., social interaction).

Social-Avoidance Compared to social-escape contingencies, comparatively little behavioral research has been conducted on human behavior maintained by social-avoidance contingencies (see Dymond & Roche, 2009; LeDoux, Moscarello, Sears, & Campese, 2016). However, avoidance behavior has been extensively studied in the context of various anxiety disorders, including social-anxiety disorder (for recent treatments, see Eaton, Bienvenu, & Miloyan, 2018; Krypotos, Effting, Kindt, & Beckers, 2015). Social-anxiety disorder affects a sizable portion of the American populations, with roughly a 9.1% lifetime prevalence in adolescent individuals (NIMH, 2017). Generally, social-anxiety disorder involves the experience of excessive fear elicited by specific social stimuli or situations and is characterized in part by avoidance of the fear-eliciting social situations (APA, 2013).

Avoidance of social situations is thought to contribute to the development and maintenance of social anxiety (and anxiety disorders, in general) in at least two ways. First, social avoidance often results in the individual coming into minimal contact with fear-eliciting conditioned stimuli (CS). Because the individual has limited opportunity to experience the CS(s) in the absence of the unconditioned stimuli (US), extinction of the CS-US association(s) is prevented (see Vervliet & Indekeu, 2015). Second, very brief, intermittent exposure to fear-eliciting CSs (as one is likely to see in individuals who avoid those USs) may *increase* the fear-eliciting properties of the CS (i.e., through a process termed fear *incubation*; Eysenck, 1968; see also Bersh, 1980). Based on these observations, exposure-based treatment approaches for anxiety disorders are effective in part because they explicitly arrange extinction of avoidance behavior by exposing the participant to the fear-eliciting CS(s) for prolonged periods of time in the absence of the US (for review, see Cooper, Clifton, & Feeny, 2017; NCCMH, 2013). Nevertheless, challenging behavior may be the product of avoidance learning and constitutes a potential function that may be uncovered during functional assessment.

Automatic Reinforcement

Thus far in the chapter we have discussed socially mediated forms of reinforcement (e.g., attention, tangible, and escape) of which challenging behavior can be a function. However, the section that follows will highlight the identification of reinforcers that are thought to be produced by challenging behavior itself and are thus not socially mediated (Vaughn & Michael, 1982). That is, we will discuss what has been termed automatic or nonsocial reinforcement (Wacker, Berg, Harding, & Cooper-Brown, 2011).

Similar to reinforcers mediated by social contingencies, automatic reinforcers can be further categorized as positive or negative. *Positive-automatic* reinforcement is described as reinforcement that provides the individual with preferred stimulation or elicits a physical sensation (Rapp & Vollmer, 2005). For example, a student may twirl her hair between her fingers during a lecture because it produces a desirable sensation in her scalp and/or fingers. Conversely, *negative-automatic* reinforcement is described as a mechanism for reducing non-preferred/aversive stimulation or physical discomfort. For example, a child may scratch a bug bite to reduce the itching sensation. However, with both forms of automatic reinforcement, the consequences of behavior occur within the individual and are largely unobservable—one cannot observe, with the naked eye, another person's sensory experiences. Thus, given the difficulty with accurately or definitively identifying these reinforcing consequences, simply using the umbrella term "automatic" is most common and will be used in the current chapter when describing this class of reinforcers.

As described above, functions of challenging behavior are established during functional assessment by observing and/or manipulating various environmental variables and recording the occurrence or non-occurrence of challenging behavior (Roane et al., 2019). This method of identifying functional relations lends itself well to the assessment of socially mediated forms of reinforcement. However, the inability to manipulate or observe automatic reinforcers results in challenges to identifying functional relations and developing effective treatments based specifically on this class of consequences (Vollmer, 1994). Despite this shortcoming, the use of functional assessment methodology still has utility for identifying automatic functions of challenging behavior. In functional analysis (Iwata et al., 1982/1994), for example, automatic reinforcement is tested for by removing all forms of social reinforcement in an alone or ignore test condition. If challenging behavior persists in the absence of any social contingencies (i.e., in the alone or ignore condition) and/or across all test and control conditions, it may be concluded that challenging behavior is automatically maintained (Iwata et al., 1982/1994; Mason & Iwata, 1990; Querim et al., 2013). Based on the reviews by Hanley et al. (2003) and Beavers et al. (2013), 16.3% of cases in the published literature were found to display patterns of challenging behavior during functional analyses that indicated the influence of automatic reinforcement on the occurrence of challenging behavior.

The occurrence of challenging behavior in the alone or ignore condition of a functional analysis, but the absence of challenging behavior in all other conditions, may lead one to question whether or not social events are in fact functionally related to the occurrence of challenging behavior. Stated another way, if the social antecedent events presented are associated with the absence of challenging behavior, then can it not be concluded that challenging behavior is mediated by social contingencies? Although this question may be a reasonable one, we must consider two procedural details that complicate clear interpretation. First, if challenging behavior never occurs in a given test condition(s), then the behavior never contacts the programmed social contingencies which is necessary for establishing a functional relationship. Second, if the antecedent arrangement in a given test condition(s) affects the occurrence of challenging behavior, then competing sources of reinforcement or punishment may be present that influence challenging behavior. For example, access to and engagement with certain stimuli (e.g., toys) during relevant test conditions may compete with an individual's motivation to engage in challenging behavior because they already have access to an alternative source of reinforcement. Alternatively, an individual may engage in challenging behavior in the attention-test condition and contact contingent attention. This attention may serve as a punisher for the target behavior resulting in the individual refraining from engaging in the target behavior during future attention sessions. Thus, the presence of the target behavior during the alone or ignore condition, in the absence of any other potential sources of competing reinforcement or punishment, leads most straightforwardly to the conclusion of maintenance by automatic reinforcement.

The conclusion regarding the influence of automatic reinforcement on target behavior is derived somewhat differently when the behavior is observed to occur across all test and control conditions within a functional analysis. Given this pattern of responding, it does not appear as though the antecedent social events present across conditions provide alternative sources of reinforcement or punishment. Furthermore, and perhaps more importantly, the behavior contacts social consequences in all test conditions aside from the alone or ignore condition, yet we do not observe differentiated responding. This lack of differentiated responding persists even in the control condition, during which the social variables are available independent of behavior. Thus, we can readily conclude that the presence of the programmed social variables do not directly affect the occurrence or non-occurrence of the target behavior. For interested readers, please refer to Hagopian, Rooker, and Zarcone (2015) for further classification of automatically maintained SIB based on distinctive patterns displayed during functional analyses.

One concern with conducting a comprehensive functional analysis to confirm suspected automatic reinforcement is prolonged assessment duration, which may delay the onset of effective treatment. This consideration may be particularly important if the targeted behavior is one that may result in significant harm or injury to the individual (e.g., self-injury) or others (e.g., aggression). In an effort to help mitigate this concern, Querim et al. (2013) proposed a screening procedure for more rapid identification of behavior maintained by automatic reinforcement. That is, the authors suggested implementing a series of alone or ignore conditions when automatic reinforcement is hypothesized. If the targeted behavior persists across sessions, one can conclude maintenance by automatic reinforcement and initiate treatment development. However, if the behavior is not maintained across sessions, then additional assessment procedures may be necessary to identify the relevant maintaining variables of the targeted behavior (Querim et al., 2013).

Multiple Control and Combined Contingencies

Throughout this chapter we have discussed each function of challenging behavior in isolation. However, it is possible that challenging behavior may have more than one function or serve multiple purposes for the individual. That is, challenging behavior may be sensitive to and controlled by more than one source of reinforcement either separately or together. Take for instance a child that becomes aggressive in a classroom setting. The teacher may provide multiple consequences for engaging in aggressive behavior. For example, they may reprimand the child (social-positive reinforcement [attention]), remove the child from the classroom (social-negative reinforcement [escape]), or allow the child to access a preferred tangible items to help them calm down (social-positive reinforcement [tangible]). Thus, it is possible that a child may initially learn to engage in aggressive behavior to escape academic work. Over time, however, she or he may also learn to engage in aggressive behavior to obtain teacher attention and preferred tangible items. Based on the reviews by Hanley et al. (2003) and Beavers et al. (2013) challenging behavior was found to have more than one function in 18.9% of the cases reviewed. Thus, in the following sections we will discuss challenging behavior that has more than one function (i.e., multiply controlled), as well as challenging behavior that may be maintained by combined contingencies (e.g., escape-to-tangible).

Within the literature, there have been a number of reports indicating that challenging behavior can be maintained by more than one source of reinforcement (e.g., Day, Horner, & O'Neill, 1994; Neidert, Iwata, & Dozier, 2005; Scheithauer, Mevers, Call, & Shrewsbury, 2017). For example, Neidert et al. (2005) conducted functional analyses of challenging behavior (i.e., SIB and aggression) displayed by two young children, both of whom were diagnosed with a developmental disability. Results of the functional analyses showed that both children's challenging behavior was maintained by both social-positive reinforcement (attention) and social-negative reinforcement (escape). Accordingly, the authors designed and evaluated two function-based treatments that addressed each function of challenging behavior individually, which produced socially significant reductions in challenging behavior.

As described above, functional-assessment outcomes are not constrained to only one set of contingencies. Challenging behavior may occur under a variety of different stimulus conditions and produce a number of different consequences for which challenging behavior may be a function. Furthermore, there may be times in which challenging behavior is not a function of one isolated contingency but rather a function of a combined contingency. Combined functions can be described as an interactive effect where two or more contingencies simultaneously affect challenging behavior, above and beyond the effects produced by any of the single contingencies alone (Fisher et al., 2016).

Hanley et al. (2014) offered an alternative approach to functional analysis, termed interview-informed synthesized contingency analysis (IISCA), in which brief indirect and descriptive assessments are used to inform a single test and control condition that combined all reported contingencies suspected to influence challenging behavior. For example, the test condition might consist of restricting access to preferred tangible items, presenting academic work sheets, and diverting attention away from the individual. Then, contingent on challenging behavior, access to the tangible item and attention would be presented as the academic work sheets are simultaneously removed, creating a combined social-positive and -negative reinforcement contingency. The control condition, for which levels of challenging behavior in the test condition are compared, provides noncontingent access to tangible items and attention in the absence of academic work. This approach has been employed a number of times and shown to produce clear functional relations between challenging behavior and combined contingencies (e.g., Jessel, Hanley, & Ghaemmaghami, 2016).

Although this approach can be effective in terms of designing a combined test and control condition that produce differentiated levels of challenging behavior, it falls short in terms of providing evidence that challenging behavior is truly a function of the combined contingency, rather than any one contingency in isolation. That is, there is no relative control to test for an interactive effect or the dependency between challenging behavior and the combined contingency (see Gail in Hanley et al., 2014, for one exception). To test for an interactive effect, one must compare a test condition that combines the relevant independent variables with control conditions that isolates each of the variables (Barlow & Hersen, 1984). For example, Mueller, Sterling-Turner, and Moore (2005) and Sarno et al. (2011) conducted functional analyses of four school-aged children's challenging behavior that tested for escape and attention in isolation. Results indicated that the function of each child's challenging behavior, across both studies, was to escape academic demands. The attention condition did not produce differential levels of challenging behavior when compared with the control condition. Then, in a follow-up functional analysis, they compared the levels of challenging behavior across an isolated escape condition and an escape-to-attention condition that combined the contingencies. Under this arrangement, an interactive effect was observed with the majority of participants. That is, there were elevated levels of challenging behavior in the escape-to-attention condition relative to the escape and control condition for three of the four participants.

Therefore, at times, challenging behavior may be maintained or exacerbated by a combined contingency relative to an isolated contingency. However, to more directly compare the combined (i.e., IISCA) and isolated (i.e., standard functional analysis) approaches to functional analysis, Fisher et al. (2016) conducted a within-subject comparison with five children that displayed severe forms of challenging behavior (e.g., SIB and aggression). Results illustrated that four of the five participants' pattern of responding was consistent with the notion that isolated contingencies independently reinforced challenging behavior and none of the participants showed a response pattern that would suggest their challenging behavior was solely a function of a combined contingency. Nevertheless, within functional assessment, combined contingencies may occur and have the potential to maintain challenging behavior in the natural environment.

Idiosyncratic Functions

As noted previously, functions of challenging behavior are defined by the environmental events that contribute to the occurrence and maintenance of behavior. Although those particular events can be classified across broad categories of reinforcement as described above, there are times in which idiosyncratic functions may emerge. Again, from a functional perspective, challenging behavior is learned and the circumstances that precipitate learning are unique to the individual. Thus, although there are common situations that are functionally related to challenging behavior, the exact situations may be slightly different from individual to individual. Those situations sometimes depart from the common functions of challenging behavior described thus far.

Schlichenmeyer, Roscoe, Rooker, Wheeler, and Dube (2013) conducted a systematic review of the literature on idiosyncratic variables that affect functional analysis outcomes. In this review, a range of antecedents and consequences were described that diverge from the typical functional analysis procedures. Below, each of these idiosyncratic variables are outlined in Table 3.1. Although describing each of these studies is beyond the scope of this chapter, an example is provided.

Hausman, Kahng, Farrell, and Mongeon (2009) describe an idiosyncratic function of challenging behavior (i.e., SIB, aggression, property destruction) in a 9-year-old girl with intellectual and developmental disabilities. The authors began by conducting a functional analysis that tested for social-positive reinforcement in the form of attention, social-negative reinforcement in the form of escape from academic and daily living demands, and automatic reinforcement. Each of these test conditions was compared with a control condition that consisted of noncontingent attention, high-preferred toys, and the absence of demands. In general outcomes were undifferentiated and the authors were unable to determine a function. However, parental report revealed that challenging behavior tended to occur when she was blocked from engaging in ritualistic behaviors (i.e., opening and closing doors). Thus, a functional analysis was designed to assess this possibility.

Here, Hausman et al. (2009) designed a test condition in which therapists would manipulate the session room door on a fixed-time 30 s schedule. Contingent on challenging behavior, the participant was permitted to engage in ritualistic behavior (i.e., opening the door and propping it open with a doorstop). This condition was

Table 3.1 Range of stimulus parameters assessed

Stimulus parameter	First author (publication year)
Social-negative reinforcement	
Antecedent events	
Specific type of task	Butler and Luiselli (2007), Roscoe, Rooker, Pence, and Longworth (2009)
Aspects of task (difficulty, preference, amount)	Boelter et al. (2007), Call, Wacker, Ringdahl, Cooper-Brown, and Boelter (2004), Moore and Edwards (2003), Ebanks and Fisher (2003)
Instructional style (tone)	Borrero, Vollmer, and Borrero (2004)
Instructional style (prompt type or delay)	Tiger, Fisher, Toussaint, and Kodak (2009), Ebanks and Fisher (2003)
Instructional style (wording)	Northup, Kodak, Lee, and Coyne (2004)
Level of social attention	Call, Wacker, Ringdahl, Cooper-Brown, and Boelter (2004), Moore and Edwards (2003)
Client location	Le and Smith (2002)
Continuous attention	Hagopian, Wilson, and Wilder (2001), Tiger, Fisher, Toussaint, and Kodak (2009)
Walking	Volkert, Lerman, Call, and Trosclair-Lasserre (2009)
Transitions	McCord, Thomson, and Iwata (2001)
Social-positive reinforcement	
Antecedent events	
Therapist leaves room	Edwards, Magee, and Ellis (2002)
Attending to another's problem behavior	Kuhn, Hardesty, and Luczynski (2009)
Combine motivating operations	Call, Wacker, Ringdahl, and Boelter (2005), Dolezal and Kurtz (2010)
Therapist consumes edible item (tangible)	Kuhn, Hardesty, and Luczynski (2009)
Assign ownership (tangible)	Kuhn, Hardesty, and Luczynski (2009)
Consequent events	
Specific type of attention	Kodak, Northrup, and Kelley, (2007)
Attention delivered by a specific person	Tiger, Fisher, Toussaint, and Kodak (2009)
Alternative behavior	Hagopian, Bruzek, Bowman, and Jennett (2007)
Ritualistic behavior	Falcomata, Roane, Feeney, and Stephenson (2010), Hausman, Kahng, Farrell, and Mongeon (2009)
Walks	Ringdahl, Christensen, and Boelter (2009)
Wheelchair movement	DeLeon, Kahng, Rodriguez-Catter, Sveinsdóttir, and Sadler (2003)
Preferred conversations	Roscoe, Kindle, and Pence (2010)
Restraint materials	Rooker and Roscoe (2005)
Active play (tangible)	McLaughlin et al. (2003)
High preference or low preference (tangible)	Mueller, Wilczynski, Moore, Fusilier, and Trahant (2001), Wilder, Harris, Reagan, and Rasey (2007)

(continued)

Table 3.1 (continued)

Stimulus parameter	First author (publication year)
Music (tangible)	Carey and Halle (2002)
Peer attention	Skinner, Veerkamp, Kamps, and Andra (2009), Flood, Wilder, Flood, and Masuda (2002)
Combine consequences	Mann and Mueller (2009)
Automatic reinforcement	
Include leisure items in alone condition	Carter, Devlin, Doggett, Harber, and Barr (2004), Tiger, Hanley, and Bessette (2006)
Contextual variables	
Noise	McCord, Iwata, Galensky, Ellingson, and Thomson (2001)
Illness	Carter (2005)
Rapport	McLaughlin and Carr (2005)
Settings	Lang et al. (2008, 2009, 2010)
Therapist	English and Anderson (2004), Huete and Kurtz (2010), McAdam, DiCesare, Murphy, and Marshall (2004), Butler and Luiselli (2007)

then compared with a control condition in which the door was not manipulated by the therapist. During this analysis, no challenging behavior was observed in the control condition and elevated levels of challenging occurred during the test condition. It should be noted that it is difficult to directly determine if challenging behavior was maintained by access to the ritual (social-positive reinforcement), causing the therapists to stop manipulating the door (social-negative reinforcement), or both. Nevertheless, the study illustrates that in some cases idiosyncratic functions of challenging behavior can occur.

Conclusion

Throughout this chapter we have discussed the various reinforcement contingencies of which challenging behavior has been shown to be a function. The overall goal of the chapter was to describe how these functions of challenging behavior are defined and established in functional assessment. Across all forms of functional assessment, the goal is to determine the antecedent conditions that evoke challenging behavior and the consequences that maintain it. Based on informant report (i.e., indirect assessment), direct observation (i.e., descriptive assessment), or carefully controlled experimental analyses that manipulate those antecedent and consequent variables (i.e., functional analysis), the function(s) of challenging behavior may be established by identifying systematic patterns in responding.

Establishing and classifying challenging behavior based on its environmental determinants is a hallmark of behavior-analytic service delivery and is particularly useful in terms of treatment development. By identifying the function(s) of challenging behavior, the reinforcement contingency responsible for the occurrence of the behavior can be modified and functionally equivalent alternative responses can be taught and reinforced (Fisher et al., 2016; Fisher & Bouxsein, 2011; Vollmer & Athens, 2011; Vollmer, Iwata, Zarcone, Smith, & Mazaleski, 1993). For example, if it is determined that challenging behavior is a function of caregiver attention, then in treatment, caregivers may stop providing attention contingent on challenging behavior (i.e., extinction). Instead, they may deliver attention contingent on a socially appropriate behavior (i.e., differential reinforcement) or on a time-based schedule (i.e., noncontingent reinforcement). Detailing each of these function-based treatments for challenging behavior is beyond the scope of this chapter. It is important for the reader to recognize, however, that by establishing a functional relation between challenging behavior and the environment, function-matched treatments can be prescribed.

References

American Psychiatric Association (APA). (2013). *Diagnostic and statistical manual of mental disorders* (5th ed.). Arlington, VA: Author.

Barlow, D. H., & Hersen, M. (1984). *Single case experimental designs: Strategies for studying behavior change* (2nd ed.). New York, NY: Pergamon.

Beavers, G. A., Iwata, B. A., & Lerman, D. C. (2013). Thirty years of research on the functional analysis of problem behavior. *Journal of Applied Behavior Analysis, 46*, 1–21. https://doi.org/10.1002/jaba.30

Berg, W. K., Peck, S., Wacker, D. P., Harding, J., McComas, J., … Brown, K. (2000). The effects of presession exposure to attention on the results of assessments of attention as a reinforcer. *Journal of Applied Behavior Analysis, 33*, 463–477. https://doi.org/10.1901/jaba.2000.33-463

Bersh, P. J. (1980). Eysenck's theory of incubation: A critical analysis. *Behaviour Research and Therapy, 18*, 11–17. https://doi.org/10.1016/0005-7969(80)90064-9

Bijou, S. W., Peterson, R. F., & Ault, M. H. (1968). A method to integrate descriptive and experimental field studies at the level of data and empirical concepts. *Journal of Applied Behavior Analysis, 1*, 175–191. https://doi.org/10.1901/jaba.1968.1-175

Bloom, S. E., Iwata, B. A., Fritz, J. N., Roscoe, E. M., & Carreau, A. B. (2011). Classroom application of a trial-based functional analysis. *Journal of Applied Behavior Analysis, 44*, 19–31. https://doi.org/10.1901/jaba.2011.44-19

Boelter, E. W., Wacker, D. P., Call, N. A., Ringdahl, J. E., Kopelman, T., & Gardner, A. W. (2007). Effects of antecedent variables on disruptive behavior and accurate responding in young children in outpatient settings. *Journal of Applied Behavior Analysis, 40*(2), 321–326. https://doi.org/10.1901/jaba.2007.51-06

Borrero, C. S., Vollmer, T. R., & Borrero, J. C. (2004). Combining descriptive and functional analysis logic to evaluate idiosyncratic variables maintaining aggression. *Behavioral Interventions: Theory & Practice in Residential & Community-Based Clinical Programs, 19*, 247–262. https://doi.org/10.1002/bin.176

Bowman, L. G., Fisher, W. W., Thompson, R. H., & Piazza, C. C. (1997). On the relation of mands and the function of destructive behavior. *Journal of Applied Behavior Analysis, 30*, 251–265. https://doi.org/10.1002/jaba.23

Butler, L. R., & Luiselli, J. K. (2007). Escape-maintained problem behavior in a child with autism: Antecedent functional analysis and intervention evaluation of noncontingent escape and instructional fading. *Journal of Positive Behavior Interventions, 9*, 195–202. https://doi.org/10.1177/10983007070090040201

Call, N. A., Wacker, D. P., Ringdahl, J. E., & Boelter, E. W. (2005). Combined antecedent variables as motivating operations within functional analyses. *Journal of Applied Behavior Analysis, 38*, 385–389. https://doi.org/10.1901/jaba.2005.51-04

Call, N. A., Wacker, D. P., Ringdahl, J. E., Cooper-Brown, L. J., & Boelter, E. W. (2004). An assessment of antecedent events influencing noncompliance in an outpatient clinic. *Journal of Applied Behavior Analysis, 37*, 145–157. https://doi.org/10.1901/jaba.2004.37-145

Carey, Y. A., & Halle, J. W. (2002). The effect of an idiosyncratic stimulus on self-injurious behavior during task demands. *Education and Treatment of Children*, 131–141. https://www.jstor.org/stable/42900520

Carr, E. G. (1977). The motivation of self-injurious behavior: A review of some hypotheses. *Psychological Bulletin, 84*(4), 800. https://doi.org/10.1037/0033-2909.84.4.800

Carr, E. G., Newsom, C. D., & Binkoff, J. A. (1976). Stimulus control of self-destructive behavior in a psychotic child. *Journal of Abnormal Child Psychology, 4*, 139–153.

Carter, S. L., Devlin, S., Doggett, R. A., Harber, M. M., & Barr, C. (2004). Determining the influence of tangible items on screaming and handmouthing following an inconclusive functional analysis. *Behavioral Interventions, 19*, 51–58. https://doi.org/10.1002/bin.150

Carter, S. L. (2005). An empirical analysis of the effects of a possible sinus infection and weighted vest on functional analysis outcomes of self-injury exhibited by a child with autism. *Journal of Early and Intensive Behavior Intervention, 2*, 252–258. http://dx.doi.org/10.1037/h0100318

Castillo, M. I., Clark, D. R., Schaller, E. A., Donaldson, J. M., DeLeon, I. G., & Kahng, S. (2018). Descriptive assessment of problem behavior during transitions of children with intellectual and developmental disabilities. *Journal of Applied Behavior Analysis, 51*, 99–117. https://doi.org/10.1002/jaba.430

Cataldo, M. F., Kahng, S. W., DeLeon, I. G., Martens, B. K., Friman, P. C., & Cataldo, M. (2012). Behavioral principles, assessment, and therapy. In M. L. Batshaw, N. J. Roizen, & G. R. Lotrecchiano (Eds.), *Children with disabilities* (7th ed., pp. 579–597). Baltimore, MD: Paul H. Brookes Publishing Co..

Cooper, A. A., Clifton, E. G., & Feeny, N. C. (2017). An empirical review of potential mediators and mechanisms of prolonged exposure therapy. *Clinical Psychology Review, 56*, 106–121. https://doi.org/10.1016/j.cpr.2017.07.003

Cooper, J. O., Heron, T. E., & Heward, W. L. (2007). *Applied behavior analysis* (2nd ed.). Upper Saddle River, NJ: Pearson Prentice Hall.

Cooper, L. J., Wacker, D. P., Thursby, D., Plagmann, L. A., Harding, J., Millard, T., & Derby, M. (1992). Analysis of the effects of task preferences, task demands, and adult attention on child behavior in outpatient and classroom settings. *Journal of Applied Behavior Analysis, 25*, 823–840. https://doi.org/10.1901/jaba.1992.25-823

Day, H. M., Horner, R. H., & O'Neill, R. E. (1994). Multiple functions of problem behaviors: Assessment and intervention. *Journal of Applied Behavior Analysis, 27*(2), 279–289. https://doi.org/10.1901/jaba.1994.27-279

DeLeon, I. G., & Iwata, B. A. (1996). Evaluation of a multiple-stimulus presentation format for assessing reinforcer preferences. *Journal of Applied Behavior Analysis, 29*, 519–533. https://doi.org/10.1901/jaba.1996.29-519

DeLeon, I. G., Kahng, S., Rodriguez-Catter, V., Sveinsdóttir, I., & Sadler, C. (2003). Assessment of aberrant behavior maintained by wheelchair movement in a child with developmental disabilities. *Research in Developmental Disabilities, 24*, 381–390. https://doi.org/10.1016/S0891-4222(03)00056-8

Derby, K. M., Wacker, D. P., Peck, S., Sasso, G., DeRaad, A., Berg, W., … Ulrich, S. (1994). Functional analysis of separate topographies of aberrant behavior. *Journal of Applied Behavior Analysis, 27*, 267–278. https://doi.org/10.1901/jaba.1994.27-26

Dolezal, D. N., & Kurtz, P. F. (2010). Evaluation of combined-antecedent variables on functional analysis results and treatment of problem behavior in a school setting. *Journal of Applied Behavior Analysis, 43*, 309–314. https://doi.org/10.1901/jaba.2010.43-309

Durand, V. M., & Crimmins, D. B. (1988). Identifying the variables maintaining self-injurious behavior. *Journal of Autism and Developmental Disorders, 18*, 99–117. https://doi.org/10.1007/BF02211821

Dymond, S., & Roche, B. (2009). A contemporary behavior analysis of anxiety and avoidance. *The Behavior Analyst, 32*, 7–27. https://doi.org/10.1007/bf03392173

Eaton, W. W., Bienvenu, O. J., & Miloyan, B. (2018). Specific phobias. *Lancet Psychiatry, 5*, 678–686. https://doi.org/10.1016/S2215-0366(18)30169-X

Ebanks, M. E., & Fisher, W. W. (2003). Altering the timing of academic prompts to treat destructive behavior maintained by escape. *Journal of Applied Behavior Analysis, 36*, 355–359. https://doi.org/10.1901/jaba.2003.36-355

Eckert, T. L., Martens, B. K., & DiGennaro, F. D. (2005). Increasing the accuracy of functional assessment methods: Describing antecedent-behavior-consequence relations using conditional probabilities. *School Psychology Review, 34*, 520–528. https://doi.org/10.1080/02796015.2005.12088013

Edwards, W. H., Magee, S. K., & Ellis, J. (2002). Identifying the effects of idiosyncratic variables on functional analysis outcomes: A case study. *Education and Treatment of Children, 25*, 317–330. https://www.jstor.org/stable/42899708

English, C. L., & Anderson, C. M. (2004). Effects of familiar versus unfamiliar therapists on responding in the analog functional analysis. *Research in developmental disabilities, 25*, 39–55. https://doi.org/10.1016/j.ridd.2003.04.002

Erchul, W. P., & Martens, B. K. (2010). *School consultation: Conceptual and empirical bases of practice* (3rd ed.). New York, NY: Springer.

Eysenck, H. J. (1968). A theory of the incubation of anxiety/fear responses. *Behaviour Research and Therapy, 6*, 309–321. https://doi.org/10.1016/0005-7967(68)90064-8

Fahmie, T. A., Iwata, B. A., Harper, J. M., & Querim, A. C. (2013). Evaluation of the divided attention condition during functional analyses. *Journal of Applied Behavior Analysis, 46*, 71–78. https://doi.org/10.1002/jaba.20

Falcomata, T. S., Roane, H. S., Feeney, B. J., & Stephenson, K. M. (2010). Assessment and treatment of elopement maintained by access to stereotypy. *Journal of Applied Behavior Analysis, 43*, 513–517. https://doi.org/10.1901/jaba.2010.43-513

Fisher, W. W. (2001). Functional analysis of precurrent contingencies between mands and destructive behavior. *The Behavior Analyst Today, 2*, 176–181. https://doi.org/10.1037/h0099937

Fisher, W. W., & Bouxsein, K. (2011). Developing function-based reinforcement procedures for problem behavior. In W. W. Fisher, C. C. Piazza, & H. S. Roane (Eds.), *Handbook of applied behavior analysis* (pp. 335–347). New York, NY: Guilford.

Fisher, W. W., Greer, B. D., Romani, P. W., Zangrillo, A. N., & Owen, T. M. (2016). Comparisons of synthesized and individual reinforcement contingencies during functional analysis. *Journal of Applied Behavior Analysis, 49*, 596–616. https://doi.org/10.1002/jaba.314

Fisher, W. W., Piazza, C. C., Bowman, L. G., & Amari, A. (1996). Integrating caregiver report with a systematic choice assessment to enhance reinforcer identification. *American Journal on Mental Retardation, 101*, 15–25.

Fisher, W. W., Piazza, C. C., Bowman, L. G., Hagopian, L. P., Owens, J. C., & Slevin, I. (1992). A comparison of two approaches for identifying reinforcers for persons with severe and profound disabilities. *Journal of Applied Behavior Analysis, 25*, 491–498. https://doi.org/10.1901/jaba.1992.25-491

Flood, W. A., Wilder, D. A., Flood, A. L., & Masuda, A. (2002). Peer-mediated reinforcement plus prompting as treatment for off-task behavior in children with attention deficit hyperactivity disorder. *Journal of Applied Behavior Analysis, 35*, 199–204. https://doi.org/10.1901/jaba.2002.35-199

Gabor, A. M., Fritz, J. N., Roath, C. T., Rothe, B. R., & Gourley, D. A. (2016). Caregiver preference for reinforcement-based interventions for problem behavior maintained by positive reinforcement. *Journal of Applied Behavior Analysis, 49*, 215–227. https://doi.org/10.1002/jaba/286

Gardner, A. W., Wacker, D. P., & Boelter, E. W. (2009). An evaluation of the interaction between quality of attention and negative reinforcement with children who display escape-maintained problem behavior. *Journal of Applied Behavior Analysis, 42*, 343–348. https://doi.org/10.1901/jaba.2009.42-343

Geiger, K. B., Carr, J. E., & LeBlanc, L. A. (2010). Function-based treatments for escape-maintained problem behavior: A treatment-selection model for practicing behavior analysts. *Behavior Analysis in Practice, 3*, 22–32. https://doi.org/10.1007/BF03391755

Greer, B. D., Neidert, P. L., Dozier, C. L., Payne, S. W., Zonneveld, K. L. M., & Harper, A. M. (2013). Functional analysis and treatment of problem behaviors in early education classrooms. *Journal of Applied Behavior Analysis, 46*, 289–295. https://doi.org/10.1002/jaba.10

Hagopian, L. P., Bruzek, J. L., Bowman, L. G., & Jennett, H. K. (2007). Assessment and treatment of problem behavior occasioned by interruption of free-operant behavior. *Journal of Applied Behavior Analysis, 40*, 89–103. https://doi.org/10.1901/jaba.2007.63-05

Hagopian, L. P., Rooker, G. W., & Zarcone, J. R. (2015). Delineating subtypes of self-injurious behavior maintained by automatic reinforcement. *Journal of Applied Behavior Analysis, 48*, 523–543. https://doi.org/10.1002/jaba.236

Hagopian, L. P., Wilson, D. M., & Wilder, D. A. (2001). Assessment and treatment of problem behavior maintained by escape from attention and access to tangible items. *Journal of Applied Behavior Analysis, 34*, 229–232. https://doi.org/10.1901/jaba.2001.34-229

Hanley, G. P., Iwata, B. A., & McCord, B. E. (2003). Functional analysis of problem behavior: A review. *Journal of Applied Behavior Analysis, 36*, 147–185. https://doi.org/10.1901/jaba.2003.36-147

Hanley, G. P., Jin, C. S., Vanselow, N. R., & Hanratty, L. A. (2014). Producing meaningful improvements in problem behavior of children with autism via synthesized analyses and treatments. *Journal of Applied Behavior Analysis, 47*, 16–36. https://doi.org/10.1002/jaba.106

Harper, J. M., Iwata, B. A., & Camp, E. M. (2013). Assessment and treatment of social avoidance. *Journal of Applied Behavior Analysis, 46*, 147–160. https://doi.org/10.1002/jaba.18

Hausman, N., Kahng, S., Farrell, E., & Mongeon, C. (2009). Idiosyncratic functions: Severe problem behavior maintained by access to ritualistic behaviors. *Education and Treatment of Children, 32*, 77–87. https://doi.org/10.1353/etc.0.0051

Holehan, K. M., Dozier, C. L., Diaz de Villegas, S. C., Jess, R. L., Goddard, K. S., & Foley, E. A. (2020). A comparison of isolated and synthesized contingencies in functional analyses. *Journal of Applied Behavior Analysis*. https://doi.org/10.1002/jaba.700

Huete, J. M., & Kurtz, P. F. (2010). Therapist effects on functional analysis outcomes with young children. *Research in Developmental Disabilities, 31*, 804-810. https://doi.org/10.1016/j.ridd.2010.02.005

Iwata, B. A., DeLeon, I. G., & Roscoe, E. M. (2013). Reliability and validity of the functional analysis screening tool. *Journal of Applied Behavior Analysis, 46*, 271–284. https://doi.org/10.1002/jaba.31

Iwata, B. A., Dorsey, M. F., Slifer, K. J., Bauman, K. E., & Richman, G. S. (1994). Toward a functional analysis of self-injury. *Journal of Applied Behavior Analysis, 27*, 197–209. https://doi.org/10.1901/jaba.1194.27-197. (Reprinted from *Analysis and Intervention in Developmental Disabilities, 2*, 3–20, 1982).

Jessel, J., Hanley, G. P., & Ghaemmaghami, M. (2016). Interview-informed synthesized contingency analyses: Thirty replications and reanalysis. *Journal of Applied Behavior Analysis, 49*, 576–595. https://doi.org/10.1002/jaba.316

Kazdin, A. E. (1977). Artifact, bias, and complexity of assessment: The ABCs of reliability. *Journal of Applied Behavior Analysis, 10*, 141–150. https://doi.org/10.1901/jaba.1977.10-141

Kazdin, A. E. (2011). *Single-case research designs: Methods for clinical and applied settings* (2nd ed.). New York, NY: Oxford University Press.

Kodak, T., Northup, J., & Kelley, M. E. (2007). An evaluation of the types of attention that maintain problem behavior. *Journal of Applied Behavior Analysis, 40*, 167–171. https://doi.org/10.1901/jaba.2007.43-06

Kuhn, D. E., Hardesty, S. L., & Luczynski, K. (2009). Further evaluation of antecedent social events during functional analysis. *Journal of Applied Behavior Analysis, 42*, 349–353. https://doi.org/10.1901/jaba.2009.42-349

Krypotos, A., Effting, M., Kindt, M., & Beckers, T. (2015). Avoidance learning: A review of theoretical models and recent developments. *Frontiers in Behavioral Neuroscience, 9*, 189. https://doi.org/10.3389/fnbeh.2015.00189

Lang, R., Davis, T., O'Reilly, M., Machalicek, W., Rispoli, M., Sigafoos, J., ... & Regester, A. (2010). Functional analysis and treatment of elopement across two school settings. *Journal of Applied Behavior Analysis, 43*, 113–118. https://doi.org/10.1901/jaba.2010.43-113

Lang, R., O'Reilly, M., Lancioni, G., Rispoli, M., Machalicek, W., Chan, J. M., ... & Franco, J. (2009). Discrepancy in functional analysis results across two settings: Implications for intervention design. *Journal of Applied Behavior Analysis, 42*, 393–397. https://doi.org/10.1901/jaba.2009.42-393

Lang, R., O'Reilly, M., Machalicek, W., Lancioni, G., Rispoli, M., & Chan, J. M. (2008). A preliminary comparison of functional analysis results when conducted in contrived versus natural settings. *Journal of Applied Behavior Analysis, 41*, 441–445. https://doi.org/10.1901/jaba.2008.41-441

Lang, R., van der Werff, M., Verbeek, K., Didden, R., Davenport, K., ... Lancioni, G. (2014). Comparison of high and low preferred topographies of contingent attention during discrete trial training. *Research in Autism Spectrum Disorders, 8*, 1279–1286. https://doi.org/10.1016/j.rasd.2014.06.012

Le, D. D., & Smith, R. G. (2002). Functional analysis of self-injury with and without protective equipment. *Journal of Developmental and Physical Disabilities, 14*, 277–290. https://doi.org/10.1023/A:1016028522569

LeDoux, J. E., Moscarello, J., Sears, R., & Campese, V. (2016). The birth, death and resurrection of avoidance: A reconceptualization of a troubled paradigm. *Molecular Psychiatry, 22*, 24–36. https://doi.org/10.1038/mp.2016.166

Lerman, D. C., & Iwata, B. A. (1993). Descriptive and experimental analyses of variables maintaining self-injurious behavior. *Journal of Applied Behavior Analysis, 26*(3), 293–319. https://doi.org/10.1901/jaba.1993.26-293

Lovaas, O. I., & Simmons, J. Q. (1969). Manipulation of self-destruction in three retarded children. *Journal of Applied Behavior Analysis, 2*, 143–157. https://doi.org/10.1901/jaba.1969.2-143

Love, J. R., Carr, J. E., & LeBlanc, L. A. (2009). Functional assessment of problem behavior in children with autism spectrum disorders: A summary of 32 outpatient cases. *Journal of Autism and Developmental Disorders, 39*, 363–372. https://doi.org/10.1007/s10803-008-0633-z

Mace, F. C., & Lalli, J. S. (1991). Linking descriptive and experimental analyses in the treatment of bizarre speech. *Journal of Applied Behavior Analysis, 24*(3), 553–562. https://doi.org/10.1901/jaba.1991.24-553

Mann, A. J., & Mueller, M. M. (2009). False positive functional analysis results as a contributor of treatment failure during functional communication training. *Education and Treatment of Children, 32*, 121–149. https://doi.org/10.1353/etc.0.0044

Martens, B. K., & Ardoin, S. P. (2010). Disruptive behavior problems. In G. G. Peacock, R. A. Ervin, E. J. Daly, & K. W. Merrell (Eds.), *Practical handbook of school psychology: Effective practices for the 21st century* (pp. 157–174). New York, NY: Guilford Press.

Martens, B. K., DiGennaro, F. D., Reed, D. D., Szczech, F. M., & Rosenthal, B. D. (2008). Contingency space analysis: An alternative method for identifying contingent relations from observational data. *Journal of Applied Behavior Analysis, 41*(1), 69–81. https://doi.org/10.1901/jaba.2008.41-69

Martens, B. K., Witt, J. C., Daly, E. J., & Vollmer, T. R. (1999). Behavior analysis: Theory and practice in educational settings. In C. R. Reynolds & T. B. Gutkin (Eds.), *The handbook of school psychology* (pp. 638–663). New York, NY: Wiley.

Mason, S. A., & Iwata, B. A. (1990). Artifactual effects of sensory-integrative therapy on self-injurious behavior. *Journal of Applied Behavior Analysis, 23*, 361–370. https://doi.org/10.1901/jaba.1990.23-361

Matson, J. L., & Vollmer, T. R. (1995). *User's guide: Questions about behavioral function (QABF)*. Baton Rouge, LA: Scientific Publishers.

McAdam, D. B., DiCesare, A., Murphy, S., & Marshall, B. (2004). The influence of different therapists on functional analysis outcomes. *Behavioral Interventions, 19*, 39–44. https://doi.org/10.1002/bin.148

McComas, J. J., Moore, T., Dahl, N., Hartman, E., Hoch, J., & Symons, F. (2009). Calculating contingencies in natural environments: Issues in the application of sequential analysis. *Journal of Applied Behavior Analysis, 42*, 413–423. https://doi.org/10.1901/jaba.2009.42-413

McCord, B. E., Iwata, B. A., Galensky, T. L., Ellingson, S. A., & Thomson, R. J. (2001). Functional analysis and treatment of problem behavior evoked by noise. *Journal of Applied Behavior Analysis, 34*, 447–462. https://doi.org/10.1901/jaba.2001.34-447

McCord, B. E., Thomson, R. J., & Iwata, B. A. (2001). Functional analysis and treatment of self-injury associated with transitions. *Journal of Applied Behavior Analysis, 34*, 195–210. https://doi.org/10.1901/jaba.2001.34-195

McLaughlin, D. M., & Carr, E. G. (2005). Quality of rapport as a setting event for problem behavior: Assessment and intervention. *Journal of Positive Behavior Interventions, 7*, 68–91. https://doi.org/10.1177/10983007050070020401

McLaughlin, T. F., Derby, K. M., Gwinn, M., Taitch, H., Bolich, B., Weber, K. P., ... & Williams, R. L. (2003). The effects of active and violent play activities on brief functional analysis outcomes. *Journal of Developmental and Physical Disabilities, 15*, 93–99. https://doi.org/10.1023/A:1022846515596

Miltenberger, R. G. (2012). *Behavior modification: Principles and procedures.* Belmont, CA: Thomson Wadsworth.

Moore, J. W., & Edwards, R. P. (2003). An analysis of aversive stimuli in classroom demand contexts. *Journal of Applied Behavior Analysis, 36*, 339–348. https://doi.org/10.1901/jaba.2003.36-339

Morris, S. L., & Vollmer, T. R. (2019). Assessing preference for types of social interaction. *Journal of Applied Behavior Analysis, 52*, 1064–1075. https://doi.org/10.1002/jaba.597

Mueller, M. M., Sterling-Turner, H. E., & Moore, J. W. (2005). Towards developing a classroom-based functional analysis condition to assess escape-to-attention as a variable maintaining problem behavior. *School Psychology Review, 34*, 425–431. https://doi.org/10.1080/02796015.2005.12086296

Mueller, M. M., Wilczynski, S. M., Moore, J. W., Fusilier, I., & Trahant, D. (2001). Antecedent manipulations in a tangible condition: Effects of stimulus preference on aggression. *Journal of Applied Behavior Analysis, 34*, 237–240. https://doi.org/10.1901/jaba.2001.34-237

National Collaborating Centre for Mental Health (NCCMH). (2013). *Social anxiety disorder: Recognition, assessment and treatment.* Leicester, UK: British Psychological Society.

National Institute of Mental Health (NIMH). (2017, November). *Social anxiety disorder.* Retrieved from: https://www.nimh.nih.gov/health/statistics/social-anxiety-disorder.shtml

Ndoro, V. W., Hanley, G. P., Tiger, J. H., & Heal, N. A. (2006). A descriptive assessment of instruction-based interactions in the preschool classroom. *Journal of Applied Behavior Analysis, 39*, 79–90. https://doi.org/10.1901/jaba.2006.146-04

Neidert, P. L., Iwata, B. A., & Dozier, C. L. (2005). Treatment of multiply controlled problem behavior with procedural variations of differential reinforcement. *Exceptionality, 13*, 45–53. https://doi.org/10.1207/s15327035ex1301_6

Northup, J., Kodak, T., Lee, J., & Coyne, A. (2004). Instructional influences on analogue functional analysis outcomes. *Journal of Applied Behavior Analysis, 37*, 509–512. https://doi.org/10.1901/jaba.2004.37-509

O'Neil, R. E., Horner, R. H., Albin, R. W., Storey, K., & Sprague, J. R. (1990). *Functional analysis of problem behavior: A practical guide.* Sycamore, IL: Sycamore Publishing.

O'Neill, R. E., Horner, R. H., Albin, R. W., Sprague, J. R., Storey, K., & Newton, J. S. (1997). *Functional assessment and program development for problem behavior: A practical handbook.* Pacific Grove, CA: Brooks/Cole.

Owen, T. M., Fisher, W. W., Akers, J. S., Sullivan, W. E., Falcomata, T. S., ... Zangrillo, A. N. (2020). Treating destructive behavior reinforced by increased caregiver compliance with the participant's mands. *Journal of Applied Behavior Analysis, 53*, 1494–1513. https://doi.org/10.1002/jaba.674

Pace, G. M., Ivancic, M. T., Edwards, G. L., Iwata, B. A., & Page, T. J. (1985). Assessment of stimulus preference and reinforcer value with profoundly retarded individuals. *Journal of Applied Behavior Analysis, 18*(3), 249–255. https://doi.org/10.1901/jaba.1985.18-249

Querim, A. C., Iwata, B. A., Roscoe, E. M., Schlichenmeyer, K. J., Ortega, J. V., & Hurl, K. E. (2013). Functional analysis screening for problem behavior maintained by automatic reinforcement. *Journal of Applied Behavior Analysis, 46*, 47–60. https://doi.org/10.1002/jaba.26

Rapp, J. T., & Vollmer, T. R. (2005). Stereotypy: A review of behavioral assessment and treatment. *Research in Developmental Disabilities, 26*, 527–547. https://doi.org/10.1016/j.ridd.2004.11.005

Ringdahl, J. E., Christensen, T. J., & Boelter, E. W. (2009). Further evaluation of idiosyncratic functions for severe problem behavior: Aggression maintained by access to walks. *Behavioral Interventions: Theory & Practice in Residential & Community-Based Clinical Programs, 24*, 275–283. https://doi.org/10.1002/bin.289

Roane, H. S., Sullivan, W. E., Martens, B. K., & Kelley, M. E. (2019). Behavioral treatments for individuals with developmental disabilities. In M. L. Batshaw, N. J. Roizen, & L. Pelligrino (Eds.), *Children with developmental disabilities* (8th ed.). Baltimore, MD: Brookes Publishing.

Roane, H. S., Vollmer, T. R., Ringdahl, J. E., & Marcus, B. A. (1998). Evaluation of a brief stimulus preference assessment. *Journal of Applied Behavior Analysis, 31*, 605–620. https://doi.org/10.1901/jaba.1998.31-605

Rooker, G. W., & Roscoe, E. M. (2005). Functional analysis of self-injurious behavior and its relation to self-restraint. *Journal of Applied Behavior Analysis, 38*, 537–542. https://doi.org/10.1901/jaba.2005.12-05

Roscoe, E. M., Kindle, A. E., & Pence, S. T. (2010). Functional analysis and treatment of aggression maintained by preferred conversational topics. *Journal of Applied Behavior Analysis, 43*, 723–727. https://doi.org/10.1901/jaba.2010.43-723

Roscoe, E. M., Rooker, G. W., Pence, S. T., & Longworth, L. J. (2009). Assessing the utility of a demand assessment for functional analysis. *Journal of Applied Behavior Analysis, 42*, 819–825. https://doi.org/10.1901/jaba.2009.42-819

Sarno, J. M., Sterling, H. E., Mueller, M. M., Dufrene, B., Tingstrom, D. H., & Olmi, D. J. (2011). Escape-to-attention as a potential variable for maintaining problem behavior in the school setting. *School Psychology Review, 40*, 57–71. https://doi.org/10.1080/02796015.2011.12087728

Scheithauer, M. C., Mevers, J. E. L., Call, N. A., & Shrewsbury, A. N. (2017). Using a test for multiply-maintained self injury to develop function-based treatments. *Journal of Developmental and Physical Disabilities, 29*(3), 443–460. https://doi.org/10.1007/s10882-017-9535-3

Schlichenmeyer, K. J., Roscoe, E. M., Rooker, G. W., Wheeler, E. E., & Dube, W. V. (2013). Idiosyncratic variables that affect functional analysis outcomes: A review (2001–2010). *Journal of Applied Behavior Analysis, 46*, 339–348. https://doi.org/10.1002/jaba.12

Skinner, B. F. (1953). *Science and human behavior*. New York, NY: Macmillan.

Skinner, J. N., Veerkamp, M. B., Kamps, D. M., & Andra, P. R. (2009). Teacher and peer participation in functional analysis and intervention for a first grade student with attention deficit hyperactivity disorder. *Education and Treatment of Children, 32*, 243–266. https://doi.org/10.1353/etc.0.0059

Sullivan, W. E., Saini, V., DeRosa, N. M., Craig, A. R., Ringdahl, J. E., & Roane, H. S. (2020). Measurement of nontargeted problem behavior during investigations of resurgence. *Journal of Applied Behavior Analysis, 53*, 249–264. https://doi.org/10.1002/jaba.589

Tiger, J. H., Fisher, W. W., Toussaint, K. A., & Kodak, T. (2009). Progressing from initially ambiguous functional analyses: Three case examples. *Research in Developmental Disabilities, 30*, 910–926. https://doi.org/10.1016/j.ridd.2009.01.005

Tiger, J. H., Hanley, G. P., & Bessette, K. K. (2006). Incorporating descriptive assessment results into the design of a functional analysis: A case example involving a preschooler's hand mouthing. *Education and Treatment of Children*, 107–123. https://www.jstor.org/stable/42899872

Touchette, P. E., MacDonald, R. F., & Langer, S. N. (1985). A scatter plot for identifying stimulus control of problem behavior. *Journal of Applied Behavior Analysis, 18*, 343–351. https://doi.org/10.1901/jaba.1985.18-343

Vaughn, M. E., & Michael, J. L. (1982). Automatic reinforcement: An important but ignored concept. *Behavior, 10*, 127–127.

Vervliet, B., & Indekeu, E. (2015). Low-cost avoidance behaviors are resistant to fear extinction in humans. *Frontiers in Behavioral Neuroscience, 9*, 351. https://doi.org/10.3389/fnbeh.2015.00351

Vollmer, T. R. (1994). The concept of automatic reinforcement: Implications for behavioral research in developmental disabilities. *Research in Developmental Disabilities, 15*, 187–207. https://doi.org/10.1016/0891-4222(94)90011-6

Vollmer, T. R., & Athens, E. (2011). Developing function-based extinction procedures for problem behavior. In W. W. Fisher, C. C. Piazza, & H. S. Roane (Eds.), *Handbook of applied behavior analysis* (pp. 317–334). New York, NY: Guilford.

Vollmer, T. R., Iwata, B. A., Zarcone, J. R., Smith, R. G., & Mazaleski, J. L. (1993). The role of attention in the treatment of attention-maintained self-injurious behavior: Noncontingent reinforcement and differential reinforcement of other behavior. *Journal of Applied Behavior Analysis, 26*, 9–21. https://doi.org/10.1901/jaba.1993.26-9

Volkert, V. M., Lerman, D. C., Call, N. A., & Trosclair-Lasserre, N. (2009). An evaluation of resurgence during treatment with functional communication training. *Journal of Applied Behavior Analysis, 42*, 145–160. https://doi.org/10.1901/jaba.2009.42-145

Wacker, D. P., Berg, W. K., Harding, J. W., & Cooper-Brown, L. J. (2011). Functional and structural approaches to behavioral assessment of problem behavior. In W. W. Fisher, C. C. Piazza, & H. S. Roane (Eds.), *Handbook of applied behavior analysis* (pp. 335–347). New York, NY: Guilford Press.

Wilder, D. A., Harris, C., Reagan, R., & Rasey, A. (2007). Functional analysis and treatment of noncompliance by preschool children. *Journal of Applied Behavior Analysis, 40*, 173–177. https://doi.org/10.1901/jaba.2007.44-06

Part II
Assessment

Chapter 4
Populations and Problems Evaluated with Functional Assessment

Geraldine Leader, Mia Casburn, Leanne Maher, Chiara Ferrari, Katie Naughton, Taylor R. Wicks, and Arlene Mannion

Introduction

Functional assessment is defined as "a process of identifying functional relationships between environmental events and the occurrence or nonoccurrence of a target behavior" (Dunlap et al., 1993, p. 275). The purpose of functional assessment is to identify environmental events that reliably predict and maintain challenging behavior (CB) (McIntosh, Brown, & Borgmeier, 2008; Steege, Pratt, Wickerd, Guare, & Watson, 2019). Functional assessment has most commonly been conducted in clinical settings with individuals who have developmental disabilities exhibiting severe forms of CB including self-injurious behavior (SIB), aggression, and disruptive behaviors (Hanley, Iwata, & McCord, 2003). The focus of this chapter is to review the literature on the range of CB and populations for whom functional assessment has been used.

The first part of this chapter will review the different populations commonly evaluated with functional assessment. These populations include the following: autism spectrum disorder (ASD), intellectual disability (ID), Emotional Behavioral Disorder, Attention-deficit/hyperactivity disorder (AD/HD), Fragile X Syndrome, Angelman Syndrome, Prader-Willi Syndrome, Smith-Magenis Syndrome, Lesch-Nyhan Syndrome, Acquired Brain Injury, Typically Developing Children, Children at Risk of Developmental Disabilities, Children with Prenatal Drug Exposure, and Children who use Wheelchairs. The second part of this chapter will focus on the

G. Leader (✉) · M. Casburn · L. Maher · C. Ferrari · K. Naughton · T. R. Wicks · A. Mannion
National University of Ireland, Galway, Ireland

Irish Centre for Autism and Neurodevelopmental Research, School of Psychology, National University of Ireland, Galway, Ireland
e-mail: Geraldine.leader@nuigalway.ie

© Springer Nature Switzerland AG 2021
J. L. Matson (ed.), *Functional Assessment for Challenging Behaviors and Mental Health Disorders*, Autism and Child Psychopathology Series,
https://doi.org/10.1007/978-3-030-66270-7_4

specific behaviors exhibited by these populations, including the following: aggression, SIB, stereotypy, bizarre speech, skin picking, hand mouthing, feeding problems, elopement, noncompliance and disruptive behavior, multiple topographies of behavior, sleep problems, and happiness behaviors.

Populations Evaluated with Functional Assessment

Autism Spectrum Disorder

Autism spectrum disorder (ASD) is a neurodevelopmental disorder characterized by persistent deficits in social communication and social interaction in combination with restricted, repetitive patterns of behavior, interests, or activities (American Psychiatric Association, 2013). Individuals with ASD often engage in CB that interferes with their quality of life. The most common challenging behaviors (CBs) assessed in individuals with ASD are aggression, property destruction, SIB, stereotypy, and tantrums (Devlin, Healy, Leader, & Reed, 2008; Leader & Mannion, 2016; Liddon, Zarcone, Pisman, & Rooker, 2016; Machalicek et al., 2010; O'Reilly et al., 2010; Kern, 1997). Other behaviors include elopement, flopping, inappropriate vocalizations, verbal protesting, pica, and spitting (O'Reilly, Edrisinha, Sigafoos, Lancioni, & Andrews, 2006; Olive, Lang, & Davis, 2008).

CBs are often assessed through functional assessments. A large number of studies showed the effectiveness of functional analysis (FA) in identifying the maintaining functions of CB displayed by individuals with ASD in both applied and school settings (Falcomata & Gainey, 2014; Falcomata, Muething, Gainey, Hoffman, & Fragale, 2013; Fragale, Rojeski, O'Reilly, & Gevarter, 2016; Olive et al., 2008; Rose & Beaulieu, 2019; Sasso et al., 1992; Scalzo & Davis, 2017; Smith, Carr, & Moskowitz, 2016). Additional studies suggested the importance of individualizing functional analyses (FAs) in order to both identify multiple functions of CB (LaBelle & Charlop-Christy, 2002) and incorporate specific establishing operations in the FA test conditions (Strohmeier, Murphy, & O'Connor, 2017). Machalicek et al. (2009, 2010) also showed the effectiveness of FAs with videoconferencing equipment to identify the functions of aggression, SIB, property disruption, flopping, and stereotypy in children with ASD in a classroom setting. However, Hausman, Kahng, Farrell, and Mongeon (2009) showed that when CBs are idiosyncratic in nature, FAs may be inconclusive and further analysis to evaluate more idiosyncratic functions might be necessary. Although effective, FAs have a number of limitations including the length of time, the high level of expertise required, and the reinforcement of CB. For this reason, alternatives and variations of FAs have been investigated to identify CB displayed by children with ASD.

The length of FAs has been addressed with the implementation of shorter test conditions in Brief Functional Analyses (BFA). Several studies showed the effectiveness of BFA in identifying the maintaining functions of CB displayed by children with ASD (Kelly, Ax, Allen, & Maguire, 2015; Roberts-Gwinn, Luiten, Derby, Johnson, & Weber, 2001). The limitation of reinforcing CB during the implementation of FAs can be addressed with the implementation of manding analysis (MA). LaRue et al. (2011) showed the effectiveness of MA in identifying the maintaining functions of CB. The analysis involved reinforcement contingent on mands rather than CB in four individuals with ASD. Studies also suggested the benefits of using a trial-based functional analysis (TBFA) to investigate the maintaining functions of CB of individuals with ASD compared to traditional FAs. TBFA does not require the repeated reinforcement of CB, and it is conducted in shorter time than FAs (LaRue et al., 2010; Larkin, Hawkins, & Collins, 2016).

Studies also found a high correspondence between Questions About Behavioral Function (QABF; Matson &Vollmer (1995) and FAs in the analysis of function of CB displayed by individuals with ASD (Healy, Brett, & Leader, 2013; Watkins & Rapp, 2013). Devlin, Healy, Leader, and Hughes (2011) also found the QABF and Functional Analysis Screening Tool-Revised (FAST-R) effective in identifying the maintaining functions of CB displayed by children with ASD. Herman, Healy, and Lydon (2018) showed the effectiveness of an Interview-Informed Synthesized Contingency Analysis to identify the function of flopping in one child with ASD in a school setting. Studies showed the effectiveness of descriptive observational assessment in identifying the maintaining functions of CB displayed by individuals with ASD (Carr & Carlson, 1993; Toogood, Boyd, Bell, & Salisbury, 2011). Tarbox et al. (2009) showed that descriptive assessments did not identify clear maintaining functions of CB when compared to indirect assessments and experimental FAs, which led to conclusive functions. Martens, Gertz, de Lacy Werder, and Rymanowski (2010) showed the correspondence of Contingency Space Analysis of behavior-consequence recordings with the results of FAs under naturalistic test conditions for three children with ASD. Discrete-trial functional analysis was also found to be an effective experimental methodology to identify the maintaining functions of CB in natural routines (Schmidt, Drasgow, Halle, Martin, & Bliss, 2014).

Although there are a wide variety of FA methodologies, the most common identified functions of CB displayed by individuals with ASD are attention and escape from demand, followed by self-stimulation and access to preferred food or toys (Matson et al., 2011). CBs displayed by individuals with ASD are often maintained by multiple functions, and studies showed that function-based interventions are more effective when the maintaining variables are identified through FAs (Heyvaert, Saenen, Campbell, Maes, & Onghena, 2014).

Intellectual Disability

Intellectual disability (ID) is seen as a disorder with onset during the developmental period that includes both intellectual and adaptive functioning deficits in conceptual, social, and practical domains (American Psychiatric Association, 2013). Between 10% and 15% of individuals with ID present with CB (Emerson et al.,

2001; Lowe et al., 2007). In the adult ID population, prevalence estimates for SIB are 15% (Kahng, Iwata, & Lewin, 2002) and 10–24% for aggressive behavior (Crocker et al., 2006). Regarding the prevalence of behavior functions for people with ID, previous research has identified that SIB and stereotypy are more likely to be maintained by automatic reinforcement (Chung & Cannella-Malone, 2010; Delgado-Casas, Navarro, Garcia-Gonzalez-Gordon, & Marchena, 2014) and aggressive behavior is more likely maintained by social positive or negative rein-forcement (Britton, Carr, Landaburu, & Romick, 2002; Delgado-Casas et al., 2014; Emerson et al., 1996; Hanley, Piazza, Fisher, & Maglieri, 2005; Ellingson, Miltenberger, Stricker, Galensky, & Garlinghouse, 2000; Rispoli et al., 2011, Smith & Churchill, 2002; Vollmer et al., 1998). Data from other studies, however, have identified higher percentages of cases of SIB as maintained by social positive and/ or negative reinforcement (Hanley et al., 2003; Hetzroni & Roth, 2003; O'Reilly et al., 2008; Smith & Churchill, 2002; Wacker et al., 1998; Wacker et al., 1990).

Previous literature has also identified that CB may be maintained by a combina-tion of social positive, social negative, and automatic reinforcement (Lloyd & Kennedy, 2014; Matson & Boisjoli, 2007; Scheithauer, Cariveau, Call, Ormand, & Clark, 2016). In some cases, the function of CB has been found to vary by topogra-phy. For example, Derby et al. (1994) identified stereotypy to be maintained by automatic reinforcement and SIB to be maintained by social positive or social nega-tive reinforcement for two individuals with ID. Similarly, Delgado-Casas et al. (2014) identified SIB to be maintained by both automatic reinforcement and social positive reinforcement across three participants with ID. For one participant in par-ticular, aggression was maintained by negative reinforcement, social attention, and tangible positive reinforcement. Their SIB was maintained by automatic reinforce-ment, and stereotypy was maintained by social attention and tangible positive reinforcement.

Hall (2005) examined the outcomes of descriptive, experimental, and informant-based methods of FA for four individuals with ID presenting with CB. Results indi-cated that the descriptive and experimental assessments were concordant in only one of the four cases, while informant-based and experimental assessments were concordant in three of the four cases. For example, the experimental and informant-based assessment identified an escape function for SIB, while the descriptive assess-ment identified attention. Results suggested that information from descriptive assessments may not be useful adjunct to experimental assessment. In order to accu-rately identify CB in ID, recent research has shown promise in training nonprofes-sionals in learning to carry out a FA and implementing the information gained from the FA into effective behavioral interventions (Tassé, 2006).

Emotional Behavioral Disorder

Emotional Behavioral Disorder (EBD) is a broad term used to describe a range of CB observed in individuals that would often be characteristic of the presence of a disability (Kavale, Forness, & Mostert, 2005). Although attempts to define EBD in research have been difficult, certain characteristics are assessed as part of a diagnosis (Kavale et al., 2005): (1) Incompetence when forming and sustaining relationships; (2) Learning difficulties due to factors outside of intellectual or health problems; (3) Consistent and abnormal behaviors and feelings in normal situations; (4) Consistent development of fears and physical symptoms related to personal and professional problems; and (5) General low mood and feelings of depression or sadness. Individuals diagnosed with EBD usually display behavior pertaining to at least one of the characteristics above, which result in problems with development and interpersonal relationships (Poulou, 2013). Often EBD is associated with other subdisorders, for example, AD/HD.

CB associated with EBD are often studied and treated in the context of a FA. Flanagan and DeBar (2018) conducted a TBFA to identify the idiosyncratic functions of CB in a 10-year-old boy with an EBD. The CB under analysis were vocal disruptions, physical aggression, and falling on the floor/crawling. Indirect and experimental assessments of CB were conducted to identify the conditions favorable to the FA. The TBFA involved trials of ten varying conditions. FA results showed that the CB was maintained by attention and escape from demands. This study provides evidence to support the use of trial-based FAs in the analysis of CB in EBD.

Attention-Deficit/Hyperactivity Disorder

Attention-deficit/hyperactivity disorder (AD/HD) is the most common neurodevelopmental disorder diagnosed in childhood (Perou et al., 2013) and is characterized by chronic symptoms of inattention, impulsivity, and/or hyperactivity that lead to functional impairment experienced in multiple settings (American Psychiatric Association, 2013). Kodak, Grow, and Northup (2004) conducted a FA with a 5-year-old girl with AD/HD in a summer school setting to identify the maintaining function of elopement during a kickball game. Elopement was operationally defined as running more than 1 m away from the kicking area or designated base when it was not functional to the game. The FA included attention, escape, and control conditions. Results of the FA showed that the duration of elopement was consistently high in the attention condition and was always low in the escape and control conditions. A subsequent treatment consisting of noncontingent attention and time-out was used to eliminate elopement during the kickball game.

Fragile X Syndrome

Fragile X Syndrome (FRAX) is caused by a change in the DNA sequence of the Fragile X Mental Retardation 1 (FMR1) gene, which results in a wide range of intellectual disabilities and is often associated with different disorders such as ASD (Hagerman, 2008; Newman, Leader, Chen, & Mannion, 2015). Kurtz, Chin, Robinson, O'Connor, and Hagopian (2015) investigated the use of FA in understanding the function of CB in children with FRAX. FA conditions of attention, demand, tangible, alone, and play were implemented. Results found CB to be primarily maintained by escape from demands and access to tangibles.

Monlux, Pollard, Rodriquez, and Hall (2019) used FA in a population diagnosed with FRAX when investigating the efficiency of telehealth to uncover functions of and treat CB. Results indicated escape from academic demands, escape from transition demands, access to tangibles, and attention as the primary functions behind CB. These results were then used to implement treatments via telehealth. Machalicek et al. (2014) examined the function of CB in 12 participants with FRAX under attention, social avoidance, demand, tangible, and play conditions. They found escape from demands and/or escape from social interactions as maintaining functions in eight participants and access to preferred items in nine participants. Three participants showed attention as a maintaining factor.

Angelman Syndrome

Angelman Syndrome (AS) is a clinical, neurogenetic disorder, affecting approximately 1 in 12,000–20,000 people (Buckley, Dinno, & Weber, 1998; Galván-Manso et al., 2002). Symptoms of the disorder include craniofacial abnormalities, an ataxic gait, limbic weakness, seizures, decreased cognitive functioning, lack of communication, hyperactivity, inappropriate laughter, and a perceived happy demeanor (Adams, Horsler, Mount, & Oliver, 2015; Holland, Whittington, & Butler, 2002; Williams et al., 1995).

Studies have used FA to assess the functions of CB in participants with AS. Conditions similar to Iwata, Dorsey, Slifer, Bauman, and Richman (1994) were implemented for both of the following studies (Radstaake et al., 2013; Radstaake, Didden, Oliver, Allen, & Curfs, 2012). Radstaake et al. (2012) found attention, access to tangibles, and demand as maintaining factors of CB, and results showed the presence of precursors before nearly all incidences of CB. Similarly, Radstaake et al. (2013) found attention and access to tangibles to be primary maintaining factors for CB in participants and identified precursor behavior in one of the three participants.

Strachan et al. (2009) conducted experimental FAs of CB in 12 children with AS. The target behavior being observed was aggression, with 10 of 12 participants displaying aggressive behaviors. Results indicated that one participant showed attention as a maintaining factor of CB, three showed social interaction, and two showed escape as a maintaining factor. Based on these results, the authors suggested that in their sample, aggression may serve as a means to maintain and initiate social contact.

Prader-Willi Syndrome

Prader-Willi syndrome (PWS) is a rare genetic disorder consisting of several implications to metabolic, endocrine, neurologic systems, with behavior and intellectual difficulties (Gutierrez & Mendez, 2020). PWS is characterized by hypotonia, feeding difficulties, and hyperphagia and can lead to morbid obesity (Gutierrez & Mendez, 2020). Functional assessment has been used to identify the maintaining functions of CB associated with food displayed by individuals with PWS. Lambert et al. (2019) used latency-based FA in a clinical setting to investigate the functions of food stealing behaviors of a 7 year-old girl with PWS. Results of the FA revealed that food stealing was maintained by contingent access to food. As part of a function-based intervention, differential reinforcement (DR) procedures combined with a token board and schedule thinning were implemented. The intervention was successful in teaching the participant to wait for small portions of food across longer timeframes, eliminating food stealing behaviors, and creating family inclusion during mealtime.

Didden, Korzilius, and Curfs (2007) used FA to investigate the association of skin-picking with compulsive behavior and SIB in 119 children with PWS. Two rating scales were distributed to the participants' parents to investigate behavioral and operant functions of skin-picking while collecting data on SIB and compulsive behaviors. QABF was used to assess functions of skin-picking. FA results showed that skin-picking was primarily reinforced by nonsocial and intrinsic consequences in 70% of the sample. The authors hypothesized that skin-picking is negatively reinforced by tension and arousal reduction. Therefore, skin-picking may be treated using relaxation training, anxiety and anger management, and teaching coping strategies in dealing with psychological stressors.

Smith-Magenis Syndrome

Smith-Magenis Syndrome (SMS) is a rare neurobehavioral disorder characterized by a recognizable pattern of physical, behavioral, and developmental features. It is caused by particular genetic changes on chromosomal region 17p11.2, which contains the gene RAI1 (Juyal et al., 1996). A diagnosis of SMS is associated with high levels of CB, specifically SIB, and aggression toward others (Arron, Oliver, Berg, Moss, & Burbidge, 2011; Sloneem, Oliver, Udwin, & Woodock, 2011). Hodnett, Scheithauer, Call, Mevers, and Miller (2018) assessed and treated severe CB exhibited by two children with SMS. The primary target behaviors of the first participant, a 13 year old male, were SIB, disruptive behavior, and disrobing. The primary target behaviors of the second participant, a four-year-old female, were SIB, aggression, and disruptive behavior. For both participants, the function of CB was identified through a FA. All sessions started with a multielement design. If rates of CB were variable across conditions, a pairwise design was employed. If no CB was observed, the caregivers of the participants were incorporated into the FA. Control, escape, attention, tangible, and alone (the first participant only) conditions were conducted.

The first participant, the 13-year-old male, engaged in consistently higher rates of CB in the escape condition when compared to the control. Inconsistent rates of CB were observed in the tangible and attention conditions. In a pairwise design, elevated rates of CB were observed in the tangible condition. Initially, in the attention pairwise analysis, high rates were observed that decreased to stable rates, suggesting that the CB of the participants was not maintained by access to attention. It was concluded that the participant's CB was maintained by escape from demands and access to tangible items. The second participant engaged in no CB during the initial FA with the therapist. However, elevated rates of CB were observed in the tangible and attention conditions when her mother conducted the FA. It was determined that the participant's CB was maintained by access to attention and tangible items.

Torres-Viso, Strohmeier, and Zarcone (2018) conducted a FA of the relation between mands and CB. The participant was a 12-year-old female diagnosed with ASD and SMS. The mands involved requests from others to change their body positioning or proximity or rearrange items back to their original position. For example, her mother's legs could only sometimes be crossed or her father could not stand at certain windows. When her parents did not comply with these demands, she would exhibit CB. A multielement FA was conducted in which the role of social positive reinforcement in the form of access to an individual's attention, divided attention, and toys contingent on CB was evaluated. Social negative reinforcement in the form of escape from demands and automatic reinforcement was also evaluated in which her behavior was ignored. The results of FA confirmed the relation between CB and mand compliance, indicating that CB was maintained by other's compliance with mands for rearrangement.

Lesch-Nyhan Syndrome

Obi (1997) designed a function-based intervention to decrease the occurrences of SIB and the use of wrist restraints in a 24 year-old adult with Lesch-Nyhan Syndrome. The target behavior under analysis was SIB, which was operationally defined as banging his head and hands on different objects such as wall, bed rails, or Plexiglass screen, finger biting, and flipping out of his wheelchair. A semistructured behavioral interview was conducted with the participant, and a simple questionnaire and direct observation was completed by the staff as part of the functional assessment process. Results were then analyzed in a concurrent analysis, which identified negative reinforcement in the form of avoidance of anxiety contingent on the absence of restraints as the maintaining function. From the functional assessment results, a 4-phase intervention was successfully designed and delivered to decrease the restraint time and the occurrences of SIB.

Acquired Brain Injury

Rahman, Oliver, and Alderman (2010) conducted a descriptive FA investigating the CB exhibited by nine adults with acquired brain injury (ABI). The target behaviors were operationally defined under aggression as "physical aggression", "property destruction", "SIB", and " verbal aggression". The descriptive FA involved observation of the participants in their natural environment, and data was collected using a coding system on a personal computer. A concurrent analysis was conducted to assess the likelihood that environmental events occurred prior to the target behaviors. A sequential analysis was conducted to investigate the sequences in which CBs were related to appropriate environmental events. The two analyses were compared, and 88% of concordance was found. The overall findings showed that the CB displayed by the adults with ABI occurred in a functional, orderly, and predictable way. Escape from demand and escape from social attention were identified as maintaining functions for 13 behaviors, respectively. Multiple functions were identified for five participants, and 88% of CBs were found to be significantly likely to co-occur with environmental events.

Rahman, Alderman, and Oliver (2013) investigated the effects of structured descriptive assessments in identifying the maintaining functions of CB displayed by four adult survivors of traumatic brain injury. Three participants sustained a brain injury following a road traffic accident and one participant following a suicide attempt. For three participants, the CB under analysis was aggression in the form of property destruction and physical and/or verbal aggression. The CB exhibited by the fourth participant was verbal perseveration defined as repetitive recitation of a phrase, word, or indecipherable verbalization. A hybrid approach to functional assessment and experimental FA was used to identify the functions of the target behaviors. The structured descriptive analysis involved the systematic manipulation of antecedent events typically involved in a FA but without manipulating the consequences in a structured descriptive way. The target behaviors were observed in the natural environment, in contrast to the FA methodology but characteristic of a typical functional assessment. Results from the analysis showed that escape from demand was the maintaining function for two participants, and social attention was the function for the other two participants. Results showed that structured descriptive assessment is an efficient methodology to effectively identify behavior functions in individuals with ABI.

Typically Developing Children

Arndorfer and Miltenberger (1993) reviewed literature on FA and treatment of CB in children with developmental disabilities. Informant assessment, direct observation assessment, and experimental analysis were reviewed in-depth. The implications for early childhood were discussed, and the authors revealed that because FA involves the manipulation of antecedent or consequent variables, a school psychologist or other professional would need to organize the process and instruct parents/teachers how to carry out the FA conditions. The authors revealed that practitioners in the field of early childhood special education or other areas of developmental disabilities should approach CB from a functional perspective in order to develop effective treatments.

CBs presented in young children have increased over the years, which places them at risk for developing an emotional/behavioral disorder (Conroy, Davis, Fox, & Brown, 2002). Conroy et al. (2002) examined FA of behavior and effective supports for young children with CB. A multilevel system model that outlines prevention on various levels, as well as remediation strategies that can be used to ameliorate CB exhibited by young children, was assessed. This hierarchical model consists of applying a multilevel FA and interventions when working with young children who present with CB. Conroy et al. (2002) suggested that early intervention can make a significant difference in behavioral and developmental outcomes and this model provides a framework for addressing these behaviors across three levels of prevention and intervention. The importance of addressing CB of children in early childhood settings and the incorporation of this model may prevent further development of EBD in children. This model provides a least restrictive, intrusive framework for identifying and intervening with high-risk environments and children in early childhood programs. This model may be time efficient for teachers and typically developing children.

Rispoli et al. (2015) investigated TBFA on Head Start teachers during classroom routines. The purpose of this study was to train teachers to conduct TBFA in the classroom, assess the accuracy of TBFA results by comparing function-based with nonfunction-based CB interventions, and assess teacher observations of the social validity of a TBFA in Head Start classroom setting. Three Head Start teachers and one child from each teacher's classroom were selected to participate. Data was collected on the children's CB and appropriate communication, and an A-B-A-C-D design was employed for the purpose of the study. Function-based intervention produced greater decreases in CB than the nonfunction-based intervention for in all three children. TBFA represents an important innovation for developing function-based interventions for children with challenging behavior.

Children at Risk of Developmental Disabilities

A variety of research have been conducted for children who may be at risk of developmental disabilities and the factors that may contribute to this (Macks and Reeve, 2007). Schroeder, Richman, Abby, Courtemanche, and Oyama-Ganiko (2014) investigated the prevalence of CB in young children at risk of developmental disabilities in 17 at-risk children. SIB, stereotypy, property destruction, aggression, and tantrums as target CB were assessed using an analogue FA under play, attention, escape, and alone conditions, and the Behavior Problem Inventory was also conducted. Researchers found that most of the CBs displayed were maintained by automatic reinforcement with a minority being attributed to social reinforcement.

Children with Prenatal Drug Exposure

Very few studies focus on the analysis of CB in a population consisting of children with a history of prenatal drug exposure. Kurtz, Chin, Rush, and Dixon (2008) used FA to identify the functions of CB displayed by children who had experienced prenatal drug exposure. The participants were two toddlers under the age of 2 years that had been prenatally exposed to drugs (cocaine, heroin, alcohol) and were reported to often display various forms of CB. The CBs under analysis were aggression, SIB, and destructive behaviors. An experimental FA consisting of attention, play, tangible, and demand conditions was carried out in order to establish the variables maintaining the CB. The results showed that the CBs of both children were maintained by positive reinforcement in the form of attention from adults and access to tangible items. For one child, escape from demands was also a maintaining function of CB. Function-based interventions were then delivered based on the results of FA that were shown to be effective in reducing CB. The results showed the effectiveness of using a FA to analyze behavioral functions in children with prenatal drug exposure and to provide evidence that often CB derived from environmental factors.

Children Who Use Wheelchairs

DeLeon, Kahng, Rodriguez-Catter, Sveinsdóttir, and Sadler (2003) conducted an experimental FA in order to identify the maintaining functions of CB in a child with a developmental disability using a wheelchair. The participant was a 14-year-old boy with severe mental problems, cerebral palsy, and visual impairments. The target behavior under analysis was aggression in the form of hitting, grabbing, and pushing. Experimental FA involved seven different conditions: toy play, social attention, alone, demand, activities of daily living, social escape, and contingent wheelchair movement. The results showed movement as a positively reinforcing CB in the participant, with aggression levels rising contingent on being pushed in the wheelchair.

Behaviors and Problems Evaluated
with Functional Assessment

Aggression

Aggression is defined as a behavior that is intended to harm another person who is motivated to avoid that harm (DeWall, Anderson, & Bushman, 2012). Cariveau, Miller, Call, and Alvarez (2019) used a FA to determine whether aggression exhibited by an eight-year-old male with a diagnosis of ASD and AD/HD was maintained by termination of interruptions to repetitive behavior. A multielement FA was conducted which included attention, toy play, tangible, escape, and interruption conditions. The results of the FA demonstrated that aggression was maintained by escape from demands and termination of interruptions to repetitive behavior.

Newcomb, Wright, and Camblin (2019) examined aggressive behavior maintained by access to physical attention using two preparations of a FA. The participant was a 13-year-old male with a diagnosis of ASD who attended a private, specialized education facility due to underdeveloped communication skills and CB. The target behavior under analysis was aggression. A FA was carried out similar to procedures described by Iwata, Dorsey, Slifer, Bauman, and Richman (1994). Test conditions included in the FA were escape from demands, ignore, physical attention, nonphysical attention, and a control condition. Following the FA, a competing stimulus assessment was carried out to identify one or more stimuli that would compete with aggression. Results showed that physical attention was the maintaining function of aggression and that certain stimuli competed with it. The intervention consisted of noncontingent reinforcement (NCR) using competing stimuli, and it was successful in decreasing the occurrences of aggression.

Romani et al. (2019) focused on aggressive behavior exhibited by two children during public outings. The first participant was a 5-year-old boy with ASD and had unspecified disruptive, impulse-control, and conduct disorder. The second participant was a 12-year-old boy diagnosed with ASD, mild ID, and unspecified disruptive, impulse-control, and conduct disorder. The target behavior was aggression, and it was operationally defined as when the participant's hand or foot contacted the body of another adult resulting in the movement of an adult's body. The FA based on procedures described by Iwata et al. (1994) was conducted in a clinic setting within a multielement design. A tangible condition was added based on parent report of CB occurring when preferred activities were denied. Results of the clinic-based FAs showed that the CB displayed by the first participant was maintained by tangibles. However, the second participant did not engage in aggressive behavior neither in the clinic setting nor in the public setting, but aggressive behavior was observed when the modified tangible condition was conducted in the hospital cafeteria. Results showed that the CBs of both participants were maintained by tangibles. The intervention for both participants involved differential reinforcement of alternative (DRA) behavior, which was effective in decreasing aggressive behavior and increasing compliance to instructions.

White et al. (2011) examined aggressive and stereotyped behavior in two children diagnosed with ASD using analogue FA protocols. This study demonstrated the link between aggressive and stereotyped behavior using an extended FA protocol. The participants included two 7-year-old males diagnosed with severe ASD. The CB exhibited by the first participant consisted of aggressive behavior, which was defined as grabbing and shaking the arm of the therapist and/or biting. Stereotypical play was defined as repeatedly spinning or rocking the stacking rings. Appropriate play was defined as use of the toy as intended (i.e., sorting and stacking the rings). The second participant also exhibited aggressive behavior. For this participant, aggression was defined as grabbing the therapist or an item and pulling forcefully. When he grabbed, he also engaged in screaming (loud vocalizations above the typical conversational level). Stereotypical play was defined as nonfunctional repetitive play with the toy glove (e.g., tossing the glove from one hand to the other). A multielement FA, similar to that of Iwata, Dorsey, Slifer, Bauman, and Richman (1982); Iwata et al. (1994), was conducted. Test conditions included in the FA were attention, demand, tangible, and free play. For both participants, high rates of aggressive behavior occurred during the tangible condition, suggesting that access to the glove or ring stackers was a maintaining consequence for aggression. Data on the rates of stereotypy and appropriate play were collected during an extended FA tangible condition, where ten additional sessions were conducted. The purpose of the extended assessment was to assess the potential influence of stereotypy on the occurrence of CB in a FA tangible condition. Results revealed that once the participant was given access to the items shown to be maintaining CB, these items were then used to engage in stereotypy. These results suggested a relationship between stereotypy and socially mediated CB.

Previous research has identified that false-negative errors can occur during FAs, whereby some individuals do not engage in CB during analogue conditions (Wacker, Berg, Harding, & Cooper-Brown, 2004). One reason for this is that antecedent variables manipulated in test conditions do not function as motivating operations (Laraway, Snycerski, Michael, & Poling, 2003) and therefore do not occasion CB. O'Reilly, Lacey, and Lancioni (2000) demonstrated that combinations of antecedent variables might motivate CB in a FA. Call, Wacker, Ringdahl, and Boelter (2005) examined whether manipulating multiple antecedent variables within FA test conditions would be one means of clarifying false-negative outcomes. The participants were a 17-year-old male diagnosed with a genetic disorder resulting in ID and a seizure disorder and a 2-year 8-month-old male diagnosed with a disruptive behavior disorder. The first participant engaged in aggressive and destructive behavior in the form of throwing objects. The second participant also engaged in aggressive behavior. Aggression was defined as audible contact between an extremity and another person or displacement of an object that resulted in audible contact between that object and another person. This study used a single-antecedent FA test condition and combined antecedent test conditions within a multielement design. FA procedures included free play, attention, escape, and tangible conditions (Iwata et al., 1982, 1994). The combined-antecedent conditions for the first participant included demand and diverted attention/contingent attention. Demand and restricted tangible item/contingent escape conditions were implemented for the second participant.

For both participants, elevated rates of aggressive behavior were observed within the combined-antecedent test conditions, whereas little or no aggressive behavior was observed in the control or single-antecedent test conditions. Failure to include the combined-antecedent variables would likely have resulted in false-negative findings for these participants. Results suggested that FAs that combining selected pairs of antecedent variables may clarify outcomes when standard test conditions do not result in CB.

The majority of FAs are implemented in highly controlled, long-term inpatient settings. Northup et al. (1991) recognized that in order to provide further evidence of the utility of FA as an assessment procedure for severe CB, it is necessary to demonstrate the generalizability of the assessment procedures and to determine if a more brief version of assessment is feasible. Northup et al. (1991) conducted a brief FA on three individuals exhibiting aggressive behavior in an outpatient setting during a 90-minute period. The first participant was a 24-year-old male diagnosed with severe to profound range of ID and was nonverbal. His aggressive behavior included scratching, pinching, grabbing, hitting, and pulling hair. Participant two, 21-year-old female, was also diagnosed with severe to profound ID and was nonverbal. Her aggressive behavior consisted of pinching, hitting, and biting. The third participant was a 13-year-old female diagnosed with cerebral palsy and had moderate to severe ID. Her aggressive behavior included pinching, biting, and hitting, which have occurred daily for the past five to ten years.

This study used a multielement design, consisting of two rapidly changing reversal designs conducted in two phases: an initial analogue assessment and a contingency reversal. For the second and third participants, the analogue assessment consisted of alone, tangible, demand, and/or social attention conditions, based on the analogue conditions used by Iwata et al. (1982, 1994). For the first participant, the analogue assessment consisted of alone, escape, alone, and escape conditions. The social attention and tangible conditions were not conducted for this participant, as he was observed to be unresponsive to social interaction and tangible reinforcement (he initially laid on the classroom floor and physically resisted any attempts to engage him in activities or physical contact). Following the initial analogue assessment, all participants were observed during three additional conditions, referred to as a contingency reversal. In the first contingency reversal condition, the contingency producing the highest percentage of aggressive behavior during the analogue assessment was again presented, but the consequence was provided contingently upon the occurrence of appropriate manding rather than for aggressive behavior. Aggressive behavior was ignored for Participants 2 and 3, or graduated guidance was used to redirect the participant to task for Participant 1. This condition was followed by a control condition, which was either a complete reversal in which the condition producing the highest percentage of aggressive behavior during the initial analogue assessment was repeated (Participants 2 and 3) or the alone condition was repeated (Participant 1). The control condition was then followed by a second contingency reversal condition to form a reversal design.

During the initial analogue assessments, each of the participants displayed a greater percentage of aggressive behavior during one maintaining condition than during any other. For Participant 1, elevated rates of aggressive behavior occurred during the escape conditions. Participant 2 displayed aggressive behavior during the tangible and escape conditions. Participant 3 displayed aggressive behavior during the escape and attention conditions. During this contingency reversal phase, each participant displayed a substantial reduction in aggressive behavior and a substantial increase in alternative behavior, therefore providing a direct analysis of the equivalency of the contingency for maintaining either behavior. This demonstrated that the contingencies identified as maintaining aggressive behavior also served to reinforce an alternative, replacement behavior.

Self-Injurious Behavior

Dunkel-Jackson, Kenney, Borch, and Neveu (2018) investigated TBFA on a 9 year-old male with ASD in a school setting and evaluated the effects of a function-based intervention informed by TBFA results. CB was assessed as two TBFAs were conducted for swearing and head banging. The intervention team replicated and extended previous treatment evaluation research by using the results of the TBFAs to identify yet another function-based intervention: demand fading. Results determined that head banging and swearing were most sensitive to contingencies involving escape from challenging tasks as well as access to tangibles. These results support the effectiveness and practicality of TBFAs to assess behavioral function and the resulting behavioral approaches to reduce challenging and disruptive behavior in publicly funded school settings.

Davis et al. (2013) examined the effects of a weighted vest on aggression and SIB in young boy with ASD. The effects of the weighted vest were examined during a FA utilizing an ABAB design with an embedded multielement design. This consisted of two phases each of no vest (A) and weighted vest (B). Within each phase, alternating conditions of a FA were conducted. The FA was conducted in a manner similar to that described by Iwata et al. (1982, 1994), consisting of five conditions. The occurrences of CB (i.e., biting) were compared across phases in which a weighted vest was worn or not worn. Findings revealed that the weighted vest had no effect on levels of aggression and SIB. Undifferentiated responding occurred across conditions of the FA, which suggested that SIB was maintained by automatic reinforcement.

Healey, Ahearn, Graff, and Libby (2001) investigated chronic SIB utilizing an experimental FA conducted with a 21-year-old male with ASD and ID. A multielement FA was conducted in which several conditions alternated rapidly (attention, edible, demand, alone, play, and sensory). Based on the results of the multielement phase and the blocked assessment phases, a sensory condition was introduced to further assess whether SIB was maintained by automatic reinforcement. These results suggested that SIB was unrelated to programmed positive or negative reinforcement contingencies. The behavior appeared to be automatically reinforced; it decreased when access to alternative sensory stimuli was provided. Findings of this study related to those of Thompson and Iwata (2007) as they found that three participants' SIB was maintained by automatic reinforcement. Similar findings were found by Scheithauer, Mevers, Call, and Shrewsbury (2017) as results of the FA suggested that SIB was maintained by automatic reinforcement alone for one participant and both automatic reinforcement and physical attention for the other participant. These results were used to create function-based treatments for SIB that were successfully generalized across settings and caregivers.

O'Reilly, Sigafoos, Lancioni, Edishinha, and Andrews (2005) examined levels of engagement and SIB with a child with severe ASD using a FA methodology within a classroom setting. A series of four FAs were conducted to identify contexts in which SIB occurred in the 12-year-old boy's classroom (i.e. attention, no interaction, demand, and play). SIB was associated with academic demands and SIB rarely occurred during play and no interaction conditions of the FA. The results of an analogue FA were used to determine an individualized schedule for a child with severe ASD who exhibited severe SIB. The FA revealed that SIB did not occur under a specific schedule of activities, and therefore, the schedule of activities in the child's classroom curriculum was modified based on these results. This modified curriculum resulted in considerable reductions in SIB and increases in classroom engagement.

Vollmer, Iwata, Zarcone, Smith, and Mazaleski (1993) investigated differential reinforcement of other behavior (DRO) and noncontingent reinforcement (NCR) in three females with developmental disabilities with severe SIB. A series of conditions were presented in a multielement format to each participant (i.e. alone, attention, demand, and play). Results from the FA showed that, for each of the three participants, SIB was differentially sensitive to attention as a positive reinforcer. Findings revealed that both DRO and NCR can be effective treatment procedures for SIB that is maintained by socially mediated positive reinforcement. In contrast, Vollmer, Marcus, and LeBlanc (1994) examined interventions for three children with severe disabilities, and their findings revealed that FA results were inconclusive.

Iwata et al. (1994) focused on the identification of variables associated with the occurrence of SIB. SIB was relatively high during the alone condition in four of the participants, suggesting a form of self-stimulation as a motivational variable. Lower levels of SIB were associated with the control condition. The authors suggested that their results provide empirical evidence that SIB may be a function of different sources of reinforcement. Iwata et al. (1994) summarized 152 single-subject analyses of the reinforcing functions of SIB. Their findings revealed that social negative reinforcement accounted for the largest proportion of the sample at 38.1%. Social positive reinforcement accounted for 26.3% of cases, followed closely by automatic reinforcement at 25.7%. Overall, these studies suggest that SIB could be maintained by multiple functions.

Stereotypy

Stereotypy is defined as repetitive, invariant, and contextually inappropriate behavior that persists in the absence of socially mediated reinforcement (Rapp & Vollmer, 2005). Common examples of stereotypy are hand flapping, body rocking, toe walking, spinning objects, sniffing, immediate and delayed echolalia, and running objects across one's peripheral vision (Schreibman, Heyser, & Stahmer, 1999).

FA methodologies are often used to identify the maintaining functions of vocal stereotypy. Rapp, Patel, Ghezzi, O'Flaherty, and Titterington (2009) used FA to identify the maintaining functions of vocal stereotypy exhibited by three children with ASD. Vocal stereotypy was operationally defined as a vocal response that was not appropriate to the context, indistinguishable, or repetitive. The FA included no-interaction, attention, and demand as experimental conditions and free play as the control condition. Results suggested that vocal stereotypy exhibited by all participants was maintained by nonsocial reinforcement and a punishment procedure was used to establish stimulus control to decrease the occurrences of vocal stereotypy. Asmus, Franzese, Conroy, and Dozier (2003) conducted two FAs to identify the maintaining functions of vocal stereotypy in a 7-year-old boy with ASD. In both FAs, the participant was exposed to the same 5-minute conditions: attention, tangible, and escape as experimental conditions and free play and alone as control conditions. However, in the first FA, reinforcement was delivered contingent on the occurrence of the target behaviors, while in the second analysis, no consequence was delivered. Results from both FAs suggested that automatic reinforcement was the maintaining function of vocal stereotypy.

Belfiore, Kitchen, and Lee (2016) examined the role of a staff-delivered rule on the occurrence of stereotypic behavior of a 37-year-old female diagnosed with a severe ID. The participant engaged in repetitive, stereotypic touching of objects and people. A multielement design was used to assess stereotypy variability across four experimental conditions: attention, rule and attention, rule only, and a control condition. Data of stereotypy behavior during all analogue FA sessions were collected using a 10 second partial interval recording procedure for continuous 15 minute sessions. The data from the FA yielded a percentage of intervals of stereotypy occurring within two consecutive 10 second intervals of a controlled environmental event. Results from this analysis showed that the percentage of intervals in which stereotypy behavior occurred was greater within the experimental condition where a rule statement was embedded with contingent attention.

Previous research has identified that stereotypy is most commonly served by automatic reinforcement functions. Automatic reinforcement is reinforcement that is not mediated by the deliberate action of another person (Vaughan & Michael, 1982). Wilke et al. (2012) used indirect FAs across 53 children and adolescents with

ASD and found that 90% of the stereotypic behavior appeared to be maintained by automatic reinforcement. Watkins and Rapp (2013) also employed indirect functional assessment and found similar results whereby six participants diagnosed with ASD presented with stereotypy behavior that was maintained by automatic reinforcement. Similar results using experimental FAs procedures have also been found in the literature (Athens, Vollmer, Sloman, & Pipkin, 2008; Britton et al., 2002; Brusa & Richman, 2008; Doughty, Anderson, Doughty, Williams, & Saunders, 2007; Neely, Rispoli, Gerow, & Ninci, 2015; Rapp et al., 2009; Wilder, Kellum, & Carr, 2000).

Bizarre Speech

Bizarre or maladaptive speech is common across both individuals with developmental disabilities and psychiatric populations (Mace & Lalli, 1991). There have only been two experimental studies that were performed that analyze the connection between maladaptive speech and reinforcement contingencies with individuals with schizophrenia and ASD (Durand & Crimmins, 1988, Mace & Lalli, 1991). Mace and Lalli (1991) identified contingencies made from bizarre statements. The participant was a 46-year-old adult male, Mitch, with moderate ID and a history of epilepsy. Due to his maladaptive speech behavior, he had trouble initiating conversations, he would often self-talk, and say unrelated statements in conversation (Mace & Lalli, 1991). During a food preparation task, Mitch made attention-oriented comments. The researchers investigated how Mitch acted within a group setting, being interrupted and uninterrupted by the experimenter. Mitch's interactions were recorded and placed into a number of categories such as interaction, no interaction, task, and alone and their subsequent events and social disapproval, no staff/client response, positive interaction, tangible reinforcement, and task disengagement (Mace & Lalli, 1991).

The data from the first experiment backed the two hypotheses presented, which were supported by the findings from Mitch's maladaptive speech; bizarre speech was positively reinforced by attention, but it was negatively reinforced by escape-task related demands (Mace & Lalli, 1991). The data from the second experiment showed that manipulation of the consequences of Mitch's bizarre speech culminated in a large level of maladaptive vocalizations during the social disapproval subsequent event (Mace & Lalli, 1991). It was determined from this data that Mitch's behavior and speech were provoked by others at his group home (Mace & Lalli, 1991).

Skin Picking

Skin picking is a common SIB, among those with developmental disabilities. Skin picking can be categorized as different repetitive manners. Although it seems relatively mundane, skin picking can pose a lot of health problems. Of a survey conducted by Wilhelm, Deckersbach, and Keuthen (2003) about skin picking, over 90% of participants recorded that they experienced tissue damage, 61% recorded infections, and 45% of participants recorded deep craters in the skin as a result of their skin picking. As it is normally designated as a relatively rare behavior, with the pervasiveness of skin picking only being seen in about 2–4 percent of those with ASD, there are little to no effective treatment approaches (Griesemer, 1978; Gupta, Gupta, & Haberman, 1987).

A competing stimulus assessment and FA were used in both phases of the study to identify effective types of treatments to be delivered in various formats to those with ASD. It investigated which format of item delivery was to reduce skin picking the most using noncontingent access to items in session durations, such as different types of toys (Clay et al., 2018). Molly was a 12-year-old girl diagnosed with ASD who also exhibited covert SIB and skin picking specifically that would occur daily (Clay et al., 2018). The FA was modeled on the FA performed by Iwata et al. (1982, 1994). The first phase focused specifically on the FAs used in the study. A multielement design was implemented in the form of a 5-minute session where Molly was introduced to five different conditions: ignore, play, attention, escape, or play with no items (Clay et al., 2018). These sessions relied on Molly's engagement with the stimulus provided or not provided by a therapist. This would either result in a SIB or would prevent the behavior from occurring. The phases that followed were competing stimulus assessment and treatment evaluation, respectively. It was determined that Molly's SIB was maintained by automatic reinforcement and not socially mediated reinforcement (Clay et al., 2018). Noncontingent access to a singular item proved to be the most effective way of decreasing skin picking. Play items that were removed during the 5-minute sessions showed an 11% increase in SIB (Clay et al., 2018). When the reversal design was introduced and play items were reintroduced into the room, skin picking decreased to a 2.5% mean interval, from a previous 14% (Clay et al., 2018). A positive automatic function for SIB is observed for Molly (Clay et al., 2018). Most importantly, out of the toys provided, a BopIt© had the highest mean percent interval of engagement and the lowest mean percent interval for SIB (Clay et al., 2018). The introduction of competing stimuli allowed for Molly's SIB, or her skin picking, to decrease.

Hand Mouthing

Hand mouthing is a type of stereotypical behavior and is categorized by inserting the hand, or a finger, past the plane of the lips. The behavior continues by proceeding to bite or suck on the body part or allowing it to remain with the mouth agape for long durations of time (Canella, O'Reilly, & Lancioni, 2006). This behavior can bring harm to the individual, creating problems such as scarring, skin breakage, and even a hematoma. It also allows for maladaptive social behavior.

Cannella-Malone and O'Reilly (2014) focused on five individuals with ID and hand mouthing. All participants were 21 or younger and presented with different disorders such as epilepsy, speech disorders, and ASD. The study had two purposes, both derived from a previous paper by Goh et al. (1995). Cannella-Malone and O'Reilly (2014) investigated reinforcement properties to determine if sensory stimulation would automatically maintain hand mouthing and to examine if other function-matched substitutes would produce reinforcement, such as a switch or button (Cannella-Malone & O'Reilly, 2014; Goh et al., 1995). An analogue FA was performed within the study to confirm that hand mouthing was maintained by automatic reinforcement (Cannella-Malone & O'Reilly, 2014). Toys, vibrating items, and switches/buttons were provided for the five participants to play with during the 15-minute observation sessions without consequence. When a preferred item was obtained that could be manipulated by the hands, hand mouthing decreased extensively. It was determined that this was a predominant reinforcer. However, for those who were provided with substitute reinforcements, the stimulus was not preferred. Automatically maintained behaviors can be influenced by items that match sensory contingencies, but by using preintervention, researchers would be able to decrease the automatic maladaptive behavior by outlining an intervention tailored to the participant.

The relationship between Gastro-Esophageal Reflux Disorder (GERD) and hand mouthing was the primary focus of the following research. In Study 1 of Swender, Matson, Mayville, Gonzalez, and McDowell (2006), there were 60 participants in total; 30 who engaged in frequent hand mouthing and 30 who did not. Participants were matched with each other within 1 year of age, level of disability, and gender to keep a control. The only aspect that differed was the diagnosis; a positive diagnosis referred to a participant who had been diagnosed with GERD by a physician. After analyzation of the data, it was determined that GERD occurred in those who hand mouthed more frequently than those who did not (Swender et al., 2006). In Study 2 of Swender et al. (2006), the same 30 participants who frequently hand mouthed participated again. The QABF was used, where responses are divided into tangible, attention, escape, physical, and nonsocial (Paclawskyj, Matsol, Rush, Smalls, & Vollmer, 2000). It was found by researchers that those who hand mouthed scored highest in the nonsocial subscale of the QABF than the other subscales with no other significant results (Swender et al., 2006). Those who participated in the autonomous maladaptive behavior of hand mouthing had an increased chance, by 36.7%, of receiving a GERD diagnosis and being categorized as nonsocial than other possible subscales.

Feeding Problems

Feeding problems are defined as the inability or refusal to orally consume adequate nutritional, hydration, or caloric intake in the amounts required to thrive results in negative nutritional, developmental, social, and psychological consequences (Babbitt et al., 1994). Feeding problems have been identified as a common issue among individuals with ASD and other populations (Leader, Tuohy, Chen, Mannion, & Gilroy, 2020).

Sprague, Flannery, and Szidon (1998) conducted a FA of feeding problems in a 13-year-old female with severe ID and cerebral palsy. The participant engaged in high levels of spitting and whining following bites of food. A preliminary functional assessment was conducted by interviewing the family and classroom staff regarding the participant's eating problems at home and at school. Based on these observations, two separate FAs were conducted in a lunchtime setting to detect the influence of trainer attention and pace of eating. In the first analysis, the participant was assessed under two eating conditions to detect the differential effect of trainer attention for CB versus a no attention condition. Results from this analysis identified attention was not a maintaining factor. A second analysis examined the reinforcing effects of food on trainer paced eating, and student paced eating (SR spoon grasping) and tangible (food) reinforcement for CB. Results from this analysis identified that CB was highest when access to food was contingent on CB and lowest when contingent on the participant grasping the spoon. The intervention of reinforcement for spoon grasping and a 10 second removal of food following CB resulted in reduction of spitting and whining during meals.

Girolami and Scotti (2001) compared the results of the analogue FA with those with less direct methods of assessments including interviews, questionnaires, and descriptive observations with three children with a history of mealtime behavior problems. Participants were a 32-month-old female with congenital bilateral perisylvian syndrome, a 32-month-old female with Down Syndrome and a 28-month-old male. The CB exhibited included pushing or slapping away the hand of the feeder, throwing food, crying and screaming excessively during mealtimes, and refusing to eat food. A standard analogue FA was conducted to determine each child's preferred and nonpreferred foods. The FA conditions included attention, demand, tangible toy, tangible food, alone, and control. Prior to this, the clinician interviewed the parents of the children with the FA interview Form (FAIF; O'Neill, Horner, Albin, Storey, & Sprague, 1990) and had parents complete the Motivation Assessment Scale (MAS; Durand & Crimmins, 1988). Direct observation by the clinician (i.e., A-B-C observations at a mealtime setting) and a food preference assessment were then conducted. Results from the analogue FA indicated that the primary function of food refusal for the first two participants was escape from food presentation and mealtime demands. For the third participant, contingent access to toys and attention were the maintaining variables. These analogue results were highly consistent with other forms of functional assessment data, including interviews, questionnaires, and direct observations, demonstrating the feasibility, and concurrent validity, of conducting an analogue FA of mealtime behaviors.

Wacker et al. (1996) investigated the effects meal schedule and quantity had on displays of CB in two children with developmental disabilities. The first participant was a 2 years, 2 months old male, diagnosed with severe to profound developmental delays. He had a visual impairment, was not ambulatory, and displayed severe SIB in the form of hand biting, eye gouging, and head banging. The primary behavior of concern was eye gouging, which had caused retinal damage and severe bruising around both eyes. The second participant, a 7 years 6 months old female, was diagnosed with Rett-like syndrome and severe ID. She was nonambulatory and had severe SIB and feeding problems. She also displayed SIB in the form of hand biting and continuous stereotypy in the form of placing her hands on her face.

For the first participant, a brief FA that alternated contingent attention and free play conditions was conducted within a multielement design. In order to assess the effects of meal schedule on his behavior, high and low levels of noncontingent parent attention were alternated within a multielement design, whereby the analysis was conducted under two conditions, before his meal and after his meal. For the second participant, contingent attention, free play, and alone conditions were counterbalanced three times each within a multielement design. In order to assess the quantity of food eaten on her behavior, two phases were conducted using a reversal design. Phase 1 consisted of eating three meals each day compared to eating six meals each day to evaluate the effects of food quantity on SIB and crying during free-play conditions. Phase 2 consisted of comparing the effects of eating six meals with no meals on SIB and crying behavior. Free play was replaced with a DRO treatment package in which attention and toys were provided if the participant did not engage in SIB for 5 seconds. Phase 3 included four follow-up probes, two at 4 months and another two at 6 months.

For the first participant, results suggested that SIB, which was identified by the FA as being maintained by attention, was also correlated with the schedule of meals. Differences in SIB occurred across the two social conditions, but only after a meal. Crying, however, was correlated almost exclusively with meal schedule and was not associated with the social conditions. Crying occurred frequently before a meal but rarely after a meal, irrespective of high or low levels of attention.

Based on the FA for the second participant, results suggested that SIB was not maintained by social reinforcement. Results for Phase 1 of the assessment indicated that SIB and crying occurred more often during the three-meal sequence (Conditions 1 and 3) than during the six-meal sequence (Conditions 2 and 4) in free-play sessions. Crying and SIB appeared to be correlated. Results from Phase 2 suggested that crying and SIB were related to gastric discomfort, rather than to food satiation only. When this was evaluated further, both SIB and crying occurred more frequently during the no-meal condition than during the six-meal condition. Results from the follow-up probes indicated that SIB occurred at low frequencies and showed a decreasing trend over time and crying also occurred infrequently.

Elopement

Elopement is when an individual runs away from or leaves a supervised area (Boyle & Adamson, 2017), which can be a dangerous and challenging problem. Elopement compromises the safety of people with disabilities at disproportionately high rates (Phillips, Briggs, Fisher, & Greer, 2018). Neidert, Iwata, Dempsey, and Thomason-Sassi (2013) conducted TBFAs in which latency was the index of elopement for two students. Participants were two males aged 21 and 22-years-old who had a profound ID diagnosis. The FA consisted of three test conditions: ignore, attention, and demand, as well as a control condition. A reversal design was used for Participant 1's assessment where he was exposed to each condition until stable levels of responding were observed. A pairwise test-control design was used for Participant 2's assessment, where test conditions were presented sequentially, as in a reversal design, but were altered with the control condition within each phase in a multielement design. Elopement was maintained by social positive reinforcement as it continued to occur in the attention condition, in which the therapist provided contingent attention but did not allow the behavior to occur.

Boyle, Keenan, Forck, and Curtis (2019) conducted a FA on the elopement of a child and evaluated a treatment that did not include blocking. The participant was a 6 year-old girl with ASD. A multielement FA was conducted using the following conditions; demand, attention, play, and ignore. This study entailed a FA of elopement and successfully decreased elopement through the use of a rule and without the need for blocking. Elopement during the FA occurred in all test conditions, which suggests that it was maintained by multiple contingencies (escape and attention), perhaps including automatic reinforcement. These findings are comparable to those of Piazza et al. (1997) as they conducted multielement FAs on three children who displayed elopement and found that behavior was maintained by a variety of functions.

Lang et al. (2010) assessed the elopement of a 4-year-old child with Asperger syndrome using a FA. This study evaluated the influence of assessment setting on the analysis and treatment of elopement. Separate FAs and corresponding interventions were compared in two school settings; classroom and resource room. Elopement was assessed during 5-minute individual sessions across play, attention, escape, and tangible conditions. FAs indicated that elopement was maintained by access to attention in the resource room and obtaining a preferred activity in the classroom. Attention and tangible-based interventions were compared in an alternating treatment design in both settings. These results replicated previous research that suggested that setting can influence FA results and that such an influence is relevant to intervention design.

Noncompliance and Disruptive Behavior

Noncompliance (NC) is defined as a passive maladaptive behavior when it involves refusing to follow an instruction or direction within a specific time frame and as an active maladaptive behavior when it involves behaviors such as crying, aggression, or self-injurious (Ekas, McDonald, Pruitt, & Messinger, 2017). Factors that can interfere with the function of NC are communication difficulties, lack of comprehension, lack of motivation, or high response effort (Kleinsinger, 2003). Disruptive behavior (DB) is defined as a maladaptive behavior that includes angry outbursts, irritability, and oppositional, noncompliant, and aggressive behaviors (Petrovic & Scholl, 2018). Examples of disruptive behaviors include throwing materials, leaving the activity area, screaming, kicking, flopping, crying, and property destruction (Waters, Lerman, & Hovanetz, 2009).

Several studies showed the effectiveness of FAs and their variations in identifying the maintaining functions of NC and DB in the form of aggression and property destruction. Reed, Ringdahl, Wacker, Barretto, and Andelman (2005) used FA with attention, tangibles escape, and play conditions with two children aged 8 and 10 years who were referred for their CB. FA results showed that CB was maintained by escape from demand. The function-based intervention consisted of differential negative reinforcement of alternative behavior (DNRA), which was delivered alone and in combination with lean and dense fixed-time schedules of reinforcement on CB and appropriate behavior.

Waters, Lerman, and Hovanetz (2009) used brief FA with two 6-year-old boys with ASD who were reported to engage in transition DB in multiple settings. The brief FAs consisted of three different transitions including pretransition, the transition itself, and post-transition activity. Results of the FA showed that the DB was maintained by avoidance of nonpreferred activities and access to preferred activities. As part of the function-based intervention, results showed that DRO was effective in reducing the occurrences of CB with or without the presence of visual schedules.

Schmidt, Shanholtzer, Mezhoudi, Scherbak, and Kahng (2014) investigated the utility of BFA with a 14-year-old boy with PDD-NOS and mild ID. Target behaviors were operationally defined as physical aggression, verbal aggression, and disruption. The study consisted of three phases: FA, brief experimental analysis of different intervention procedures, and an extended treatment evaluation. Results suggested that the highest occurrences of CB occurred during subtraction. In the second phase, a brief experimental analysis was conducted to investigate the effectiveness of five procedures on reducing the occurrences of CB and increase compliance during subtraction problems. Each condition lasted 5 minutes and involved cover-copy-compare, DRA for compliance, DRA for appropriate communication, the use of choices, and a number line. Results showed when the participant used a number line, no CB was emitted, while he exhibited high rates of problems behavior across all the other conditions. In the third phase, stimulus fading and differential reinforcement procedures were implemented to promote independence from the number line while attempting to maintain low rates of CB.

Studies also investigated whether the setting in which a FA is conducted influences the results, and incongruent results have been found. Lang et al. (2008) conducted two FAs with a 12-year-old girl and a 7-year-old girl with ASD who were referred for the frequency and intensity of the CB exhibited in school. For both participants, the target behaviors under analysis were operationally defined as dropping to the floor, aggression, elopement, and head hitting. Two FAs were conducted for each participant to investigate the maintaining functions of the CB in an assessment room and in the classroom. Both FAs included the same 5-minute conditions: attention and escape with play as control condition. For one participant, the two FAs identified the same functions of attention and escape from demand in both settings. For the second participant, the FA conducted in the classroom did not provide clear results, while the FA conducted in the assessment room identified attention and escape as maintaining functions. The results showed a discrepancy between settings, suggesting that if idiosyncratic controlling stimuli are absent in the setting, the analysis may fail to yield conclusive results.

Other studies suggested a good applicability of FA with ID across different settings while showing high variability in the functions identified. Cooper et al. (1992) conducted a two-study analysis to evaluate two slightly different variations of experimental FA in the assessment of CB in an outpatient clinic and classroom. The purpose was to identify variables to facilitate appropriate behavior. In the first study, participants were 10 children between the ages of 6 and 14 years in an outpatient clinic, while in the second study, participants were two 8 and 9-year-old boys within the mild range of ID and histories of noncompliant behaviors in class. The target behaviors were problems with conduct such as noncompliance, aggression, and opposition at home or school. Slightly different brief FAs were conducted in the two studies but with both the same conditions: task preference, task demand, and adult attention as experimental conditions in an outpatient clinic and school setting, respectively. Results of the first study showed that one child engaged in appropriate behavior during task preference, three children showed improved behavior when changes were made to the task demand condition, and four showed improved behavior after changes were made in the adult attention conditions.

Studies also showed the effectiveness of functional behavioral assessment (FBA) in identifying the maintaining functions of NC and DB. Luiselli and Sobezenski (2017) used FBA to identify the maintaining functions of frequency of bathroom requests and the duration of bathroom visits of a 22-year-old woman with ASD and ID. The FBA included direct observation, review of the baseline data, and FA interviews with the participant's care providers. The results of FBA suggested that the CB was maintained by negative reinforcement in the form of escape from demand. The intervention included activity scheduling and cuing, demand-fading and cuing, and duration-fading. The function-based intervention was effective in decreasing both frequency and duration of the bathroom visits.

Reese, Richman, Belmont, and Morse (2005) conducted functional behavioral assessment interviews to investigate the maintaining functions of DB. Parents of 23 children with ASD and 23 typically developing children completed the assessment process. The Functional Assessment Interview (O'Neill et al., 1997) was conducted with caregivers in which they were asked to define the disruptive behaviors and describe the situations in which they occurred. Results suggested that escape from demand, positive reinforcement in the form of social attention, and tangibles were the maintaining functions of disruptive behaviors for typically developing children and girls with ASD. However, disruptive behaviors displayed by boys with ASD were found to be maintained by escape from demands that interfere with repetitive behavior, access to tangibles used in repetitive routines, or to avoid idiosyncratically aversive stimuli. The findings suggested that disruptive behaviors occur with high variability between functions and populations and suggested the importance of considering the role of gender in disorders when conducting an FBA.

Multiple Typographies of Problem Behavior

Matson et al. (2011) reviewed 173 studies that used FA as a method in addressing problem behaviors. They found that SIB and aggression tended to be the most studied forms of CB and where multiple typographies of behavior were assessed with two or three being the most common. Rojahn, Zaja, Turygin, Moore, and Van Ingen (2012) conducted a FA that investigated whether behavior categories or behavior topographies determine behavioral function. Participants consisted of 115 adults with ID and a history of CB. SIB and stereotyped and aggressive behaviors were the focus in this study. The QABF was used to establish the functions of each CB. The results of this study showed that aggression, SIB, and stereotypy tended to be maintained by negative social reinforcement. SIB and stereotypy were shown to be maintained by automatic positive reinforcement. Behavior categories were found to be far more determining of behavioral function than behavior topographies.

Bell and Fahmie (2018) emphasized using FA to analyze multiple topographies of CB by examining the function of primary behavioral topographies alongside topographies that would be viewed as secondary or less influential. Participants consisted of three young children under the age of six with ASD. A primary topography was identified for each child (aggression, chin-hitting, and biting) alongside less extreme secondary topographies (vocal disruptions and stereotypy). A visual analysis was carried out to predict the function of secondary topographies of CB and was followed by a FA consisting of ignore, attention, play, escape, and tangible conditions to test the accuracy of predictions. Results showed a high consistency between the predictions of the functions of CB and the results of the FA. There was an indication that aggression tended to be maintained by social functions with vocal disruptions being sensitive to escape. Stereotypy tended to be maintained by automatic reinforcement in one participant and social reinforcement in another. Biting was maintained by escape and access to tangibles. This study provided support for the use of a FA to analyze both primary and secondary topographies of CB and may be useful for clinicians who are under time restraints.

Call et al. (2017) presented the issue that often carrying out FAs of various topographies of CB can be controversial as it could potentially cause interaction effects resulting in an increase of CB as opposed to being beneficial. Call et al. (2017) investigated whether conducting a FA of CB may lead to an increase in the behavior outside of a FA setting. Participants consisted of six children chosen from a day-treatment clinic where they had been admitted due to their history of CB. Target CB consisted of aggression, disruptive behaviors, and SIB. CBs were assessed both within and outside of the FA setting under escape, attention, and tangible conditions. The functions of each behavior varied per person between escape, access to tangibles, and attention. The results were found to be idiosyncratic with CB being both increased, decreased, and unaffected outside of the FA setting depending on the individual.

Following on from the hypothesis that conducting a FA of CB may cause carry-over effects, Davis, Durand, Fuentes, Dacus, and Blenden (2014) investigated the effect that a school-based FA may have on subsequent classroom behavior. They investigated five children all diagnosed with a disability, who had been identified through teacher reports as frequently displaying multiple topographies of CB. Each child displayed at least one CB in the forms of aggression, screaming, verbal protest, throwing, and pinching. The procedure involved a FA of CB in an academic setting followed by observations of subsequent behavior. The FA involved four conditions which lasted 10 minutes each, attention, tangible, demand, and play. Results found that CB in participants both immediately after the analysis and in the following days showed no significant increase. This provides evidence that FA procedures do not negatively influence subsequent CB in children and supports the use of FAs in school settings to assess and treat behavior.

Derby et al. (2000) investigated the idea that individuals often display multiple topographies of CB that may each hold varying functions. They present an alternative approach to understanding the multiple topographies of an individual's behavior that does not involve carrying out individual FAs for each. Their method involved conducting a single FA of numerous CBs and analyzing the results as part of an aggregated graph, also consisting of separate topographies. Participants were 48 individuals with severe ID who had a history of multiple topographies of severe CB. Target behaviors consisted of SIB, aggression, destruction, and disruptive behaviors. FA sessions consisted of multiple conditions in which behavior was assessed, escape, attention, alone, tangible, and a control condition. The results of the FA suggested that often individuals display numerous topographies of CB, and these may be maintained by multiple contingencies. The authors acknowledged that this method of analyzing behavioral functions may not be as definitive as conducting several individual analyses; however, the purpose was to reduce time taken for clinicians using FAs to analyze multiple topographies of CB.

Derby et al. (1994) investigated the idea that separate typographies of behavior are maintained by the same reinforcing factors. Their methods involved two brief and two extended FAs to understand the functions of distinct topographies of CB. Participants for the extended analyses consisted of a 23-year-old man and a six-year-old girl with IDs and histories of CB. Participants for the brief analyses were a 28-year-old woman and a 12-year-old boy with IDs. Target behaviors were aggression, SIB, and stereotypy. Conditions for the FAs were divided attention, noncontingent, alone, high sensory, tangible, escape, and social attention. Behaviors were analyzed both together and separately. An important finding was found during the brief FA where functions of a behavior were not identified when analyzed as part of an aggregate, whereas when each target behavior was plotted separately, more functions were identified. This study provided an important contribution to the area of FA in that it emphasized the importance of being wary of results when viewing an aggregate analysis and shows the efficiency of viewing target behaviors separately in order to get more accurate perspectives on the function of CB.

Matson and Boisjoli (2007) discussed the difficulties presented to researchers when attempting to identify a single maintaining factor of CB in individuals with ID. They emphasized that often functions of an individual's CB can be manifold and referred to the lack of studies investigating the possibility of multiple factors being present. The QABF was implemented by researchers in order to identify the maintaining factors of CB in 88 participants with an ID. Each participant had a history of SIBs and/or aggression. The authors found that in the vast majority of cases, the CB of individuals with an ID was maintained by multiple functions as opposed to a single definite function. They emphasized the importance of clinicians in taking the possibility of multiple maintaining factors into account when using FA to understand CB.

Hagopian, Contrucci, Long, and Rush (2005) discussed the challenges that often occur when implementing functional communication training (FCT) in individuals with ID, following the use of FA in the identification of maintaining variables of CB. Researchers conducted a successful FA that effectively identified the functions of CB in three individuals diagnosed with ID and ASD. Participants were assessed under four experimental conditions; social attention, tangible, toy play, and demand. Within the target CB of SIB, aggression, and disruption, it was shown that attention and access to tangibles were the primary factors maintaining CB in participants. Results also showed that the presence of reinforcing stimuli allowed for an enhancement in FCT success and caused a significant reduction in CB. Hagopian, Fisher, Thibault-Sullivan, Acquisto, and LeBlanc (1998) incorporated the use of FCT as a treatment procedure following FA, basing their treatments on the functions of problem behavior identified from FAs of each of their participants.

Hagopian, Bruzek, Bowman, and Jennett (2007) carried out FAs on multiple topographies of CB of two participants diagnosed with ASD. CB of interest consisted of aggression, SIB, and disruption. Analyses were carried out within multiple conditions; attention, tangible, demand, ignore, and control. However, researchers found these to be inconclusive with a lack of CB being shown in 16 of 18 sessions. In order to overcome the inconclusive nature of these results, a subsequent interruption analysis was conducted, which involved conditions in which participants were interrupted from what they were doing and given 'do' or 'don't' demands to follow. Results showed that CB occurred at high rates during the interruption analysis, indicating that an interruption and demand to engage in a different activity caused CB to occur more frequently. A second FA was administered to assess the CB of a

12-year-old girl with ASD and cerebral palsy with frequent aggressive behaviors. Little to no instances of CB were reported during the analysis. An interruption analysis taking the same form as previously described was then conducted with instances of aggressive behavior occurring frequently, providing further evidence for interruption with a demand as a reinforcer for CB.

Wacker et al. (2013) investigated the efficiency of using telehealth when conducting FAs of CB in individuals with ASD. Participants consisted of 20 children diagnosed with ASD with a history of displaying multiple topographies of CB in the forms of aggression, SIB, disruption, and/or destruction. FA procedures were implemented by the parents of participants, and they had been trained by a qualified behavioral consultant via telehealth. The parents were brought into a room in a clinic and given information from a consultant via telehealth about the various conditions and situations that would be implemented during the FAs. Parents implemented the FAs within the conditions of attention, escape, tangibles, and free play based on the direction given by professionals via telehealth. The results showed that identification of the function of CB was successful through telehealth communication with multiple functions being identified in each child. The results of this study are vital for the field of behavioral analysis as they support the practice of implementing FAs via telehealth, meaning that distance, travel costs, and other obstructing factors may be eliminated in the analysis and treatment of individuals with ID.

Patel, Carr, Kim, Robles, and Eastridge (2000) conducted FAs and other subsequent antecedent assessments in order to investigate the sensory qualities that maintain CB. Participants consisted of a 10-year-old male with ASD displaying rapid tongue movements and a 30-year-old male with ID, fetal alcohol syndrome, and a history of SIB. An experimental FA consisting of various conditions (attention, escape/avoidance, no interaction, and control) was conducted to identify the maintaining factors of the individuals' CB. Results showed that both behaviors were maintained independent of the social environment, showing that CB derived from automatic reinforcement. An antecedent assessment allowed interpretation of the nature of sensory stimuli maintaining CB in both participants. Results of this assessment indicated that rapid tongue movements were significantly reduced when auditory stimulation was present, suggesting audition as a maintaining factor. SIB was reduced in the presence of another form of tactile stimulation (forehead stimulation reduced head-banging). These results provided evidence supporting a strategy within FA that allowed for the assessment and treatment of various topographies of CB maintained by sensory stimulation.

Often, when individuals with IDs display severe symptoms of CB, it may be necessary for them to be kept under restraint to prevent them from injuring themselves or others. The use of restraint to reduce CB can be controversial and may cause stress or impose danger to those involved. Petursson and Eldivek (2018) discussed how it may often be difficult for carers to reduce time spent in restraint for individuals with disabilities due to the severity or continued prevalence of CB. They suggested the use of FA and FCT as a method of reducing CB and the amount of time individuals need to be kept in restraint. A FA with multiple conditions (alone, demand, attention, and control) was carried out to identify the functions behind precursors and CB in a 30-year-old man with ASD. The individual's aggressive behavior and SIB were the focus of assessment. Results showed that CB and precursors were highly prevalent in three of the demand conditions with CB appearing to be maintained by escape from demands. Following the FA, FCT was then implemented in order to teach the individual to use an alternative response and reduce CB.

Asmus et al. (1999) carried out a study with the purpose of recognizing an efficient method of identifying maintaining factors of CB in individuals with ID. Emphasis was placed on the investigation of the presence of task instructions as a maintaining factor of CB. Participants were three children diagnosed with an ID and had a history of multiple CB. The focus was different for each participant with a range of CB being assessed, including aggression, SIB, disruption, and destruction. The investigation was composed of multiple phases all serving different functions. Phase 1 involved an analysis of antecedents in order to identify if task instructions precede instances of CB. Results from this phase showed that participants tended to display more CB following being presented with a task instruction and less instances when task instruction was not applied. Phase 2 involved investigating if the participants' behavior varied with changes in therapist, setting, and task instruction. Results showed that regardless of who presented task instructions or what the context was participants consistently displayed CB, therefore eliminating confounding variables and providing evidence for task instruction as a maintaining factor of CB. Phase 3 consisted of a FA of CB to determine if negative reinforcement was a maintaining factor. Results confirmed this hypothesis showing that for two of the participants CB were maintained by negative reinforcement. This study provided significant results that add to the ever-growing research into the use of FA to analyze CB and the various functions that maintain this.

Karsh, Repp, Dahlquist, and Munk (1995) carried out FAs and multielement interventions of CB in three individuals with ID. CB in participants included pinching, shouting, hitting, kicking, pulling other people's hair, falling on the floor, and yelling. The FAs were carried out in a natural setting without any prescribed conditions in order to identify the function of each CB. Results showed that two of the three participants engaged in CB when given instructions to carry out a task, especially when this task required active as opposed to passive responses. The third participant showed CB during toileting, and these proved to be almost nonexistent in the absence of demands. Following these FAs, interventions for each participant were developed that were based on the premise that participant's CBs are a means of escape from various environmental antecedents. These were proven to be successful with instances of CB reducing significantly in each child following intervention.

Marcus and Vollmer (1996) investigated the efficiency of noncontingent reinforcement based on FA in the reduction of CB. Participants consisted of three individuals with histories of CB seeking assessment and treatment. An initial brief FA was carried out to determine the function of CB in the form of aggression, SIB, and disruption. The results of this showed that each participant's CBs were maintained by positive reinforcement in the form of access to tangible items. Based on these FA results, further experiments were carried out using noncontingent reinforcement and differential reinforcement of alternative behavior. Vollmer, Roane, Ringdahl, and Marcus (1999) used FA in conjunction with differential reinforcement of alternative behavior.

Marcus, Swanson, and Vollmer (2001) carried out a study that investigated the efficiency of parent training in reducing CB following FA. Participants consisted of four children with ID and histories of CB in the form of tantrums and/or aggression. A FA was implemented in order to identify the function of CB in participants to later allow for the development of treatment practices. Results of this analysis showed that for two of the participants, CB occurred in the demand condition and was maintained by escape. Another participant showed that their CB was reinforced by contingent access to materials. The last participant displayed CB under multiple reinforcers, the dominant of these being during self-care activities and in instances when their mother's attention was elsewhere. The results of these FAs were then used to develop parental training procedures to allow parents to implement interventions and reduce CB.

O'Reilly, Lacioni, King, Lally, and Nic Dhomhnaill (2000) investigated the use of brief experimental functional assessments in identifying idiosyncratic variables associated with multiple CB. Participants consisted of two individuals with ID with target CB involving hitting, pinching, SIB, and property destruction. Parents were trained to carry out the brief functional assessments, which consisted of attention, demand, noncontingent attention, and diverted attention conditions. Researchers found that CB for both participants was apparent in the diverted attention condition, which consisted of participants' parents placing their attention onto a third person in the room. This provides evidence that CB can be maintained by low levels of or diverted parental attention.

O'Reilly et al. (2012) demonstrated how often FA is used as a first step in gathering information that is later used in the development and implementation of intervention practices. Their focus was on the efficiency of implementing an antecedent communication intervention to reduce CB. An initial FA was carried out in order to establish the function of CB in three students with varying developmental disorders. Multiple topographies of behavior were examined including elopement, yelling, flopping, head slapping, and biting. FA conditions consisted of demand, attention, tangible, and play. Results of the FA indicated that for all three participants, CB was maintained by access to tangible items. This was then used to develop antecedent communication interventions.

Peck et al. (1996) investigated choice-making behavior in children with developmental disabilities who had frequent CB. Their study consisted of multiple analyses serving various functions, one of which was a FA. Participants consisted of five children with developmental disabilities and different CB such as pulling medical tubes and leads connected to them, food refusal, SIB, tantrums, noncompliance, and aggression. Each participant's FA consisted of different conditions to fit the needs and behaviors of each. Results showed that for three participants low attention was a maintaining factor for CB, one participant showed high demand as a maintaining factor, and escape was identified as a maintaining factor in the final participant.

Piazza, Adelinis, Hanley, Goh, and Delia (2000) carried out a study with a purpose to extend on previous literature surrounding matched stimuli to three dissimilar CB. They wished to identify the effect of matched stimuli on automatically reinforced CB. A FA was conducted in order to identify if certain behaviors were maintained by automatic reinforcement. Participants were three individuals with a previous diagnosis of intellectual and behavioral disorders. The target behaviors of interest were dangerous behavior, saliva play, and hand-mouthing. The FA consisted of multiple conditions; social attention, alone, toy play, demand, and tangible. Results found that for the first participant, dangerous behavior was most frequent in the alone condition, the second participant showed increases of saliva play across all experimental conditions, and the final participant also displayed increased levels of hand-mouthing across all conditions. The results from all three participants suggest automatic reinforcement as a maintaining factor for CB.

Petursdottir, Esch, Sautter, and Stewart (2010) conducted an archival study that examined the different types of CB that occur and later conducted a FA of participants to determine functions of these behaviors. They wished to identify the primary topographies of CB and their functions. The initial assessment involved 174 participants with ID who were found to display a total of 536 CBs. The assessment showed that the most frequented behaviors were physical aggression, verbal aggression, noncompliance, property destruction, inappropriate verbal and social behavior, and SIB, in this order. A FA showed that for 53.2% of behaviors, only a single maintaining function was identified and 41% seemed to show multiple functions. The most common function of CB identified was attention with aggression and SIB being the most common behaviors usually assessed.

Research studies have conducted FAs of multiple topographies of CB followed by extinction procedures (Richman, Wacker, Asmus, & Casey, 1998; Richman, Wacker, Asmus, Casey, & Andelman, 1999). Tucker, Sigafoos, and Bushell (1998) carried out a study involving FA of CB and suggested that analyzing the conditions associated with low rates of CB as well as those in which the behavior is maintained may be beneficial to treatment and intervention. Call, Pabico, and Lomas (2009) used FA to establish escape and attention as maintaining factors of CB in children with ID. Research has investigated different ways of establishing functions maintaining multiple topographies of CB and contrasted varying methods (Camp, Iwata, Hammond, & Bloom, 2009; Potoczak, Carr, & Michael, 2007).

Sleep Problems

McLay, France, Blampied, and Hunter (2019) conducted a study to investigate the effectiveness of functional behavioral assessment in identifying the maintaining functions of sleep problems in two children with ASD. The participants were a 4- and 10-year-old nonverbal children who were referred for sleep problems by their parents, and they both engaged in vocal stereotypy. The target behaviors under assessment for the first participant were frequent curtain calls and frequent and prolonged night-wakings. The CBs exhibited by the second child were bedtime resistance, delayed sleep onset latency, frequent curtain calls, frequent and prolonged night-wakings, and unwanted co-sleeping. The FBA consisted of a clinical interview with the parents, the Sleep Assessment Treatment Tool (SATT), sleep diaries, and videosomnography (VSG). Results of the FBA showed that all target behaviors were maintained by at least two functions, and it suggested that vocal stereotypy was an active component of the CB. In the intervention phase, function-based procedures were conducted in the attempt to decrease sleep problems. Results showed a decrease in the frequency and duration of the night awakenings for each participant and reduction of curtain calls for one of the children.

Happiness Behaviors

Although FAs have been primarily been used to identify controlling environmental variables of CB, there is emerging literature suggesting the effectiveness of FA methodologies in identifying the maintaining functions of positive and prosocial behaviors. Thomas, Charlop, Lim, and Gumaer (2019) used TBFA to conduct a concurrent analysis of Happiness Behaviors (HB) and CB displayed by four children with ASD. HB included smiling, grinning, and laughing, while CB included yelling and screaming. The TBFA consisted of four conditions with a control and test trial per each condition: attention, escape, tangible, and ignore. The TBFA included contingent reinforcement for CB, but no consequence was delivered contingent on HB. Overall, the results of the FA showed that CB occurred most often in the tangible test conditions, while the respective tangible control conditions showed high percentages of HB, suggesting the pattern of an inverse relationship between CB and HB. However, results also showed that HB occurred at high percentages during the control attention conditions. The concurrent information gathered during the TBFA was used for subsequent treatment analyses that resulted effective in both decreasing CB and increasing HB. This study showed that using FA to identify controlling variables of HB in addition to CB can provide valuable information that could be masked or hidden with the use of a traditional FA. This study showed that measures of HB identified within FA can be used to support the implementation of effective behavioral interventions to decrease CB and increase appropriate and positive ones (Table 4.1).

Conclusion

FA has widely been used to identify the environmental variables that predict and maintain severe CB displayed by individuals with developmental disorders. This chapter provided a descriptive analysis of how FA methodologies have been used to identify the maintaining functions of CB across different populations and

Table 4.1 Summary of populations and behaviors evaluated with functional assessment

Authors	Population	N	Age	Behavior	Type of functional assessment used	Function identified
Asmus et al. (1999)	ID	3	P1: 3-year-old P2: 4-year-old P3: 5-year-old	P1: SIB, aggression, destruction, and disruption. P2: Aggression, destruction, and disruption. P3: SIB, aggression, destruction, and disruption	Multielement FA	Two participants showed negative reinforcement as a maintaining factor. In all participants, the presence of a task instruction increased problem behavior.
Asmus et al. (2003)	ASD & language impairment	1	7-year-old	CB1: Stereotypical vocalizations CB2: Disruptive behavior	Multielement FA	CB1: Automatic reinforcement, CB2: Tangibles & Escape from demands
Athens et al. (2008)	ASD & Down Syndrome	1	11-year-old	Stereotypy including loud, repetitive, noncontextual verbalizations & repetitive, loud, and unintelligible vocalizations	Multielement FA	Automatic reinforcement
Belfiore et al. (2016)	Severe ID	1	37-year-old	Stereotypic touching of objects & people	Multielement FA	Rule + attention

Authors	Population	N	Age	Behavior	Type of functional assessment used	Function identified
Bell and Fahmie (2018)	ASD	3	P1: 4-year-old P2: 4-year-old P3: 5-year-old	P1: Physical aggression (primary typography), vocal disruption, and property destruction P2: Chin-hitting (primary typography) and motor stereotypy P3: Biting (primary typography)	Multielement FA	P1: Escape & access to tangibles P2: Automatic reinforcement P3: Access to tangibles and social reinforcement
Boyle and Adamson (2017)	ASD	1	6-year-old	Elopement	An indirect assessment using the Functional Analysis Screening Tool (FAST) & Multielement FA	Multiple contingencies, possibly including automatic reinforcement
Britton et al. (2002)	ID & ASD	3	P1: 28-year-old P2: 26-year-old P3: 8-year-old	P1: Head rocking P2: Face rubbing P3: Repetitive hand movements	Multielement FA	Automatic reinforcement
Brusa and Richman (2008)	ASD	1	8-year-old	Stereotypy behavior including shaking objects, & string play	Multielement FA	Automatic reinforcement
Call et al. (2005)	P1: Genetic disorder resulting in ID & seizure disorder P2: Disruptive behavior disorder	2	P1: 17-year-old P2: 2-year 8-month-old	P1: Aggressive and destructive behavior in the form of throwing objects. P2: Aggressive behavior	Multielement FA	P1: Demands & diverted attention/ contingent attention P2: Demands & restricted tangibles item/contingent escape conditions

(continued)

Table 4.1 (continued)

Authors	Population	N	Age	Behavior	Type of functional assessment used	Function identified
Call et al. (2017)	Aggression, disruptive behavior, SIB, dropping, hair pulling, pica, & spitting	6	Ranged between 5–13-years-old	Aggression, disruptive behavior, SIB, dropping, hair pulling, pica, & spitting.	Descriptive FA	Escape, access to tangibles, & attention.
Call et al. (2009)	P1: ASD P2: Cerebral palsy & ID	2	P1: 6-year-old P2: 14-year-old	P1: Aggression, SIB, & disruptive behavior P2: Aggression, SIB, disruptive behavior, & swearing	Multielement FA	P1: Attention & escape P2: Escape
Camp et al. (2009)	Developmental disabilities	7	16–54-years-old	SIB & property destruction	Multielement FA	Automatic reinforcement, escape, & attention
Canella et al. (2006)	ID	33	1–4-years-old	Hand mouthing	Intervention & FA	Automatic reinforcement
Canella-Malone & O'Reilly (2014)	ID, Rett syndrome, ASD, and cerebral palsy	5	P1: 6-year-old P2:12-year-old P3:11-year-old P4: 19-year-old P5: 21-year-old	Hand mouthing	Multielement FA	Automatic reinforcement
Cariveau et al. (2019)	ASD & AD/HD	1	8-year-old	Aggressive behavior	Multielement FA	Escape from demands & termination of interruptions to repetitive behavior
Carr and Carlson (1993)	ASD	3	P1: 18-year-old P2: 17-year-old P3: 16-year-old	Aggression, property destruction, SIB, & tantrum behavior	FBA	Escape from demands & tangibles

Authors	Population	N	Age	Behavior	Type of functional assessment used	Function identified
Chung and Cannella-Malone (2010)	P1: Multiple disabilities P2: Multiple disabilities P3: ASD & ID P4: Multiple disabilities	4	P1: 11-year-old P2: 14-year-old P3: 11-year-old P4: 16-year-old	P1: Stereotypy behavior including chair scratching P2: Stereotypy behavior including shirt biting P3: Stereotypy behavior including putting one or both of her hands into her pants and between her pants and her diaper P4: Stereotypy behavior including teeth tapping & knuckle clapping	Multielement FA & a pre-session access analysis, & a treatment analysis	Automatic reinforcement
Clay et al. (2018)	ASD	1	12-year-old	Skin picking	CSA, reverse FA, & multielement FA	Automatic reinforcement
Cooper et al. (1992)	AD/HD, anxiety disorder, conduct disorder, developmental motor dyscoordination, developmental reading and language disorders, learning disorders, mild ID, mixed developmental disorder, & Oppositional Defiant Disorder (ODD)	10	Ranged between 6 and 14-years-old	Noncompliance, aggression, & opposition	BFA	Escape from demands, Tangibles, & Adult attention

(continued)

Table 4.1 (continued)

Authors	Population	N	Age	Behavior	Type of functional assessment used	Function identified
Davis et al. (2013)	ASD	1	9-year-old	Aggression & SIB	Multielement design embedded within an ABAB design	Automatic reinforcement
Davis et al. (2014)	ID	5	Ranged between 6 and 10-years-old	SIB, aggression, and destruction	Multielement FA	Attention, escape from demands & access to tangibles
DeLeon et al. (2003)	Mental problems, cerebral palsy, & visual impairments	1	14-year-old	SIB, aggression, & disruptive behavior	Multielement FA	Wheelchair movement
Delgado-Casas et al. (2014)	P1: ASD & profound ID P2: ASD & profound ID P3: ASD & severe ID P4: Down syndrome, profound ID, & Obsessive Compulsive Disorder (OCD) traits	4	P1: 42-year-old P2: 33-year-old P3: 43 -year-old P4: 40 -year-old	P1: SIB, aggression, & disruptive behavior P2: SIB, aggression, & stereotypy behavior P3: SIB & disruptive behavior P4: SIB & aggression	Multielement FA	P1: Social attention, self-stimulation, & escape from task demands P2: Social attention, self-stimulation, & tangibles P3: Social attention, self-stimulation, & escape P4: Negative reinforcement

Authors	Population	N	Age	Behavior	Type of functional assessment used	Function identified
Derby et al. (1994)	ID	4	P1: 23-year old P2: 6-year-old P3: 28-year-old P4: 12-year-old	Aggression, SIB, & stereotypy	Multielement FA	P1: Automatic & sensory reinforcers P2: Automatic & sensory reinforcers P3: Automatic function & negative reinforcement P4: Attention
Derby et al. (2000)	ID	48	Ranged between 3 and 32-years-old	SIB, aggression, destruction, & dangerous acts	Multielement FA	Different reinforcement contingencies, e.g. attention, escape, and tangibles
Devlin et al. (2011)	ASD	4	P1: 6-year-old P2: 11-year-old P3: 10-year-old P4: 9-year-old	Aggression, stamping feet, crying, & SIB	P1: QABF P2: Multielement FA P3: Multielement FA P4: FAST-R.	P1: Escape from demands & tangibles P2: Escape from demands P3: Escape from demand & tangibles P4: Escape from demand & tangibles
Didden et al. (2007)	Prader-Willi Syndrome (PWS)	119	4–49-years-old	Skin-picking	QABF	Nonsocial & intrinsic consequences

(continued)

Table 4.1 (continued)

Authors	Population	N	Age	Behavior	Type of functional assessment used	Function identified
Doughty et al. (2007)	P1: Severe ID, profound deafness, & legal blindness P2: Profound ID & Down syndrome P3: Severe ID & bipolar disorder	3	P1: 45-year-old P2: 40-year-old P3: 54-year-old	P1: Stereotypy including hand, & arm flapping P2: Stereotypy including finger manipulation P3: Stereotypy including repetitive line drawing	Multielement FA	Automatic reinforcement
Dunkel-Jackson et al. (2018)	ASD	1	9-year-old	Swearing & head banging	QABF, ABC checklist, & TBFA	Escape from challenging tasks & access to tangibles
Durand and Crimmins (1988)	ASD	1	9-year-old	Psychotic speech	Multielement FA	Reduction of behavior

Authors	Population	N	Age	Behavior	Type of functional assessment used	Function identified
Ellingson et al. (2000)	P1: ID & cerebral palsy P2: ID & Angelman syndrome P3: ID	3	P1: 19-year-old P2: 18-year-old P3: 12-year-old	P1: Disruptive behaviors including hand pounding on flat surfaces P2: Aggression including head butting, hitting, & kicking P3: Disruptive behavior including hand pounding, kicking, rocking, leaving the immediate work area and wandering about the immediate area, and pushing and throwing materials	Descriptive assessment using a questionnaire and interview format, & direct observation using an ABC checklist	Attention
Emerson et al. (1996)	Severe learning disabilities	3	P1: 8-year-old P2: 13-year-old P3: 11-year-old	SIB & aggression	Time-based lag sequential analysis	Socially mediated negative reinforcement involving escape from demands and social contact & automatic reinforcement
Falcomata et al. (2013)	ASD	2	P1: 7-year-old P2: 12-year-old	P1: Aggression & disruptive behavior P2: Aggression & SIB	Multielement FA	P1: Attention, escape, & tangibles P2: Escape & tangibles
Falcomata and Gainey (2014)	ASD	1	4-year-old	SIB	Multielement FA	Escape, tangibles, & attention

(continued)

Table 4.1 (continued)

Authors	Population	N	Age	Behavior	Type of functional assessment used	Function identified
Flanagan and DeBarr (2018)	Emotional behavioral disorder (EBD)	1	10-year-old	Vocal disruptions, physical aggression, and falling on the floor/crawling	Trial-based FA	Attention & escape from demands
Fragale et al. (2016)	ASD	4	P1: 9-year-old P2: 5-year-old P3: 4-year-old P4: 4-year-old	P1: SIB including head slapping & biting P2: Elopement, flopping, & whining P3: Vocal protesting, physical protesting, aggression, & elopement P4: Elopement	Multielement FA	Tangibles
Girolami and Scotti (2001)	P1: Congenital bilateral perisylvian syndrome P2: Down syndrome P3: Language & feeding difficulties	3	P1: 32-months-old P2: 32-months-old P3: 28-months-old	P1: Pushing/slapping away the hand of the parent feeding her, throwing food, and crying and screaming P2: Vomiting, gagging, refusal of solid food, screaming crying, throwing food, and turning her head away from food during mealtimes P3: Throwing food, crying during mealtimes, & food refusal	Multielement FA	P1: Escape from food presentation & mealtime demands P2: Escape from food presentation & mealtime demands P3: Access to toys & attention

Authors	Population	N	Age	Behavior	Type of functional assessment used	Function identified
Hagopian et al. (2007)	ASD	3	P1: 12-year-old P2: 6-year-old P3: 12-year-old	P1: SIB & disruption P2: SIB, aggression, & throwing objects P3: Aggression	Multielement FA	Inconclusive results of the FA
Hagopian et al. (2005)	ID & ASD	3	P1: 13-year-old P2: 12-year-old P3: 7-year-old	P1: SIB, aggression, & disruption P2: SIB, aggression, and disruption P3: Aggression	Multielement FA	P1: Social attention P2: Access to preferred items P3: Access to verbal and physical attention, & access to tangibles items
Hagopian et al. (1998)	ID & Behavior Disorders	21	Ranged between 2 and 16-years-old	SIB, aggression, & property destruction	Multielement FA	Escape, attention, demands, & tangibles

(continued)

Table 4.1 (continued)

Authors	Population	N	Age	Behavior	Type of functional assessment used	Function identified
Hall (2005)	ID	4	P1: 29-year-old P2: 51-year-old P3: 31-year-old P4: 31-year-old	P1: Pica, which included the ingestion of toilet tissue, pages of magazines, plaster, threads, pegs, and stones P2: SIB including head-banging, throat-pulling, arm-pulling, face-scratching, & hair-pulling P3: Aggression including hitting and grabbing support-staff and pulling at their hair P4: Aggression including hitting or kicking support-staff, or pulling at their hair	Direct observations, multielement FA, & QABF	P1: Nonsocial reinforcement & attention P2: Escape & attention P3: Attention P4: Attention & tangibles
Hanley et al. (2005)	P1: Moderate ID, ASD, & a seizure disorder P2: Mild to moderate ID, AD/HD, & ODD	2	P1: 5-year-old P2: 8-year-old	P1: SIB, aggression, & disruptive behavior P2: SIB, aggression, & pica	Multielement FA	P1: Attention P2: Attention & escape
Hausman et al. (2009)	ASD, cerebral palsy, & moderate ID	1	9-year-old	SIB, aggression, property destruction, & ritualistic behaviors	Multielement FA	Automatic reinforcement (access to ritualistic behaviors)

Authors	Population	N	Age	Behavior	Type of functional assessment used	Function identified
Healy et al. (2013)	ASD	32	Ranged between 6 and 19-years-old	CB1: Aggressive/ destructive behavior CB2: SIB CB3: stereotypy	QABF & Multielement FA	CB1: Escape from demands, & tangibles CB2: Automatic reinforcement & escape from demands CB3: Automatic reinforcement
Herman et al. (2018)	ASD & ODD	1	4.6-year-old	Flopping	An open-ended interview and brief direct observation informed an Interview-Informed Synthesized Contingency Analysis (IISCA)	Escape from demands & tangibles

(continued)

Table 4.1 (continued)

Authors	Population	N	Age	Behavior	Type of functional assessment used	Function identified
Hetzroni and Roth (2003)	P1: Moderate ID P2: Moderate ID P3: Severe ID & Cri-du-chat syndrome P4: Moderate ID & Down syndrome P5: Severe ID	5	P1: 14-year-old P2: 12-year-old P3: 16-year-old P4: 19-year-old P5: 19-year-old	P1: Tugging a staff member, pulling his pants down, pulling and biting classroom peers, and screaming P2: Pushing, pinching, spitting, and pulling the hair of peers and staff P3: Aggressive behaviors including pushing and throwing items, running away from the classroom, and SIB that included lying on the floor while head banging P4: Crying, laughing, passivity, ignoring, putting head on table, & siting under the table P5: Sitting on the floor while banging his head, screaming, jumping on chairs, and manipulating pieces of paper	Descriptive assessment & direct observation	P1: Attention & request for assistance P2: Attention & request for assistance P3: Escape from activity P4: Escape from task demands & general refusal to communicate with staff P5: Attention & request for assistance

Authors	Population	N	Age	Behavior	Type of functional assessment used	Function identified
Hodnett et al. (2018)	Smith-Magenis syndrome	2	P1: 13-year-old P2: 4-year-old	P 1: SIB, disruptive behavior, & disrobing P 2: SIB, aggression, & disruptive behavior	Multielement FA	P1: Escape from demands & access to tangibles items P2: Access to attention & tangible items
Iwata et al. (1994)	ID	9	Ranged between 1.5 and 17.5-years-old	SIB	Multielement FA	SIB may come from different sources of reinforcement
Karsh et al. (1995)	P1: ASD P2: Developmental delay, cerebral palsy, and dysarthria P3: Developmentally disabled and seizure disorder	3	P1: 11-year-old. P2: 11-year-old. P3: 7-year-old.	P1: Yelling, crying, pinching, & hitting P2: Crying, kicking, hitting, & pulling hair P3: Crying, whining, kicking, struggling, falling on the floor, & grabbing	Multielement FA	P1: Problem behaviors reinforced by instructions to carry out an active task P2: Problem behaviors reinforced by instructions to carry out an active task P3: Problem behaviors reinforced by toileting demands
Kelly et al. (2015)	ASD	3	P1: 9-year-old P2: 11-year-old P3: 11-year-old	P1: SIB & crying P2: Task refusal, nonresponsiveness, & negative statements P3: Task refusal, nonresponsiveness, negative statements about task, & property destruction	Descriptive assessments & multielement FA	P1: Escape from demands P2: Attention & escape from demands P3: Attention & escape from demands

(continued)

Table 4.1 (continued)

Authors	Population	N	Age	Behavior	Type of functional assessment used	Function identified
Kern (1997)	ASD	1	15-year-old	CB1: SIB CB2: Aggression	Multielement FA	CB1:Tangibles CB2: Escape from demands
Kern and Vorndran (2000)	ID	1	11-year-old	Flopping	ABC data	Tangibles (preferred activities) & adult attention
Kodak et al. (2004)	AD/HD	1	5-year-old	Elopement	Multielement FA	Verbal & physical attention
Kurtz, Chin, Robinson, O'Connor and Hagopian (2015)	Fragile X syndrome	9	Ranging from 6–15-years old	SIB, destructive behaviors, & aggression.	Multielement FA.	Escape from demands & access to tangibles.
Kurtz et al. (2008)	Children with prenatal drug exposure	2	P1: 10-month-old P2: 22-month-old	P1: SIB, aggressive behavior, & severe tantrums P2: SIB, aggressive, & disruptive behavior	Multielement FA	Attention, tangibles, & escape
LaBelle and Charlop-Christy (2002)	ASD	3	P1: 9-year and 6-month-old P2: 8-year and 6-month-old P3: 8-year and 8-month-old	P1: Disruptive behavior, aggression, & throwing objects P2: Inappropriate vocalizations P3: Disruptive behaviors	Individualized multielement FA	Attention, escape, tangibles, & automatic reinforcement
Lambert et al. (2019)	PWS	1	7-year-old	Food stealing	Latency-based FA	Differential reinforcement
Lang et al. (2008)	ASD	2	P1: 7-year-old P2: 12-year-old	Dropping to the floor, aggression, elopement, & head hitting	Multielement FA	Attention & escape from demands

Authors	Population	N	Age	Behavior	Type of functional assessment used	Function identified
Lang et al. (2010)	Asperger syndrome	1	4-year-old	Elopement	Multielement FA	Attention & tangibles
Larkin et al. (2016)	ASD	3	P1: 7-year-old P2: 4-year-old P3: 5-year-old	P1: Loud vocalizations & elopement P2: Elopement & flopping P3: Inappropriate vocalizations & aggression	TBFA	P1: Escape from demands & adult attention P2: Tangibles P3: Tangibles
LaRue et al. (2010)	ASD	5	P1: 9-year-old P2: 8-year-old P3: 20-year-old P4: 29-year-old P5: 4-year-old	Aggression, SIB, disruption, spitting, stereotypy, and vocalizations	Multielement FA & TBFA	P1: Tangibles P2: Tangibles P3: Tangibles P4: Escape from demands (multielement FA) tangibles (TBFA) P5: Automatic
LaRue et al. (2011)	ASD & ID	4	P1: 7-year-old P2: 24-yearold P3: 15-year-old P4: 10-year-old	P1: Inappropriate vocalization P2: SIB P3: SIB P4: Aggression & SIB	Multielement FA & Manding analysis (MA)	P1: Escape from demands & tangibles P2: Social attention P3: Social attention P4: Social attention & tangibles (secondary)

(continued)

Table 4.1 (continued)

Authors	Population	N	Age	Behavior	Type of functional assessment used	Function identified
Liddon et al. (2016)	ASD & ID	110	Ranged between 1 and above 21-years-old	SIB, aggression, & property destruction	Multielement FA & anecdotal information	ASD only group: Automatic reinforcement (58.9%) & access to activities/items (29.4%) ASD + ID group: Access to activities/items (61.4%) & automatic reinforcement (42.2%)
Luiselli and Sobezenski (2017)	ASD and ID	1	22-year-old	Bathroom visits	Functional Analysis Interview (FAI)	Escape from demands
Mace and Lalli (1991)	ID & Epilepsy	1	46-year-old	Bizarre speech	Multielement FA	Positive & negative reinforcement
Machalicek et al. (2009)	ASD & ID	2	P1: 7-year-old P2: 11-year-old	Aggression, property destruction, SIB, & flopping	FA using videoconferencing equipment	Escape from demand & attention
Machalicek et al. (2010)	ASD	6	Ranging from 5 to 9-years-old	Aggression, SIB, & stereotypy	Multielement FA using video tele-conferencing	Unknown
Machalicek et al. (2014)	Fragile X syndrome	12	Ranging from 27–51-years old	Aggression, SIB, & disruptive behavior.	Multielement FA.	Escape from demands and escape from social interactions and attention.

Authors	Population	N	Age	Behavior	Type of functional assessment used	Function identified
Marcus and Vollmer (1996)	P1: Down syndrome, language delay, & speech articulation difficulties P2: ID P3: ASD	3	P1: 5-year old P2: 4-year-old P3: 5-year-old	P1: SIB, aggression, & disruptive behavior P2: Aggression P3: SIB, aggression, & disruptive behavior	Multielement FA	Tangibles
Marcus et al. (2001)	ID & Speech delays	4	Unknown	Tantrums & aggressive behavior	Multielement FA	Escape, tangibles, & attention
Martens et al. (2010)	ASD	3	P1: 4.5-year-old P2: 5.5-year-old P3: 4-year-old	P1: Aggression & inappropriate vocalizations P2: Noncompliant behavior & inappropriate vocalizations P3: Inappropriate vocalizations	Multielement FA & Contingency Space Analysis (CSA)	P1: Attention P2: Escape P3: Automatic reinforcement
Matson and Boisjoli (2007)	ID	88	Mean = 49.13	SIB & aggression	QABF	Both behaviors were all found to have multiple maintaining functions

(continued)

Table 4.1 (continued)

Authors	Population	N	Age	Behavior	Type of functional assessment used	Function identified
McLay et al. (2019)	ASD	2	P1: 4-year and 2-month-old P2: 10-year and 10-month-old	P1: Frequent curtain calls & frequent and prolonged night-wakings P2: Bedtime resistance, delayed sleep onset delay, and frequent curtain calls, frequent and prolonged night-wakings, & unwanted co-sleeping	Sleep Assessment Treatment Tool (SATT), parent-reported sleep diaries, & videosomnography(VSG)	Multiple functions: Parental attention, Automatic Reinforcement, & Tangibles
Monlux, Pollard, Rodriquez and Hall (2019)	Fragile X syndrome	10	Ranging from 3–10-years old	SIB, aggression, & destructive behaviors.	Multielement FA via telehealth.	Escape from academic demands, escape from transition demands, and access to tangibles and attention.
Neely et al. (2015)	ASD & severe ID	2	P1: 8-year-old P2: 7-year-old	P1: Repetitive rocking & bouncing P2: Repetitive arm swinging & head touching	Multielement FA	Automatic reinforcement
Neidert et al. (2013)	Profound ID	2	P1: 21-year-old P2: 22-year-old	Elopement	Multielement FA	Social-positive reinforcement
Newcomb et al. (2019)	ASD	1	13-year-old	Aggressive behavior, property destruction, & loud vocalizations	Multielement FA & CSA	Access to physical attention

Authors	Population	N	Age	Behavior	Type of functional assessment used	Function identified
Northup et al. (1991)	P1: ID P2: ID P3: ID & cerebral palsy	3	P1: 24-year-old P2: 21-year-old P3: 13-year-old	P1: Aggressive behavior including scratching, pinching, grabbing, hitting, and pulling hair P2: Aggressive behavior including pinching, hitting and biting & SIB consisting of face-slapping and self-pinching P3: Aggressive behavior including pinching, biting, and hitting	Multielement FA consisting of two rapidly changing reversal designs conducted in two phases: an initial analogue assessment & a contingency reversal	P1: Escape P2: Escape & tangibles P3: Escape & attention
Obi (1997)	Lesch-Nyhan syndrome	1	24-year-old	SIB	FBA including a semistructured interview with participant, questionnaire with staff, & ABC data	Avoidance of anxiety contingent on the absence of restraints
O'Reilly et al. (2005)	ASD	1	12-year-old	SIB	Multiseries FA	Antecedent intervention in positive behavioral support plans through scheduled activities
O'Reilly et al. (2006)	ASD	1	20-year-old	Bizarre speech & elopement	Multielement FA	Attention
O'Reilly et al. (2008)	ASD	3	P1: 16-years-old P2: 22-years-old P3: 25-years-old	Challenging behavior	Multielement FA	Attention or tangible items

(continued)

Table 4.1 (continued)

Authors	Population	N	Age	Behavior	Type of functional assessment used	Function identified
O'Reilly et al. 2010	ASD	10	Ranged between 4 and 8-years-old	SIB, aggression, inappropriate vocalizations, and stereotypy	Multielement FA	Automatic reinforcement (8 Participants) Reinforcement (multiple sources) (2 Participants)
O'Reilly et al. (2012)	Developmental disorders	3	P1: 5-year-old P2: 9-year-old P3: 5-year-old	P1: Elopement, yelling, & flopping P2: Head slaps & biting P3: Elopement, yelling, & flopping	Multielement FA	Tangibles
O'Reilly, Lacey, & Lancioni (2000)	Williams syndrome	1	5-years and 2-months	Aggressive behavior	Multielement FA	Aversiveness of task demand
O'Reilly, Lacioni, et al. (2000)	ID	2	P1: 22-year-old P2: 9-year-old	P1: Pushing & pinching P2: Property destruction & SIB	Multielement FA	Attention, especially when parents were interacting with another person
Olive et al. (2008)	ASD	1	4-year-old	Screaming, running from the table, placing materials in mouth, lying on the floor, or shouting "no!"	Multielement FA & FBA	Attention
Patel et al. (2000)	P1: ASD P2: ID & fetal alcohol syndrome	2	P1: 10-year-old P2: 30-year-old	P1: Rapid tongue movements P2: SIB	Multielement FA	P1: Auditory stimulation P2: Tactile stimulation

Authors	Population	N	Age	Behavior	Type of functional assessment used	Function identified
Peck et al. (1996)	Developmental disabilities	5	P1: 22-months-old P2: 16-months-old P3: 3-year-old P4: 4-year-old P5: 2-year-old	Pulling and chewing medical tubes and wires, food refusal, SIB, noncompliance, & aggressive behavior	Multielement FA, FCT, & choice making analysis	Low attention, high demands, & escape
Petursdottir et al. (2010)	ID	174	Under 18: 46 Adults: 128	Physical aggression, verbal aggression, noncompliance, property destruction, inappropriate verbal and social behavior, and SIB	Multielement FA	Attention accounted for 62.9% of behaviors, escape, and access to tangibles
Petursson & Eldivek (2018)	ASD	1	30-year-old	Aggression & SIB	Multielement FA	Escape from demands
Piazza et al. (1997)	P1: Moderate ID, ASD, AD/HD, & a seizure disorder P2: Severe ID, ASD, bipolar disorder, & AD/HD P3: Cerebral palsy, a seizure disorder, & learning and speech delays	3	P1: 10-year-old P2: 11-year-old P3: 4-year-old	Elopement	Multielement FA	P1: Access to tangibles P2: Attention & ignore conditions P3: Attention

(continued)

Table 4.1 (continued)

Authors	Population	N	Age	Behavior	Type of functional assessment used	Function identified
Piazza et al. (2000)	P1: AD/HD P2: AD/HD P3: ID	3	P1: 6-year-old P2: 8-year-old P3: 17-year-old	P1: Dangerous behavior, aggression, disruption, & SIB P2: Saliva play, aggression, disruption, & SIB P3: SIB	Multielement FA	Automatic reinforcement
Potoczak et al. (2007)	P1: Down syndrome P2: ASD P3: No diagnosis P4: AD/HD	4	P1: 9-year-old P2: 7-year-old P3: 8-year-old P4: 17-year-old	P1: Refusal to reply and/or participate P2: Grabbing/tearing materials and refusal to participate P3: Grabbing/tearing materials and out-of-seat behavior P4: Refusal to reply & out-of-seat behavior	Multielement FA	Escape from demands
Radstaake et al. (Radstaak et al. 2013)	Angelman syndrome	3	P1: 7-year-old P2: 15-year-old P3: 6-year-old	SIB, hurting/pinching others, biting, throwing, and hair-pulling.	Multielement FA	Attention, escape & access to tangibles.
Radstaake, Didden, Oliver, Allen and Curfs (Radstaak et al. 2012)	Angelman syndrome	4	Ranged from 5–18-years-old.	Hitting other people, hair-pulling, saliva-play, disruption, and throwing items.	Multielement FA	Attention, access to tangibles and demand.
Rahman et al. (2010)	Acquired Brain Injury (ABI)	9	Ranged between 30 and 59-years-old	Physical aggression, property destruction, self-injury, and verbal aggression	Descriptive FA	Escape from demands, Escape from social attention & multiple functions

Authors	Population	N	Age	Behavior	Type of functional assessment used	Function identified
Rahman et al. (2013)	ABI	4	P1: 60-year-old P2: 49-year-old P3: 45-year-old P4: 50-year-old	P1: Aggression P2: Aggression P3: Aggression P4: Verbal perseveration	Structured descriptive assessment	P1: Escape from demand P2: Escape from demands P3: Social attention P4: Social attention
Rapp et al. (2009)	ASD	3	P1: 8-year-old P2: 8-year-old P3: 5-year-old	Vocal stereotypy	Multielement FA	Automatic reinforcement
Richman et al. (1998)	ID & ASD	1	27-year-old	Disruptive behavior & SIB (finger picking)	Multielement FA	Escape & automatic reinforcement
Reed et al. (2005)	P1: ASD, moderate ID, & seizure disorder P2: ODD, AD/HD, & mild ID	2	P1: 8-year-old P2: 10-year-old	P1: Property destruction, noncompliance, aggression, & disruptive behaviors P2: Aggression & noncompliance	Multielement FA	Escape from demands
Reese et al. (2005)	Typically developing & ASD	23 ASD 23 typically developing	Unknown	Disruptive behavior	Multielement FA	Girls with ASD and typically developing: escape from demands, attention, & tangibles Boys with ASD: Access to tangibles & escape from demands

(continued)

Table 4.1 (continued)

Authors	Population	N	Age	Behavior	Type of functional assessment used	Function identified
Richman et al. (1999)	P1: ID & AD/HD P2: Developmental delays & ASD P3: ID & AD/HD	3	P1: 8-year-old P2: 4-year-old P3: 6-year-old	P1: Stereotypic movements, facial tics, disruptive, & aggressive behaviors P2: Aggression P3: Disruptive behavior	Multielement FA	P1: Access to tangibles items & attention P2: Escape, attention, & tangibles P3: Escape
Rispoli et al. (2011)	Severe ID & Cerebral Palsy	1	5-year-old	Hitting others & throwing objects	Multielement FA	Attention & demands
Rispoli et al. (2015)	Not specified	3	P1: 4-year-old P2: 4-year-old P3: 3-year-old	Challenging behavior	TBFA	Access to tangibles
Roberts-Gwinn et al. (2001)	ASD	1	11-year-old	Aggression, disrobing, & elopement	BFA	Automatic reinforcement
Rojahn et al. (2012)	ID & Developmental Disabilities	115	Ranged between 20 and 73-years-old	SIB and stereotyped & aggressive behaviors	QABF	Aggression: attention and escape SIB & stereotypy: self-stimulation & escape
Romani et al. (2019)	P1: ASD, unspecified disruptive, impulse-control, & conduct disorder P2: ASD, mild ID, unspecified disruptive, impulse-control, & conduct disorder	2	P1: 5-year-old P2: 12-year-old	Aggression	Multielement FA	Tangible reinforcement

Authors	Population	N	Age	Behavior	Type of functional assessment used	Function identified
Rose and Beaulieu (2019)	ASD	2	P1: 3-year-10-month old P2: 5-year-11-month old	P1: Vocal protests P2: Vocal protesting, aggression, and environmental destruction	FBA & Multielement FA	Tangibles & attention
Sasso et al. (1992)	ASD	2	P1: 7.5-year-old P2: 13-year-old	P1: Aggression, loud vocalizations, and noncompliance P2: Aggression in the form of hitting, pinching, scratching, and kicking & stereotypy in the form of hand waving and rocking	Multielement FA	Escape from demands
Scalzo and Davis (2017)	ASD	4	P1: 4-year-old P2: 5-year-old P3: 4-year-old P4: 12-year-old	P1: Crying P2: Screaming P3: Aggression P4: Aggression	Functional assessment interview & multielement FA	Tangibles
Scheithauer et al. (2016)	ASD, AD/HD, conduct disorder, disruptive behavior disorder, & development delay	24	Ranged between 3 and 18-years-old	Aggression, disruptive behavior, elopement, inappropriate vocalizations, SIB, & spitting	Multielement FA	Escape, tangibles, attention, & automatic reinforcement

(continued)

Table 4.1 (continued)

Authors	Population	N	Age	Behavior	Type of functional assessment used	Function identified
Scheithauer et al. (2017)	ASD	2	P1: 12-year-old P2: 9-year-old	P1: SIB including hand-to-head, hand-to-body, head-to-surface, & shoulder-to-head hits P2: SIB including head-to-surface, hand-to-head, body-to-surface (specifically wrists), and hand-to-body hits	Multielement FA	P1: Automatic & social reinforcement P2: Automatic reinforcement
Schmidt, Drasgow, et al. (2014)	P1: ASD & Profound ID P2: ASD & Profound ID P3: ASD, severe ID, depressive disorder—not otherwise specified, & psychotic disorder—not otherwise specified	3	P1: 9-year-old P2: 10-year-old P3: 15-year old	P1: Food stealing & aggression P2: Food stealing & aggression P3: Aggression, inappropriate touching, & cursing/sexual statements	Discrete-trial Functional Analysis (DTFA)	P1: Tangible-edible & escape P2: Tangible-edible P3: Attention
Schmidt, Shanholtzer, et al. (2014)	Mild ID	1	14-year-old	Physical aggression, verbal aggression, & disruptive behaviors	Multielement FA	Escape from demands
Schroeder et al. (2014)	Children at risk of developmental disabilities	17	Ranged between 17 and 41-month-old	SIB, stereotypy, property destruction, aggression, and tantrums	Multielement FA, & the Behavior Problem Inventory	70% maintained by automatic reinforcement and 22% maintained by escape from demands

Authors	Population	N	Age	Behavior	Type of functional assessment used	Function identified
Smith et al. (2016)	ASD	3	P1: 28-year-old P2: 9-year-old P3: 14-year-old	P1: SIB P2: Aggression & tantrums P3: Tantrums	FBA & Multielement FA	Escape from demands & fatigue
Smith and Churchill (2002)	Profound ID	4	P1: 41-year-old P2: 53-year-old P3: 35-year-old P4: 52-year-old	P1: SIB P2: SIB P3: Aggression P4: SIB	Multielement FA	P1: Demands P2: Demands P3: Attention P4: Demands
Sprague et al. (1998)	Severe ID & cerebral palsy	1	13-year-old	Feeding problems including spitting & whining following bites of food	Preliminary FA, attention analysis, & differential reinforcement analysis	Access to food
Strachan, Shaw. Burrow, Horsler, Allen and Oliver (2009)	Angelman syndrome	12	Ranged between 4 and 16-year-old.	Aggression.	Multielement FA	Attention, social interaction & escape.
Strohmeier et al. (2017)	ASD	1	12-year-old	Self-injury, aggression, & disruption	Parent conducted combined establishing operations (EO) FA	Tangibles & escape from demands
Swender et al. (2006)	ID	60	Range between 21 and 79-years-old	Hand mouthing	Behavioral multielement FA & QABF	GERD was more likely under nonsocial conditions

(continued)

Table 4.1 (continued)

Authors	Population	N	Age	Behavior	Type of functional assessment used	Function identified
Tarbox et al. (2009)	ASD	7	Range between 3 and 9-years-old	P1: Aggression P2: Tantrums P3: Property destruction P4: Whining P5: Stereotypy P6: Verbal protesting P7: Stereotypy	Indirect assessment, descriptive assessment, & multielement FA	P1: Escape from demands P2: Tangibles P3: Attention & escape from demands P4: Escape from demands P5: Escape from demands P6: Tangibles P7: Automatic reinforcement
Thompson and Iwata (2007)	ASD	12	Range between 30 and 52-years-old	SIB & aggression	Multielement FA	Access to tangible (3 Participants) Attention (3 Participants) Escape from demands (3 Participants) Automatic reinforcement (3 Participants)
Torres-Viso et al. (2018)	SMS & ASD	1	12-year-old	Mands	Multielement FA	Others' compliance with mands for rearrangement

Authors	Population	N	Age	Behavior	Type of functional assessment used	Function identified
Toogood et al. (2011)	ASD & Severe ID	1	32-year-old	CB1: Aggression, SIB & Property disruption CB2: Stereotypy CB3: Skin-picking CB4: Vocalization	FBA	CB1: Attention & escape from demands CB2: Automatic reinforcement CB3: Automatic reinforcement CB4: Attention
Tucker et al. (1998)	ID	2	P1: 18-year-old P2: 13-year-old	P1: Screaming & property disruption P2: Aggression & grabbing	Multielement FA	P1: Access to tangibles P2: Social attention
Vollmer et al. (1999)	ID	3	P1: 17-year-old P2: 16-year-old P3: 4-year-old	P1: SIB & aggression P2: SIB P3: Aggression	Multielement FA	P1: Escape P2: Materials P3: Escape
Vollmer et al. (1993)	P1: Profound ID P2: Severe ID P3: Profound ID	3	P1: 32-year-old P2: 40-year-old P3: 42-year-old	P1: SIB including head hitting, body hitting, & head banging P2: Hand mouthing P3: SIB including head banging & head hitting	Multielement FA	Attention
Vollmer et al. (1994)	Severe disabilities	3	P1: 3-year-old P2: 3-year-old P3: 4-year-old	SIB & hand mouthing	Multielement FA	P1: Access to tangibles P2: Access to tangibles P3: Unknown

(continued)

Table 4.1 (continued)

Authors	Population	N	Age	Behavior	Type of functional assessment used	Function identified
Vollmer et al. (1998)	P1: Severe ID P2: Moderate ID & severe hearing loss P3: Moderate ID	3	P1: 22-year-old P2: 6-year-old P3: 16-year-old	P1: Aggression n in the form of hitting other people & pinching P2: Disruptive, SIB, & tantrum behavior P3: Aggression including hitting others	Multielement FA	P1: Escape From social proximity P2: Positive reinforcement in the form of attention P3: Escape from instructional proximity
Wacker et al. (1990)	P1: ASD, severe to profound ID, & a seizure disorder P2: Phenylketonuria & Profound ID P3: Severe to profound ID	3	P1: 7-year-old P2: 30-year-old P3: 9-year-old	P1: SIB including hand-biting P2: Stereotypy including body-rocking P3: Aggression including slapping & biting others	Multielement FA	P1: Positive reinforcement P2: Automatic reinforcement P3: Attention
Wacker et al. (1998)	P1: Severe to profound developmental delays P2: Rett-like syndrome & severe ID	2	P1: 2 year 2 months old P2: 7-year-6 months old	P1: SIB in the form of hand-biting, eye-gouging, & head banging P2: SIB & feeding problems	Multielement FA	P1: Parent attention P2: Automatic reinforcement
Wacker et al. (2013)	ASD	20	Ranged between 18 and 83-months-old	Aggression, SIB, destruction, and disruption.	Multielement FA	90% of participants showed a social function, 13 participants showed an escape function, and 2 showed a tangible function

Authors	Population	N	Age	Behavior	Type of functional assessment used	Function identified
Waters et al. (2009)	ASD	2	P1: 6-year-old P2: 6-year-old	P1: Aggression P2: Aggression & disruption	BFA	Escape from demands (nonpreferred activities and transition) & tangibles (preferred activities)
Watkins and Rapp (2013)	ASD	6	Ranged between 9 and 19-years-old	Repetitive, SIB, & stereotypy behavior	QABF	Automatic reinforcement
White et al. (2011)	ASD	2	P1: 7-year-old P2: 7-year-old	Aggressive & stereotypy behavior	Multielement FA	P1: Access to tangibles P2: Access to tangibles
Wilder et al. (2000)	ID	1	30-year-old	Stereotypy behavior	Multielement FA	Automatic reinforcement
Wilke et al. (2012)	ASD	53	Ranged between 30 and 204 months	Stereotypy behavior	QABF	Automatic reinforcement

Multi element FA Experimental Functional Analysis, *FBA* Functional Behavioral Assessment, *QABF* Questions About Behavioral Function, *BFA* Brief Functional Analysis, and *TBFA* Trial-Based Functional Analysis topographies of behavior. This chapter focused on how the different types of FA methodologies are used across different developmental disorders and other populations, while taking into consideration the disorder, the topography of the CB, details on the FA methodology conducted, the maintaining functions of CB identified with it, and the function-based interventions designed based on the FA results. In describing the use of FA, how different types of FA are used with specific topographies of behavior were discussed, outlining the different operational definitions of CB, characteristics of the populations displaying the CB, possible variables that should be taken into consideration when assessing specific topographies of behavior, the FA methodologies used, and the functions identified with the FA.

Conducting a FA is the first crucial step to design an intervention that can successfully decrease CB in both clinical and outpatient settings. In addition, because every CB has a maintaining function, it is important that the functions identified through FA are used to design a function-based intervention that can functionally replace the CB with an appropriate one whenever the function allows the behavior to be replaced. Analyzing the use of FA across different populations and topographies allows clinicians to consider additional controlling variables that can add value and reliability to the use of FA while better guiding its implementation. Interventions designed and delivered following the implementation of FAs increase the likelihood that the intervention will be successful in decreasing CB while improving the quality of life of individuals.

References

Adams, D., Horsler, K., Mount, R., & Oliver, C. (2015). Brief report: A longitudinal study of excessive smiling and laughing in children with Angelman syndrome. *Journal of Autism and Developmental Disorders, 45*(8), 2624–2627.

American Psychiatric Association. (2013). *Diagnostic and statistical manual of mental disorders (DSM-5)*. Arlington, VA: American Psychiatric Publishing.

Arndorfer, R. E., & Miltenberger, R. G. (1993). Functional assessment and treatment of challenging behavior: A review with implications for early childhood. *Topics in Early Childhood Special Education, 13*(1), 82–105.

Arron, K., Oliver, C., Moss, J., Berg, K., & Burbidge, C. (2011). The prevalence and phenomenology of self-injurious and aggressive behaviour in genetic syndromes. *Journal of Intellectual Disability Research, 55*(2), 109–120.

Asmus, J. M., Franzese, J. C., Conroy, M. A., & Dozier, C. L. (2003). Clarifying functional analysis outcomes for disruptive behaviors by controlling consequence delivery for stereotypy. *School Psychology Review, 32*(4), 624–630.

Asmus, J. M., Wacker, D. P., Harding, J., Berg, W. K., Derby, K. M., & Kocis, E. (1999). Evaluation of antecedent stimulus parameters for the treatment of escape-maintained aberrant behavior. *Journal of Applied Behavior Analysis, 32*(4), 495–513.

Athens, E. S., Vollmer, T. R., Sloman, K. N., & Pipkin, C. S. P. (2008). An analysis of vocal stereotypy and therapist fading. *Journal of Applied Behavior Analysis, 41*(2), 291–297.

Babbitt, R. L., Hoch, T. A., Coe, D. A., Cataldo, M. F., Kelly, K. J., Stackhouse, C., & Perman, J. A. (1994). Behavioral assessment and treatment of pediatric feeding disorders. *Journal of Developmental and Behavioral Pediatrics, 15*(4), 278–291.

Belfiore, P. J., Kitchen, T., & Lee, D. L. (2016). Functional analysis of maladaptive behaviors: Rule as a transitive conditioned motivating operation. *Research in Developmental Disabilities, 49*, 100–107.

Bell, M. C., & Fahmie, T. A. (2018). Functional analysis screening for multiple topographies of problem behavior. *Journal of Applied Behavior Analysis, 51*(3), 528–537.

Boyle, M. A., & Adamson, R. M. (2017). Systematic review of functional analysis and treatment of elopement (2000–2015). *Behavior Analysis in Practice, 10*(4), 375–385.

Boyle, M. A., Keenan, G., Forck, K. L., & Curtis, K. S. (2019). Treatment of elopement without blocking with a child with autism. *Behavior Modification, 43*(1), 132–145.

Britton, L. N., Carr, J. E., Landaburu, H. J., & Romick, K. S. (2002). The efficacy of noncontingent reinforcement as treatment for automatically reinforced stereotypy. *Behavioral Interventions: Theory & Practice in Residential & Community-Based Clinical Programs, 17*(2), 93–103.

Brusa, E., & Richman, D. (2008). Developing stimulus control for occurrences of stereotypy exhibited by a child with autism. *International Journal of Behavioral Consultation and Therapy, 4*(3), 264–269.

Buckley, R. H., Dinno, N., & Weber, P. (1998). Angelman syndrome: Are the estimates too low? *American Journal of Medical Genetics, 80*(4), 385–390.

Call, N. A., Pabicio, R. S., & Lomas, J. E. (2009). Use of latency to problem behavior to evaluate demands for inclusion in functional analysis. *Journal of Applied Behavior Analysis, 42*(3), 723–728.

Call, N. A., Reavis, A. R., Clark, S. B., Parks, N. A., Cariveau, T., & Muething, C. S. (2017). The effects of conducting a functional analysis on problem behavior in other settings: A descriptive study on potential interaction effects. *Behavior Modification, 41*(5), 609–625.

Call, N. A., Wacker, D. P., Ringdahl, J. E., & Boelter, E. W. (2005). Combined antecedent variables as motivating operations within functional analyses. *Journal of Applied Behavior Analysis, 38*(3), 385–389.

Camp, E. M., Iwata, B. A., Hammond, J. L., & Bloom, S. E. (2009). Antecedent versus consequent events as predictors of problem behavior. *Journal of Applied Behavior Analysis, 42*(2), 469–483.

Canella, H. I., O'Reilly, M. F., & Lancioni, G. E. (2006). Treatment of hand mouthing in individuals with severe to profound developmental disabilities: A review of the literature. *Research in Developmental Disabilities, 27*(5), 529–544.

Cannella-Malone, H. R., & O'Reilly, M. F. (2014). Clinical report: A replication of the analysis of the reinforcing properties of hand mouthing. *Journal of Developmental and Physical Disabilities, 26*(5), 543–548.

Cariveau, T., Miller, S. J., Call, N. A., & Alvarez, J. (2019). Assessment and treatment of problem behavior maintained by termination of interruptions. *Developmental Neurorehabilitation, 22*(3), 203–208.

Carr, E. G., & Carlson, J. I. (1993). Reduction of severe behavior problems in the community using a multicomponent treatment approach. *Journal of Applied Behavior Analysis, 26*(2), 157–172.

Chung, Y. C., & Cannella-Malone, H. I. (2010). The effects of presession manipulations on automatically maintained challenging behavior and task responding. *Behavior Modification, 34*(6), 479–502.

Clay, C. J., Clohisy, A. M., Ball, A. M., Haider, A. F., Schmitz, B. A., & Kahng, S. (2018). Further evaluation of presentation format of competing stimuli for treatment of automatically maintained challenging behavior. *Behavior Modification, 42*(3), 382–397.

Conroy, M. A., Davis, C. A., Fox, J. J., & Brown, W. H. (2002). Functional assessment of behavior and effective supports for young children with challenging behaviors. *Assessment for Effective Intervention, 27*(4), 35–47.

Cooper, L. J., Wacker, D. P., Thursby, D., Plagmann, L. A., Harding, J., Millard, T., & Derby, M. (1992). Analysis of the effects of task preferences, task demands, and adult attention on child behavior in outpatient and classroom settings. *Journal of Applied Behavior Analysis, 25*(4), 823–840.

Crocker, A. G., Mercier, C., Lachapelle, Y., Brunet, A., Morin, D., & Roy, M. E. (2006). Prevalence and types of aggressive behaviour among adults with intellectual disabilities. *Journal of Intellectual Disability Research, 50*(9), 652–661.

Davis, T. N., Dacus, S., Strickland, E., Copeland, D., Chan, J. M., Blenden, K., & Christian, K. (2013). The effects of a weighted vest on aggressive and self-injurious behavior in a child with autism. *Developmental Neurorehabilitation, 16*(3), 210–215.

Davis, T. N., Durand, S., Fuentes, L., Dacus, S., & Blenden, K. (2014). The effects of a school-based functional analysis on subsequent classroom behavior. *Education and Treatment of Children, 37*(1), 95–110.

DeLeon, I. G., Kahng, S., Rodriguez-Catter, V., Sveinsdóttir, I., & Sadler, C. (2003). Assessment of aberrant behavior maintained by wheelchair movement in a child with developmental disabilities. *Research in Developmental Disabilities, 24*(5), 381–390.

Delgado-Casas, C., Navarro, J. I., Garcia-Gonzalez-Gordon, R., & Marchena, E. (2014). Functional analysis of challenging behavior in people with severe intellectual disabilities. *Psychological Reports, 115*(3), 655–669.

Derby, K., Wacker, D., Peck, S., Sasso, G., DeRaad, A., Berg, W., & Ulrich, S. (1994). Functional analysis of separate topographies of aberrant behavior. *Journal of Applied Behavior Analysis, 27*(2), 267–278.

Derby, K. M., Hagopian, L., Fisher, W. W., Richman, D., Augustine, M., Fahs, A., & Thompson, R. (2000). Functional analysis of aberrant behavior through measurement of separate response topographies. *Journal of Applied Behavior Analysis, 33*(1), 113–117.

Devlin, S., Healy, O., Leader, G., & Hughes, B. M. (2011). Comparison of behavioral intervention and sensory-integration therapy in the treatment of challenging behavior. *Journal of Autism and Developmental Disorders, 41*(10), 1303–1320.

Devlin, S., Healy, O., Leader, G., & Reed, P. (2008). The analysis and treatment of problem behavior evoked by auditory stimulation. *Research in Autism Spectrum Disorders, 2*(4), 671–680.

DeWall, C. N., Anderson, C. A., & Bushman, B. J. (2012). Aggression. In I. Weiner (Ed.), Handbook of psychology (2nd ed., Vol. 5, pp. 449–466). H. Tennen & J. Suls (Eds.), Personality and social psychology. New York: Wiley.

Didden, R., Korzilius, H., & Curfs, L. M. (2007). Skin-picking in individuals with Prader-Willi syndrome: Prevalence, functional assessment, and its comorbidity with compulsive and self-injurious behaviours. *Journal of Applied Research in Intellectual Disabilities, 20*(5), 409–419.

Doughty, S. S., Anderson, C. M., Doughty, A. H., Williams, D. C., & Saunders, K. J. (2007). Discriminative control of punished stereotyped behavior in humans. *Journal of the Experimental Analysis of Behavior, 87*(3), 325–336.

Dunkel-Jackson, S. M., Kenney, K., Borch, S., & Neveu, C. N. (2018). Case report: Intervention evaluation of trial-based functional analyses in school. *Journal on Developmental Disabilities, 23*(2), 55–65.

Dunlap, G., Kern, L., Deperczel, M., Clarke, S., Wilson, D., Childs, K. E., … Falk, G. D. (1993). Functional analysis of classroom variables for students with emotional and behavioral disorders. *Behavioral Disorders, 18*(4), 275–291.

Durand, V. M., & Crimmins, D. B. (1988). Identifying the variables maintaining self-injurious behavior. *Journal of Autism and Developmental Disorders, 18*(1), 99–117.

Ekas, N. V., McDonald, N. M., Pruitt, M. M., & Messinger, D. S. (2017). Brief report: The development of compliance in toddlers at-risk for autism spectrum disorder. *Journal of Autism and Developmental Disorders, 47*(4), 1239–1248.

Ellingson, S. A., Miltenberger, R. G., Stricker, J., Galensky, T. L., & Garlinghouse, M. (2000). Functional assessment and intervention for challenging behaviors in the classroom by general classroom teachers. *Journal of Positive Behavior Interventions, 2*(2), 85–97.

Emerson, E., Kiernan, C., Alborz, A., Reeves, D., Mason, H., Swarbrick, R., & Hatton, C. (2001). The prevalence of challenging behaviors: A total population study. *Research in Developmental Disabilities, 22*(1), 77–93.

Emerson, E., Reeves, D., Thompson, S., Henderson, D., Robertson, J., & Howard, D. (1996). Time-based lag sequential analysis and the functional assessment of challenging behavior. *Journal of Intellectual Disability Research, 40*(3), 260–274.

Falcomata, T. S., & Gainey, S. (2014). An evaluation of noncontingent reinforcement for the treatment of challenging behavior with multiple functions. *Journal of Developmental and Physical Disabilities, 26*(3), 317–324.

Falcomata, T. S., Muething, C. S., Gainey, S., Hoffman, K., & Fragale, C. (2013). Further evaluations of functional communication training and chained schedules of reinforcement to treat multiple functions of challenging behavior. *Behavior Modification, 37*(6), 723–746.

Flanagan, T. F., & DeBar, R. M. (2018). Trial-based functional analyses with student identified with an emotional and behavioral disorder. *Behavioral Disorders, 43*(4), 423–435.

Fragale, C., Rojeski, L., O'Reilly, M., & Gevarter, C. (2016). Evaluation of functional communication training as a satiation procedure to reduce challenging behavior in instructional environments for children with autism. *International Journal of Developmental Disabilities, 62*(3), 139–146.

Galván-Manso, M., Campistol, J., Monros, E., Poo, P., Vernet, A. M., Pineda, … Sanmartí, F. X. (2002). Angelman syndrome: Physical characteristics and behavioral phenotype in 37 patients with confirmed genetic diagnosis. *Revista de Neurologia, 35*(5), 425–429.

Girolami, P. A., & Scotti, J. R. (2001). Use of analog functional analysis in assessing the function of mealtime behavior problems. *Education and Training in Mental Retardation and Developmental Disabilities, 36*(2), 207–223.

Goh, H. L., Iwata, B. A., Shore, B. A., DeLeon, I. G., Lerman, D. C., Ulrich, S. M., & Smith, R. G. (1995). An analysis of the reinforcing properties of hand mouthing. *Journal of Applied Behavior Analysis, 28*(3), 269–283.

Griesemer, R. D. (1978). Emotionally triggered diseases in dermatological practice. *Psychiatric Annals, 8*(8), 49–56.

Gupta, M. A., Gupta, A. K., & Haberman, H. F. (1987). Psoriasis and psychiatry: An update. *General Hospital Psychiatry, 9*(3), 157–166.

Gutierrez, M. A. F., & Mendez, M. D. (2020). Prader-Willi syndrome. In *StatPearls* [internet]. StatPearls Publishing.

Hagerman, P. J. (2008). The fragile X prevalence paradox. *Journal of Medical Genetics, 45,* 498–499.

Hagopian, L. P., Bruzek, J. L., Bowman, L. G., & Jennett, H. K. (2007). Assessment and treatment of problem behavior occasioned by interruption of free-operant behavior. *Journal of Applied Behavior Analysis, 40*(1), 89–103.

Hagopian, L. P., Contrucci Kuhn, S. A., Long, E. S., & Rush, K. S. (2005). Schedule thinning following communication training: Using competing stimuli to enhance tolerance to decrements in reinforcer density. *Journal of Applied Behavior Analysis, 38*(2), 177–193.

Hagopian, L. P., Fisher, W. W., Thibault Sullivan, M., Acquisto, J., & LeBlanc, L. A. (1998). Effectiveness of functional communication training with and without extinction and punishment: A summary of 21 inpatient cases. *Journal of Applied Behavior Analysis, 31*(2), 211–235.

Hall, S. S. (2005). Comparing descriptive, experimental and informant-based assessments of problem behaviors. *Research in Developmental Disabilities, 26*(6), 514–526.

Hanley, G. P., Iwata, B. A., & McCord, B. E. (2003). Functional analysis of problem behavior: A review. *Journal of Applied Behavior Analysis, 36*(2), 147–185.

Hanley, G. P., Piazza, C. C., Fisher, W. W., & Maglieri, K. A. (2005). On the effectiveness of and preference for punishment and extinction components of function-based interventions. *Journal of Applied Behavior Analysis, 38*(1), 51–65.

Hausman, N., Kahng, S., Farrell, E., & Mongeon, C. (2009). Idiosyncratic functions: Severe problem behavior maintained by access to ritualistic behaviors. *Education and Treatment of Children, 32*(1), 77–87.

Healey, J. J., Ahearn, W. H., Graff, R. B., & Libby, M. E. (2001). Extended analysis and treatment of self-injurious behavior. *Behavioral Interventions: Theory & Practice in Residential & Community-Based Clinical Programs, 16*(3), 181–195.

Healy, O., Brett, D., & Leader, G. (2013). A comparison of experimental functional analysis and the Questions About Behavioral Function (QABF) in the assessment of challenging behavior of individuals with autism. *Research in Autism Spectrum Disorders, 7*(1), 66–81.

Herman, C., Healy, O., & Lydon, S. (2018). An interview-informed synthesized contingency analysis to inform the treatment of challenging behavior in a young child with autism. *Developmental Neurorehabilitation, 21*(3), 202–207.

Hetzroni, O. E., & Roth, T. (2003). Effects of a positive support approach to enhance communicative behaviors of children with mental retardation who have challenging behaviors. *Education and Training in Developmental Disabilities, 38*, 95–105.

Heyvaert, M., Saenen, L., Campbell, J. M., Maes, B., & Onghena, P. (2014). Efficacy of behavioral interventions for reducing problem behavior in persons with autism: An updated quantitative synthesis of single-subject research. *Research in Developmental Disabilities, 35*(10), 2463–2476.

Hodnett, J., Scheithauer, M., Call, N. A., Mevers, J. L., & Miller, S. J. (2018). Using a functional analysis followed by differential reinforcement and extinction to reduce challenging behaviors in children with Smith-Magenis syndrome. *American Journal on Intellectual and Developmental Disabilities, 123*(6), 558–573.

Holland, A., Whittington, J., & Butler, J. (2002). Prader-Willi and Angelman syndromes: From childhood to adult life. In P. Howlin & O. Udwin (Eds.), *Outcomes in neurodevelopmental and genetic disorders* (pp. 220–240). Cambridge: Cambridge University Press.

Iwata, B. A., Dorsey, M. F., Slifer, K. J., Bauman, K. E., & Richman, G. S. (1982). Toward a functional analysis of self-injury. *Analysis and Intervention in Developmental Disabilities, 2*(1), 3–20.

Iwata, B. A., Dorsey, M. F., Slifer, K. J., Bauman, K. E., & Richman, G. S. (1994). Toward a functional analysis of self-injury. *Journal of Applied Behavior Analysis, 27*(2), 197–209.

Juyal, R. C., Figuera, L. E., Hauge, X., Elsea, S. H., Lupski, J. R., Greenberg, F., & Patel, P. I. (1996). Molecular analyses of 17p11.2 deletions in 62 Smith-Magenis syndrome patients. *American Journal of Human Genetics, 58*(5), 998–1007.

Kahng, S., Iwata, B. A., & Lewin, A. B. (2002). Behavioral treatment of self-injury, 1964 to 2000. *American Journal on Mental Retardation, 107*(3), 212–221.

Karsh, K. G., Repp, A. C., Dahlquist, C. M., & Munk, D. (1995). In vivo functional assessment and multi-element interventions for problem behaviors of students with disabilities in classroom settings. *Journal of Behavioral Education, 5*(2), 189–210.

Kavale, K. A., Forness, S. R., & Mostert, M. P. (2005). Defining emotional or behavioral disorders: The quest for affirmation. In P. Garner, F. Yuen, P. Clough, & T. Pardeck (Eds.), *Handbook of emotional and behavioral difficulties* (pp. 38–49). London: Sage.

Kelly, A. N., Axe, J. B., Allen, R. F., & Maguire, R. W. (2015). Effects of presession pairing on the challenging behavior and academic responding of children with autism: Effects of presession pairing. *Behavioral Interventions, 30*(2), 135–156.

Kern, L. (1997). Analysis and intervention with two topographies of challenging behavior exhibited by a young woman with autism. *Research in Developmental Disabilities, 18*(4), 275–287.

Kern, L., & Vorndran, C. M. (2000). Functional assessment and intervention for transition difficulties. *Journal of the Association for Persons with Severe Handicaps, 25*(4), 212–216.

Kleinsinger, F. (2003). Understanding noncompliant behavior: Definitions and causes. *The Permanente Journal, 7*(4), 18–21.

Kodak, T., Grow, L., & Northup, J. (2004). Functional analysis and treatment of elopement for a child with attention deficit hyperactivity disorder. *Journal of Applied Behavior Analysis, 37*(2), 229–232.

Kurtz, P. F., Chin, M. D., Robinson, A. N., O'Connor, J. T., & Hagopian, L. P. (2015). Functional analysis and treatment of problem behavior exhibited by children with fragile X syndrome. *Research in Developmental Disabilities, 35*(7), 1694–1704.

Kurtz, P. F., Chin, M. D., Rush, K. S., & Dixon, D. R. (2008). Treatment of challenging behavior exhibited by children with prenatal drug exposure. *Research in Developmental Disabilities, 29*(6), 582–594.

LaBelle, C. A., & Charlop-Christy, M. H. (2002). Individualizing functional analysis to assess multiple and changing functions of severe behavior problems in children with autism. *Journal of Positive Behavior Interventions, 4*(4), 231–241.

Lambert, J. M., Parikh, N., Stankiewicz, K. C., Houchins-Juarez, N. J., Morales, V. A., Sweeney, E. M., & Milam, M. E. (2019). Decreasing food stealing of child with Prader-Willi syndrome through function-based differential reinforcement. *Journal of Autism and Developmental Disorders, 49*(2), 721–728.

Lang, R., Davis, T., O'Reilly, M., Machalicek, W., Rispoli, M., Sigafoos, J., & Regester, A. (2010). Functional analysis and treatment of elopement across two school settings. *Journal of Applied Behavior Analysis, 43*(1), 113–118.

Lang, R., O'Reilly, M., Machalicek, W., Lancioni, G., Rispoli, M., & Chan, J. M. (2008). A preliminary comparison of functional analysis results when conducted in contrived versus natural settings. *Journal of Applied Behavior Analysis, 41*(3), 441–445.

Laraway, S., Snycerski, S., Michael, J., & Poling, A. (2003). Motivating operations and terms to describe them: Some further refinements. *Journal of Applied Behavior Analysis, 36*(3), 407–414.

Larkin, W., Hawkins, R. O., & Collins, T. (2016). Using trial-based functional analysis to design effective interventions for students diagnosed with autism spectrum disorder. *School Psychology Quarterly, 31*(4), 534–547.

LaRue, R. H., Lenard, K., Weiss, M. J., Bamond, M., Palmieri, M., & Kelley, M. E. (2010). Comparison of traditional and trial-based methodologies for conducting functional analyses. *Research in Developmental Disabilities, 31*(2), 480–487.

LaRue, R. H., Sloman, K. N., Weiss, M. J., Delmolino, L., Hansford, A., Szalony, J., ... Lambright, N. M. (2011). Correspondence between traditional models of functional analysis and a functional analysis of manding behavior. *Research in Developmental Disabilities, 32*(6), 2449–2457.

Leader, G., & Mannion, A. (2016). Challenging behaviors. In J. L. Matson (Ed.), *Handbook of assessment and diagnosis of autism spectrum disorder* (pp. 209–232). Cham: Springer.

Leader, G., Tuohy, E., Chen, J. L., Mannion, A., & Gilroy, S. P. (2020). Feeding problems, gastrointestinal symptoms, challenging behavior and sensory issues in children and adolescents with autism spectrum disorder. *Journal of Autism and Developmental Disorders, 50*, 1401–1410.

Liddon, C. J., Zarcone, J. R., Pisman, M., & Rooker, G. W. (2016). Examination of behavioral flexibility and function of severe challenging behavior in individuals with autism and intellectual disability. *International Journal of Developmental Disabilities, 62*(3), 167–173.

Lloyd, B. P., & Kennedy, C. H. (2014). Assessment and treatment of challenging behaviour for individuals with intellectual disability: A research review. *Journal of Applied Research in Intellectual Disabilities, 27*(3), 187–199.

Lowe, K., Allen, D., Jones, E., Brophy, S., Moore, K., & James, W. (2007). Challenging behaviours: Prevalence and topographies. *Journal of Intellectual Disability Research, 51*(8), 625–636.

Luiselli, J. K., & Sobezenski, T. (2017). Escape-motivated bathroom visits: Effects of activity scheduling, cuing, and duration-fading in an adult with intellectual disability. *Clinical Case Studies, 16*(5), 417–426.

Mace, F. C., & Lalli, J. S. (1991). Linking descriptive and experimental analyses in the treatment of bizarre speech. *Journal of Applied Behavior Analysis, 24*(3), 553–562.

Machalicek, W., McDuffie, A., Oakes, A., Ma, M., Thurman, A. J., Rispoli, M. J., & Abbeduto, L. (2014). Examining the operant function of challenging behavior in young males with fragile X syndrome: A summary of 12 cases. *Research in Developmental Disabilities, 35*(7), 1694–1704.

Machalicek, W., O'Reilly, M., Rispoli, M., Davis, T., Lang, R., Franco, J., & Chan, J. (2010). Training teachers to assess the challenging behaviors of students with autism using video tele-conferencing. *Education and Training in Autism and Developmental Disabilities, 45*, 203–215.

Machalicek, W., Shogren, K., Lang, R., Rispoli, M., O'Reilly, M. F., Franco, J. H., & Sigafoos, J. (2009). Increasing play and decreasing the challenging behavior of children with autism during recess with activity schedules and task correspondence training. *Research in Autism Spectrum Disorders, 3*(2), 547–555.

Macks, R. J., & Reeve, R. E. (2007). The adjustment of non-disabled siblings of children with autism. *Journal of Autism and Developmental Disorders, 37*(6), 1060–1067.

Marcus, B. A., Swanson, V., & Vollmer, T. R. (2001). Effects of parent training on parent and child behavior using procedures based on functional analysis. *Behavioral Interventions, 16*(2), 87–104.

Marcus, B. A., & Vollmer, T. R. (1996). Combining noncontingent reinforcement and differential reinforcement schedules as treatment for aberrant behavior. *Journal of Applied Behavior Analysis, 29*(1), 43–51.

Martens, B. K., Gertz, L. E., de Lacy Werder, C. S., & Rymanowski, J. L. (2010). Agreement between descriptive and experimental analyses of behavior under naturalistic test conditions. *Journal of Behavioral Education, 19*(3), 205–221.

Matson, J. L., & Boisjoli, J. A. (2007). Multiple versus single maintaining factors of challenging behaviors as assessed by the QABF for adults with intellectual disabilities. *Journal of Intellectual and Developmental Disability, 32*(1), 39–44.

Matson, J. L., Kozlowski, A. M., Worley, J. A., Shoemaker, M. E., Sipes, M., & Horovitz, M. (2011). What is the evidence for environmental causes of challenging behaviors in persons with intellectual disabilities and autism spectrum disorders? *Research in Developmental Disabilities, 32*(2), 693–698.

Matson, J. L., Sipes, M., Horovitz, M., Worley, J. A., Shoemaker, M. E., & Kozlowski, A. M. (2011). Behaviors and corresponding functions addressed via functional assessment. *Research in Developmental Disabilities, 32*(2), 625–629.

Matson, J. L., & Vollmer, T. R. (1995). *User's guide: Questions about behavioral function (QABF).* Baton Rouge, LA: Scientific Publishers.

McIntosh, K., Brown, J. A., & Borgmeier, C. J. (2008). Validity of functional behavior assessment within a response to intervention framework: Evidence, recommended practice, and future directions. *Assessment for Effective Intervention, 34*(1), 6–14.

McLay, L., France, K., Blampied, N., & Hunter, J. (2019). Using functional behavioral assessment to treat sleep problems in two children with autism and vocal stereotypy. *International Journal of Developmental Disabilities, 65*(3), 175–184.

Monlux, K. D., Pollard, J. S., Bujanda Rodriguez, A. Y., & Hall, S. S. (2019). Telehealth delivery of function-based behavioral treatment for problem behaviors exhibited by boys with fragile X syndrome. *Journal of Autism and Developmental Disorders, 49*(6), 2461–2475.

Neely, L., Rispoli, M., Gerow, S., & Ninci, J. (2015). Effects of antecedent exercise on academic engagement and stereotypy during instruction. *Behavior Modification, 39*(1), 98–116.

Neidert, P. L., Iwata, B. A., Dempsey, C. M., & Thomason-Sassi, J. L. (2013). Latency of response during the functional analysis of elopement. *Journal of Applied Behavior Analysis, 46*(1), 312–316.

Newcomb, E. T., Wright, J. A., & Camblin, J. G. (2019). Assessment and treatment of aggressive behavior maintained by access to physical attention. *Behavior Analysis: Research and Practice, 19*(3), 222.

Newman, I., Leader, G., Chen, J. L., & Mannion, A. (2015). An analysis of challenging behavior, comorbid psychopathology, and Attention-Deficit/Hyperactivity Disorder in Fragile X Syndrome. *Research in Developmental Disabilities, 38*, 7–17.

Northup, J., Wacker, D., Sasso, G., Steege, M., Cigrand, K., Cook, J., & DeRaad, A. (1991). A brief functional analysis of aggressive and alternative behavior in an outclinic setting. *Journal of Applied Behavior Analysis, 24*(3), 509–522.

O'Reilly, M., Fragale, C., Gainey, S., Kang, S., Koch, H., Shubert, J., ... Van Der Meer, L. (2012). Examination of an antecedent communication intervention to reduce tangibly maintained challenging behavior: A controlled analog analysis. *Research in Developmental Disabilities, 33*(5), 1462–1468.

O'Reilly, M., Rispoli, M., Davis, T., Machalicek, W., Lang, R., Sigafoos, J., ... Didden, R. (2010). Functional analysis of challenging behavior in children with autism spectrum disorders: A summary of 10 cases. *Research in Autism Spectrum Disorders, 4*(1), 1–10.

O'Reilly, M., Sigafoos, J., Lancioni, G., Edrisinha, C., & Andrews, A. (2005). An examination of the effects of a classroom activity schedule on levels of self-injury and engagement for a child with severe autism. *Journal of Autism and Developmental Disorders, 35*(3), 305–311.

O'Reilly, M. F., Edrisinha, C., Sigafoos, J., Lancioni, G., & Andrews, A. (2006). Isolating the evocative and abative effects of an establishing operation on challenging behavior. *Behavioral Interventions, 21*(3), 195–204.

O'Reilly, M. F., Lacey, C., & Lancioni, G. E. (2000). Assessment of the influence of background noise on escape-maintained problem behavior and pain behavior in a child with Williams syndrome. *Journal of Applied Behavior Analysis, 33*(4), 511–514.

O'Reilly, M. F., Lacioni, G. E., King, L., Lally, G., & Nic Dhomhnaill, O. (2000). Using brief assessments to evaluate aberrant behavior maintained by attention. *Journal of Applied Behavior Analysis, 33*(1), 109–122.

O'Reilly, M. F., Sigafoos, J., Lancioni, G., Rispoli, M., Lang, R., Chan, J., & Langthorne, P. (2008). Manipulating the behavior-altering effect of the motivating operation: Examination of the influence on challenging behavior during leisure activities. *Research in Developmental Disabilities, 29*(4), 333–340.

Obi, C. (1997). Restraint fading and alternate management strategies to treat a man with Lesch–Nyhan syndrome over a 2-year period. *Behavioral Interventions, 12*(4), 195–202.

Olive, M. L., Lang, R. B., & Davis, T. N. (2008). An analysis of the effects of functional communication and a voice output communication aid for a child with autism spectrum disorder. *Research in Autism Spectrum Disorders, 2*(2), 223–236.

O'Neill, R. E., Horner, R. H., Albin, R. W., Sprague, J. R., Storey, K., & Newton, J. S. (1997). *Functional assessment of problem behavior: A practical assessment guide* (2nd ed.). Pacific Grove, CA: Brooks/Cole Publishing.

O'Neill, R. E., Horner, R. H., Albin, R. W., Storey, K., & Sprague, J. R. (1990). *Functional analysis of problem behavior: A practical assessment guide*. Sycamore, IL: Sycamore Publishing Company.

Paclawskyj, T. R., Matsol, J. L., Rush, K. S., Smalls, Y., & Vollmer, T. R. (2000). Questions about behavioral function (QABF): A behavioral checklist for functional assessment of aberrant behavior. *Research in Developmental Disabilities, 21*(3), 223–229.

Patel, M. R., Carr, J. E., Kim, C., Robles, A., & Eastridge, D. (2000). Functional analysis of aberrant behavior maintained by automatic reinforcement: assessments of specific sensory reinforcers. *Research in Developmental Disabilities, 21*(5), 393–407.

Peck, S. M., Wacker, D. P., Berg, W. K., Cooper, L. J., Brown, K. A., Richman, D., ... Millard, T. (1996). Choice-making treatment of young children's severe behavior problems. *Journal of Applied Behavior Analysis, 29*(3), 263–290.

Perou, R., Bitsko, R. H., Blumberg, S. J., Pastor, P., Ghandour, R. M., Gfroerer, J. C., & Huang, L. N. (2013). Mental health surveillance among children–United States, 2005–2011. *Morbidity and Mortality Weekly Report, 62*(Suppl. 2), 1–35.

Petrovic, M. A., & Scholl, A. T. (2018). Why we need a single definition of disruptive behavior. *Cureus, 10*(3), e2339.

Petursdottir, A. I., Esch, J. W., Sautter, R. A., & Kelise, K. S. (2010). Characteristics and Hypothesized Functions of Challenging Behavior in a Community-Based Sample. *Education and Training in Autism and Developmental Disabilities, 45*(1), 81–93.

Petursson, P. I., & Eldevik, S. (2018). Functional analysis and communication training to reduce problem behavior and time in restraint: A case study. *Behavior Analysis: Research and Practice, 19*(1), 114–122.

Phillips, L. A., Briggs, A. M., Fisher, W. W., & Greer, B. D. (2018). Assessing and treating elopement in a school setting. *Teaching Exceptional Children, 50*(6), 333–342.

Piazza, C. C., Adelenis, J. D., Hanley, G. P., Goh, H., & Delia, M. D. (2000). An evaluation of the effects of matched stimuli on behaviors maintained by automatic reinforcement. *Journal of Applied Behavior Analysis, 33*(1), 13–17.

Piazza, C. C., Hanley, G. P., Bowman, L. G., Ruyter, J. M., Lindauer, S. E., & Saiontz, D. M. (1997). Functional analysis and treatment of elopement. *Journal of Applied Behavior Analysis, 30*(4), 653–672.

Potoczak, K., Carr, J. E., & Michael, J. (2007). The effects of consequence manipulation during functional analysis of problem behavior maintained by negative reinforcement. *Journal of Applied Behavior Analysis, 40*(4), 719–724.

Poulou, M. S. (2013). Emotional and behavioral difficulties in preschool. *Journal of Child and Family Studies, 24*(2), 225–236.

Radstaak, M., Didden, R., Lang, R., O'Reilly, M., Sigafoos, J., Lancioni, G. E., … Curfs, L. M. G. (2013). Functional analysis and functional communication training in the classroom for three children with Angelman syndrome. *Journal of Developmental and Physical Disabilities, 25*(1), 49–63.

Radstaak, M., Didden, R., Oliver, C., Allen, D., & Curfs, L. M. G. (2012). Functional analysis and functional communication training in individuals with Angelman syndrome. *Developmental Neurorehabilitation, 15*(2), 91–104.

Rahman, B., Alderman, N., & Oliver, C. (2013). Use of the structured descriptive assessment to identify possible functions of challenging behaviour exhibited by adults with brain injury. *Neuropsychological Rehabilitation, 23*(4), 501–527.

Rahman, B., Oliver, C., & Alderman, N. (2010). Descriptive analysis of challenging behaviours shown by adults with acquired brain injury. *Neuropsychological Rehabilitation, 20*(2), 212–238.

Rapp, J. T., Patel, M. R., Ghezzi, P. M., O'Flaherty, C. H., & Titterington, C. J. (2009). Establishing stimulus control of vocal stereotypy displayed by young children with autism. *Behavioral Interventions: Theory & Practice in Residential & Community-Based Clinical Programs, 24*(2), 85–105.

Rapp, J. T., & Vollmer, T. R. (2005). Stereotypy I: A review of behavioral assessment and treatment. *Research in Developmental Disabilities, 26*(6), 527–547.

Reed, G. K., Ringdahl, J. E., Wacker, D. P., Barretto, A., & Andelman, M. S. (2005). The effects of fixed-time and contingent schedules of negative reinforcement on compliance and aberrant behavior. *Research in Developmental Disabilities, 26*(3), 281–295.

Reese, R. M., Richman, D. M., Belmont, J. M., & Morse, P. (2005). Functional characteristics of disruptive behavior in developmentally disabled children with and without autism. *Journal of Autism and Developmental Disorders, 35*(4), 419–428.

Richman, D. M., Wacker, D. P., Asmus, J. M., & Casey, S. D. (1998). Functional analysis and extinction of different behavior problems exhibited by the same individual. *Journal of Applied Behavior Analysis, 31*(3), 475–478.

Richman, D. M., Wacker, D. P., Asmus, J. M., Casey, S. D., & Andelman, M. (1999). Further analysis of problem behavior in response class hierarchies. *Journal of Applied Behavior Analysis, 32*(3), 269–283.

Rispoli, M., Ninci, J., Burke, M. D., Zaini, S., Hatton, H., & Sanchez, L. (2015). Evaluating the accuracy of results for teacher implemented trial-based functional analyses. *Behavior Modification, 39*(5), 627–653.

Rispoli, M., O'Reilly, M., Lang, R., Sigafoos, J., Mulloy, A., Aguilar, J., & Singer, G. (2011). Effects of language of implementation on functional analysis outcomes. *Journal of Behavioral Education, 20*(4), 224–232.

Roberts-Gwinn, M. M., Luiten, L., Derby, K. M., Johnson, T. A., & Weber, K. (2001). Identification of competing reinforcers for behavior maintained by automatic reinforcement. *Journal of Positive Behavior Interventions, 3*(2), 83–87.

Rojahn, J., Zaja, R. H., Turygin, N., Moore, L., & Van Ingen, D. J. (2012). Functions of maladaptive behavior in intellectual and developmental disabilities: Behavior categories and topographies. *Research in Developmental Disabilities, 33*(6), 2020–2027.

Romani, P. W., Donaldson, A. M., Ager, A. J., Peaslee, J. E., Garden, S. M., & Ariefdjohan, M. (2019). Assessment and treatment of aggression during public outings. *Education and Treatment of Children, 42*(3), 345–359.

Rose, J. C., & Beaulieu, L. (2019). Assessing the generality and durability of interview-informed functional analyses and treatment. *Journal of Applied Behavior Analysis, 52*(1), 271–285.

Sasso, G. M., Reimers, T. M., Cooper, L. J., Wacker, D., Berg, W., Steege, M., … Allaire, A. (1992). Use of descriptive and experimental analyses to identify the functional properties of aberrant behavior in school settings. *Journal of Applied Behavior Analysis, 25*(4), 809–821.

Scalzo, R., & Davis, T. N. (2017). Analysis of behavioral indicators as a measure of satiation. *Behavior Modification, 41*(2), 308–322.

Scheithauer, M., Cariveau, T., Call, N. A., Ormand, H., & Clark, S. (2016). A consecutive case review of token systems used to reduce socially maintained challenging behavior in individuals with intellectual and developmental delays. *International Journal of Developmental Disabilities, 62*(3), 157–166.

Scheithauer, M. C., Mevers, J. E. L., Call, N. A., & Shrewsbury, A. N. (2017). Using a test for multiply maintained self-injury to develop function-based treatments. *Journal of Developmental and Physical Disabilities, 29*(3), 443–460.

Schmidt, J. D., Drasgow, E., Halle, J. W., Martin, C. A., & Bliss, S. A. (2014). Discrete-trial functional analysis and functional communication training with three individuals with autism and severe problem behavior. *Journal of Positive Behavior Interventions, 16*(1), 44–55.

Schmidt, J. D., Shanholtzer, A., Mezhoudi, N., Scherbak, B., & Kahng, S. (2014). The utility of a brief experimental analysis for problem behavior maintained by escape from demands. *Education and Treatment of Children, 37*(2), 229–247.

Schreibman, L., Heyser, L., & Stahmer, A. (1999). Autistic disorder: Characteristics and behavioral treatment. In *Challenging behavior of persons with mental health disorders and severe disabilities* (pp. 39–63). Washington, DC: American Association of Mental Retardation.

Schroeder, S. R., Richman, D. M., Abby, L., Courtemanche, A. B., & Oyama-Ganiko, R. (2014). Functional analysis outcomes and comparison of direct observations and informant rating scales in the assessment of severe behavior problems of infants and toddlers at-risk for developmental delays. *Journal of Developmental and Physical Disabilities, 26*(3), 325–334.

Sloneem, J., Oliver, C., Udwin, O., & Woodcock, K. A. (2011). Prevalence, phenomenology, aetiology and predictors of challenging behaviour in Smith-Magenis syndrome. *Journal of Intellectual Disability Research, 55*(2), 138–151.

Smith, C. E., Carr, E. G., & Moskowitz, L. J. (2016). Fatigue as a biological setting event for severe problem behavior in autism spectrum disorder. *Research in Autism Spectrum Disorders, 23*, 131–144.

Smith, R. G., & Churchill, R. M. (2002). Identification of environmental determinants of behavior disorders through functional analysis of precursor behaviors. *Journal of Applied Behavior Analysis, 35*(2), 125–136.

Sprague, J., Flannery, B., & Szidon, K. (1998). Functional analysis and treatment of mealtime problem behavior for a person with developmental disabilities. *Journal of Behavioral Education, 8*(3), 381–392.

Steege, M. W., Pratt, J. L., Wickerd, G., Guare, R., & Watson, T. S. (2019). *Conducting school-based functional behavioral assessments: A practitioner's guide*. New York: Guilford Publications.

Strachen, R., Shaw, R., Burrow, C., Horsler, K., Allen, D., & Oliver, C. (2009). Experimental functional analysis of aggression in children with Angelman syndrome. *Research in Developmental Disabilities, 30*(5), 1095–1106.

Strohmeier, C. W., Murphy, A., & O'Connor, J. T. (2017). Parent-informed test-control functional analysis and treatment of problem behavior related to combined establishing operations. *Developmental Neurorehabilitation, 20*(4), 247–252.

Swender, S. L., Matson, J. L., Mayville, S. B., Gonzalez, M. L., & McDowell, D. (2006). A functional assessment of hand mouthing among persons with severe and profound intellectual disability. *Journal of Intellectual and Developmental Disability, 31*(2), 95–100.

Tarbox, J., Wilke, A. E., Najdowski, A. C., Findel-Pyles, R. S., Balasanyan, S., Caveney, A. C., … Tia, B. (2009). Comparing indirect, descriptive, and experimental functional assessments of challenging behavior in children with autism. *Journal of Developmental and Physical Disabilities, 21*(6), 493–514.

Tassé, M. J. (2006). Functional behavioural assessment in people with intellectual disabilities. *Current Opinion in Psychiatry, 19*(5), 475–480.

Thomas, B. R., Charlop, M. H., Lim, N., & Gumaer, C. (2019). Measuring happiness behavior in functional analyses of challenging behavior for children with autism spectrum disorder. *Behavior Modification*. https://doi.org/10.1177/0145445519878673

Thompson, R. H., & Iwata, B. A. (2007). A comparison of outcomes from descriptive and functional analyses of problem behavior. *Journal of Applied Behavior Analysis, 40*(2), 333–338.

Toogood, S., Boyd, S., Bell, A., & Salisbury, H. (2011). Self-injury and other challenging behaviour at intervention and ten years on: A case study. *Tizard Learning Disability Review, 16*(1), 18–29.

Torres-Viso, M., Strohmeier, C. W., & Zarcone, J. R. (2018). Functional analysis and treatment of problem behavior related to mands for rearrangement. *Journal of Applied Behavior Analysis, 51*(1), 158–165.

Tucker, M., Sigafoos, J., & Bushell, H. (1998). Analysis of conditions associated with low rates of challenging behaviour in two adolescents with multiple disabilities. *Behavior Change, 15*(2), 126–139.

Vaughan, M., & Michael, J. (1982). Automatic reinforcement: An important but ignored concept. *Behavior, 10*(2), 217–227.

Vollmer, T. R., Iwata, B. A., Zarcone, J. R., Smith, R. G., & Mazaleski, J. L. (1993). The role of attention in the treatment of attention-maintained self-injurious behavior: Noncontingent reinforcement and differential reinforcement of other behavior. *Journal of Applied Behavior Analysis, 26*(1), 9–21.

Vollmer, T. R., Marcus, B. A., & LeBlanc, L. (1994). Treatment of self-injury and hand mouthing following inconclusive functional analyses. *Journal of Applied Behavior Analysis, 27*(2), 331–344.

Vollmer, T. R., Progar, P. R., Lalli, J. S., Van Camp, C. M., Sierp, B. J., Wright, C. S., … Eisenschink, K. J. (1998). Fixed-time schedules attenuate extinction-induced phenomena in the treatment of severe aberrant behavior. *Journal of Applied Behavior Analysis, 31*(4), 529–542.

Vollmer, T. R., Roane, H. S., Ringdahl, J. E., & Marcus, B. A. (1999). Evaluating treatment challenges with differential reinforcement of alternative behavior. *Journal of Applied Behavior Analysis, 32*(1), 9–23.

Wacker, D., Berg, W., Harding, J., & Cooper-Brown, L. (2004). Use of brief experimental analyses in outpatient clinic and home settings. *Journal of Behavioral Education, 13*(4), 213–226.

Wacker, D., Steege, M., Northup, J., Sasso, G., Berg, W., Reimers, T., & Donn, L. (1990). A component analysis of functional communication training across three topographies of severe behavior problems. *Journal of Applied Behavior Analysis, 23*(4), 417–429.

Wacker, D. P., Berg, W. K., Harding, J. W., Derby, K. M., Asmus, J. M., & Healy, A. (1998). Evaluation and long-term treatment of aberrant behavior displayed by young children with disabilities. *Journal of Developmental and Behavioral Pediatrics, 19*(4), 260–266.

Wacker, D. P., Harding, J., Cooper, L. J., Derby, K. M., Peck, S., Asmus, J., & Brown, K. A. (1996). The effects of meal schedule and quantity on problematic behavior. *Journal of Applied Behavior Analysis, 29*(1), 79–87.

Wacker, D. P., Lee, J. F., Padilla-Dalmau, Y. C., Kopelman, T. G., Lindgren, S. D., Kuhle, J., … Waldron, D. B. (2013). Conducting functional analyses of problem behavior via telehealth. *Journal of Applied Behavior Analysis, 46*(1), 31–46.

Waters, M. B., Lerman, D. C., & Hovanetz, A. N. (2009). Separate and combined effects of visual schedules and extinction plus differential reinforcement on problem behavior occasioned by transitions. *Journal of Applied Behavior Analysis, 42*(2), 309–313.

Watkins, N., & Rapp, J. T. (2013). The convergent validity of the questions about behavioral function scale and functional analysis for problem behavior displayed by individuals with autism spectrum disorder. *Research in Developmental Disabilities, 34*(1), 11–16.

White, P., O'Reilly, M., Fragale, C., Kang, S., Muhich, K., Falcomata, T., … Lancioni, G. (2011). An extended functional analysis protocol assesses the role of stereotypy in aggression in two young children with autism spectrum disorder. *Research in Autism Spectrum Disorders, 5*(2), 784–789.

Wilder, D. A., Kellum, K. K., & Carr, J. E. (2000). Evaluation of satiation-resistant head rocking. *Behavioral Interventions: Theory & Practice in Residential & Community- Based Clinical Programs, 15*(1), 71–78.

Wilhelm, S., Deckersbach, T., & Keuthen, N. (2003). Self-injurious skin picking: Clinical characteristics, assessment methods, and treatment modalities. *Brief Treatment and Crisis Intervention, 3*(2), 249–260.

Wilke, A. E., Tarbox, J., Dixon, D. R., Kenzer, A. L., Bishop, M. R., & Kakavand, H. (2012). Indirect functional assessment of stereotypy in children with autism spectrum disorders. *Research in Autism Spectrum Disorders, 6*(2), 824–828.

Williams, C. A., Angelman, H., Clayton-Smith, J., Driscoll, D. J., Hendrickson, J. E., Knoll, J. H. M., … Zori, R. T. (1995). Angelman syndrome: Consensus for diagnostic criteria. *American Journal of Medical Genetics, 56*(2), 237–238.

Chapter 5
Nature, Prevalence, and Characteristics of Challenging Behaviors in Functional Assessment

Rebekka C. W. Strand, Oda M. Vister, Sigmund Eldevik, and Svein Eikeseth

Introduction

Research has shown that individuals with a diagnosis of Autism Spectrum Disorder (ASD) and individuals with Intellectual Disabilities (ID) are at a higher risk of developing challenging behavior as compared other populations (Emerson et al., 2001; Holden & Gitlesen, 2006; Jang, Dixon, Tarbox, & Granpeesheh, 2011; Matson & Kozlowski, 2011; Murphy, Healy, & Leader, 2009; Simó-Pinatella et al., 2017). Behaviors typically classified as challenging are aggression, tantrums, hand mouthing, property destruction, stereotypic behaviors (SB), and self-injurious behaviors (SIB) (Emerson et al., 2001; Hong, Dixon, Stevens, Burns, & Linstead, 2018; Matson & Kozlowski, 2011). These behaviors may be damaging or life-threatening to the individual and/or to others. They are considered socially unacceptable, may result in an inability to socialize with peers and social stigma (Chezan, Gable, McWhorter, & White, 2017; Hong et al., 2018; Matson & Kozlowski, 2011; Matson & Nebel-Schwalm, 2007).

Challenging behavior may be defined as "culturally abnormal behavior(s) of such intensity, frequency or duration that the physical safety of the person or others is placed in serious jeopardy, or behavior which is likely to seriously limit or deny access to the use of ordinary community facilities" (Emerson & Einfeld, 2011, p. 7).

There are several ways to assess challenging behaviors. A common way is to use standardized assessment instruments to measure the presence and absence of different topographies of challenging behavior. Examples are the Aberrant Behavior Checklist (Aman, Singh, Stewart, & Field, 1985; Brinkley et al., 2007; Farmer & Aman, 2017), Behavior Problems Inventory (Rojahn, Matson, Lott, Esbensen, & Smalls, 2001), Overt Aggression Scale (OAS; Hellings et al., 2005), and Autism

R. C. W. Strand · O. M. Vister · S. Eldevik · S. Eikeseth (✉)
Department of Behavioral Science, Oslo Metropolitan University, Oslo, Norway
e-mail: sigmund.eldevik@oslomet.no; seikeset@oslomet.no

© Springer Nature Switzerland AG 2021
J. L. Matson (ed.), *Functional Assessment for Challenging Behaviors and Mental Health Disorders*, Autism and Child Psychopathology Series,
https://doi.org/10.1007/978-3-030-66270-7_5

Spectrum Disorders – Behavior Problems for Children (ASD – BPC; Matson, Gonzalez, & Rivet, 2008). However, few instruments are available to assess challenging behaviors in young children. Matson and Nebel-Schwalm (2007) argued that challenging behavior has not been considered important when diagnosing children with ASD and that there is a growing need to assess a broad range of challenging behaviors in this population. One assessment instrument, the ASD-BPC can reliably assess challenging behavior in children with ASD (Matson et al., 2008). However, more research is needed to develop reliable and valid instruments to assess challenging behavior in young children.

To understand the function of challenging behaviors and to allow function-based treatments, several assessments instruments have been developed. Instruments to assess the function of challenging behavior are the Motivation Assessment Scale (MAS; Durand & Crimmins, 1988) and the Questions about Behavioral Function (QABF; Matson et al., 2005; Matson & Wilkins, 2009; Singh et al., 2009).

In the Functional Assessment (FA) literature, dating back to the 1970s and 1980s, (Horner, 1994; Howlin et al., 1973; Iwata, Dorsey, Slifer, Bauman, & Richman, 1982), there are a multitude of studies addressing challenging behavior. Over the past three decades, major advances have been made in the FA of challenging behavior and in function-based interventions (Borrero & Borrero, 2008; Dunlap & Fox, 2011; Neidert, Dozier, Iwata, & Hafen, 2010; O'Reilly et al., 2010). Matson et al., (2011) found that the most reported functions of challenging behaviors are attention and escape.

They also found that challenging behaviors commonly have multiple functions (Bell & Fahmie, 2018; Matson et al., 2011). Similarly, Hong et al. (2018) found that escape was the most common function of challenging behavior in a sample of 3216 individuals. Hong et al. (2018) also found that function-based treatment generally results in 80–90% reduction in challenging behavior. Currently, FA based on applied behavior analysis is considered the treatment of choice for identifying the functions and treatment for challenging behavior (Bawazeer, Alhammadi, & Kelly, 2019; Hurl, Wightman, Haynes, & Virues-Ortega, 2016; Matson & Minshawi, 2007). It is no longer a question as to whether function-based treatments of challenging behavior are effective; it is a discussion of how to make it more accessible, efficient, and adaptable (Denis, Van den Noortgate, & Maes, 2011; Hanley, Jin, Vanselow, & Hanratty, 2014; Hong et al., 2018; Iwata et al., 1994; Jessel, Hanley, & Ghaemmaghami, 2019; Matson et al., 2011).

The literature is not clear on what type of challenging behavior that is most commonly reported in the FA literature (Hong et al., 2018; Murphy, Healy, & Leader, 2009). According to Matson et al. (2011), the most common topography of challenging behavior in the FA literature is aggressive behavior and SIB. However, Jang et al., (2011), found SB more prevalent, and Horner, Carr, Strain, Todd, and Reed (2002) found that tantrums and aggression were more commonly reported. Also, research has shown that most individuals with ASD exhibit more than one form of challenging behavior, but that in most cases one of these behaviors is more frequent than the others (Stevens et al., 2017).

The Prevalence in Literature

Researchers have shown that challenging behavior is relatively common in individuals with ASD and ID compared to typical developed individuals. Overall, the prevalence of challenging behavior among this population has been estimated to be between 10% and 15% (Didden et al., 2012; Emerson et al., 2001; Holden & Gitlesen, 2006; Lowe et al., 2007).

McCarthy et al. (2010) showed that individuals with both ID and ASD were more likely to engage in challenging behavior than individuals with ID. In this study, 87.9% of the participants engaged in challenging behavior. The participants were referrals for assessments. Studies on individuals with ASD have shown prevalence rates between 64.3% and 94% (Jang et al., 2011; McTiernan, Leader, Healy, & Mannion, 2011; Murphy et al., 2009). These samples consisted of participants who were receiving a form of therapy; this may explain the high rates of challenging behavior.

In this chapter, we describe most common types of challenging behavior, their definitions, topography, functions, and risk factors. In addition, the various effects of frequency and intensity will be reviewed. We will focus on aggressive behavior, SIB, and SB.

Aggressive Behavior

Aggression poses a significant challenge to caregivers, clinicians, and the individual affected (Baker, Blacher, Crnic, & Edelbrock, 2002). For example, individuals with ASD or ID who exhibit high levels of aggressive behaviors are more likely to become hospitalized (Mandell, 2008) and to be treated with psychotropic medication. Aggression may also limit independence, community engagement, and the possibility of forming social relationships (Benson & Aman, 1999).

Definition According to the Cambridge English Dictionary, aggression is defined as spoken or physical behavior that is threatening or involves harm to someone or something. When examining the literature on aggressive behavior in ASD and ID, Farmer and Aman (2011) noted that there is a lack of terminological consensus among researchers, partly because the label "aggression" is emotionally charged and involves moral and social judgments. Because of this, many have been reluctant to use the word aggressive, and this has led to the use of other types of labels with similar meanings such as explosive behavior, disruptive, or maladaptive behavior (Farmer & Aman, 2011).

Parke and Slaby (1983, p. 50) defined aggressive behavior as "behavior that is aimed at harming or injuring another person," which suggests some sort of intent. Similarly, Hartrup (2005) defined aggressive behavior as "intentional harm doing". As Farmer and Aman (2011) argues, these definitions have an attribution of intent. However, it is difficult to measure "intent." They suggest that paying special attention to the subtypes of aggressive behavior may solve the issue of intent. Another problem with the term "intent" is that individuals with ASD or ID to various extent lack the ability to understand other people's perspective, and it is difficult to "intend harm" if empathy or perspective-taking-skills are deficient.

Several articles avoid this problem by not explicitly defining aggression, and instead detail the effects of aggressive behavior on quality of life (Brosnan & Healy, 2011; Hill et al., 2014).

Fitzpatrick, Srivorakiat, Wink, Pedapati, and Erickson (2016) provided a definition of aggression and replaced "intent" with likelihood: "behavior that is threatening or likely to cause harm and may be verbal (e.g., threatening or cursing at another person) or physical (e.g., hitting, biting, or throwing objects at another person) (p. 1525). They also noted that a person with ASD or ID may demonstrate one form of aggressive behavior or many, with variable frequency, intensity, and duration.

Topography Matson and Rivert (2008) studied a group of 161 adults with ASD or PDD-NOS and 159 matched controls with ID. Using the Autism Spectrum Disorder – Behavior Problems for Adults (ASD – BPA; Matson, Terlonge, & González, 2006), the most frequent topography of aggressive behavior was yelling or shouting at others (29%), followed by physical aggression towards others (27.4%), property destruction (24.2%), banging on objects (22.6%), kicking objects (19.4%), throwing objects at others (16.1%), and ripping cloths (11.3%). The participants with PDD-NOS and the participants with ID scored significantly less frequent on these measures except from the categories "aggression towards other" and "ripping cloths". On these categories, there were no significant differences across diagnostic groups. Also, frequency of challenging behaviors increased with severity of ASD symptoms (Matson & Rivet, 2008).

Using Children's Scale for Hostility and Aggression: Reactive/Proactive (C-SHARP), Farmer and Aman (2011) assessed 121 individuals with ASD and 244 individuals with ID. The participants were between 3 and 21 years of age. The C-SHARP comprises five empirically derived subscales: Verbal Aggression, Bullying, Covert Aggression, Hostility, and Physical Aggression. Results showed that the participants with ASD scored significantly higher compared to the ID group on three of the subscales: Bullying, Hostility, and Physical Aggression. The items with the highest overall score were; Reacts impulsively (70.1%), Hot-headed (63.6%), and Slow to cool off (55%). Within the ASD group, children with Asperger's disorder were rated significantly higher on verbal aggressive behaviors than children with ASD (Farmer & Aman, 2011).

Frequency and intensity Research indicates that rates of aggressive behavior may be higher in individuals with ASD compared to typically developing peers and those with other developmental disabilities (Farmer & Aman, 2011; Matson & Rivet, 2008). Individuals with ASD and comorbid ID are more frequently aggressive as compared to individuals with ID alone (McClintock, Hall, & Oliver, 2003; Tsakanikos, Costello, Holt, Sturmey, & Bouras, 2007).

Prevalence When considering individuals with ASD, research has reported variable aggression prevalence rates. Kanne and Mazurek (2011) found that 56% of individuals with ASD ($N = 1380$) directed aggression toward caregivers and 32% directed aggression toward noncaregivers. The high-prevalence rate may be related to the definition of aggressive behavior. Other studies found a lower prevalence of aggression in ASD. Scores in the clinically significant range for aggression on the Child Behavior Checklist (CBCL:ref) were found in 22.5% of young children diagnosed with autistic disorder (Hartley, Sikora, & McCoy, 2008). In a population of adults with ASD and comorbid ID, 15–18% were found to engage in aggression toward others (Matson & Rivet, 2008).

Several studies have been conducted on the prevalence rate among individuals with ID (e.g., Cooper et al., 2009b; Emerson et al., 2001; Holden & Gitlesen, 2006; Pavlović, Žunić-Pavlović, & Glumbić, 2013; Ruddick, Davies, Bacarese-Hamilton, & Oliver, 2015; Simó-Pinatella et al., 2017). The reported prevalence rate has differed from 6.4% (Holden & Gitlesen, 2006) to 71.5% (Simó-Pinatella et al., 2017). Severity of ID has been associated with higher prevalence rates of aggressive behavior (Holden & Gitlesen, 2006; McTiernan et al., 2011). The studies report a great deal of variation in the prevalence of aggression in ID. More studies are therefore needed.

One study only included participants with ASD who received a form of intervention/treatment. They report that 56.3% of the participants showed aggressive behavior (McTiernan et al., 2011). It is likely that participants who receive a form a therapy show higher rates of aggressive behavior compared to those who do not.

In a sample of individuals with learning disability, the prevalence rate was 54% for aggression (Lowe et al., 2007). The rate is similar to what has been reported for both individuals with ID and ASD. The highest reported prevalence rate is among individuals with a genetic syndrome (Angelman, Cornelia de Lange, Cri du Chat, Fragile X, Lowe, Prader-Willi, & Smith Magenis) ranging from 52.8% to 85% (Arron, Oliver, Moss, Berg, & Burbidge, 2011; Newman, Leader, Chen, & Mannion, 2015). Only a few studies have been conducted on the prevalence rates in genetic syndromes and the prevalence rates vary. It is therefore difficult to give good estimates for the prevalence rates.

Function of Aggressive Behavior Newcomer and Lewis (2004) found that interventions informed by an FA are more effective than those that are not. When FA is not conducted, clinicians run the risk of applying inappropriate treatment and potentially worsening behavior. Healey, Brett, and Leader (2013) used the Questions about Behavioral Function (QABF) and experimental functional analysis to identify the function of aggressive behavior in individuals diagnosed with ASD. They found that aggressive behavior in most cases was maintained by escape and access to tangibles. Dawson, Matson, and Cherry (1998) examined aggression in adults (between 22 and 58 years old) with ASD, PDD-NOS, and profound intellectual disability. Using the QABF, they found that aggression was primarily maintained by attention for all three diagnostic groups. They suggest that the function of aggressive behavior may be associated with the particular maladaptive behavior displayed rather than diagnostic category.

Roscoe, Kindle, and Pence (2010) found that an initial FA did not yield conclusive outcomes and that modifications to conditions were necessary to determine the function of aggression in a 13-year-old girl diagnosed with pervasive developmental disorder. A preference assessment of conversational topics was conducted to identify topics that were highly preferred. After high-preferred and low-preferred conversation topics were included as conditions in the FA, results showed that social attention containing the highly preferred conversation topics maintained the aggressive behavior.

Reese, Richman, Belmont, and Morse (2005) conducted functional behavioral assessment interviews with parents of 23 children with ASD and 23 controls without ASD. Participants were pair-matched for CA, developmental age, and sex. The interviews suggested that control children's disruptive behavior typically functioned to gain attention or items, or to escape demands. This was also true for girls with ASD. For boys with ASD, disruptive behavior more often functioned to gain or maintain access to ritualistic or repetitive behaviors, or to avoid idiosyncratically aversive sensory stimuli (e.g., ordinary household noises). The authors argue that when conducting functional behavioral assessments, it is important to consider behavioral characteristics that are associated with sex and specific disorders or syndromes (Reese et al., 2005).

Embregts, Didden, Schreuder, Huitink, and Nieuwenhuijzen (2009) examined behavioral function for aggressive behavior in 87 individuals with moderate to borderline intellectual disability who lived in a residential facility. They used the QABF, and results show that in most cases aggression was maintained by attention, tangibles, or escape, or avoidance from aversive situations.

Research assessing the function of aggressive behavior is not conclusive, and hence, more research is needed to address this important topic. As it stands now, research suggests that aggression typically is maintained by social reinforcement in the form of access to tangibles and attention, or by escape from aversive situations. Sometimes, however, automatic reinforcement is involved, such as when aggressive behavior results in access to stereotyped and ritualistic behaviors. In the one study comparing different diagnostic categories of ASD, PDD-NOS, and profound intellectual disability, no difference in behavioral function across diagnosis was detected.

Risk factors Research has shown that aggression is associated with poor outcomes in ASD (Fitzpatrick et al., 2016). In contrast to findings in the typically developing population, gender has not been found to predict aggression in ASD (Farmer et al., 2015; Hartley et al., 2008). Also, social factors such as marital status and level of parent education, which have been associated with aggression in the typically developing population, do not predict of aggression in individuals with ASD (Kanne & Mazurek, 2011).

Language ability, IQ, and adaptive functioning predict aggression (Dominick, Davis, Lainhart, Tager-Flusberg, & Folstein, 2007; Sikora, & McCoy, 2008). Other studies, however, have reported different results. In a sample of 1380 children and adolescents with ASD, neither severity of ASD symptoms, intellectual functioning, or adaptive functioning were associated with aggression (Kanne & Mazurek, 2011).

Specific behaviors seem to be better predictors of aggression. In a large sample of individuals with ASD ($N = 1584$), Mazurek et al. (2013) found that self-injurious behavior, sleep problems, and sensory issues were strong predictors of aggression. Also, comorbid anxiety has been shown to be correlated with aggression in ASD (Gotham et al., 2013; Panju et al., 2015), and low and high levels of social anxiety predicted aggression in individuals with high-functioning ASD (Pugliese et al., 2013). Cognitive inflexibility, or an inability to shift attentional focus, has also been associated with aggression (Pugliese et al., 2014).

A number of factors are associated with aggressive behaviors in individuals with ID (Stith et al., 2009). These factors are lower cognitive ability, female gender, not living with a family carer, not having Down syndrome, having attention-deficit hyperactivity disorder, and having urinary incontinence (Cooper et al., 2009b; Kim, van den Bogaard, Nijman, Palmstierna, and Embregts (2018). Cooper et al. (2009b) found that over a quarter of the participants with ID and aggressive behavior gained full remission in the short to medium term, with others gaining partial remission. Nevertheless, there is much to learn about the etiology and maintenance of aggressive behavior in this population as well as for the ASD population.

Adverse consequences Aggression is associated with a number of negative outcomes for individuals with ASD and ID (Kanne & Mazurek, 2011). These behaviors include impaired social relationships (Benson & Aman, 1999; Luiselli, 2009), higher risk of being placed in restrictive school or residential settings (Dryden-Edwards & Combrinck-Graham, 2010,), increased risk of being victimized (Smith et al., 2009), and the use of physical intervention (Dagnan & Weston, 2006). Aggressive behaviors can also contribute to school provider burnout leading to probable impact on the quality of education (Otero-López et al., 2009). Aggression also contributes to negative outcomes for caregivers, including increased stress levels (Neece, Green, & Baker, 2012), financial difficulties, lack of support services, and negative impact on day-to-day family life and well-being (Hodgetts, Nicholas, & Zwaigenbaum, 2013). Clearly, addressing aggressive behavior is pivotal to improving outcomes for individuals with ASD and ID and their caregivers (Fitzpatrick et al., 2016). Interventions informed by FA are an effective technology for achieving this goal.

Self-Injurious Behavior

SIB is perhaps the most devastating type of challenging behavior (Rattaz, Michelon, & Baghdadli, 2015). In contrast to aggressive behavior, where the challenging behavior is directed against other people or someone's property, SIB is directed against the individual who is engaging in the behavior.

Definition SIB has been defined as "Behavior that produces or has the capacity to produce tissue damage to the individual's own body." (Smith, Vollmer, & St Peter Pipkin, 2007, p. 188). Arguably, this definition does not take into the account that an instance of hitting oneself in the head once, for example, could be the result of an unlucky accident. Each time the behavior is repeated, however, the likelihood that the behavior occurs by chance is reduced. Hence, it has been argued that the definition should include repetitiveness. Tate and Baroff (1966, p. 281) argue for this as they describe SIB as "... a series of self-injurious responses (SIRs) that are repetitive and sometimes rhythmical..."

Conscious suicidal intents and behaviors evoked by sexual arousal as defined by Winchel and Stanley (1991), have typically been excluded when defining SIB in the FA literature (Winchel & Stanley, 1991). Weiss (2003) argued that acts associated with suicide, sexual arousal, or socially sanctioned practices are distinct from the behavior observed in people with ASD and ID. It has therefore been agreed that these behaviors should not be defined as SIB (Minshawi, Hurwitz, Morriss, & McDougle, 2015; Rojahn, Whittaker, Hoch, & González, 2007; Smith et al., 2007; Tate & Baroff, 1966).

Some have argued for including the degree of damage caused by the behavior when defining SIB, as some high-frequent repetitive behaviors might cause minor tissue damage (such as light nail biting) whereas other high-frequency behaviors could result in damage that needs immediate medical attention (such as when someone is hitting their head on a metal- edged table; Minshawi et al., 2015). On the other hand, this could exclude some types of SIB that might not cause harmful consequences to the individual in the short-term, but might potentially do so in the long-term, such as pica, vomiting, and rumination (Matson, 2012, p. 27). Assessing the severity of the SIB is very important when designing interventions. Certain dangerous forms of SIB may require immediate attention and perhaps sometimes more restrictive interventions. However, including a specific scale in the definition of SIB may be troublesome and limiting, and should therefore be discussed further.

Recently, Morano, Ruiz, Hwang, Wertalik, Moeller, Karal, and Mulloy (2017) proposed a similar definition to Yates (2004) in that self-injurious behavior must be deemed socially unacceptable. They defined SIB as "... behaviors that cause unintentional, self-inflicted, socially unacceptable physical injury to the individual's own body". This definition, however, does not include anything about repetitive behavior, it also refers to some sort of intention which might be misleading, but including socially unacceptability in the definition may be important, and should be considered in further research.

Recently, Huisman, Mulder, Kuijk, Kersholt, van Eeghen, Leenders, Balkom, Oliver, Piening, and Jennekam (2018) discussed the prevalence of SIB in genetic syndromes. They proposed a definition of SIB based on definitions by Tate and Baroff (1966) and Wolff, Hazlett, Lightbody, Reiss, and Piven (2013) using the following criteria for a definition of SIB: the behavior is directed towards the body, the actor himself-herself exhibits the behavior, reoccurrence, topography, chronometrics, severity, and exclusion of intention of suicide or sexual arousal. Based on this, Huisman et al. (2018) proposed the following definition "non-accidental behavior resulting in demonstrable, self-inflicted physical injury, without intent of suicide or sexual arousal. Typically, the behavior is repetitive and persistent." With the inclusion of chronometrics, topography, and severity, this definition is precise and clear. However, measuring the difference between nonaccidental and accidental behavior can complicate the measurement of SIB, and this dimension of Huisman et al.'s (2018) definition needs to be researched further.

For the purpose of this chapter, we define SIB as *repetitive behavior resulting in demonstrable, self-inflicted physical injury, without intent of suicide or sexual arousal.*

Topography In the FA literature, there are numerous behaviors described that fall within the definition of SIB. Most commonly described are head banging or hitting, self-biting, scratching, body banging or hitting, hair or nail pulling, inserting in orifice, and picking, rubbing, poking ears, eyes, and/or skin, and/or a combination of two or more of these (Baghdadli, Pascal, Grisi, & Aussilloux, 2003; Hong et al., 2018; Huisman et al., 2018; Iwata et al., 1994; Kurtz et al., 2003; Minshawi et al., 2015; Morano et al., 2017; Murphy, Hall, Oliver, & Kissi-Debra, 1999). Less common is pica, mouthing, crushing or snapping neck, vomiting/rumination, excessive drinking, and air swallowing (Huisman et al., 2018). The topography of SIB only describes the forms and visual aspect of the behavior however, a behavior like scratching could in one instance only affect the individual with light white marks on their skin, but if the frequency or intensity of the scratching increases, the scratching may lead to bloody open scars that may cause deadly infections.

Frequency and Intensity Summers et al. (2017) suggested that frequency and intensity are on a continuum, ranging from mild and infrequent to severe and chronic. In other words, frequency and intensity are highly correlated with the severity of SIB and the consequences the behavior has for the individual. The measure of frequency and intensity of SIB has been used for defining severity (Oliver, Petty, Ruddick, & Bacarese-Hamilton, 2012). Poppes, Putten, and Vlaskamp (2010) found that SIB typically occurs daily or weekly in individuals with ASD. The higher the frequency or/and intensity of SIB, the more likely it is that the behavior will have severe consequences for the individual.

In some ways, frequency and severity of SIB are synonymous. However, there is also low-frequency, but very high-intensity SIB, which can be just as severe as high-frequency SIB. It will always be important to look at each type of SIB and measure both the intensity and frequency when assessing its severity. The social significance of SIB is an important aspect, which is not always included when analyzing data. But, in some cases this may be just as important.

Function of SIB Iwata et al. (1994) summarized data from 152 single-subject analysis of the reinforcing function of SIB. They found that the largest proportion of their sample, 38.1%, exhibited SIB under negative reinforcement (to escape from aversive stimuli). Further, positive reinforcement, access to food or materials, accounted for 26.3% of their sample. Automatic reinforcement accounted for 25.7% and multiple controlling variables accounted for the rest, 5.3%. These are similar to the results reported by Matson et al., (2011) and Hong et al., (2018).

Prevalence and SIB Risk Factors in ASD and ID Research has shown that the populations with ASD and ID are at a higher risk for developing SIB at some point in their lifetime compared to the general population (Baghdadli et al., 2003; Cooper et al., 2009a; Dimian et al., 2017; Duerden, Oatley, Mak-Fan, McGrath, Taylor, Szatmari, & Roberts, 2012). Erturk, Machalicek, and Drew (2018) found that between 4% and 53% of children with ASD or developmental disabilities have engaged in at least a single topography of SIB.

There are a number of risk factors for SIB in the ASD and ID populations (Baghdadli et al., 2003; Barnard-Brak, Rojahn, Richman, Chesnut, & Wei, 2015; Cooper et al., 2009a; Duerden et al., 2012; Erturk et al., 2018; Kozlowski, Matson, & Rieske, 2012; Matson & Rivet, 2008; Murphy et al., 2009; Sigafoos, Arthur, & O'Reilly, 2003). For the purpose of this chapter, we discuss the risk factors that have been the most frequently reported in the literature, and the prevalence of these risk factors in the population with ASD and/or ID.

ASD Diagnosis A comorbid diagnosis of ID increases the risk of SIB in individuals with ASD (Matson & LoVullo, 2008). Furthermore, McTiernan, Leader, Healy, and Mannion (2011) studied the relationship between IQ and SIB in 174 children with ASD. They found that about half of the children with SIB had a lower IQ. These children also had higher severity and frequency of SIB. Dimian et al. (2017) studied 235 infants to examine if the presence of SIB, proto-SIB (i.e., potentially SIB topographies not causing tissue damage), and lower developmental functioning at age 12 months, could predict SIB in 2-year-old children at high familiar risk of ASD. They found that the presence of SIB, proto-SIB, and lower developmental functioning significantly predicted SIB at 24 months. They also found that children who received a diagnosis of ASD at 24 months had 1.85 times higher risk of developing SIB than those who did not receive the diagnosis.

For individual with ASD, the prevalence of SIB varies from 27.4% to 53% (Akram, Batool, Rafi, & Akram, 2017; Baghdadli et al., 2003; Dominick et al., 2007; Jang et al., 2011; Soke et al., 2016), with one study including participants that were receiving a form of intervention/treatment (48.9%, McTiernan et al., 2011).

Severity of ASD Symptoms Rattaz et al. (2015) found a strong correlation between the severity of ASD symptoms and the severity of SIB when studying 153 children with ASD. They also found that severity of ASD symptoms in childhood predicted the development of SIB in adolescence. The prevalence of the SIB seems to be higher among individuals with a higher degree of ASD (Baghdadli et al., 2003). However, only a few studies have divided the participants into groups depending on the severity. It is therefore difficult to know how the degree of ASD is affecting the prevalence rate of SIB. More research is therefore needed.

Severity of ID Studies on the prevalence of SIB among individuals with ID indicate that SIB occurs approximately in 10 to 12% of this population (Bienstein & Nussbeck, 2009; Emerson et al., 2001; Holden & Gitlesen, 2006; Lowe et al., 2007; van Ingen, Moore, Zaja, & Rojahn, 2010), ranging from 4% to 47.2% (Emerson et al., 2001; Holden & Gitlesen, 2006; Ruddick et al., 2015; Simó-Pinatella et al., 2017). The prevalence seems to vary depending on the severity of the diagnosis, with higher prevalence among individuals with a more severe ID (McClintock et al., 2003). As with ASD, there is a strong correlation between the severity of ID and the severity of SIB. Tureck, Matson, Cervantes, and Konst (2014) found that 25% of those with profound ID exhibited SIB as compared to only 4% in the individuals with a mild ID.

ASD vs. ID As mentioned above, the prevalence of SIB in the ID population is reported to be between 10% and 12%. This is generally lower than in the population with ASD, where the prevalence of SIB is reported to be between 27.4% and 53%. Individuals with ASD are therefore at a higher risk of developing SIB compared to persons with ID. Individuals with ASD frequently also are diagnosed with ID. It is therefore important to account for both when assessing the prevalence of SIB (Erturk et al., 2018). Furthermore, Tureck, Matson, and Beighley (2013) found that individuals with both ID and ASD have significantly higher rates of SIB than those with only one of the diagnosis.

Stereotypic Behavior Matson, Hamilton, Duncan, Bamburg, Smiroldo, Anderson, Baglio, Williams, and Kirkpatrick-Sanchez (1997) found that the participants with ID were more likely to show SIB and SB. They also found SB to be related to ASD. Furthermore, Oliver et al. (2012) found that high-frequency repetitive behavior was associated with a 16 times greater risk of severe self-injury and a 12 times higher risk of developing severe challenging behavior. Barnard-Brak et al. (2015) measured SB in 1871 children and adults with ID, and they found that 69% of the participants with SB developed SIB later on. They also found that certain topographies of SB (body rocking and yelling) seemed to predict specific forms of SIB (self-biting, head hitting, body hitting, self-pinching, and hair-pulling).

These studies show that it is important to study and target SB as a preventive treatment for SIB. Also, due to the correlation between SB and SIB, treatments of SIB should involve function-based interventions to reduce stereotyped behaviors (Matson & Lovullo, 2008; Morano et al., 2017). By targeting both SIB and repetitive behaviors, risks of increased SIB in the future may be reduced (Chezan et al., 2017).

Genetic syndromes We have found very few studies on the prevalence of SIB in genetic syndromes (Angelman, Cornelia de Lange, Cri du Chat, Fragile X, Lowe, Prader-Willi, and Smith Magenis). The prevalence rate ranges from 55.8% to 80% (Arron et al., 2011; Newman et al., 2015; Symons, Clark, Hatton, Skinner, & Bailey, 2003). Lowe et al. (2007) conducted a study on individuals with learning disability and found that 35% of the participants engaged in at least one form of SIB. SIB seems to be more common among individuals with a genetic syndrome than among individuals diagnosed with ASD, ID, or learning disability. However, more studies are needed to get better prevalence numbers for SIB in various genetic syndromes.

Age There has been conflicting evidence regarding the relation between age and SIB (Baghdadli et al., 2003; Murphy et al., 2009). Although there is a discrepancy in the literature, recent studies suggest no significant relationship between age and SIB (Matson et al., 2010; Murphy et al., 2009).

Gender Kozlowski et al. (2012) found that gender had no effect on the rates of challenging behavior in 391 children with and without ASD, who were between the age of 2 and 17 years. However, further research is needed on the relation between gender and SIB.

Adaptive Behavior There are reasons to argue that individuals with low-adaptive behavior are at a higher risk at developing SIB. Baghdadli et al. (2003) found that deficits in living skills were risk factors for SIB. Arguably, there is a correlation between the prevalence of SIB and low- adaptive functioning, but this could also be because low-adaptive functioning usually is correlated with low-intellectual functioning and perhaps even severity of diagnostic symptoms. Hence, more research is needed to assess which of these factors are related strongest (if any) to SIB.

Adverse Consequences of SIB Sadly, there are major adverse consequences of SIB, not only for the individuals affected, but also for their loved ones, and other people around them. In addition to the serious health risks, such as debilitating injuries, there are a number of other adverse consequences, both physical and social. One of the physical and social risks is that individuals with SIB are more likely to be in and out of hospitals, which in turn could expose them to other illnesses and/or make them isolated from their peers (Harwell & Bradley, 2019). Another adverse consequence is that individuals exhibiting SIB are more likely to be placed on heavy medication, which may produce severe side effects. They are also at a higher risk of being placed in restraints due to the severity of their behavior. The necessities and the consequences of restraints in treating SIB have been a hot topic of discussion (Elshalabi, 2015; Lundström, Antonsson, Karlsson, & Graneheim, 2011).

It is more likely that an individual with SIB will be isolated from society due to their SIB being socially unacceptable and physically restraining. The families of individuals with SIB are also at a higher risk for financial difficulties because of the cost of treatment and hospital visits (Denis et al., 2011). SIB is not only costly for the affected individuals and their families; but SIB also provides a financial burden to society. We were not able to find current estimates of the costs of treating SIB. In 1989, the cost of SIB in the US amounted to a staggering $100,000 per year per person (The National Institutes of Health, 1989).

Stereotypic Behavior

Stereotypical Behaviors in ASD and ID

One form of challenging behavior can be subsumed under the heading stereotyped behavior. Stereotyped behaviors are also referred to as "movements, acts, stereotypies, autisms, self-stimulatory behaviors, idiosyncratic mannerisms, and blindisms" (Rojahn & Sisson, 1990). Stereotyped behavior is one of two core criteria for a diagnosis of ASD, but it can also be seen in individuals with a number of other diagnoses and in most typical functioning individuals. In the context of this book chapter, we will only focus on SB that are challenging in the sense that the behaviors create problems and make daily life functioning difficult for the individual or the environment.

The definition of SB varies in scope. ICD-11 (World Health Organization, 2018) has a broad definition of SB in ASD: "a range of restricted, repetitive, and inflexible patterns of behavior and interests." However, in DSM-5 (American Psychiatric Association, 2013), SB is limited to: "Stereotyped or repetitive motor movements, use of objects, or speech (e.g., simple motor stereotypies, lining up toys or flipping objects, echolalia, idiosyncratic phrases)". This is one of four criteria listed under the heading: *"Restricted, repetitive patterns of behavior, interests, or activities"*. The other three criteria are *"Insistence on sameness, inflexible adherence to routines, or ritualized patterns of verbal or nonverbal behavior"*, *"Highly restricted, fixated interests that are abnormal in intensity or focus"*, and, *"Hyper- or hyperactivity to sensory input or unusual interests in sensory aspects of the environment"*. In DSM-5, two of these four categories of stereotypies need to be current or to be observed in the individual's history in order to fulfill the stereotypy criteria in the diagnosis of ASD. It is perhaps a matter of debate whether all of these categories can be subsumed under the heading stereotyped behaviors.

An analysis of verb terms used to describe the topography of SB in the published literature revealed an almost 40% overlap with obsessive behavior (e.g., lining insisting, flapping, repeating, touching). However, research has shown that the four categories found in the DSM-5 criteria often have the same function. Most commonly automatic reinforcement (Hong et al., 2018; Wilke et al., 2012), and therefore it can be useful to label them all as SB in clinical practice.

Prevalence and Topography

Since SB is a necessary criterion for a diagnosis of ASD, the prevalence rate should be 100%. However, the literature reports prevalence rates for SB between 27% and 92%. (McTiernan et al., 2011; Murphy et al., 2009; Simó-Pinatella et al., 2017). These studies include both participants with ID or ASD, and participants who were receiving a form of therapy. The large variation in prevalence rates may also reflect variations in how SB was defined (e.g., sometimes only including stereotypical movements and not other stereotypies such as gazing or insistence of sameness). For ID, the prevalence rates are reported at 55%.

Typical forms of SB for ASD include body rocking, hand/object mouthing, flapping hands, finger movements, repetitive vocalizations, grunting, humming, gazing at hands, objects, or lights (American Psychiatric Association, 2013). In one study, over 50 different categories of SB were described (LaGrow & Repp, 1984). Other topographies mentioned as examples in the DSM-5 include *"extreme distress at small changes, difficulties with transitions, rigid thinking patterns, greeting rituals, need to take same route or eat food every day"*, *"strong attachment to or preoccupation with unusual objects, excessively circumscribed or perseverative interest"*, and, *"apparent indifference to pain/temperature, adverse response to specific sounds or textures, excessive smelling or touching of objects, visual fascination with lights or movement"*.

SB is not only seen in ASD. But the manifestation may differ between individuals with ASD and individuals with ID. Higher occurrence, number, and variety of motor stereotypies are reported in children with ASD, in particular those children with lower nonverbal IQ scores, compared to a group of children with intellectual disability. Gazing at fingers and objects was only seen in children with ASD (Goldman et al., 2009).

Stereotypical Behaviors in Genetic Disorders: Prevalence and Topography

While the presence of SB is not a diagnostic criterion, it can be seen in a number of other DSM-5/ICD11 diagnoses. Moss, Oliver, Arron, Burbidge, and Berg (2009) used the term "Repetitive Behavior" and the Repetitive Behavior Questionnaire (RBQ; Moss & Oliver, 2008) to measure the form and prevalence rate of SB in a number of genetic syndromes. The items on the RBQ overlap strongly with the four DSM-5 criteria we subsumed under the heading SB above, indeed the RBQ was validated against the Autism Screening Questionnaire (Berument, Rutter, Lord, Pickles, & Bailey, 1999). The RBQ has five subscales: Stereotyped Behavior, Compulsive Behavior, Restricted Preferences, Repetitive Speech, and Insistence of Sameness. The study found that the topography of SB varied across syndromes, but some topographies were more common in certain syndromes. Fragile-X showed higher levels of hand-stereotypies, lining of objects, restricted conversation, preference for routines, and echolalia. Angelman's syndrome had low levels of specificity for repetitive behaviors, in contrast to some previous studies which have reported high levels of hand flapping (Summers et al., 1995). Very specific and unique stereotypies were reported in Cri-de-Chat and Smith-Magenis syndromes. Attachment to objects was reported in 67% of the individuals with Cri-de-Chat syndrome and attachment to people in 68% of the individuals with Smith-Magenis syndrome (Moss et al., 2009). Individuals with Lowe syndrome had high prevalence of lining up and hand stereotypies, whereas individuals with Cornelia de Lange had higher levels of tidying and lining up (Moss et al., 2009). In Prader-Willi syndrome, higher levels of hoarding and a preference for routine were reported along with repetitive questioning. Of note is that this study also included a heterogenous intellectual disability group (Down, Aicardi, Hypomelanosis, Landau Kleffner, Lennox

Gastrout, Miller Deikar, Pierre Robin, Rett and Soto syndromes, Cerebral Palsy, and Trisomy). In this group, there were no distinctive patterns of SB (Moss et al., 2009).

Stereotypical Behavior in Other Mental Health Disorders

There are a number of other diagnoses where SB is a necessary requirement. In common for most of these is that the diagnosis should only be used if the behaviors cannot be better explained by other neurodevelopmental disorders (such as ASD) and that it cannot be caused by the physiological effects of a substance or a neurological condition.

Stereotyped Movement Disorder (with or without self-injury) is placed under neurodevelopmental disorder both in the DSM-5 and ICD-11 (Stein & Woods, 2014). The behavior topographies overlap with those seen in ASD and ID (including body rocking, head banging, nail biting, tics, hand waving, and mouthing an object). There is no test that can be done set the diagnoses, but a thorough medical examination is recommended. Stereotypic Movement Disorder is most common in children with intellectual disability. In addition, both the ICD-11 and the DSM-5 have a cluster of diagnoses under the heading obsessive compulsive and related disorders (OCRD). In ICD-11, Obsessive Compulsive Disorder and the diagnosis Body-Focused Repetitive Behaviors (including trichotillomania and skin-picking) disorder are placed here. In DSM-5, trichotillomania and skin-picking are included under the OCRD cluster; however, the diagnosis Body-Focused Repetitive Behaviors are placed under the heading other specified forms of OCRD.

The prevalence for each of these conditions is reported to be between 1% and 2% (Harvard Medical School, 2007). The behaviors have some common features – regardless of how they are categorized. They are typically hard to stop, and they can result in injury (infections, bald spots, scarring). They cause distress and impair daily life functioning. The most promising treatment for all of these conditions is based on behavior analysis and includes habit reversal and forced exposure.

Limitations

The studies conducted on challenging behavior have resulted in different prevalence rates among individuals with ASD, ID, learning disability, and genetic syndromes. Challenging behavior can be divided into several subcategories: attacking others, destruction, aggression, SIB, stereotypes, and other destructive or disruptive behaviors. Studies have looked at different aspects of challenging behaviors when researching prevalence rate. This gives us an overview of the different aspects of challenging behaviors that are more likely to occur within the population, for example, SIB compared to aggressive behavior. However, studies have used different instruments to measure the same subcategory. This makes it difficult to compare the results. For example, Baghdadli et al. (2003) used a questionnaire about episodes of SIB where the behavior was rated as present or absent and in terms of its severity on a scale. McTiernan et al. (2011) used The Behavior Problem Inventory (BPI-01; Rojahn et al., 2001) to assess SIB, stereotypic, and aggressive/destructive behavior. The different instruments used may explain some of the differences in the reported prevalence rates. Future research should focus on developing a common methodology for studying the prevalence rates of challenging behaviors in ASD, ID, learning disability, and genetic syndromes.

Another limitation is that studies have analyzed and used different definitions of challenging behavior. The studies have focused on different aspect of challenging behavior. For example, Kanne & Mazurek (2011) looked at aggressive behavior towards caregivers and towards others, while Holden and Gitlesen (2006) looked at attacking others. Different definitions make it somewhat difficult to compare the results and make it more difficult to get a complete picture of the prevalence rates of challenging behavior. Again, future research should focus on developing common definitions. This would give us more information about the likelihood of challenging behavior associated with different diagnoses and will help us get a better understanding of the risk factors (Table 5.1).

Conclusion

In this chapter, we have reviewed the prevalence, nature, and characteristics of challenging behavior in individuals with ASD and/or ID and other mental health disorders. New studies have found some interesting results since the last published version of this chapter. For example; although aggressive behavior, SIB, and SB are challenging behaviors they all appear, in general, to have different functions, even though the topographies sometimes overlap. There are also ongoing discussions on the definitions of SIB and SB that take the measurement of these behaviors towards functional assessments (Hong et al., 2018).

There is a growing amount of studies published on the prevalence and associated factors of challenging behavior in children and adults with ASD and/or ID. However, due to the different definitions and measurement of challenging behavior, the rates of prevalence and associated factors vary. Although these new findings are steps towards a better understanding of challenging behavior, there are still disagreements and limitations such as, the definition of aggressive behavior. Despite this, it is clear that those individuals with ASD and/or ID are at risk for developing challenging behavior, and that these behaviors also add a "severity" to the diagnosis of ASD (Matson & Rivet, 2008).

The risk factors associated with challenging behavior are many. It is unclear to what extent these risk factors are a cause for challenging behavior. In spite of this, there is a strong correlation between ASD and/or ID and challenging behavior. Moreover, the risk of developing challenging behavior is particularly high in individuals with ASD and/or ID compared to other groups, and the adverse consequences that come with these behaviors are severe not only for the individual but

Table 5.1 A summary of studies showing prevalence rates for Challenging Behaviors

Disability	Prevalence rates	Procedure	Participants (N)	Country	Setting	Reference
Challenging behavior						
Intellectual Disability (ID)	10–15%	The Individual Schedule	Total population study	UK	Service setting	Emerson et al. (2001)
	11.1%	Challenging behavior survey: Individual schedule (simplified version)	Total population study (N – 904)	Norway – Hedmark	n.p.	Holden and Gitlesen (2006)
Autism Spectrum Disorder (ASD) (received intervention)	94%	Autism Spectrum Disorder– Behavior Problems	84	US	Service setting (CARD ABA)	Jang et al. (2011)
	93.7%	Behavior problems Inventory	174	Ireland	n.p.	McTiernan et al. (2011)
	64.3%	The Behavior Problems Inventory	157	Ireland	n.p.	Murphy et al. (2009)
Aggressive behavior						
ID	9.8%	C21st Health Check	1023	UK	n.p.	Cooper et al. (2009b)
	7%	The Individual Schedule	Total population study	UK	Service setting	Emerson et al. (2001)
	6.4%	Challenging behavior survey: Individual schedule (simplified version)	Total population study (N = 904)	Norway – Hedmark	n.p.	Holden and Gitlesen (2006)
	62%	Children's Scale of Hostility and Aggression: Reactive-Proactive Behavior Scale	100	Serbia	School	Pavlović et al. (2013)
	10.8%	Behavior Scale	94.3	UK	School	Ruddick et al. (2015)
	71.5%	Challenging Behavior Prevalence in Educational Settings: School Information	205	Spain	School	Simó-Pinatella et al. (2017)

(continued)

Table 5.1 (continued)

Disability	Prevalence rates	Procedure	Participants (N)	Country	Setting	Reference
ASD		Challenging Behavior Prevalence in Educational Settings: Individual Information				
	32.7%	The Atypical Behavior Patterns Questionnaire	67	US	Boston CPEA site	Dominick et al. (2007)
	22.5%	Child Behavior Checklist	605	US	Home	Hartley et al. (2008)
	56% towards caregivers 32% noncaregivers	Autism Diagnostic Interview—Revised	1380	US	n.p.	Kanne and Mazurek (2011)
ASD (received intervention/treatment)	56.3%	Behavior problems Inventory	174	Ireland	n.p.	McTiernan et al. (2011)
	15–18% towards others	Autism Spectrum Disorders – Behavior Problems for Adults with Intellectual Disabilities	298	US	Service setting	Matson and Rivet (2008)
Genetic Syndromes	52.8% aggression physical	The Challenging Behavior Questionnaire	797	US, UK, Ireland	Different associations	Arron et al. (2011)
	85%	The Behavior Problems Inventory – Short Form	47	n.p	Online forums and support groups	Newman et al. (2015)
Self-injurious behavior						
ID	4%	The Individual Schedule	Total population study	UK	Service setting	Emerson et al. (2001)
	4.4%	Challenging behavior survey: Individual schedule (simplified version)	Total population study ($N = 904$)	Norway – Hedmark	n.p.	Holden and Gitlesen (2006)

	5.3%	Behavior scale	94.3	UK	School	Ruddick et al. (2015)
	42.7%	Challenging Behavior Prevalence in Educational Settings: School Information	205	Spain	School	Simó-Pinatella et al. (2017)
		Challenging Behavior Prevalence in Educational Settings: Individual Information				
ASD	30%	Inventory of statements about self-injury	83	Pakistan	School	Akram et al. (2017)
	53%	Questionnaire about Self-Injury Behavior	222	France	n.p.	Baghdadli et al. (2003)
	32.7%	The Atypical Behavior patterns Questionnaire	67	US	Boston CPEA site	Dominick et al. (2007)
	27.7%	Health records	Total population study ($n = 8065$)	US	n.p.	Soke et al. (2016)
ASD (received intervention/ treatment)	48.9%	Behavior problems Inventory	174	Ireland	n.p.	McTiernan et al. (2011)
Genetic Syndromes	55.8%	The Challenging Behavior Questionnaire	797	US, UK, Ireland	Different associations	Arron et al. (2011)
	80%	The Behavior Problems Inventory – Short Form	47	n.p.	Online forums and support groups	Newman et al. (2015)
Stereotyped						
ID	55.3%	Challenging Behavior Prevalence in Educational Settings: School Information	205	Spain	School	Simó-Pinatella et al. (2017)

(continued)

Table 5.1 (continued)

Disability	Prevalence rates	Procedure	Participants (N)	Country	Setting	Reference
		Challenging Behavior Prevalence in Educational Settings: Individual Information				
ASD (received intervention/treatment)	92%	Behavior Problems Inventory	174	Ireland	n.p.	McTiernan et al. (2011)
	27%	The Behavior Problems Inventory	157	Ireland	n.p.	Murphy et al. (2009)
Genetic syndromes	1.8–71.1%	Repetitive Behavior Questionnaire	797	UK, US, Ireland	Support groups	Moss et al. (2009)
	100%	The Behavior Problems Inventory – Short Form	47	n.p.	Online forums and support groups	Newman et al. (2015)
Mental Health Disorders – Obsessive-Compulsive-Related Disorders (OCRD)	1–2%	National Comorbidity Survey	9282	US	Contact representative sample	Harvard Medical School (2007)

n.p. not provided

also for family and careers (Barnard-Brak et al., 2015; Rattaz et al., 2015; Dimian et al., 2017; Simó-Pinatella et al., 2017).

Function-based treatments and other treatments based on applied behavior analysis for CB continue to show good effects. For the clinician, it seems more important to assess the function of CB and stay abreast with the behavior analytic research, than it is to further discuss topographical definition of CB (Denis et al., 2011; Hong et al., 2018; Iwata et al., 1994; Matson, Shoemaker, et al., 2011).

References

Akram, B., Batool, M., Rafi, Z., & Akram, A. (2017). Prevalence and predictors of non suicidal self-injury among children with autism spectrum disorder. *Pakistan Journal of Medical Sciences, 33*, 1225–1229. https://doi.org/10.12669/pjms.335.12931

Aman, M. G., Singh, N. N., Stewart, A. W., &Field, C. J. (1985). The aberrant behavior checklist: A behavior-rating scale for the assessment of treatment effects. *American Journal of Mental Deficiency.*

American Psychiatric Association. (2013). *Diagnostic and statistical manual of mental disorders (DSM-5®).* American Psychiatric Pub.

Arron, K., Oliver, C., Moss, J., Berg, K., & Burbidge, C. (2011). The prevalence and phenomenology of self-injurious and aggressive behaviour in genetic syndromes. *Journal of Intellectual Disability Research, 55*, 109–120. https://doi.org/10.1111/j.1365-2788.2010.01337.x

Baghdadli, A., Pascal, C., Grisi, S., & Aussilloux, C. (2003). Risk factors for self-injurious behaviours among 222 young children with autistic disorders. *Journal of Intellectual Disability Research, 47*, 622–627. https://doi.org/10.1046/j.1365-2788.2003.00507.x

Baker, B. L., Blacher, J., Crnic, K. A., & Edelbrock, C. (2002). Behavior problems and parenting stress in families of three-year-old children with and without developmental delays. *American Journal on Mental Retardation, 107*, 433–444. https://doi.org/10.1352/0895-8017(2002)107%3c0433:BPAPSI%3e2.0.CO;2

Barnard-Brak, L., Rojahn, J., Richman, D. M., Chesnut, S. R., & Wei, T. (2015). Stereotyped behaviors predicting self-injurious behavior in individuals with intellectual disabilities. *Research in Developmental Disabilities, 36*, 419–427. https://doi.org/10.1016/j.ridd.2014.08.017

Bawazeer, A., Alhammadi, M., and Kelly, M. (2019). Functional behavior assessment for challenging behavior in individuals with Autism. Bok eller artikkel?

Bell, M. C., & Fahmie, T. A. (2018). Functional analysis screening for multiple topographies of problem behavior. *Journal of Applied Behavior Analysis, 51*, 528–537. https://doi.org/10.1002/jaba.462

Benson, B. A., & Aman, M. G. (1999). Disruptive behavior disorders in children with mental retardation. In H. C. Quay & A. E. Hogan (Eds.), *Handbook of disruptive behavior disorders* (pp. 559–578). Boston, MA: Springer. https://doi.org/10.1007/978-1-4615-4881-2_26

Berument, S. K., Rutter, M., Lord, C., Pickles, A., & Bailey, A. (1999). Autism screening questionnaire: Diagnostic validity. *The British Journal of Psychiatry, 175*, 444–451. https://doi.org/10.1192/bjp.175.5.444

Bienstein, P., & Nussbeck, S. (2009). Reliability of a German version of the questions about behavioral function (QABF) scale for self-injurious behavior in individuals with intellectual disabilities. *Journal of Mental Health Research in Intellectual Disabilities, 2*, 249–260. https://doi.org/10.1080/19315860903061809

Borrero, C. S., & Borrero, J. C. (2008). Descriptive and experimental analyses of potential precursors to problem behavior. *Journal of Applied Behavior Analysis, 41*, 83–96. https://doi.org/10.1901/jaba.2008.41-83

Brinkley, J., Nations, L., Abramson, R. K., Hall, A., Wright, H. H., Gabriels, R., ... Cuccaro, M. L. (2007). Factor analysis of the aberrant behavior checklist in individuals with autism spectrum disorders. *Journal of Autism and Developmental Disorders, 37*, 1949–1959. https:// doi.org/10.1007/s10803-006-0327-3

Brosnan, J., & Healy, O. (2011). A review of behavioral interventions for the treatment of aggression in individuals with developmental disabilities. *Research in Developmental Disabilities, 32*, 437–446. https://doi.org/10.1016/j.ridd.2010.12.023

Chezan, L. C., Gable, R. A., McWhorter, G. Z., & White, S. D. (2017). Current perspectives on interventions for self-injurious behavior of children with autism spectrum disorder: A systematic review of the literature. *Journal of Behavioral Education, 26*, 293–329. https://doi. org/10.1007/s10864-017-9269-4

Cooper, S. A., Smiley, E., Allan, L. M., Jackson, A., Finlayson, J., Mantry, D., & Morrison, J. (2009a). Adults with intellectual disabilities: Prevalence, incidence and remission of self-injurious behaviour, and related factors. *Journal of Intellectual Disability Research, 53*, 200–216. https://doi.org/10.1111/j.1365-2788.2008.01060.x

Cooper, S. A., Smiley, E., Jackson, A., Finlayson, J., Allan, L., Mantry, D., & Morrison, J. (2009b). Adults with intellectual disabilities: Prevalence, incidence and remission of aggressive behaviour and related factors. *Journal of Intellectual Disability Research, 53*, 217–232. https://doi. org/10.1111/j.1365-2788.2008.01127.x

Dagnan, D., & Weston, C. (2006). Physical intervention with people with intellectual disabilities: The influence of cognitive and emotional variables. *Journal of Applied Research in Intellectual Disabilities, 19*, 219–222. https://doi.org/10.1111/j.1468-3148.2005.00262.x

Dawson, J. E., Matson, J. L., & Cherry, K. E. (1998). An analysis of maladaptive behaviors in persons with Autism, PDD-NOS, and mental retardation. *Research in Developmental Disabilities, 19*, 439–448. https://doi.org/10.1016/S0891-4222(98)00016-X

Denis, J., Van den Noortgate, W., & Maes, B. (2011). Self-injurious behavior in people with profound intellectual disabilities: A meta-analysis of single-case studies. *Research in Developmental Disabilities, 32*, 911–923. https://doi.org/10.1016/j.ridd.2011.01.014

Didden, R., Sturmey, P., Sigafoos, J., Lang, R., O'Reilly, M. F., & Lancioni, G. E. (2012). Nature, prevalence, and characteristics of challenging behavior. In *Functional assessment for challenging behaviors* (pp. 25–44). New York, NY: Springer. https://doi.org/10.1007/978-1-4614-3037-7_3

Dimian, A. F., Botteron, K. N., Dager, S. R., Elison, J. T., Estes, A. M., Pruett, J. R., Schultz, R. T., Zwaigenbaum, L., Piven, J., Wolff, J. J., & Ibis Network. (2017). Potential risk factors for the development of self-injurious behavior among infants at risk for autism spectrum disorder. *Journal of Autism and Developmental Disorders, 47*(5), 1403–1415. https://doi.org/10.1007/s10803-017-3057-9

Dominick, K. C., Davis, N. O., Lainhart, J., Tager-Flusberg, H., & Folstein, S. (2007). Atypical Behaviors in children with Autism and children with a history of language impairment. *Research in Developmental Disabilities, 28*, 145–162. https://doi.org/10.1016/j.ridd.2006.02.003

Duerden, E. G., Oatley, H. K., Mak-Fan, K. M., McGrath, P. A., Taylor, M. J., Szatmari, P., & Roberts, S. W. (2012). Risk factors associated with self-injurious behaviors in children and adolescents with autism spectrum disorders. *Journal of Autism and Developmental Disorders, 42*(11), 2460–2470. https://doi.org/10.1007/s10803-012-1497-9. PMID: 22422338.

Dunlap, G., & Fox, L. (2011). Function-based interventions for children with challenging behavior. *Journal of Early Intervention, 33*, 333–343. https://doi.org/10.1177/1053815111429971

Durand, V. M., & Crimmins, D. B. (1988). Identifying the variables maintaining self-injurious behavior. *Journal of Autism and Developmental Disorders, 18*, 99–117. https://doi.org/10.1007/BF02211821

Dryden-Edwards, R. C., & Combrinck-Graham, L. (Eds.). (2010). *Developmental disabilities from childhood to adulthood: What works for psychiatrists in community and institutional settings*. Johns Hopkins University Press, Baltimore. ISBN: 978-0801894183

Elshalabi, R. S. (2015). Uncontrollable behavior and restraints policy analysis. *Middle East Journal of Nursing, 9*. https://doi.org/10.5742/mejn.2015.92650

Embregts, P. J. C. M., Didden, R., Schreuder, N., Huitink, C., & van Nieuwenhuijzen, M. (2009). Aggressive behavior in individuals with moderate to borderline intellectual disabilities who live in a residential facility: An evaluation of functional variables. *Research in Developmental Disabilities, 30,* 682–688. https://doi.org/10.1016/j.ridd.2008.04.007

Emerson, E., Kiernan, C., Alborz, A., Reeves, D., Mason, H., Swarbrick, R., ... Hatton, C. (2001). The prevalence of challenging behaviors: A total population study. *Research in Developmental Disabilities, 22,* 77–93. https://doi.org/10.1016/S0891-4222(00)00061-5

Emerson, E., & Einfeld, S. L. (2011). *Challenging behaviour.* Cambridge: Cambridge University Press.

Erturk, B., Machalicek, W., & Drew, C. (2018). Self-injurious behavior in children with developmental disabilities: A systematic review of behavioral intervention literature. *Behavior Modification, 42,* 498–542. https://doi.org/10.1177/0145445517741474

Farmer, C. A., & Aman, M. G. (2011). Aggressive behavior in a sample of children with autism spectrum disorders. *Research in Autism Spectrum Disorders, 5,* 317–323. https://doi.org/10.1016/j.rasd.2010.04.014

Farmer, C., & Aman, M. G. (2017). Aberrant behavior checklist. In: Volkmar F. (Eds.), *Encyclopedia of Autism Spectrum Disorders.* Springer, New York, NY. https://doi.org/10.1007/978-1-4614-6435-8_1632-3

Farmer, C., Butter, E., Mazurek, M. O., Cowan, C., Lainhart, J., Cook, E. H., ... Aman, M. (2015). Aggression in children with autism spectrum disorders and a clinic-referred comparison group. *Autism, 19*(3), 281–291. https://doi.org/10.1177/1362361313518995

Fitzpatrick, S. E., SrivorakiatL., Wink, L. K., Pedapati, E. V., &Erickson, C. A. (2016). Aggression in autism spectrum disorder: presentation and treatment options. Doi:https://doi.org/10.2147/NDT.S84585.

Goldman, S., Wang, C., Salgado, M. W., Greene, P. E., Kim, M., & Rapin, I. (2009). Motor stereotypies in children with autism and other developmental disorders. *Developmental Medicine & Child Neurology, 51,* 30–38. https://doi.org/10.1111/j.1469-8749.2008.03178.x

Gotham, K., Bishop, S. L., Hus, V., Huerta, M., Lund, S., Buja, A., ... & Lord, C. (2013). Exploring the relationship between anxiety and insistence on sameness in autism spectrum disorders. *Autism Research, 6,* 33–41.

Hanley, G. P., Jin, C. S., Vanselow, N. R., & Hanratty, L. A. (2014). Producing meaningful improvements in problem behavior of children with autism via synthesized analyses and treatments. *Journal of Applied Behavior Analysis, 47,* 16–36. https://doi.org/10.1002/jaba.106

Hartley, S. L., Sikora, D. M., & McCoy, R. (2008). Prevalence and risk factors of maladaptive behaviour in young children with autistic disorder. *Journal of Intellectual Disability Research, 52,* 819–829. https://doi.org/10.1111/j.1365-2788.2008.01065.x

Hartup, W. (2005). The development of aggression: Where do we stand? In R. Tremblay, W. Hartup, & J. Archer (Eds.), *The developmental origins of aggression* (pp. 83–106). New York: Guilford Press.

Harvard Medical School. (2007). National Comorbidity Survey (NCSSC). (2020, March 15). Retrieved from https://www.hcp.med.harvard.edu/ncs/index.php. Data Table 2: 12-month prevalence DSM-IV/WMH-CIDI disorders by sex and cohort.

Harwell, C., & Bradley, E. (2019). Caring for children with autism in the emergency department. *Pediatric Annals, 48,* e333–e336. https://doi.org/10.3928/19382359-20190725-01

Healy, O., Brett, D., & Leader, G. (2013). A comparison of experimental functional analysis and the questions about behavioral function (QABF) in the assessment of challenging behavior of individuals with autism. *Research in Autism Spectrum Disorders, 7,* 66–81. https://doi.org/10.1016/j.rasd.2012.05.006

Hellings, J. A., Nickel, E. J., Weckbaugh, M., McCarter, K., Mosier, M., & Schroeder, S. R. (2005). The overt aggression scale for rating aggression in outpatient youth with autistic disorder: Preliminary findings. *The Journal of Neuropsychiatry and Clinical Neurosciences, 17,* 29–35.

Hill, A. P., Zuckerman, K. E., Hagen, A. D., Kriz, D. J., Duvall, S. W., Van Santen, J., ... Fombonne, E. (2014). Aggressive behavior problems in children with autism spectrum disorders: Prevalence and correlates in a large clinical sample. *Research in Autism Spectrum Disorders, 8,* 1121–1133. https://doi.org/10.1016/j.rasd.2014.05.006

Hodgetts, S., Nicholas, D., & Zwaigenbaum, L. (2013). Home sweet home? Families' experiences with aggression in children with autism spectrum disorders. *Focus on Autism and Other Developmental Disabilities, 28*, 166–174. https://doi.org/10.1177/1088357612472932

Holden, B., & Gitlesen, J. P. (2006). A total population study of challenging behaviour in the county of Hedmark, Norway: Prevalence, and risk markers. *Research in Developmental Disabilities, 27*, 456–465. https://doi.org/10.1016/j.ridd.2005.06.001

Hong, E., Dixon, D. R., Stevens, E., Burns, C. O., & Linstead, E. (2018). Topography and function of challenging behaviors in individuals with autism spectrum disorder. *Advances in Neurodevelopmental Disorders, 2*, 206–215. https://doi.org/10.1007/s41252-018-0063-7

Horner, R. H. (1994). Functional assessment: contributions and future directions. *Journal of Applied Behavior Analysis, 27*, 401–404. https://doi.org/10.1901/jaba.1994.27-401

Horner, R. H., Carr, E. G., Strain, P. S., Todd, A. W., & Reed, H. K. (2002). Problem behavior. Interventions for Young Children with Autism: A Research Synthesis. *Journal of Autism and Developmental Disorders, 32*, 423–446. https://doi.org/10.1023/A:1020593922901

Howlin, P., Marchant, R., Rutter, M., Berger, M., Hersov, L., & Yule, W. (1973). A home-based approach to the treatment of autistic children. *Journal of Autism and Childhood Schizophrenia, 3*, 308–336. https://doi.org/10.1007/BF01538540

Huisman, S., Mulder, P., Kuijk, J., Kerstholt, M., van Eeghen, A., Leenders, A., … Hennekam, R. (2018). Self-injurious behavior. *Neuroscience & Biobehavioral Reviews, 84*, 483–491.

Hurl, K., Wightman, J., Haynes, S. N., & Virues-Ortega, J. (2016). Does a pre-intervention functional assessment increase intervention effectiveness? A meta-analysis of within-subject interrupted time-series studies. *Clinical Psychology Review, 47*, 71–84.

Iwata, B. A., Dorsey, M. F., Slifer, K. J., Bauman, K. E., & Richman, G. S. (1982). Toward a functional analysis of self-injury. *Analysis and Intervention in Developmental Disabilities, 2*, 3–20. https://doi.org/10.1016/0270-4684(82)90003-9

Iwata, B. A., Pace, G. M., Dorsey, M. F., Zarcone, J. R., Vollmer, T. R., Smith, R. G., … Willis, K. D. (1994). The functions of self-injurious behavior: An experimental-epidemiological analysis. *Journal of Applied Behavior Analysis, 27*, 215–240. https://doi.org/10.1901/jaba.1994.27-215

Jang, J., Dixon, D. R., Tarbox, J., & Granpeesheh, D. (2011). Symptom severity and challenging behavior in children with ASD. *Research in Autism Spectrum Disorders, 5*, 1028–1032. https://doi.org/10.1016/j.rasd.2010.11.008

Jessel, J., Hanley, G. P., & Ghaemmaghami, M. (2019). On the standardization of the functional analysis. *Behavior Analysis in Practice, 13*, 1–12. https://doi.org/10.1007/s40617-019-00366-1

Kanne, S. M., & Mazurek, M. O. (2011). Aggression in children and adolescents with ASD: Prevalence and risk factors. *Journal of Autism and Developmental Disorders, 41*, 926–937. https://doi.org/10.1007/s10803-010-1118-4

Kim, J. H. M., van den Bogaard, Nijman, H. L. I., Palmstierna, T., & Embregts, P. J. C. M. (2018). Characteristics of aggressive behavior in people with mild to borderline intellectual disability and co-occurring psychopathology. *Journal of Mental Health Research in Intellectual Disabilities, 11*, 124–142. https://doi.org/10.1080/19315864.2017.1408726

Kozlowski, A. M., Matson, J. L., & Rieske, R. D. (2012). Gender effects on challenging behaviors in children with autism spectrum disorders. *Research in Autism Spectrum Disorders, 6*, 958–964. https://doi.org/10.1016/j.rasd.2011.12.011

Kurtz, P. F., Chin, M. D., Huete, J. M., Tarbox, R. S., O'Connor, J. T., Paclawskyj, T. R., & Rush, K. S. (2003). Functional analysis and treatment of self-injurious behavior in young children: A summary of 30 cases. *Journal of Applied Behavior Analysis, 36*, 205–219. https://doi.org/10.1901/jaba.2003.36-205

LaGrow, S. J., & Repp, A. C. (1984). Stereotypic responding: a review of intervention research. *American Journal of Mental Deficiency, 88*, 595–609. PMID: 6377896.

Lowe, K., Allen, D., Jones, E., Brophy, S., Moore, K., & James, W. (2007). Challenging behaviours: Prevalence and topographies. *Journal of Intellectual Disability Research, 51*, 625–636. https://doi.org/10.1111/j.1365-2788.2006.00948.x

Luiselli, J. K. (2009). *Applied behavior analysis for children with autism spectrum disorders* (Aggression and noncompliance) (pp. 175–187). Berlin, Germany: Springer.

Lundström, M. O., Antonsson, H., Karlsson, S., & Graneheim, U. H. (2011). Use of physical restraints with people with intellectual disabilities living in Sweden's group homes. *Journal of Policy and Practice in Intellectual Disabilities, 8*, 36–41. https://doi.org/10.1111/j.1741-1130.2011.00285.x

Mandell, D. S. (2008). Psychiatric hospitalization among children with autism spectrum disorders. *Journal of Autism and Developmental Disorders, 38*, 1059–1065. https://doi.org/10.1007/s10803-007-0481-2

Matson, J. L., Hamilton, M., Duncan, D., Bamburg, J., Smiroldo, B., Anderson, S., Baglio, C., Williams, D., & Kirkpatrick-Sanchez, S. (1997). Characteristics of stereotypic movement disorder and self-injurious behavior assessed with the Diagnostic Assessment for the Severely Handicapped (DASH-II). *Research in Developmental Disabilities, 18*(6), 457–469. https://doi.org/10.1016/S0891-4222(97)00022-X

Matson, J. L., Mayville, S. B., Kuhn, D. E., Sturmey, P., Laud, R., & Cooper, C. (2005). The behavioral function of feeding problems as assessed by the questions about behavioral function (QABF). *Research in Developmental Disabilities, 26*, 399–408. https://doi.org/10.1016/j.ridd.2004.11.008

Matson, J. L., & Minshawi, N. F. (2007). Functional assessment of challenging behavior: Toward a strategy for applied settings. *Research in Developmental Disabilities, 28*, 353–361.

Matson, J. L., & Nebel-Schwalm, M. (2007). Assessing challenging behaviors in children with autism spectrum disorders: A review. *Research in Developmental Disabilities, 28*, 567–579. https://doi.org/10.1016/j.ridd.2006.08.001

Matson, J. L., & Rivet, T. T. (2008). The effects of severity of autism and PDD-NOS symptoms on challenging behaviors in adults with intellectual disabilities. *Journal of Developmental and Physical Disabilities, 20*, 41–51. https://doi.org/10.1007/s10882-007-9078-0

Matson, J. L., Gonzalez, M. L., & Rivet, T. T. (2008). Reliability of the autism spectrum disorder-behavior problems for children (ASD-BPC). *Research in Autism Spectrum Disorders, 2*, 696–706. https://doi.org/10.1016/j.rasd.2008.02.003

Matson, J. L., & LoVullo, S. V. (2008). A review of behavioral treatments for self-injurious behaviors of persons with autism spectrum disorders. *Behavior Modification, 32*, 61–76. https://doi.org/10.1177/0145445507304581

Matson, J. L., & Wilkins, J. (2009). Factors associated with the questions about behavior function for functional assessment of low- and high-rate challenging behaviors in adults with intellectual disability. *Behavior Modification, 33*, 207–219. https://doi.org/10.1177/0145445508320342

Matson, J. L., Fodstad, J. C., Mahan, S., & Rojahn, J. (2010). Cutoffs, norms and patterns of problem behaviours in children with developmental disabilities on the Baby and Infant Screen for Children with aUtIsm Traits (BISCUIT-Part 3). *Developmental Neurorehabilitation, 13*(1), 3–9. https://doi.org/10.3109/17518420903074887

Matson, J. L., & Kozlowski, A. M. (2011). The increasing prevalence of autism spectrum disorders. *Research in Autism Spectrum Disorders, 5*, 418–425. https://doi.org/10.1016/j.rasd.2010.06.004

Matson, J. L., Kozlowski, A. M., Worley, J. A., Shoemaker, M. E., Sipes, M., & Horovitz, M. (2011). What is the evidence for environmental causes of challenging behaviors in persons with intellectual disabilities and autism spectrum disorders? *Research in Developmental Disabilities, 32*, 693–698. https://doi.org/10.1016/j.ridd.2010.11.012

Matson, J. L., Shoemaker, M. E., Sipes, M., Horovitz, M., Worley, J. A., & Kozlowski, A. M. (2011). Replacement behaviors for identified functions of challenging behaviors. *Research in Developmental Disabilities, 32*, 681–684. https://doi.org/10.1016/j.ridd.2010.11.014

Matson, J. L. (2012). *Functional assessment for challenging behaviors*. New York: Springer.

Mazurek, M. O., Kanne, S. M., & Wodka, E. L. (2013). Physical aggression in children and adolescents with autism spectrum disorders. *Research in Autism Spectrum Disorders, 7*, 455–465. https://doi.org/10.1016/j.rasd.2012.11.004

McCarthy, J., Hemmings, C., Kravariti, E., Dworzynski, K., Holt, G., Bouras, N., & Tsakanikos, E. (2010). Challenging behavior and co-morbid psychopathology in adults with intellectual disability and autism spectrum disorders. *Research in Developmental Disabilities, 31*, 362–366. https://doi.org/10.1016/j.ridd.2009.10.009

McClintock, K., Hall, S., & Oliver, C. (2003). Risk markers associated with challenging behaviours in people with intellectual disabilities: A meta-analytic study. *Journal of Intellectual Disability Research, 47*, 405–416. https://doi.org/10.1046/j.1365-2788.2003.00517.x

McTiernan, A., Leader, G., Healy, O., & Mannion, A. (2011). Analysis of risk factors and early predictors of challenging behavior for children with autism spectrum disorder. *Research in Autism Spectrum Disorders, 5*, 1215–1222. https://doi.org/10.1016/j.rasd.2011.01.009

Minshawi, N. F., Hurwitz, S., Morriss, D., & McDougle, C. J. (2015). Multidisciplinary assessment and treatment of self-injurious behavior in autism spectrum disorder and intellectual disability: Integration of psychological and biological theory and approach. *Journal of Autism and Developmental Disorders, 45*, 1541–1568. https://doi.org/10.1007/s10803-014-2307-3

Morano, S., Ruiz, S., Hwang, J., Wertalik, J. L., Moeller, J., Karal, M. A., & Mulloy, A. (2017). Meta-analysis of single-case treatment effects on self-injurious behavior for individuals with autism and intellectual disabilities. *Autism & Developmental Language Impairments, 2*, 2396941516688399. https://doi.org/10.1177/2396941516688399

Moss, J., & Oliver, C. (2008). The Repetitive Behaviour Scale. Manual for administration and scorer interpretation. University of Birmingham.

Moss, J., Oliver, C., Arron, K., Burbidge, C., & Berg, K. (2009). The prevalence and phenomenology of repetitive behavior in genetic syndromes. *Journal of Autism and Developmental Disorders, 39*, 572–588. https://doi.org/10.1007/s10803-008-0655-6

Murphy, G., Hall, S., Oliver, C., & Kissi-Debra, R. (1999). Identification of early self-injurious behavior in young children with intellectual disability. *Journal of Intellectual Disability Research, 43*, 149–163. https://doi.org/10.1046/j.1365-2788.1999.00183.x

Murphy, O., Healy, O., & Leader, G. (2009). Risk factors for challenging behaviors among 157 children with autism spectrum disorder in Ireland. *Research in Autism Spectrum Disorders, 3*, 474–482. https://doi.org/10.1016/j.rasd.2008.09.008

Neece, C. L., Green, S. A., & Baker, B. L. (2012). Parenting stress and child behavior problems: A transactional relationship across time. *American Journal on Intellectual and Developmental Disabilities, 117*, 48–66. https://doi.org/10.1352/1944-7558-117.1.48

Neidert, P. L., Dozier, C. L., Iwata, B. A., & Hafen, M. (2010). Behavior analysis in intellectual and developmental disabilities. *Psychological Services, 7*, 103. https://doi.org/10.1037/a0018791

Newcomer, L. L., & Lewis, T. J. (2004). Functional behavioral assessment: An investigation of assessment reliability and effectiveness of function-based interventions. *Journal of Emotional and Behavioral Disorders, 12*, 168–181. https://doi.org/10.1177/10634266040120030401

Newman, I., Leader, G., Chen, J. L., & Mannion, A. (2015). An analysis of challenging behavior, comorbid psychopathology, and attention-deficit/hyperactivity disorder in fragile X syndrome. *Research in Developmental Disabilities, 38*, 7–17. https://doi.org/10.1016/j.ridd.2014.11.003

Oliver, C., Petty, J., Ruddick, L., & Bacarese-Hamilton, M. (2012). The association between repetitive, self-injurious and aggressive behavior in children with severe intellectual disability. *Journal of Autism and Developmental Disorders, 42*(6), 910–919. https://doi.org/10.1007/s10803-011-1320-z

O'Reilly, M., Rispoli, M., Davis, T., Machalicek, W., Lang, R., Sigafoos, J., … Didden, R. (2010). Functional analysis of challenging behavior in children with autism spectrum disorders: A summary of 10 cases. *Research in Autism Spectrum Disorders, 4*, 1–10. https://doi.org/10.1016/j.rasd.2009.07.001

Otero-López, J. M., Castro, C., Villardefrancos, E., & Santiago, M. J. (2009). Job dissatisfaction and burnout in secondary school teachers: student's disruptive behaviour and conflict management examined. *European Journal of Education and Psychology, 2*(2), 99–111.

Panju, S., Brian, J., Dupuis, A., Anagnostou, E., & Kushki, A. (2015). Atypical sympathetic arousal in children with autism spectrum disorder and its association with anxiety symptomatology. *Molecular Autism, 6*(1), 64.

Parke, R., & Slaby, R. (1983). The development of aggression. In P. Mussen & E. Hetherington (Eds.), *Handbook of child psychology: Socialization, personality, and social development* (Vol. 4, pp. 547–641). New York: Wiley.

Pavlović, M., Žunić-Pavlović, V., & Glumbić, N. (2013). Students' and teachers' perceptions of aggressive behaviour in adolescents with intellectual disability and typically developing adolescents. *Research in Developmental Disabilities, 34*, 3789–3797. https://doi.org/10.1016/j. ridd.2013.07.035

Poppes, P., Van der Putten, A. J. J., & Vlaskamp, C. (2010). Frequency and severity of challenging behaviour in people with profound intellectual and multiple disabilities. *Research in Developmental Disabilities, 31*, 1269–1275. https://doi.org/10.1016/j.ridd.2010.07.017

Pugliese, C. E., White, B. A., & White, S. W. (2013). Social Anxiety Predicts Aggression in Children with ASD: Clinical Comparisons with Socially Anxious and Oppositional Youth. *Journal of Autism and Developmental Disorders, 43*, 1205–1213. https://doi.org/10.1007/ s10803-012-1666-x

Pugliese, C. E., Fritz, M. S., & White, S. W. (2014). The role of anger rumination and autism spectrum disorder-linked perseveration in the experience of aggression in the general population. *Autism, 19*(6), 704–712. https://doi.org/10.1177/1362361314548731

Rattaz, C., Michelon, C., & Baghdadli, A. (2015). Symptom severity as a risk factor for self injurious behaviors in adolescents with autism spectrum disorders. *Journal of Intellectual Disability Research, 59*, 730–741. https://doi.org/10.1111/jir.12177

Reese, R. M., Richman, D. M., Belmont, J. M., & Morse, P. (2005). Functional characteristics of disruptive behavior in developmentally disabled children with and without Autism. *Journal of Autism and Developmental Disorders, 35*, 419–428. https://doi.org/10.1007/ s10803-005-5032-0

Rojahn, J., & Sisson, L. A. (1990). Stereotyped behavior. In J. L. Matson (Ed.), *Handbook of behavior modification with the mentally retarded*. Boston, MA: Applied Clinical Psychology. Springer.

Rojahn, J., Matson, J. L., Lott, D., Esbensen, A. J., & Smalls, Y. (2001). The behavior problems inventory: An instrument for the assessment of self-injury, stereotyped behavior, and aggression/destruction in individuals with developmental disabilities. *Journal of Autism and Developmental Disorders, 31*, 577–588. https://doi.org/10.1023/A:1013299028321

Rojahn, J., Whittaker, K., Hoch, T. A., & González, M. L. (2007). Assessment of self injurious and aggressive behavior. *International Review of Research in Mental Retardation, 34*, 281–319. https://doi.org/10.1016/S0074-7750(07)34009-3

Roscoe, E. M., Kindle, A. E., & Pence, S. T. (2010). Functional analysis and treatment of aggression maintained by preferred conversational topics. *Journal of Applied Behavior Analysis, 43*, 723–727. https://doi.org/10.1901/jaba.2010.43-723

Ruddick, L., Davies, L., Bacarese-Hamilton, M., & Oliver, C. (2015). Self-injurious, aggressive and destructive behaviour in children with severe intellectual disability: Prevalence, service need and service receipt in the UK. *Research in Developmental Disabilities, 45*, 307–315. https://doi.org/10.1016/j.ridd.2015.07.019

Sigafoos, J., Arthur, M., & O'Reilly, M. (2003). Challenging behavior and developmental disability. (1st ed.) Wiley.

Singh, A. N., Matson, J. L., Mouttapa, M., Pella, R. D., Hill, B. D., & Thorson, R. (2009). A critical item analysis of the QABF: Development of a short form assessment instrument. *Research in Developmental Disabilities, 30*, 782–792. https://doi.org/10.1016/j.ridd.2008.11.001

Smith, R. G., Vollmer, T. R., and St Peter Pipkin, C. (2007). Functional approaches to assessment and treatment of problem behavior in persons with Autism and related disabilities. Autism spectrum disorders: Applied behavior analysis, evidence, and practice (pp. 187–234).

Smith, C. E., Fischer, K. W., & Watson, M. W. (2009). Toward a refined view of aggressive fantasy as a risk factor for aggression: interaction effects involving cognitive and situational variables. *Aggressive Behavior, 35*(4), 313–323. https://doi.org/10.1002/ab.20307. PMID: 19373900.

Simó-Pinatella, D., Mumbardó-Adam, C., Montenegro-Montenegro, E., Cortina, A., Mas, J. M., Baqués, N., & Adam-Alcocer, A. L. (2017). Prevalence and risk markers of challenging behavior among children with disabilities. *Advances in Neurodevelopmental Disorders, 1*, 158–167. https://doi.org/10.1007/s41252-017-0022-8

Soke, G. N., Rosenberg, S. A., Hamman, R. F., Fingerlin, T., Robinson, C., Carpenter, L., … DiGuiseppi, C. (2016). Brief report: Prevalence of self-injurious behaviors among children with autism spectrum disorder – A population-based study. *Journal of Autism and Developmental Disorders, 46*, 3607–3614. https://doi.org/10.1007/s10803-016-2879-1

Stein, D. J., & Woods, D. W. (2014). Stereotyped movement disorder in ICD-11. *Brazilian Journal of Psychiatry, 36*, 65–68.

Stevens, E., Atchison, A., Stevens, L., Hong,E., Granpeesheh, D., Dixon, D., &Linstead, E. (2017). A cluster analysis of challenging behaviors in autism spectrum disorder. In machine learning and applications (ICMLA), 2017 I.E. 16th international conference on (to appear). doi: https://doi.org/10.1109/ICMLA.2017.00-85.

Stith, S. M., Liu, T., Davies, L. C., Boykin, E. L., Alder, M. C., Harris, J. M., … Dees, J. E. M. E. G. (2009). Risk factors in child maltreatment: A meta-analytic review of the literature. *Aggression and Violent Behavior, 14*, 13–29. https://doi.org/10.1016/j.avb.2006.03.006

Summers, J. A., Allison, D. B., Lynch, P. S., & Sandier, L. (1995). Behaviour problems in Angelman syndrome. *Journal of Intellectual Disability Research, 39*(2), 97–106. https://doi.org/10.1111/j.1365-2788.1995.tb00477.x

Summers, J., Shahrami, A., Cali, S., D'Mello, C., Kako, M., Palikucin-Reljin, A., Savage, M., Shaw, O., & Lunsky, Y. (2017). Self-Injury in autism spectrum disorder and intellectual disability: Exploring the role of reactivity to pain and sensory input. *Brain Sciences, 7*(11), 140. https://doi.org/10.3390/brainsci7110140. PMID: 29072583; PMCID: PMC5704147.

Symons, F. J., Clark, R. D., Hatton, D. D., Skinner, M., & Bailey, D. B. (2003). Self-injurious behavior in young boys with fragile X syndrome. *American Journal of Medical Genetics, 118A*, 115–121. https://doi.org/10.1002/ajmg.a.10078

Tate, B. G., & Baroff, G. S. (1966). Aversive control of self-injurious behavior in a psychotic boy. *Behavior Research and Therapy, 4*, 281–287. https://doi.org/10.1016/0005-7967(66)90024-6

Tsakanikos, E., Costello, H., Holt, G., Sturmey, P., & Bouras, N. (2007). Behaviour management problems as predictors of psychotropic medication and use of psychiatric services in adults with autism. *Journal of Autism and Developmental Disorders, 37*, 1080–1085. https://doi.org/10.1007/s10803-006-0248-1

Tureck, K., Matson, J. L, & Beighley, J. S. (2013). An investigation of self-injurious behaviors in adults with severe intellectual disabilities. *Research in Developmental Disabilities, 34*(9), 2469–2474. https://doi.org/10.1016/j.ridd.2013.05.022

Tureck, K., Matson, J. L., Cervantes, P., & Konst, M. J. (2014). An examination of the relationship between autism spectrum disorder, intellectual functioning, and comorbid symptoms in children. *Research in Developmental Disabilities, 35*(7), 1766–1772. https://doi.org/10.1016/j.ridd.2014.02.013

National Institutes of Health. (1989). *Treatment of Destructive Behaviors in Persons with Developmental Disabilities (Consensus development conference statement)* (Vol. 7(9)). Bethesda: Author.

Van Ingen, D. J., Moore, L. L., Zaja, R. H., & Rojahn, J. (2010). The behavior problems inventory (BPI-01) in community-based adults with intellectual disabilities: Reliability and concurrent validity vis-à-vis the Inventory for Client and Agency Planning (ICAP). *Research in Developmental Disabilities, 31*, 97–107. https://doi.org/10.1016/j.ridd.2009.08.004

Weiss, J. A. (2003). Self-injurious behaviours in autism: A literature review. York Space. http://hdl.handle.net/10315/33094

Wilke, A. E., Tarbox, J., Dixon, D. R., Kenzer, A. L., Bishop, M. R., & Kakavand, H. (2012). Indirect functional assessment of stereotypy in children with autism spectrum disorders. *Research in Autism Spectrum Disorders, 6*, 824–828. https://doi.org/10.1016/j.rasd.2011.11.003

Winchel, R. M., & Stanley, M. (1991). Self-injurious behavior: A review of the behavior and biology of self-mutilation. *The American Journal of Psychiatry*. https://doi.org/10.1176/ajp.148.3.306

Wolff, J. J., Hazlett, H. C., Lightbody, A. A., Reiss, A. L., & Piven, J. (2013). Repetitive and self-injurious behaviors: Associations with caudate volume in autism and fragile X syndrome. *Journal of Neurodevelopmental Disorders, 5*, 12. https://doi.org/10.1186/1866-1955-5-12

World Health Organization. (2018). *International Classification of Diseases for Mortality and Morbidity Statistics* (11th Revision). Retrieved from https://icd.who.int/browse11/l-m/en

Yates, T. M. (2004). The developmental psychopathology of self-injurious behavior: Compensatory regulation in posttraumatic adaptation. *Clinical Psychology Review, 24*(1), 35–74, https://doi.org/10.1016/j.cpr.2003.10.001

Chapter 6
Research on Challenging Behaviors and Functional Assessment

Matthew J. O'Brien and Nicole M. Hendrix

Introduction

Numerous theories have been posited on the etiology of challenging behavior, ranging from neurobiological models (e.g., Willner, 2015) to explanations informed by genetics (e.g., Oliver et al., 2013) and psychopathology (e.g., Emerson, 2001). However, no model has been studied as extensively or led to more successful treatment approaches for challenging behavior than the operant learning model, which explains behavior as a result of the environmental stimuli that evoke and maintain or reinforce such behavior (Matson et al., 2011). It is this model that is the basis for functional behavioral assessment (FBA), the methods and procedures used to understand the variables maintaining challenging behavior and the heart of this text. Although the earliest methods of FBA date back more than 50 years (Bijou, Peterson, & Ault, 1968; Lovaas, Freitag, Gold, & Kassorla, 1965) and development of comprehensive models of experimental analysis (i.e., functional analysis) date back more than 35 years (Iwata, Dorsey, Slifer, Bauman, & Richman, 1982/1994), research over the past few decades has advanced FBA technologies and provided insight into exact and efficient methods. This chapter provides an overview of recent research advances on FBA methods for challenging behavior, including enhancements to FBA efficiency and precision, usage and acceptability in research and practice, and emerging FBA practices.

M. J. O'Brien (✉)
University of Iowa Center for Disabilities and Development, University of Iowa Stead Family Children's Hospital, Iowa City, IA, USA
e-mail: matthew-j-obrien@uiowa.edu

N. M. Hendrix
Pediatric Institute with Emory University School of Medicine, Marcus Autism Center, Atlanta, GA, USA

© Springer Nature Switzerland AG 2021
J. L. Matson (ed.), *Functional Assessment for Challenging Behaviors and Mental Health Disorders*, Autism and Child Psychopathology Series,
https://doi.org/10.1007/978-3-030-66270-7_6

FBA Precision and Efficiency

FBA methods are often categorized as: (1) indirect assessment, including interviews, rating scales, or questionnaires that collect information on challenging behavior in the absence of observation; (2) descriptive assessment, in which data are collected on the occurrence of challenging behavior and environmental events preceding and following a targeted behavior without manipulation of these events; or (3) experimental or functional analysis, or the systematic introduction and withdrawal of environmental events hypothesized to influence the occurrence of a target behavior (Hanley, Iwata, & McCord, 2003). Researchers and clinicians commonly choose FBA methods based on the time it takes to conduct them, the training they require, and/or the precision of their findings. Unfortunately, time requirements and outcome precision tend to inversely covary such that the more accurate the assessment methods, the longer the assessment period. This can be particularly concerning as some challenging behaviors have the potential to cause harm when treatment is delayed or when the assessment does not lead to a clearly identified function or functions. For these reasons, there is a need for FBA methods that are expeditious and precise. Research on different FBA methods and modifications to those methods offers insight into the balance between precision and speed that each method offers.

Indirect Assessment

Indirect assessment, such as rating scales and structured interviews, generally produce results faster than other forms of FBA, often in less than 1 hour. However, in comparison to functional analyses, limited evidence supports the validity, reliability, and treatment utility of indirect measures (Dufrene, Kazmerski, & Labrot, 2017; Floyd, Phaneuf, & Wilczynski, 2005; Sturmey, 1994). Though greater attention in recent years has been given to some aspects of technical adequacy of specific instruments (e.g., *Questions about Behavioral Function*; *QABF*), Dufrene et al. (2017) concluded that most indirect measures lack systematic evaluation of their technical adequacy and they denote the limitations of using indirect assessment in isolation of other assessment methods. That is not to say that studies on indirect assessments have not demonstrated adequate validity and reliability in recent years; in fact, some studies have evidenced, for example, strong internal consistency (e.g., Embregts, Didden, Huitink, & Schreuder, 2009) and convergent validity with functional analyses (Poole, Dufrene, Sterling, Tingstrom, & Hardy, 2012). Across indirect assessments, however, more rigorous research related to technical adequacy is needed to bolster utility of these measures when used in isolation.

Indirect assessment is recommended as an initial step in the FBA process and not as a stand-alone assessment (Hanley, 2010). For instance, Iwata and others (Iwata, DeLeon, & Roscoe, 2013) designed the *Functional Analysis Screening Tool* (*FAST*), a closed-ended indirect assessment used to guide more efficient caregiver interviews as well as to identify idiosyncratic antecedent or consequent events to support the design of more efficient functional analyses. Inter-rater reliability ranging from 53.3% to 84.5% and moderate correspondence between the *FAST* and functions of challenging behavior yielded through functional analysis have been found (Iwata et al., 2013). Based upon the recent popularity of interview-informed functional analysis methods (e.g., Hanley, Jin, Vanselow, & Hanratty, 2014), increased focus on the type (e.g., closed- vs open-ended) and efficiency of the interview conducted are warranted (Fryling & Baires, 2016). Although open-ended interviews promote exploration of idiosyncratic functions and perhaps assist in building rapport (Fryling & Baires, 2016), early evidence suggests that they are restricted by the same limitations as closed-ended interviews, including moderate inter-rater reliability and weak correspondence with results of functional analyses (Saini, Ubdegrove, Biran, & Duncan, 2019).

Descriptive Assessment

Given that descriptive assessment relies upon direct observation of challenging behavior in natural environments, one might surmise that descriptive methods would offer both the benefit of increased precision over indirect methods as well as reduced assessment time when compared to functional analyses. Yet current research does not support these assumptions. In addition to studies consistently showing weak correspondence between descriptive assessments and functional analyses (Borrero & Vollmer, 2002; Lerman & Iwata, 1993; Mace & Lalli, 1991; Pence, Roscoe, Bourret, & Ahearn, 2009; Thompson & Iwata, 2007), several studies have noted greater concordance between indirect methods and functional analyses than between descriptive assessments and functional analyses (e.g., Hall, 2005; Tarbox et al., 2009). Reduced agreement may be due in part to descriptive assessments over-identifying attention as a maintaining reinforcer (St. Peter et al., 2005; Tarbox et al., 2009; Thompson & Iwata, 2007) or the high likelihood of obtaining inconclusive results that is associated with descriptive assessments (Tarbox et al., 2009). Obtaining an adequate sample of behavior can reduce the probability of inconclusive data yielded through descriptive assessment (e.g., Rooker, DeLeon, Borrero, Frank-Crawford, & Roscoe, 2015) with the inherent risk of then increasing the time devoted to assessment. Moreover, unlike functional analyses, which rely on visual inspection or standardized methods for identifying a function (Hagopian et al., 1997; Roane, Fisher, Kelley, Mevers, & Bouxsein, 2013), and rating scales, which are developed to derive a function or functions, there is no clear threshold for when a descriptive assessment should conclude.

Despite limitations associated with descriptive assessment, they continue to be employed widely in clinical practice (e.g., Floyd et al., 2005; Oliver, Pratt, & Normand, 2015; Roscoe, Phillips, Kelly, Farber, & Dube, 2015). Thus, advancement in descriptive assessment technology—such as the use of structured descriptive assessments and probability models—remains necessary. Structured descriptive assessments (e.g., Anderson & Long, 2002; Freeman, Anderson, & Scotti, 2000) provide a more targeted observation by controlling the antecedent variables, but allowing for naturally occurring consequences for the targeted behavior. A structured descriptive assessment can avoid indefinite observation and recording by programming for short observation periods across antecedent contexts. Literature is emerging on structured descriptive assessments, and some studies have found that the results of this method may match the outcomes of functional analyses (e.g., Anderson & Long, 2002; Martens et al., 2019).

Probability models (Martens, DiGennaro, Reed, Szczech, & Rosenthal, 2008; McComas et al., 2009; McKerchar & Thompson, 2004) utilize the data collected in descriptive assessments to calculate the magnitude of relationships between target behavior and environmental events. For example, Martens et al. (2008) developed a *contingency space analysis* probability method whereby the probability of a consequence or the absence of that consequence following a behavior is compared to assess the relation between the target behavior and specific consequences. Although probability models provide greater insight into the relationship between behaviors and environmental events, no research to date has evaluated whether this model leads to more rapid assessment outcomes or initiation of treatment.

Functional Analysis

A comprehensive functional analysis methodology, which was first described by Iwata and colleagues (1982/Iwata et al., 1994) has been the subject of an enormous amount of research (see review in Beavers, Iwata, & Lerman, 2013) and likely more than all other forms of FBA combined. Iwata et al.'s functional analysis provided a systematic method for empirically testing hypotheses about functional relations between behavior and environmental events. This method included tests for hypotheses that challenging behavior functioned for attention (the *social disapproval* condition), escape from a work task (the *academic demand* condition), and automatic reinforcement (the *alone* condition). Most published studies using functional analyses have continued to employ tests for attention and escape from demands, but fewer studies have incorporated a test for an automatic function (Beavers et al., 2013). Slightly fewer studies have also included a test for a tangible function (i.e., food, items, and activities); relatedly, several researchers have expressed caution about including a tangible condition due to a greater likelihood of obtaining false-positive findings (Galiatsatos & Graff, 2003; Rooker, Iwata, Harper, Fahmie, & Camp, 2011). Beyond these basic conditions, a seemingly infinite number of idiosyncratic conditions may also be included (see Schlichenmeyer, Roscoe, Rooker, Wheeler, & Dube, 2013, for a review). Antecedent modifications, such as modifying the tone used to present demands (Borrero, Vollmer, & Borrero, 2004), interrupting ritualistic behavior (Leon, Lazarchick, Rooker, & Deleon, 2013), providing attention to others (i.e., divided attention; Fahmie, Iwata, Harper, & Querim, 2013), and including a test for social avoidance (Harper, Iwata, & Camp, 2013) have been used to obtain differentiated functional analysis results. Consequence manipulations, like providing varied forms of attention (Kodak, Northup, & Kelley, 2007; Skinner, Veerkamp, Kamps, & Andra, 2009; Tiger, Fisher, Toussaint, & Kodak, 2009), and access to restraint materials (Rooker & Roscoe, 2005) or ritualistic behavior (Falcomata, Roane, Feeney, & Stephenson, 2010; Hausman, Kahng, Farrell, & Mongeon, 2009), have been incorporated as well.

The use of idiosyncratic conditions is appealing because it may increase the likelihood of differentiated results, particularly when clear results are not obtained through the standard conditions (Hagopian, Rooker, Jessel, & DeLeon, 2013); however, by including additional test conditions, the time required to complete the analysis will be extended. Additional factors that greatly contribute to the length of the assessment include the number of iterations for each test condition and the session duration. According to Beavers et al. (2013), a substantial majority of published functional analyses, since Iwata et al. have included multiple test conditions and most often those test conditions are conducted three or more times within the analysis. In fact, Roane et al. (2013) analyzed a large sample of functional analyses completed in two outpatient clinics specializing in the assessment and treatment of severe problem behavior and reported that nearly three quarters of the functional analyses analyzed included at least five sessions of each condition. Moreover, the average number of sessions conducted for all functional analyses were 33.8.

Although the original (Iwata et al. 1982/1994) functional analysis continues to be referred to as the "gold standard" of behavioral assessment, experimental analyses are less utilized than other forms of FA, in part due to the perception that a standard functional analysis requires a great deal of time and resources to conduct (Oliver et al., 2015). Fortunately, a substantial amount of research has focused on modifications and new types of functional analysis that may improve both efficiency and applicability.

Brief Functional Analysis

Early functional analysis modifications including reductions to session length and the number of sessions led to the development of the brief functional analysis (Cooper, Wacker, Sasso, Reimers, & Donn, 1990; Northup et al., 1991). The brief functional analysis was developed to support clinicians who desired an assessment with the experimental control of the standard functional analysis but practiced in time-limited outpatient clinics (Wacker, Berg, Harding, & Cooper-Brown, 2004). In the brief functional analysis, the functions of target behaviors are identified through a series of 5-minute hypothesis-driven test and control conditions that are rapidly alternated in "mini-reversals". Additional confirmation of a function or functions may be made through a contingency reversal, whereby the identified maintaining reinforcer is delivered for mands rather than the target behavior.

Research has shown that results from the brief functional analysis may be obtained in 20% to 50% less time than the standard functional analysis (e.g., Muething et al., 2017; Tincani, Castrogiavanni, & Axelrod, 1999). Moreover, the use of 5-minute sessions, as opposed to 10- or 15-minute sessions, appears to provide the same level of accuracy as analyses utilizing longer session lengths (Wallace &Iwata, 1999). Despite such benefits, studies comparing assessment outcomes of the brief functional analysis to the standard functional analysis have had mixed results. The correlation between outcomes ranges from low (Muething et al., 2017) to moderately high (Kahng & Iwata, 1999). Muething et al. (2017) examined the correspondence between brief and standard analysis results with 19 individuals who demonstrated severe challenging behavior. Correspondence between assessment methods was only 10.5% exact agreement. Future research to clarify the mixed findings on correspondence and examine what factors may contribute to low correspondence is warranted.

Trial-Based Functional Analysis

Other functional analysis variations have the potential to reduce the occurrence of target behaviors within the assessment and produce outcomes more efficiently than the standard functional analysis. Within the trial-based functional analysis (Sigafoos & Saggers, 1995), brief test sessions or trials, oftentimes 1–2 minutes in duration, are followed by control trials and are terminated at the first occurrence of the target behavior. Test and control trials tailored to all hypothesized functions are conducted for as many as ten or more blocks, and determination of behavioral function is made by comparing the percentage of test and control trials in which the target behavior occurred.

The trial-based functional analysis has been touted as a safer alternative to the standard functional analysis, but only one study has reported on the differences in challenging behavior frequency across the two types of assessment, with the trial-based functional analysis resulting in substantially fewer occurrences (i.e., Curtis et al., 2019). The trial-based approach has been reported to sometimes take longer to conduct than the standard and brief formats (Bloom, Iwata, Fritz, Roscoe, & Carreau, 2011; Curtis et al., 2019; Flanagan et al., 2019); however, the trial-based functional analysis has been conducted using trials as short as 1 minute (i.e., 30 seconds each for a test component and a corresponding control component; Kodak, Fisher, Paden, & Dickes, 2013) and as few as three trials (McDonald, Moore, & Anderson, 2012). Accordingly, when conducted in a brief manner, the trial-based functional analysis, consisting of fewer trials and shorter trial duration, has the potential to produce rapid results. Comparisons of the results of trial-based and standard functional analyses have ranged from moderate to high correspondence (Bloom et al., 2011; Curtis et al., 2019; Flanagan et al., 2019; LaRue et al., 2010).

Latency-Based Functional Analysis

Like the trial-based functional analysis, the latency-based functional analysis (Thomason-Sassi, Iwata, Neidert, & Roscoe, 2011) terminates sessions at the first occurrence of a target behavior. By limiting each session to one instance of the target behavior, the time necessary to complete an analysis may be reduced. Latency-based functional analyses have been posited as appropriately matched for more dangerous behaviors, such as elopement, as they allow fewer opportunities for these behaviors to occur (Boyle & Adamson, 2017). Moreover, they have been used to establish baseline performance when later evaluating function-based interventions (Caruthers, Lambert, Chazin, Harbin, & Houchins-Juarez, 2015).

In practice, concerns have emerged regarding the ability of latency-based functional analyses to effectively identify the function of challenging behavior. Recognizing their possible utility within settings in which evoking high rates of challenging behavior is not possible, Lambert et al. (2017) used latency-based functional analysis procedures with 18 participants admitted to either psychiatric or medical floors of a children's hospital. Differentiated results that corresponded with standard functional analysis results were yielded for 44.4% (or 8 of 18) of the participants, which contrasted with the high correspondence found in Thomason-Sassi et al. (2011).

Precursor Functional Analysis

The precursor functional analysis sets experimental contingencies for less severe challenging behaviors that reliably precede behaviors of greater concern, which are assumed to be functioning as earlier emerging behaviors within specific response-class hierarchies (see review in Heath & Smith, 2019). Smith and Churchill (2002) examined these procedures in comparison with standard functional analyses across four participants with severe challenging behavior. Rates of self-injury and aggression were lower in precursor functional analyses, and the standard and precursor functional analyses matched in identifying the same maintaining contingencies for the behaviors. Subsequent research has demonstrated high correspondence with standard functional analysis results (e.g., Borlase, Vladescu, Kisamore, Reeve, & Fetzer, 2017; Fritz, Iwata, Hammond, & Bloom, 2013) as well as reduced rates of challenging behaviors during assessment (e.g., Dracobly & Smith, 2012), suggesting reduced risk. Evolving practices with precursor functional analyses include devising rigorous methods of identifying these precursor behaviors, including use of conditional probabilities (e.g., Borrero & Borrero, 2008; Dracobly & Smith, 2012; Fritz et al., 2013; Langdon, Carr, & Owen-DeSchryver, 2008), and determining contexts in which precursor functional analyses may be inappropriate, including in the assessment of challenging behavior maintained by automatic reinforcement (e.g., Fahmie & Iwata, 2011).

Interview-Informed Synthesized Contingency Analysis

Another extension of the standard functional analysis—the interview-informed synthe-sized contingency analysis (IISCA)—was developed in response to limitations identi-fied by Hanley et al. (2014) with the standard functional analysis format, including resources required, possibility of harm for some participants, and reliance on generic consequences. This method thus involves combinations of putative reinforcers within the same test condition to determine the reinforcement combinations believed to be maintaining target behaviors (Hanley et al., 2014). Although more recently referred to as a specific consolidated method, it should be noted that some of the practices and func-tional analysis modifications described within the IISCA are integrated into clinical practice with more standard functional analysis procedures (e.g., Lambert et al., 2017).

The IISCA places high importance on preassessment interview and observation, which may create a somewhat longer overall assessment. Conversely, current evi-dence suggests that the IISCA identifies the maintaining reinforcers for challenging behavior in less time than is necessary for the standard functional analysis (Fisher, Greer, Romani, Zangrillo, & Owen, 2016; Jessel, Hanley, & Ghaemmaghami, 2016). Despite its efficiency, research is mixed as to whether the IISCA provides a more accurate assessment outcome than the standard functional analysis and whether it leads to more effective treatments (Fisher et al., 2016; Jessel et al., 2016; Jessel, Ingvarsson, Metras, Kirk, & Whipple, 2018).

Systematic Assessment Models

Systematic assessment models that begin with less rigorous methods and then prog-ress to more rigorous assessment tools (e.g., functional analysis) have been proposed as a way to obtain more accurate outcomes (Asmus, Vollmer, & Borrero, 2002) and/or save time and avoid unnecessary assessment (Mueller & Nkosi, 2007; Vollmer, Marcus, Ringdahl, & Roane, 1995). These models often begin with indirect methods and progress to descriptive assessments, followed by functional analyses. Vollmer et al. (1995) proposed a model for conducting functional analyses that begins with a brief functional analysis and progresses to three additional levels of extended analyses when the results fail to indicate a clear function or functions. Although this model is likely to save time when the assessment may be discontinued after the brief functional analysis, conducting assessment at each of the four levels, which may be necessary for complex behavior patterns, would likely take considerable time.

Inconclusive Outcomes

In addition to functional analysis variations, some procedural modifications have led to more rapid results, often by reducing inconclusive outcomes, producing more rapid differentiation within an analysis, or targeting idiosyncratic establishing operations not often tested in a standard functional analysis. When individuals are less sensitive to the discriminative stimuli associated with functional analysis conditions, undifferentiated responding may occur. Seeking to enhance discrimination of conditions, Conners et al. (2000) showed that by using different therapists and room colors for each condition, differentiated responding was more likely and occurred more rapidly for some individuals. Although the percentage of functional analyses published with undifferentiated outcomes remains small (Beavers et al., 2013), studies have shown that by following an initially inconclusive functional analysis with a functional analysis incorporating idiosyncratic conditions, clear results may be obtained (e.g., Hagopian et al., 2013). Accordingly, in some cases, more rapid results may be obtained by forgoing standard functional analysis conditions and testing specific putative establishing operations (EOs) in the initial analysis. Finally, a simple modification that may lead to greater assessment efficiency is the use of a fixed order of conditions rather than a random order (Hammond, Iwata, Rooker, Fritz, & Bloom, 2013). Fixed order assessment has been recommended by Hammond et al. (2013) who compared random ordering versus a fixed order (ignore, attention, play, and demand) and obtained results either faster or solely by fixed order, presumably by enhancing the EO influences on behavior.

Ongoing Visual-Inspection Procedures

Whereas efficiency often refers to reduced time, effort, or resources required to conducting a functional analysis or minimizing the time required to definitively identify the function of a target behavior, it is more likely that all these factors contribute to a net calculation of efficiency (Saini, Fisher, Retzlaff, & Keevy, 2020). As such, Saini, Fisher, and Retzlaff (2018) adapted structured ongoing visual-inspection (OVI) procedures from Roane et al. (2013) to scrutinize results as they unfold over time across the functional analysis. Specifically, they used OVI to identify the earliest point within functional analyses that differentiation between one or more test conditions and the control condition occurs, focusing on the first three sessions from each test and control condition and gradually increasing the number of sessions examined if differentiation could not be clearly identified. Saini et al. (2018) utilized this method across a randomly selected sample of 100 multielement functional analyses and found strong correspondence with interpretation on the full functional analyses (exact agreement = 93%), while relying upon 41% fewer sessions on average than the full functional analyses.

Saini et al. (2020) also extended use of OVI across functional analysis types (e.g., brief functional analyses, trial-based functional analyses, synthesized contingency analyses). OVI resulted in high concordance with interpretation using Roane et al.'s (2013) procedures across full functional analyses as well as the authors' interpretation of function within the studies. The reduction, in terms of the number of sessions required for differentiation, varied greatly within this sample. To illustrate, OVI resulted in a considerable reduction (35.4%) in the number of sessions required for demonstration of a functional relationship in the trial-based functional analyses and little reduction (4%) in the number of sessions required for brief functional analyses. OVI shows promise as a technique that may contribute to more efficient functional analyses and reduce exposure to contexts likely to evoke challenging behavior.

FBA Usage Across Populations

Most research on challenging behaviors is focused on individuals with neurodevelopmental disabilities. The foundational conceptualization of functional assessment emerged from the study of self-injury more frequently observed in these populations (e.g., Carr, 1977) and then evolved through ongoing work largely with individuals with autism spectrum disorder or intellectual disability (e.g., Matson et al., 2011; O'Reilly et al., 2010). Challenging behavior is observed at substantially higher rates in individuals with neurodevelopmental disorders as compared to individuals without disabilities (e.g., Hartley, Sikora, & McCoy, 2008; Poppes, Van der Putten, & Vlaskamp, 2010; Soke, Maenner, Christensen, Kurzius-Spencer, & Schieve, 2018), but significant variability in presentation of challenging behaviors is present. For example, the rate of challenging behavior in individuals with profound or multiple disabilities is substantially higher than the rate observed in milder disabilities (Poppes et al., 2010). It thus remains necessary to consider the application of FBA to individuals with intellectual disability—and particularly those with profound or multiple disabilities—but also to other populations for whom challenging behavior occurs and would likely benefit from FBA.

Genetic Disorders: Intersection of Biological and Behavioral Perspectives

Some research has focused on demonstrating the utility of functional analyses to guide function-based treatment for individuals with genetic disorders and challenging behavior (e.g., Hodnett, Scheithauer, Call, Mevers, & Miller, 2018; McComas, Thompson, & Johnson, 2003; Radstaake, Didden, Oliver, Allen, & Curfs, 2012; Stokes & Luiselli, 2009). While genetic disorders—such as Smith-Magenis, Cri du Chat, Prader-Willi, Lesch-Nyhan, and Angelman syndromes—are overall rare in prevalence, most are associated with intellectual disability. Moreover, some of these disorders are correlated with high rates of challenging behavior (e.g., Arron, Oliver, Moss, Berg, & Burbidge, 2011; Powis & Oliver, 2014). For example, Smith-Magenis Syndrome affects between 1 in 15,000 individuals (Laje et al., 2010) and 1 in 25,000 individuals (Greenberg et al., 1991) at birth, but rates of self-injurious and aggressive behavior may exceed 90% of individuals with the disorder (e.g., Arron et al., 2011; Sloneem, Oliver, Udwin, & Woodcock, 2011). In contrast, rates of aggression in genetic disorders like Down syndrome and Williams syndrome have consistently been found to be at or below 15% (Powis & Oliver, 2014).

Differences in rates of challenging behavior across genetic disorders suggest an interaction between phenotypic characteristics and environmental factors (e.g., Powis & Oliver, 2014). Whereas biological models highlighting phenotypic characteristics placing individuals at risk for challenging behavior would predict limited within-syndrome variability and behavioral models would predict similar prevalence rates across genetic disorders, the research on prevalence of challenging behaviors within genetic disorders instead demonstrates significant variability within and across disorders. A few attempts to blend biological and behavioral models in assessment have been proposed (e.g., Mace & Mauk, 1995), but little focus has been given to the interaction between genetic and environmental (i.e., operant) influences.

One exception is a study by Tunnicliffe and Oliver (2011), who conducted a review on operant studies with individuals diagnosed with genetic syndromes who exhibited challenging behavior. Despite the strong association of challenging behaviors with a variety of genetic conditions, challenging behaviors across individuals appeared to be highly influenced by the environment. Additionally, the authors described the possible causal pathways associated with specific syndromes. For example, they described individuals with Angelman and Smith-Magenis syndrome as having behavioral phenotypes with a predilection to seek out the attention of others, which can result in more challenging behavior to gain others' attention (i.e., an attention function). Impulsivity often observed in Soto's syndrome, reduced pain perception in Smith-Magenis syndrome, and social anxiety in fragile X syndrome are other examples of biobehavioral factors that may influence challenging behavior probabilities under certain environmental conditions. More research is needed to understand genetic-environmental interactions and to build a comprehensive biobehavioral assessment model that considers the benefits and limitations to FBA when there are strong genetic influences on behavior.

Extensions to Other Populations

Despite an ongoing need for continued research focused on how FBA can guide effective treatment for individuals with neurodevelopmental disabilities, there have been shifts in recent decades toward reaching more diverse populations. A review of the existing FBA literature reveals that the percentage of studies targeting individuals without intellectual disability more than doubled over a 10-year period, yet remains small overall (Beavers et al., 2013; Hanley et al., 2003). Given the flexibility in applying FBA procedures across behaviors, applications of FBA methods have extended in more diverse directions including substance use (e.g., Tuten, Jones, Ertel, Jakubowski, & Sperlein, 2006) and serious mental illness (e.g., Virués-Ortega & Haynes, 2005). For example, translation has begun to determine how FBA can inform treatment of adult atypical vocalizations, or delusions, hallucinations, and disorganized speech observed in disorders such as schizophrenia (e.g., Wilder, Masuda, O'Connor, & Baham, 2001) and traumatic brain injury (e.g., Travis & Sturmey, 2010).

Where more debate has occurred, it has been surrounding the extension of functional analysis to typically developing populations. Anderson and St. Peter (2013), while advocating for the use of varied FBA methods within school settings, raised concerns of extending standard functional analysis practices to typically developing children in response to Hanley (2012). Anderson and St. Peter (2013) posited that reinforcement contingencies in children without neurodevelopmental disabilities may differ from those commonly utilized in existing functional analysis research. They also noted obstacles to manipulating consequences in general education classrooms (e.g., controlling access to attention in a classroom with numerous peers) and referenced limited research supporting functional analysis of noncompliance, a frequently observed behavior in this population. Their conclusions did not discourage the use of functional analyses within the broader realm of FBA but instead cautioned direct extension from standard functional analysis literature to typically developing children in school settings as the literature builds regarding relevant applications (e.g., Flanagan & DeBar, 2018).

Usage and Acceptance of FBA Methods

FBA methods have been adopted widely, serving as best practice for varied challenging behaviors across many settings (e.g., Behavior Analyst Certification Board, 2014; Council for Children with Behavior Disorders, 2009; Epstein, Atkins, Cullinan, Kutash, & Weaver, 2008; Myers & Johnson, 2007; Rush & Frances, 2000). In school settings, FBA is required in certain circumstances under federal policy governing special education (Individuals with Disabilities Education Act [IDEA], 2004). Despite factors encouraging the use of FBA, research has shown that FBA methods are not universally employed or consistently accepted by professionals working with individuals with challenging behavior and social validity data are lacking for other stakeholders (e.g., parents and individuals being assessed; Langthorne & McGill, 2011). Further, among those who use FBA methods, there is great variability in the perception and choices of the types of FBA methods used. What follows is an overview of the research on the usage of and acceptability of FBA methods by professionals working with challenging behavior in school, clinical, and community settings.

FBA in School Settings

Most FBAs are conducted by professionals serving individuals in schools, clinics, and group homes (Beavers et al., 2013). Perhaps bolstered by the IDEA (2004) mandate, most studies on FBA usage and acceptance have focused on the school setting and school professionals. School professionals generally report a favorable view of FBA methods (Broussard & Northup, 1995; Dufrene, Doggett, Henington, & Watson, 2007; Langthorne & McGill, 2011; Nelson, Roberts, Rutherford, Mathur,

& Aaroe, 1999; O'Neill, Bundock, Kladis, & Hawken, 2015; Rispoli, Neely, Healy, & Gregori, 2016); however, perceptions vary based upon the type of FBA method and the professionals surveyed. Within the school setting, a variety of professionals may be responsible for conducting the FBAs. While Johnson, Goldberg, Hinant, and Couch (2019) found that the vast majority (90%) of FBAs were conducted in part or fully by school psychologists, a substantial number of special education teachers (45%) may also participate in the FBA process, which other studies have corroborated (Moreno, Wong-Lo, & Bullock, 2017).

Barriers to FBA usage and acceptance include the lack of training provided for school professionals and the time required to conduct FBAs and analyze the resulting data (Blood & Neel, 2007; Chitiyo & Wheeler, 2009). Studies examining training programs for teachers and school psychologists confirm that the school personnel responsible for conducting FBAs receive inadequate coursework or training on FBA procedures (Couvillon, Bullock, & Gable, 2009; Sullivan, Long, & Kucera, 2011). However, several studies have shown that when school professionals participate in training on FBA methods, there is an increase in confidence in the FBA process and greater acceptance of the procedures (e.g., Lane et al., 2015; McCahill, Healy, Lydon, & Ramey, 2014; Oakes et al., 2018). Thus, broad usage and acceptance may be dependent on whether graduate training programs for future school professionals incorporate training on FBA methods into their coursework.

Unlike the researchers conducting studies within the school setting, professionals working in the schools are far less likely to conduct functional analyses (e.g., Anderson, Rodriguez, & Campbell, 2015; Ducharme & Shecter, 2011; Gresham, 2004). In general, school professionals rate indirect assessment methods, such as functional assessment interviews, as more useful and appropriate than functional analysis or direct observation (O'Neill et al., 2015). This finding may be explained by the benefits of indirect assessment methods (i.e., simplicity, minimal time commitment, and lesser training requirements) as well as criticisms often made about functional analysis methods (i.e., disruption to classrooms and undesirable side effects; O'Neill et al., 2015; Rispoli et al., 2016).

FBA in Clinical and Community Settings

Outside of the school setting, most studies have focused on the practice of behavior analysts and other professionals who work in clinical and community settings. In an early study on FBA practices among professionals in community and residential settings, Desrochers, Hile, and Williams-Moseley (1997) conducted a survey on the usage and perceived usefulness of various FBA methods. Among more than 100 survey respondents, the majority indicated that FBAs were *very* or *extremely useful* and regularly employed in their work with challenging behavior. Most respondents reported that they frequently used indirect and descriptive assessments to conduct FBAs, and those two methods were also rated as most useful. A small number (16.8%) reported regularly including functional analysis methods as part of the

FBA process, and only three individuals identified functional analysis methods as providing the most useful information on behavioral function, making it the least used and least valued of the three types of FBA assessment methods. These results were partially replicated by Ellingson Ellingson, Miltenberger, & Long, (1999), who found that among service providers in North Dakota, FBA methods were deemed extremely useful, but more experimental methods (i.e., functional analyses conducted in controlled and natural settings) were identified as more effective.

Two recent studies shed light on current perceptions and usage among behavior analysts and other professionals who work with individuals with challenging behavior. In line with previous work (i.e., Desrochers et al., 1997; Ellingson et al., 1999), the vast majority of survey respondents in both contemporary studies reported regularly using FBA methods to develop interventions for challenging behavior (Oliver et al., 2015; Roscoe et al., 2015). Both studies also found that respondents were most likely to use descriptive assessments when conducting FBAs and substantially less likely to use functional analyses in their practice. In the study by Oliver et al. (2015), a survey of nearly 700 behavior analysts, most reported using indirect and descriptive assessments most frequently, whereas 63% of the sample reported never or rarely using functional analyses. Roscoe et al. (2015), whose sample consisted of 205 behavior analysts within the state of Massachusetts, similarly discovered that a minority (34.6%) of the sample reported regularly using functional analyses. Notably though, nearly twice as many respondents in the Roscoe et al. study indicated that functional analyses were the most informative FBA assessment method, revealing incongruence between perceptions of the value of functional analysis and actual usage among behavior analysts. In terms of the barriers to implementation of functional analyses, behavior analysts across both studies identified limited time and resources, insufficient space and materials, and administrative restrictions, which are similar to those reported by school professionals.

Future Directions in FBA Research

Extensive research demonstrating the effectiveness of FBA-based interventions has undoubtedly contributed to the acceptance and the establishment of FBA as best practice. Nonetheless, FBA practice will continue to evolve as a result of current and future research. Throughout this chapter, several promising areas of research have been noted, such as novel methods for analyzing functional analyses (Saini et al., 2020). Likewise, calls for additional research in unexplored areas have been made, such as the need for assessment models that consider genetic-environmental influences on behavior. In this section, we have chosen to highlight two areas where current FBA research is influencing the way professionals conduct FBAs now and in the future. In the first part, we focus on an assessment approach that promises to provide safer and more efficient assessment than traditional approaches. In the second part, we present research on a novel modality for conducting FBAs and training professionals that expands geographic reach of these services.

IISCA

FBA is clearly not a "one size fits all" approach to behavioral assessment. Based in part upon the practical limitations of the standard functional analysis (e.g., time obligations, prerequisite training, safety concerns), alternative functional analysis models previously described have been developed to allow greater flexibility for practitioners to conduct functional analyses under the constraints of their respective practice settings. The IISCA is the most recent alternative to the standard functional analysis, and it has garnered substantial attention in the FBA literature. In addition to promises of reduced assessment time, improved safety, and strong social validity, the IISCA approach, which involves a functional analysis with synthesized reinforcement contingencies, has been extolled by some as "one of the most prominent developments" related to the functional analysis since the publication of the Beavers et al. (2013) review (Slaton & Hanley, 2018).

The IISCA may be characterized as a comprehensive FBA model that incorporates several features not new to the FBA literature. More specifically, the IISCA process is comprised of the following components: (a) an open-ended caregiver interview with questions about the target individual's abilities, challenging behavior, contexts associated with the challenging behavior, and caregivers' responses (Hanley, 2012); (b) a brief (i.e., 15–30 minutes) observation of the target individual with probes including presentation/removal of toys and attention, as well as directives; and (c) a functional analysis informed by the interview and observation, composed of a single test condition with synthesized establishing operations and reinforcement contingencies alternated with a control condition (Hanley et al., 2014). Open-ended interviews are a common form of indirect assessment (Kelley, LaRue, Roane, & Gadaire, 2011) and descriptive assessments may be the most common FBA assessment method in practice (Oliver et al., 2015; Roscoe et al., 2015). The greatest divergence from traditional FBA methods is the use of synthesized functional analyses (including synthesized EOs and synthesized reinforcer delivery); however, synthesized approaches have been documented many times previously in the FBA literature (Slaton & Hanley, 2018).

Studies utilizing the IISCA approach have found the resulting functional analyses to be highly efficient (Curtis et al., 2019; Fisher et al., 2016; Greer, Mitteer, Briggs, Fisher, & Sodawasser, 2020; Hanley et al., 2014; Herman, Healy, & Lydon, 2018; Jessel et al., 2018; Jessel, Ingvarsson, Metras, Kirk, & Whipple, 2018; Slaton, Hanley, & Raftery, 2017). The use of an omnibus test condition incorporating multiple social functions increases the likelihood of evoking target behavior at the outset of the assessment and avoiding tests of isolated reinforcer contingencies, leading to rapid results. Researchers have even begun blending the use of synthesized conditions into already expeditious functional analysis methods, such as a synthesized trial-based approach (Curtis et al., 2019; Lloyd et al., 2015), a synthesized single-session (i.e., within session analysis ala Roane, Lerman, Kelley, & Van Camp, 1999) functional analysis approach (Jessel, Ingvarsson, Metras, Kirk, & Whipple, 2018) and a synthesized functional analysis with 3-minute sessions (Jessel, Metras, Hanley, Jessel, & Ingvarsson, 2020).

Studies employing the IISCA functional analysis to inform treatment have found the resulting treatments to be highly effective, often without substantial treatment modifications (Beaulieu, Van Nostrand, Williams, & Herscovitch, 2018; Hanley et al., 2014; Herman et al., 2018; Jessel, Ingvarsson, Metras, Kirk, & Whipple, 2018; Rose & Beaulieu, 2019; Santiago, Hanley, Moore, & Jin, 2016; Strand & Eldevik, 2018; Taylor, Phillips, & Gertzog, 2018). In addition to effective treatments, the IISCA assessment and treatment process have been associated with high social validity (Beaulieu et al., 2018; Hanley et al., 2014; Herman et al., 2018; Jessel, Ingvarsson, Metras, Kirk, & Whipple, 2018; Rose & Beaulieu, 2019; Santiago et al., 2016; Strand & Eldevik, 2018; Taylor et al., 2018) and there are indications that the IISCA assessment process and derived treatments have strong generalizability and maintenance (Rose & Beaulieu, 2019; Santiago et al., 2016).

Despite the potential benefits associated with the IISCA, some researchers have expressed concerns about the utility and imprecise nature of the IISCA. Disagreement about the utility of the IISCA is generally focused on the use of synthesized functional analysis conditions. The argument against such conditions is that by combining contingencies the researcher or practitioner may assume multiple or interactive control of the behavior being studied without ruling out the possibility of individual control by a single reinforcer (Fisher et al., 2016). For example, Fisher et al. (2016) and Greer et al. (2020) compared the outcomes of standard (single contingency) functional analyses and IISCA (i.e., synthesized) functional analyses and found that the IISCA functional analyses overidentified at least 50% of the functions implicated (i.e., false positives) when compared to standard functional analyses, suggesting that synthesized functional analysis test conditions are prone to false positives. Such outcomes may be attributable to inaccurate initial hypotheses generated from both the prefunctional analysis interview and brief observation, which have been shown to over endorse all three social functions (i.e., escape, tangible, and attention; Greer et al., 2020).

Retzlaff and colleagues (2019) also called into question whether synthesized functional analysis conditions may be more likely to result in iatrogenic effects (i.e., or to induce novel functions for challenging behavior). They hypothesized that synthesized conditions may be more susceptible to this risk because nonfunctional, yet highly preferred items are delivered on repeated occasions contingent on challenging behavior when contingencies are combined. Retzlaff and colleagues (2019) approached this hypothesis by using a translational investigation, or by having the researchers' program functions for novel responses with no history of reinforcement. Their findings indicated that the IISCA was likely to produce iatrogenic effects for an arbitrary behavior conditioned to function for a particular social reinforcer, whereas the same outcome did not follow the standard functional analysis. Concerns regarding false positives and iatrogenic effects have yet to be addressed by researchers and practitioners who employ the IISCA model.

Telehealth

Although FBAs are considered an essential precursor to developing effective treatments for challenging behavior, there is a dearth of qualified practitioners who can conduct FBAs (Zhang & Cummings, 2019) and within the school setting many professionals tasked with conducting FBAs are undertrained (Couvillon et al., 2009; Ducharme & Shecter, 2011; Sullivan et al., 2011). Moreover, highly trained practitioners tend to be located in urban/suburban areas (Mello, Urbano, Goldman, & Hodapp, 2016), leaving those located in rural areas with limited service options. The likely implication is that for some individuals in need of treatments targeting challenging behavior, the treatments may be ill-informed or simply are not developed. Recently, a potential solution to the lack of access to qualified practitioners and effective training has been offered in the form of *telehealth* and training via telecommunication technologies.

Telehealth[1] is the provision of healthcare services via electronic modalities (Institute of Medicine, 2012), and over the past decade a multitude of studies have evaluated the viability of telehealth as a modality for conducting FBA activities. The first published study using telehealth to conduct FBAs was by Barretto et al. in 2006. This study described the procedures the authors used to conduct more than 75 behavioral assessments, usually consisting of descriptive assessment and/or brief functional analyses, over a state-wide telecommunications network beginning in 1997. The Barretto research team utilized parents and school personnel to conduct the assessments in schools and community sites (e.g., Department of Human Services office), with live coaching from a behavior analyst at a remote site via a telecommunications system. Despite promise as a service and research option for conducting FBAs, the research team experienced many challenges associated with communication between the coaching and assessment sites (Wacker et al., 2016).

Further validation of telehealth as a delivery modality for FBA has been provided by a series of studies by Wacker and colleagues (Lindgren et al., 2016; Suess et al., 2014; Suess, Wacker, Schwartz, Lustig, & Detrick, 2016; Wacker et al., 2013), all of which have focused on conducting standard functional analyses with young children diagnosed with autism spectrum disorder. These studies were conducted in two phases. In the initial phase of studies (Suess et al., 2014; Suess et al., 2016; Wacker et al., 2013), caregivers conducted functional analyses in a clinic setting with coaching from a behavior analyst in a remote clinic location. Outcomes (i.e., identification of behavioral function) were similar to studies employing in-vivo assessments. In the second phase of studies (Lindgren et al., 2016; Lindgren et al., 2020), caregivers conducted the functional analyses within their homes via coaching from a behavior analyst in a remote clinic site. Once again, similar assessment results were obtained in comparison to both in-vivo and clinic-to-clinic telehealth models. Importantly, the clinic-to-home assessment and treatment model resulted in substantially lower costs than the other two models, and caregiver acceptability was statistically similar (Lindgren et al., 2016).

Other research teams have replicated and extended FBA procedures using tele-health and telecommunications strategies (Benson et al., 2018; Machalicek et al., 2016). In addition to parent-implemented functional analyses, studies have utilized graduate students and teachers to conduct functional analyses (Barretto, Wacker, Harding, Lee, & Berg, 2006; Machalicek et al., 2009). Telehealth has also been used to conduct functional analyses and develop function-based interventions for children with disabilities other than autism spectrum disorders (Benson et al., 2018; Hoffmann, Bogoev, & Sellers, 2019; Martens et al., 2019; Monlux, Pollard, Rodriguez, & Hall, 2019; Simacek, Dimian, & McComas, 2017). Researchers have employed telehealth to conduct other FBA methods, including indirect methods (e.g., caregiver interview; Benson et al., 2018; Bice-Urbach & Kratochwill, 2016; Machalicek et al., 2016; Simacek et al., 2017; Tsami, Lerman, & Toper-Korkmaz, 2019), descriptive assessments (Benson et al., 2018; Bice-Urbach & Kratochwill, 2016), and structured descriptive assessments leading to contingency space analyses (Martens et al., 2019).

Beyond providing an alternative modality for conducting FBAs, research is also exploring the capability of telecommunications as a primary means for training practitioners in FBA methods. Unlike studies that involve coaching of caregivers or others to conduct FBAs, the goal of tele-education or tele-training has focused on skill acquisition through telecommunications. Most studies have focused exclusively on training teachers (Alnemary, Wallace, Symon, & Barry, 2015; Machalicek et al., 2010); however, other school personnel, including speech and language pathologists (Frieder, Peterson, Woodward, Crane, & Garner, 2009), behavior specialists (Hoffmann et al., 2019), counselors, psychologists, and social workers (Bassingthwaite et al., 2018) have been the recipients of training. In one study, behavior analysts trained a behavior specialist in early childhood special education in FBA methods and the behavior specialist then coached parents to conduct functional analyses with their young children (Hoffmann et al., 2019), suggesting the possibility of cascading training effects in community settings. Despite several studies reporting adequate procedural fidelity for FBA implementation by trainees (Bassingthwaite et al., 2018; Frieder et al., 2009; Hoffmann et al., 2019), results have not been consistently strong. At least one study reported variable results (Alnemary et al., 2015), and another study identified weak long-term maintenance of skills (Machalicek et al., 2010).

For all the promise of conducting FBAs and training practitioners in FBA methods via telecommunications, ethical considerations have been raised and several research questions remain. Romani and Schieltz (2017) identified 23 specific ethical standards of the American Psychological Association (APA) and Behavior Analysis Certification Board (BACB) ethical codes (APA, 2010; BACB, 2014) that may be especially relevant to the delivery of telehealth services. As opposed to in-vivo assessment, the use of telehealth for conducting an FBA may require special considerations, including competence in conducting assessment procedures largely through verbal presentation, added safeguards for students or clients and those being coached to conduct the assessment, and methods for maintaining privacy and security of telehealth information, including compliance with the Health Insurance Portability and Accountability Act (HIPAA) and the Family Educational Rights and

Privacy Act (FERPA). Policy and resources drive access to telehealth as well, resulting in the same concerns of access to service that incited research on telehealth as a service modality in the first place. For instance, telehealth prerequisites include adequate equipment and internet service (see Lee et al., 2015), state rules and regulations that allow for provision of service via telehealth, and insurance coverage that includes telehealth as a reimbursable service.

Preliminary evidence encourages the use of telehealth for conducting FBAs and training individuals to conduct FBAs. Yet, research that directly compares the outcomes of FBAs and training conducted via telehealth and in-vivo is lacking. Research is also needed to determine for whom telehealth and tele-training is an appropriate modality. For example, with respect to conducting FBAs, little research has been conducted on older children and virtually no research has conducted telehealth-based FBAs with adolescents, adults, or typically developing individuals. Additionally, most studies that have provided detailed information on the therapists conducting the assessments (i.e., those being coached by a behavioral expert) have reported using parents or teachers with relatively high educational attainment (e.g., completion of a bachelor's or graduate degree), leading to questions about who might be a suitable therapist. Finally, future research on telehealth-delivered FBAs should determine whether telehealth is contraindicated for specific types of behaviors and whether more intense or severe behavior can be safely assessed and/or treated via telehealth.

[1]The term *telehealth* is often used broadly to encompass a variety of activities conducted through telecommunications, including tele-consultation, telemedicine, tele-education, and tele-research (Knutsen et al., 2016). Here, it refers only to practice and training involving FBA methods.

Conclusion

At the heart of FBA is the goal of understanding why challenging behavior occurs so that effective treatments may be developed. The operant learning model that forms the basis for FBA methodologies has not changed since first described decades ago by B.F. Skinner (1938); however, in the pursuit of furthering our understanding of challenging behavior and developing effective treatments, research has led to the development of a variety of FBA methods and demonstrated broad application across different populations, behaviors, and settings. As this chapter has detailed, research continues to explore new FBA methods and modifications to existing approaches that will yield increased precision, efficiency, and acceptability. There is little question that current and future research will promote the continued evolution of FBA and provide additional models and modifications that will allow professionals and researchers to better understand why challenging behaviors occur and develop more effective treatment options. We are also hopeful that future research will continue to contribute to broader discussions across healthcare and educational systems on the effective assessment and treatment of diverse individuals with challenging behaviors.

References

Alnemary, F., Wallace, M., Symon, J., & Barry, L. (2015). Using international videoconferencing to provide staff training on functional behavioral assessment. *Behavioral Interventions, 30*(1), 73–86.

American Psychological Association (APA). (2010). *Ethical principles of psychologists and code of conduct*. Washington, D.C.: Author.

Anderson, C. M., & Long, E. S. (2002). Use of a structured descriptive assessment methodology to identify variables affecting problem behavior. *Journal of Applied Behavior Analysis, 35*(2), 137–154.

Anderson, C. M., Rodriguez, B. J., & Campbell, A. (2015). Functional behavior assessment in schools: Current status and future directions. *Journal of Behavioral Education, 24*(3), 338–371.

Anderson, C. M., & St. Peter, C. C. (2013). Functional analysis with typically developing children: Best practice or too early to tell?: In response to Hanley (2012). *Behavior Analysis in Practice, 6*(2), 62–76.

Arron, K., Oliver, C., Moss, J., Berg, K., & Burbidge, C. (2011). The prevalence and phenomenology of self-injurious and aggressive behaviour in genetic syndromes. *Journal of Intellectual Disability Research, 55*(2), 109–120.

Asmus, J., Vollmer, T., & Borrero, J. (2002). Functional behavioral assessment: A school-based model. *Education and Treatment of Children, 25*(1), 67–90.

Barretto, A., Wacker, D. P., Harding, J., Lee, J., & Berg, W. K. (2006). Using telemedicine to conduct behavioral assessments. *Journal of Applied Behavior Analysis, 39*(3), 333–340. https://doi.org/10.1901/jaba.2006.173-04

Bassingthwaite, B., Graber, J., Weaver, A., Wacker, D., White-Staecker, D., Bergthold, S., & Judkins, P. (2018). Using tele-consultation to develop independent skills of school-based behavior teams in functional behavior assessment. *Journal of Educational and Psychological Consultation, 28*(3), 297–318.

Beaulieu, L., Van Nostrand, M., Williams, A., & Herscovitch, B. (2018). Incorporating interview-informed functional analyses into practice. *Behavior Analysis in Practice, 11*(4), 385–389.

Beavers, G. A., Iwata, B. A., & Lerman, D. C. (2013). Thirty years of research on the functional analysis of problem behavior. *Journal of Applied Behavior Analysis, 46*(1), 1–21.

Behavior Analysis Certification Board (BACB). (2014). *Professional and ethical compliance code for behavior analysts*. Littleton, CO: Author.

Behavior Analyst Certification Board. (2014). *Applied behavior analysis treatment of autism spectrum disorder: Practice guidelines for healthcare funders and managers* (2nd ed.). Littleton, CO: Author.

Benson, S., Dimian, A., Elmquist, M., Simacek, J., McComas, J., & Symons, F. (2018). Coaching parents to assess and treat self-injurious behaviour via telehealth. *Journal of Intellectual Disability Research, 62*(12), 1114–1123.

Bice-Urbach, B. J., & Kratochwill, T. R. (2016). Tele-consultation: The use of technology to improve evidence-based practices in rural communities. *Journal of School Psychology, 56*, 27–43. https://doi.org/10.1016/j.jsp.2016.02.001

Bijou, S. W., Peterson, R. F., & Ault, M. H. (1968). A method to integrate descriptive and experimental field studies at the level of data and empirical concepts. *Journal of Applied Behavior Analysis, 1*(2), 175–191.

Blood, E., & Neel, R. S. (2007). From FBA to implementation: A look at what is actually being delivered. *Education and Treatment of Children*, 67–80.

Bloom, S. E., Iwata, B. A., Fritz, J. N., Roscoe, E. M., & Carreau, A. B. (2011). Classroom application of a trial-based functional analysis. *Journal of Applied Behavior Analysis, 44*(1), 19–31.

Borlase, M. A., Vladescu, J. C., Kisamore, A. N., Reeve, S. A., & Fetzer, J. L. (2017). Analysis of precursors to multiply controlled problem behavior: A replication. *Journal of Applied Behavior Analysis, 50*(3), 668–674.

Borrero, C. S., & Borrero, J. C. (2008). Descriptive and experimental analyses of potential precursors to problem behavior. *Journal of Applied Behavior Analysis, 41*(1), 83–96.

Borrero, C. S., Vollmer, T. R., & Borrero, J. C. (2004). Combining descriptive and functional analysis logic to evaluate idiosyncratic variables maintaining aggression. *Behavioral Interventions, 19*(4), 247–262.

Borrero, J. C., & Vollmer, T. R. (2002). An application of the matching law to severe problem behavior. *Journal of Applied Behavior Analysis, 35*(1), 13–27.

Boyle, M. A., & Adamson, R. M. (2017). Systematic review of functional analysis and treatment of elopement (2000–2015). *Behavior Analysis in Practice, 10*(4), 375–385.

Broussard, C. D., & Northup, J. (1995). An approach to functional assessment and analysis of disruptive behavior in regular education classrooms. *School Psychology Quarterly, 10*(2), 151–164.

Carr, E. G. (1977). The motivation of self-injurious behavior: A review of some hypotheses. *Psychological Bulletin, 84*(4), 800–816.

Caruthers, C. E., Lambert, J. M., Chazin, K. M., Harbin, E. R., & Houchins-Juarez, N. J. (2015). Latency-based FA as baseline for subsequent treatment evaluation. *Behavior Analysis in Practice, 8*(1), 48–51.

Chitiyo, M., & Wheeler, J. J. (2009). Challenges faced by school teachers in implementing positive behavior support in their school systems. *Remedial and Special Education, 30*(1), 58–63.

Conners, J., Iwata, B. A., Kahng, S., Hanley, G. P., Worsdell, A. S., & Thompson, R. H. (2000). Differential responding in the presence and absence of discriminative stimuli during multielement functional analyses. *Journal of Applied Behavior Analysis, 33*(3), 299–308.

Cooper, L. J., Wacker, D. P., Sasso, G. M., Reimers, T. M., & Donn, L. K. (1990). Using parents as therapists to evaluate appropriate behavior of their children: Application to a tertiary diagnostic clinic. *Journal of Applied Behavior Analysis, 23*(3), 285–296.

Council for Children with Behavioral Disorders: A Division of the Council for Exceptional Children: CCBD'S Position Summary on Physical Restraint and Seclusion Procedures in School Settings: Initially Approved by the Executive Committee on 5-17-09 Revised and Approved by the Executive Committee on 7-8-09. (2009). *Beyond Behavior,19*(1), 40–41.

Couvillon, M. A., Bullock, L. M., & Gable, R. A. (2009). Tracking behavior assessment methodology and support strategies: A national survey of how schools utilize functional behavioral assessments and behavior intervention plans. *Emotional and Behavioural Difficulties, 14*(3), 215–228.

Curtis, K. S., Forck, K. L., Boyle, M. A., Fudge, B. M., Speake, H. N., & Pauls, B. P. (2019). Evaluation of a trial-based interview-informed synthesized contingency analysis. *Journal of Applied Behavior Analysis.* https://doi.org/10.1002/jaba.618

Desrochers, M. N., Hile, M. G., & Williams-Moseley, T. L. (1997). Survey of functional assessment procedures used with individuals who display mental retardation and severe problem behaviors. *American Journal of Mental Retardation, 101*(5), 535–546.

Dracobly, J., & Smith, R. (2012). Progressing from identification and functional analysis of precursor behavior to treatment of self-injurious behavior. *Journal of Applied Behavior Analysis, 45*(2), 361–374.

Ducharme, J. M., & Shecter, C. (2011). Bridging the gap between clinical and classroom intervention: Keystone approaches for students with challenging behavior. *School Psychology Review, 40*(2), 257–274.

Dufrene, B. A., Doggett, R. A., Henington, C., & Watson, T. S. (2007). Functional assessment and intervention for disruptive classroom behaviors in preschool and head start classrooms. *Journal of Behavioral Education, 16*(4), 368–388.

Dufrene, B. A., Kazmerski, J. S., & Labrot, Z. (2017). The current status of indirect functional assessment instruments. *Psychology in the Schools, 54*(4), 331–350.

Ellingson, S. A., Miltenberger, R. G., & Long, E. S. (1999). A survey of the use of functional assessment procedures in agencies serving individuals with developmental disabilities. *Behavioral Interventions: Theory and Practice in Residential & Community-Based Clinical Programs, 14*(4), 187–198.

Embregts, P. J. C. M., Didden, R., Huitink, C., & Schreuder, N. (2009). Contextual variables affecting aggressive behaviour in individuals with mild to borderline intellectual disabilities who live in a residential facility. *Journal of Intellectual Disability Research, 53*(3), 255–264.

Emerson, E. (2001). *Challenging behaviour: Analysis and intervention in people with severe intellectual disabilities*. Cambridge, UK: Cambridge University Press.

Epstein, M., Atkins, M., Cullinan, D., Kutash, K., &Weaver, R. (2008). *Reducing Behavior Problems in the Elementary School Classroom: A Practice Guide* (NCEE #2008-012). Washington, D.C.: National Center for Education Evaluation and Regional Assistance, Institute of Education Sciences, U.S. Department of Education. Retrieved from http://ies.ed.gov/ncee/ wwc/publications/practiceguides

Fahmie, T., Iwata, B., Harper, J., & Querim, A. (2013). Evaluation of the divided attention condition during functional analyses. *Journal of Applied Behavior Analysis, 46*(1), 71–78.

Fahmie, T. A., & Iwata, B. A. (2011). Topographical and functional properties of precursors to severe problem behavior. *Journal of Applied Behavior Analysis, 44*(4), 993–997.

Falcomata, T. S., Roane, H. S., Feeney, B. J., & Stephenson, K. M. (2010). Assessment and treatment of elopement maintained by access to stereotypy. *Journal of Applied Behavior Analysis, 43*(3), 513–517. https://doi.org/10.1901/jaba.2010.43-513

Fisher, W. W., Greer, B. D., Romani, P. W., Zangrillo, A. N., & Owen, T. M. (2016). Comparisons of synthesized and individual reinforcement contingencies during functional analysis. *Journal of Applied Behavior Analysis, 49*(3), 596–616.

Flanagan, T. F., & DeBar, R. M. (2018). Trial-based functional analyses with a student identified with an emotional and behavioral disorder. *Behavioral Disorders, 43*(4), 423–435.

Flanagan, T. F., DeBar, R. M., Sidener, T. M., Kisamore, A. N., Reeve, K. F., & Reeve, S. A. (2019). Teacher-implemented trial-based functional analyses with students with emotional/behavioral disorders. *Journal of Developmental and Physical Disabilities*. https://doi.org/10.1007/ s10882-019-09700-5

Floyd, R. G., Phaneuf, R. L., & Wilczynski, S. M. (2005). Measurement properties of indirect assessment methods for functional behavioral assessment: A review of research. *School Psychology Review, 34*(1), 58–73.

Freeman, K. A., Anderson, C. M., & Scotti, J. R. (2000). A structured descriptive methodology: Increasing agreement between descriptive and experimental analyses. *Education and Training in Mental Retardation and Developmental Disabilities, 35*, 55–66.

Frieder, J. E., Peterson, S. M., Woodward, J., Crane, J., & Garner, M. (2009). Tele-consultation in school settings: Linking classroom teachers and behavior analysts through web-based technology. *Behavior Analysis in Practice, 2*, 32–39.

Fritz, J. N., Iwata, B. A., Hammond, J. L., & Bloom, S. E. (2013). Experimental analysis of precursors to severe problem behavior. *Journal of Applied Behavior Analysis, 46*(1), 101–129.

Fryling, M. J., & Baires, N. A. (2016). The practical importance of the distinction between open- and closed-ended indirect assessments. *Behavior Analysis in Practice, 9*(2), 146–151.

Galiatsatos, G. T., & Graff, R. (2003). Combining descriptive and functional analyses to assess and treat screaming. *Behavioral Interventions, 18*(2), 123–138.

Greenberg, F., Guzzetta, V., de Oca-Luna, R. M., Magenis, R. E., Smith, A. C., Richter, S. F., … Lupski, J. R. (1991). Molecular analysis of the Smith-Magenis syndrome: A possible contiguous-gene syndrome associated with del(17)(p11.2). *American Journal of Human Genetics, 49*(6), 1207–1218.

Greer, B., Mitteer, D., Briggs, A., Fisher, W., & Sodawasser, A. (2020). Comparisons of standardized and interview-informed synthesized reinforcement contingencies relative to functional analysis. *Journal of Applied Behavior Analysis, 53*(1), 82–101.

Gresham, F. M. (2004). Current status and future directions of school-based behavioral interventions. *School Psychology Review, 33*(3), 326–343.

Hagopian, L. P., Fisher, W. W., Thompson, R. H., Owen-DeSchryver, J., Iwata, B. A., & Wacker, D. P. (1997). Toward the development of structured criteria for interpretation of functional analysis data. *Journal of Applied Behavior Analysis, 30*(2), 313–326.

Hagopian, L. P., Rooker, G. W., Jessel, J., & DeLeon, I. G. (2013). Initial functional analysis outcomes and modifications in pursuit of differentiation: A summary of 176 inpatient cases. *Journal of Applied Behavior Analysis, 46*(1), 88–100.

Hall, S. S. (2005). Comparing descriptive, experimental and informant-based assessments of problem behaviors. *Research in Developmental Disabilities, 26*(6), 514–526.

Hammond, J. L., Iwata, B. A., Rooker, G. W., Fritz, J. N., & Bloom, S. E. (2013). Effects of fixed versus random condition sequencing during multielement functional analyses. *Journal of Applied Behavior Analysis, 46*(1), 22–30.

Hanley, G. P. (2010). Prevention and treatment of severe problem behavior. In E. Mayville & J. Mulick (Eds.), *Behavioral foundations of autism intervention* (pp. 233–256). New York, NY: Sloman Publishing.

Hanley, G. P. (2012). Functional assessment of problem behavior: Dispelling myths, overcoming implementation obstacles, and developing new lore. *Behavior Analysis in Practice, 5*(1), 54–72.

Hanley, G. P., Iwata, B. A., & McCord, B. E. (2003). Functional analysis of problem behavior: A review. *Journal of Applied Behavior Analysis, 36*(2), 147–185.

Hanley, G. P., Jin, C. S., Vanselow, N. R., & Hanratty, L. A. (2014). Producing meaningful improvements in problem behavior of children with autism via synthesized analyses and treatments. *Journal of Applied Behavior Analysis, 47*(1), 16–36.

Harper, J., Iwata, B., & Camp, E. (2013). Assessment and treatment of social avoidance. *Journal of Applied Behavior Analysis, 46*(1), 147–160.

Hartley, S. L., Sikora, D. M., & McCoy, R. (2008). Prevalence and risk factors of maladaptive behaviour in young children with autistic disorder. *Journal of Intellectual Disability, 52*(10), 819–829.

Hausman, N., Kahng, S., Farrell, E., & Mongeon, C. (2009). Idiosyncratic functions: Severe problem behavior maintained by access to ritualistic behaviors. *Education and Treatment of Children, 32*(1), 77–87.

Heath, H., & Smith, R. G. (2019). Precursor behavior and functional analysis: A brief review. *Journal of Applied Behavior Analysis, 52*(3), 804–810.

Herman, C., Healy, O., & Lydon, S. (2018). An interview-informed synthesized contingency analysis to inform the treatment of challenging behavior in a young child with autism. *Developmental Neurorehabilitation, 21*(3), 202–207.

Hodnett, J., Scheithauer, M., Call, N. A., Mevers, J. L., & Miller, S. J. (2018). Using a functional analysis followed by differential reinforcement and extinction to reduce challenging behaviors in children with Smith-Magenis syndrome. *American Journal on Intellectual and Developmental Disabilities, 123*(6), 558–573.

Hoffmann, A. N., Bogoev, B. K., & Sellers, T. P. (2019). Using telehealth and expert coaching to support early childhood special education parent-implemented assessment and intervention procedures. *Rural Special Education Quarterly, 38*(2), 95–106. https://doi.org/10.1177/8756870519844162

Individuals with Disabilities Education Act. (2004). Retrieved from http:idea.ed.gov/

Institute of Medicine (IOM). (2012). *The role of telehealth in an evolving health care environment: Workshop summary*. Washington, D.C.: National Academy Press.

Iwata, B. A., DeLeon, I. G., & Roscoe, E. M. (2013). Reliability and validity of the functional analysis screening tool. *Journal of Applied Behavior Analysis, 46*(1), 271–284.

Iwata, B. A., Dorsey, M. F., Slifer, K. J., Bauman, K. E., & Richman, G. S. (1994). Toward a functional analysis of self-injury. *Journal of Applied Behavior Analysis, 27*, 197–209. https://doi.org/10.1901/jaba.1994.27-197. (Reprinted from Analysis and Intervention in Developmental Disabilities, 2, 3–20, 1982).

Jessel, J., Hanley, G. P., & Ghaemmaghami, M. (2016). Interview-informed synthesized contingency analyses: Thirty replications and reanalysis. *Journal of Applied Behavior Analysis, 49*(3), 576–595.

Jessel, J., Ingvarsson, E., Metras, R., Whipple, R., Kirk, H., & Solsbery, L. (2018). Treatment of elopement following a latency-based interview-informed, synthesized contingency analysis. *Behavioral Interventions, 33*(3), 271–283.

Jessel, J., Ingvarsson, E. T., Metras, R., Kirk, H., & Whipple, R. (2018). Achieving socially significant reductions in problem behavior following the interview-informed synthesized contingency analysis: A summary of 25 outpatient applications. *Journal of Applied Behavior Analysis, 51*(1), 130–157.

Jessel, J., Metras, R., Hanley, G. P., Jessel, C., & Ingvarsson, E. T. (2020). Evaluating the boundaries of analytic efficiency and control: A consecutive controlled case series of 26 functional analyses. *Journal of Applied Behavior Analysis, 53*(1), 25–43.

Johnson, A. H., Goldberg, T. S., Hinant, R. L., & Couch, L. K. (2019). Trends and practices in functional behavior assessments completed by school psychologists. *Psychology in the Schools, 56*(3), 360–377.

Kahng, S., & Iwata, B. A. (1999). Correspondence between outcomes of brief and extended functional analyses. *Journal of Applied Behavior Analysis, 32*(2), 149–160.

Kelley, M. E., LaRue, R., Roane, H. S., & Gadaire, D. M. (2011). Indirect behavioral assessments: Interviews and rating scales. In W. W. Fisher, C. C. Piazza, & H. S. Roane (Eds.), *Handbook of applied behavior analysis* (pp. 182–190). New York, NY: Guilford.

Knutsen, J., Wolfe, A., Burke, B., Hepburn, S., Lindgren, S., & Coury, D. (2016). A systematic review of telemedicine in autism spectrum disorders. *Review Journal of Autism and Developmental Disorders, 3*(4), 330–344.

Kodak, T., Fisher, W. W., Paden, A., & Dickes, N. (2013). Evaluation of the utility of a discrete-trial functional analysis in early intervention classrooms. *Journal of Applied Behavior Analysis, 46*(1), 301–306.

Kodak, T., Northup, J., & Kelley, M. E. (2007). An evaluation of the types of attention that maintain problem behavior. *Journal of Applied Behavior Analysis, 40*(1), 167–171. https://doi.org/10.1901/jaba.2007.43-064

Laje, G., Morse, R., Richter, W., Ball, J., Pao, M., & Smith, A. C. (2010). Autism spectrum features in Smith–Magenis syndrome. *American Journal of Medical Genetics Part C: Seminars in Medical Genetics, 154*(4), 456–462.

Lambert, J. M., Staubitz, J. E., Roane, J. T., Houchins-Juárez, N. J., Juárez, A. P., Sanders, K. B., & Warren, Z. E. (2017). Outcome summaries of latency-based functional analyses conducted in hospital inpatient units. *Journal of Applied Behavior Analysis, 50*(3), 487–494.

Lane, K. L., Oakes, W. P., Powers, L., Diebold, T., Germer, K., Common, E. A., & Brunsting, N. (2015). Improving teachers' knowledge of functional assessment-based interventions: Outcomes of a professional development series. *Education and Treatment of Children, 38*(1), 93–120.

Langdon, N. A., Carr, E. G., & Owen-DeSchryver, J. S. (2008). Functional analysis of precursors for serious problem behavior and related intervention. *Behavior Modification, 32*(6), 804–827.

Langthorne, P., & McGill, P. (2011). Assessing the social acceptability of the functional analysis of problem behavior. *Journal of Applied Behavior Analysis, 44*(2), 403–407.

LaRue, R. H., Lenard, K., Weiss, M. J., Bamond, M., Palmieri, M., & Kelley, M. E. (2010). Comparison of traditional and trial-based methodologies for conducting functional analyses. *Research in Developmental Disabilities, 31*(2), 480–487.

Lee, J. F., Schieltz, K. M., Suess, A. N., Wacker, D. P., Romani, P. W., Lindgren, S. D., et al. (2015). Guidelines for developing telehealth services and troubleshooting problems with telehealth technology when coaching parents to conduct functional analyses and functional communication training in their homes. *Behavior Analysis in Practice, 8*(2), 190–200. https://doi.org/10.1007/s40617-014-0031-2.

Leon, Y., Lazarchick, W., Rooker, G., & Deleon, I. (2013). Assessment of problem behavior evoked by disruption of ritualistic toy arrangements in a child with autism. *Journal of Applied Behavior Analysis, 46*(2), 507–511.

Lerman, D. C., & Iwata, B. A. (1993). Descriptive and experimental analyses of variables maintaining self-injurious behavior. *Journal of Applied Behavior Analysis, 26*(3), 293–319.

Lindgren, S., Wacker, D., Suess, A., Schieltz, K., Pelzel, K., Kopelman, T., … Waldron, D. (2016). Telehealth and autism: Treating challenging behavior at lower cost. *Pediatrics, 137*, S167–S175. https://doi.org/10.1542/peds.2015-2851

Lindgren, S., Wacker, D., Schieltz, K., Suess, A., Pelzel, K., Kopelman, T., Lee, J., Romani, P., & O'Brien, M. (2020). A randomized controlled trial of functional communication training via telehealth for young children with autism spectrum disorder. *Journal of Autism and Developmental Disorders 50*(12), 4449–4462.

Lloyd, B. P., Wehby, J. H., Weaver, E. S., Goldman, S. E., Harvey, M. N., & Sherlock, D. R. (2015). Implementation and validation of trial-based functional analyses in public elementary school settings. *Journal of Behavioral Education, 24*, 167–195. https://doi.org/10.1007/s10864-014-9217-5

Lovaas, O. I., Freitag, G., Gold, V. J., & Kassorla, I. C. (1965). Experimental studies in childhood schizophrenia: Analysis of self-destructive behavior. *Journal of Experimental Child Psychology, 2*(1), 67–84.

Mace, F. C., & Lalli, J. S. (1991). Linking descriptive and experimental analyses in the treatment of bizarre speech. *Journal of Applied Behavior Analysis, 24*(3), 553–562.

Mace, F. C., & Mauk, J. E. (1995). Bio-behavioral diagnosis and treatment of self-injury. *Mental Retardation and Developmental Disabilities Research Reviews, 1*(2), 104–110.

Machalicek, W., Lequia, J., Pinkelman, S., Knowles, C., Raulston, T., Davis, T., et al. (2016). Behavioral telehealth consultation with families of children with autism spectrum disorder. *Behavioral Interventions, 31*(3), 223–250. https://doi.org/10.1002/bin.1450.

Machalicek, W., O'Reilly, M., Chan, J. M., Lang, R., Rispoli, M., Davis, T., et al. (2009). Using videoconferencing to conduct functional analysis of challenging behavior and develop classroom behavioral support plans for students with autism. *Education and Training in Developmental Disabilities, 44*(2), 207–217.

Machalicek, W., O'Reilly, M. F., Rispoli, M., Davis, T., Lang, R., Franco, J. H., & Chan, J. M. (2010). Training teachers to assess the challenging behaviors of students with autism using video tele-conferencing. *Education and Training in Autism and Developmental Disabilities, 45*(2), 203–215.

Martens, B., DiGennaro, F., Reed, D., Szczech, F., & Rosenthal, B. (2008). Contingency space analysis: An alternative method for identifying contingent relations from observational data. *Journal of Applied Behavior Analysis, 41*(1), 69–81.

Martens, B. K., Baxter, E. L., McComas, J. J., Sallade, S. J., Kester, J. S., Caamano, M., … Pennington, B. (2019). Agreement between structured descriptive assessments and functional analyses conducted over a telehealth system. *Behavior Analysis: Research and Practice, 19*(4), 343–356.

Matson, J. L., Kozlowski, A. M., Worley, J. A., Shoemaker, M. E., Sipes, M., & Horovitz, M. (2011). What is the evidence for environmental causes of challenging behaviors in persons with intellectual disabilities and autism spectrum disorders? *Research in Developmental Disabilities, 32*(2), 693–698.

McCahill, J., Healy, O., Lydon, S., & Ramey, D. (2014). Training educational staff in functional behavioral assessment: A systematic review. *Journal of Developmental and Physical Disabilities, 26*(4), 479–505.

McComas, J. J., Moore, T., Dahl, N., Hartman, E., Hoch, J., & Symons, F. (2009). Calculating contingencies in natural environments: Issues in the application of sequential analysis. *Journal of Applied Behavior Analysis, 42*(2), 413–423.

McComas, J. J., Thompson, A., & Johnson, L. (2003). The effects of presession attention on problem behavior maintained by different reinforcers. *Journal of Applied Behavior Analysis, 36*(3), 297–307.

McDonald, J., Moore, D. W., & Anderson, A. (2012). Comparison of functional assessment methods targeting aggressive and stereotypic behaviour in a child with autism. *The Educational and Developmental Psychologist, 29*(1), 52–65.

McKerchar, P. M., & Thompson, R. H. (2004). A descriptive analysis of potential reinforcement contingencies in the preschool classroom. *Journal of Applied Behavior Analysis, 37*(4), 431–444.

Mello, M., Urbano, R., Goldman, S., & Hodapp, R. (2016). Services for children with autism spectrum disorder: Comparing rural and non-rural communities. *Education and Training in Autism and Developmental Disabilities, 51*(4), 355–365.

Monlux, K. D., Pollard, J. S., Rodriguez, A. Y. B., & Hall, S. S. (2019). Telehealth delivery of function-based behavioral treatment for problem behaviors exhibited by boys with fragile X syndrome. *Journal of Autism and Developmental Disorders, 49*(6), 2461–2475.

Moreno, G., Wong-Lo, M., & Bullock, L. M. (2017). Investigation on the practice of the functional behavioral assessment: Survey of educators and their experiences in the field. *International Journal of Emotional Education, 9*(1), 54–70.

Mueller, M. M., & Nkosi, A. (2007). State of the science in the assessment and management of severe behavior problems in school settings: Behavior analytic consultation to schools. *International Journal of Behavioral Consultation and Therapy, 3*(2), 176–202.

Muething, C. S., Call, N. A., Lomas Mevers, J., Zangrillo, A. N., Clark, S. B., & Reavis, A. R. (2017). Correspondence between the results of functional analyses and brief functional analyses. *Developmental Neurorehabilitation, 20*(8), 549–559.

Myers, S. M., & Johnson, C. P. (2007). Management of children with autism spectrum disorders. (Disease/disorder overview)(clinical report). *Pediatrics, 120*(5), 1162–1182.

Nelson, J., Roberts, M., Rutherford, R., Mathur, S., & Aaroe, L. (1999). A statewide survey of special education administrators and school psychologists regarding functional behavioral assessment. *Education & Treatment of Children, 22*(3), 267.

Northup, J., Wacker, D., Sasso, G., Steege, M., Cigrand, K., Cook, J., & DeRaad, A. (1991). A brief functional analysis of aggressive and alternative behavior in an outclinic setting. *Journal of Applied Behavior Analysis, 24*(3), 509–522.

O'Reilly, M., Rispoli, M., Davis, T., Machalicek, W., Lang, R., Sigafoos, J., … Didden, R. (2010). Functional analysis of challenging behavior in children with autism spectrum disorders: A summary of 10 cases. *Research in Autism Spectrum Disorders, 4*(1), 1–10.

Oakes, W. P., Schellman, L. E., Lane, K. L., Common, E. A., Powers, L., Diebold, T., & Gaskill, T. (2018). Improving educators' knowledge, confidence, and usefulness of functional assessment-based interventions: Outcomes of professional learning. *Education and Treatment of Children, 41*(4), 533–565.

Oliver, A. C., Pratt, L. A., & Normand, M. P. (2015). A survey of functional behavior assessment methods used by behavior analysts in practice. *Journal of Applied Behavior Analysis, 48*(4), 817–829.

Oliver, C., Adams, D., Allen, D., Bull, L., Heald, M., Moss, J., … Woodcock, K. (2013). Causal models of clinically significant behaviors in Angelman, Cornelia de Lange, Prader–Willi and Smith–Magenis syndromes. *International Review of Research in Developmental Disabilities, 44*, 167–211.

O'Neill, R. E., Bundock, K., Kladis, K., & Hawken, L. S. (2015). Acceptability of functional behavioral assessment procedures to special educators and school psychologists. *Behavioral Disorders, 41*(1), 51–66.

Pence, S. T., Roscoe, E. M., Bourret, J. C., & Ahearn, W. H. (2009). Relative contributions of three descriptive methods: Implications for behavioral assessment. *Journal of Applied Behavior Analysis, 42*(2), 425–446.

Poole, V. Y., Dufrene, B. A., Sterling, H. E., Tingstrom, D. H., & Hardy, C. M. (2012). Classwide functional analysis and treatment of preschoolers' disruptive behavior. *Journal of Applied School Psychology, 28*(2), 155–174.

Poppes, P., Van der Putten, A. J. J., & Vlaskamp, C. (2010). Frequency and severity of challenging behaviour in people with profound intellectual and multiple disabilities. *Research in Developmental Disabilities, 31*(6), 1269–1275.

Powis, L., & Oliver, C. (2014). The prevalence of aggression in genetic syndromes: A review. *Research in Developmental Disabilities, 35*(5), 1051–1071.

Radstaake, M., Didden, R., Oliver, C., Allen, D., & Curfs, L. M. (2012). Functional analysis and functional communication training in individuals with Angelman syndrome. *Developmental Neurorehabilitation, 15*(2), 91–104.

Retzlaff, B., Fisher, W., Akers, J., & Greer, B. (2019). A translational evaluation of potential iatrogenic effects of single and combined contingencies during functional analysis. *Journal of Applied Behavior Analysis, 53*(1), 67–81.

Rispoli, M., Neely, L., Healy, O., & Gregori, E. (2016). Training public school special educators to implement two functional analysis models. *Journal of Behavioral Education, 25*(3), 249–274.

Roane, H., Lerman, D., Kelley, M., & Van Camp, C. (1999). Within-session patterns of responding during functional analyses: The role of establishing operations in clarifying behavioral function. *Research in Developmental Disabilities, 20*(1), 73–89.

Roane, H. S., Fisher, W. W., Kelley, M. E., Mevers, J. L., & Bouxsein, K. J. (2013). Using modified visual-inspection criteria to interpret functional analysis outcomes. *Journal of Applied Behavior Analysis, 46*(1), 130–146.

Romani, P., & Schieltz, K. (2017). Ethical considerations when delivering behavior analytic services for problem behavior via telehealth. *Behavior Analysis: Research andPractice, 17*(4), 312–324.

Rooker, G., Iwata, B., Harper, J., Fahmie, T., & Camp, E. (2011). False-positive tangible outcomes of functional analyses. *Journal of Applied Behavior Analysis, 44*(4), 737–745.

Rooker, G. W., DeLeon, I. G., Borrero, C. S., Frank-Crawford, M. A., & Roscoe, E. M. (2015). Reducing ambiguity in the functional assessment of problem behavior. *Behavioral Interventions, 30*(1), 1–35.

Rooker, G. W., & Roscoe, E. M. (2005). Functional analysis of self-injurious behavior and its relation to self-restraint. *Journal of Applied Behavior Analysis, 38*(4), 537–542. https://doi.org/10.1901/jaba.2005.12-05

Roscoe, E. M., Phillips, K. M., Kelly, M. A., Farber, R., & Dube, W. V. (2015). A statewide survey assessing practitioners' use and perceived utility of functional assessment. *Journal of Applied Behavior Analysis, 48*(4), 830–844.

Rose, J. C., & Beaulieu, L. (2019). Assessing the generality and durability of interview-informed functional analyses and treatment. *Journal of Applied Behavior Analysis, 52*(1), 271–285. https://doi.org/10.1002/jaba.504

Rush, A. J., & Frances, A. J. (2000). Expert consensus guideline series: Treatment of psychiatric and behavioral problems in mental retardation. *American Journal of Mental Retardation, 105*(3), 159–226.

Saini, V., Fisher, W. W., & Retzlaff, B. J. (2018). Predictive validity and efficiency of ongoing visual-inspection criteria for interpreting functional analyses. *Journal of Applied Behavior Analysis, 51*(2), 303–320.

Saini, V., Fisher, W. W., Retzlaff, B. J., & Keevy, M. (2020). Efficiency in functional analysis of problem behavior: A quantitative and qualitative review. *Journal of Applied Behavior Analysis.* https://doi.org/10.1002/jaba.583

Saini, V., Ubdegrove, K., Biran, S., & Duncan, R. (2019). A preliminary evaluation of interrater reliability and concurrent validity of open-ended indirect assessment. *Behavior Analysis in Practice.* https://doi.org/10.1007/s4061

Santiago, J., Hanley, L., Moore, G., & Jin, P. (2016). The generality of interview-informed functional analyses: Systematic replications in school and home. *Journal of Autism and Developmental Disorders, 46*(3), 797–811.

Schlichenmeyer, K., Roscoe, E., Rooker, G., Wheeler, E., & Dube, W. (2013). Idiosyncratic variables that affect functional analysis outcomes: A review (2001–2010). *Journal of Applied Behavior Analysis, 46*(1), 339–348.

Sigafoos, J., & Saggers, E. (1995). A discrete-trial approach to the functional analysis of aggressive behaviour in two boys with autism. *Australia and New Zealand Journal of Developmental Disabilities, 20*(4), 287–297.

Simacek, J., Dimian, A. F., &McComas, J. J. (2017). Communication intervention for young

Skinner, B. F. (1938). *The behavior of organisms: An experimental analysis.* New York, London: D. Appletone-Century Company, Incorporated.

Skinner, B. (1938). *The behavior of organisms: An experimental analysis/by B. F. Skinner.* (The Century psychology series). New Jersey: Prentice-Hall.

Skinner, J. N., Veerkamp, M. B., Kamps, D. M., & Andra, P. R. (2009). Teacher and peer participation in functional analysis and intervention for a first grade student with attention deficit hyperactivity disorder. *Education and Treatment of Children, 32*(2), 243–266. https://doi.org/10.1353/etc.0.0059.

Slaton, J., & Hanley, G. (2018). Nature and scope of synthesis in functional analysis and treatment of problem behavior. *Journal of Applied Behavior Analysis, 51*(4), 943–973.

Slaton, J., Hanley, G., & Raftery, K. (2017). Interview-informed functional analyses: A comparison of synthesized and isolated components. *Journal of Applied Behavior Analysis, 50*(2), 252–277.

Sloneem, J., Oliver, C., Udwin, O., & Woodcock, K. A. (2011). Prevalence, phenomenology, aetiology and predictors of challenging behaviour in Smith-Magenis syndrome. *Journal of Intellectual Disability Research, 55*(2), 138–151.

Smith, R., & Churchill, R. (2002). Identification of environmental determinants of behavior disorders through functional analysis of precursor behaviors. *Journal of Applied Behavior Analysis, 35*(2), 125–136.

Soke, G. N., Maenner, M. J., Christensen, D., Kurzius-Spencer, M., & Schieve, L. A. (2018). Prevalence of co-occurring medical and behavioral conditions/symptoms among 4-and 8-year-old children with autism spectrum disorder in selected areas of the United States in 2010. *Journal of Autism and Developmental Disabilities, 48*(8), 2663–2676.

St. Peter, C. C., Vollmer, T. R., Bourret, J. C., Borrero, C. S., Sloman, K. N., & Rapp, J. T. (2005). On the role of attention in naturally occurring matching relations. *Journal of Applied Behavior Analysis, 38*(4), 429–443.

Stokes, J. V., & Luiselli, J. K. (2009). Applied behavior analysis assessment and intervention for health: Threatening self-injury (rectal picking) in an adult with Prader-Willi syndrome. *Clinical Case Studies, 8*(1), 38–47.

Strand, R. C. W., & Eldevik, S. (2018). Improvements in problem behavior in a child with autism spectrum diagnosis through synthesized analysis and treatment: A replication in an EIBI home program. *Behavioral Interventions, 33*, 102–111. https://doi.org/10.1002/bin.1505

Sturmey, P. (1994). Assessing the functions of aberrant behaviors: A review of psychometric instruments. *Journal of Autism and Developmental Disorders, 24*, 293–304.

Suess, A. N., Romani, P. W., Wacker, D. P., Dyson, S. M., Kuhle, J. L., Lee, J. F., … Waldron, D. B. (2014). Evaluating the treatment fidelity of parents who conduct in-home functional communication training with coaching via telehealth. *Journal of Behavioral Education, 23*, 34–59. https://doi.org/10.1007/s10864-013-9183-3

Suess, A. N., Wacker, D. P., Schwartz, J. E., Lustig, N., & Detrick, J. (2016). Preliminary evidence on the use of telehealth in an outpatient behavior clinic. *Journal of Applied Behavior Analysis, 49*(3), 686–692. https://doi.org/10.1002/jaba.305

Sullivan, A. L., Long, L., & Kucera, M. (2011). A survey of school psychologists' preparation, participation, and perceptions related to positive behavior interventions and supports. *Psychology in the Schools, 48*(10), 971–985.

Tarbox, J., Wilke, A. E., Najdowski, A. C., Findel-Pyles, R. S., Balasanyan, S., Caveney, A. C., … Tia, B. (2009). Comparing indirect, descriptive, and experimental functional assessments of challenging behavior in children with autism. *Journal of Developmental and Physical Disabilities, 21*(6), 493–514.

Taylor, S. A., Phillips, K. J., & Gertzog, M. G. (2018). Use of synthesized analysis and informed treatment to promote school reintegration. *Behavioral Interventions, 33*(4), 364–379. https://doi.org/10.1002/bin.1640

Thomason-Sassi, J. L., Iwata, B. A., Neidert, P. L., & Roscoe, E. M. (2011). Response latency as an index of response strength during functional analyses of problem behavior. *Journal of Applied Behavior Analysis, 44*(1), 51–67.

Thompson, R. H., & Iwata, B. A. (2007). A comparison of outcomes from descriptive and functional analyses of problem behavior. *Journal of Applied Behavior Analysis, 40*(2), 333–338.

Tiger, J. H., Fisher, W. W., Toussaint, K. A., & Kodak, T. (2009). Progressing from initially ambiguous functional analyses: Three case examples. *Research in Developmental Disabilities, 30*(5), 910–926. https://doi.org/10.1016/j.ridd.2009.01.005

Tincani, M. J., Castrogiavanni, A., & Axelrod, S. (1999). A comparison of the effectiveness of brief versus traditional functional analyses. *Research in Developmental Disabilities, 20*(5), 327–338.

Travis, R., & Sturmey, P. (2010). Functional analysis and treatment of the delusional statements of a man with multiple disabilities: A four-year follow-up. *Journal of Applied Behavior Analysis, 43*(4), 745–749.

Tsami, L., Lerman, D., & Toper-Korkmaz, O. (2019). Effectiveness and acceptability of parent training via telehealth among families around the world. *Journal of Applied Behavior Analysis, 52*(4), 1113–1129. https://doi.org/10.1002/jaba.645

Tunnicliffe, P., & Oliver, C. (2011). Phenotype–environment interactions in genetic syndromes associated with severe or profound intellectual disability. *Research in Developmental Disabilities, 32*(2), 404–418.

Tuten, M. J., Jones, H., Ertel, J., Jakubowski, J., & Sperlein, J. (2006). Reinforcement-based treatment: A novel approach to treating substance abuse during pregnancy. *Counselor Magazine, 7*(3), 22–29.

Virués-Ortega, J., & Haynes, S. N. (2005). Functional analysis in behavior therapy: Behavioral foundations and clinical application. *International Journal of Clinical and Health Psychology, 5*(3), 567–587.

Vollmer, T. R., Marcus, B. A., Ringdahl, J. E., & Roane, H. S. (1995). Progressing from brief assessments to extended experimental analyses in the evaluation of aberrant behavior. *Journal of Applied Behavior Analysis, 28*(4), 561–576.

Wacker, D., Berg, W., Harding, J., & Cooper-Brown, L. (2004). Use of brief experimental analyses in outpatient clinic and home settings. *Journal of Behavioral Education, 13*(4), 213–226.

Wacker, D. P., Lee, J. F., Dalmau, Y. C. P., Kopelman, T. G., Lindgren, S. D., Kuhle, J., et al. (2013). Conducting functional analyses of problem behavior via telehealth. *Journal of Applied Behavior Analysis, 46*(1), 31–46. https://doi.org/10.1002/jaba.29.

Wacker, D. P., Schieltz, K. M., Suess, A. N., Romani, P. W., Padilla Dalmau, Y. C., Kopelman, T. G., ... Lindgren, S. D. (2016). Telehealth. In N. N. Singh (Ed.), *Handbook of evidence-based practices in intellectual and developmental disabilities*. https://doi.org/10.1007/978-3-319-26583-4_22

Wallace, M. D., & Iwata, B. A. (1999). Effects of session duration on functional analysis outcomes. *Journal of Applied Behavior Analysis, 32*(2), 175–183.

Wilder, D. A., Masuda, A., O'Connor, C., & Baham, M. (2001). Brief functional analysis and treatment of bizarre vocalizations in an adult with schizophrenia. *Journal of Applied Behavior Analysis, 34*(1), 65–68.

Willner, P. (2015). Neurobiology of aggression. *Journal of Intellectual Disability Research, 59*, 82–92. https://doi.org/10.1111/jir.12120

Zhang, Y., & Cummings, J. (2019). Supply of certified applied behavior analysts in the United States: Implications for service delivery for children with autism. *Psychiatric Services (Washington, D.C.)*, Appips201900058.

Chapter 7
Research on Nature, Prevalence, and Characteristics in Mental Health Disorders and Functional Assessment

Jill C. Fodstad, Larrilyn Grant, Melissa A. Butler, Ann Lagges, Gabriela M. Rodríguez, and Hillary Blake

Functional assessment is a long-standing technique whereby the environmental antecedents and consequences that maintain a behavior are identified. This technique is vitally important as a first step in developing appropriate and individualized interventions that yield improved outcomes and quality of life (O'Neill, Albin, Storey, Horner, & Sprague, 2014). Functional assessment is an effective treatment development tool for externalizing behavior problems (e.g., physical aggression, noncompliance, property destruction) and for those with intellectual and developmental disabilities (Beavers, Iwata, & Lerman, 2013; Hanley, Iwata, & McCord, 2003). While literature on the use of functional assessment for other clinical populations is not as substantial, the technique has utility in cases where the individual has a diagnosis of a mental health condition.

Psychiatric disorders are as a set of mental health conditions whereby a person displays a behavioral or mental pattern that causes significant distress or impairment in personal or social functioning and is not associated with their cultural or religious beliefs (American Psychiatric Association [APA], 2013). Many psychiatric disorders can occur across the lifespan, with some being more likely to emerge in childhood and others being quite rare until adulthood. Common psychiatric

J. C. Fodstad (✉)
Indiana University School of Medicine, Indianapolis, IN, USA

Indiana University Health, Indianapolis, IN, USA

Department of Psychiatry, IU Health Neuroscience Center, Indianapolis, IN, USA
e-mail: jfodstad@iupui.edu

L. Grant
Indiana University School of Medicine, Indianapolis, IN, USA

M. A. Butler · A. Lagges · G. M. Rodríguez · H. Blake
Indiana University School of Medicine, Indianapolis, IN, USA

Indiana University Health, Indianapolis, IN, USA

© Springer Nature Switzerland AG 2021
J. L. Matson (ed.), *Functional Assessment for Challenging Behaviors and Mental Health Disorders*, Autism and Child Psychopathology Series,
https://doi.org/10.1007/978-3-030-66270-7_7

conditions include depression, anxiety, attention-deficit/hyperactivity disorder, schizophrenia, and oppositional defiant disorder. Despite each having relatively distinct symptom profiles, most conditions are characterized by a combination of abnormal thoughts, perceptions, emotions, behavior, and relationships with others. While traditional behavior analytic intervention approaches do not always recognize the influence of thought, emotions, and perceptions on one's external behavior, without a broader acceptance and understanding of the role of private events, a cohesive treatment plan for psychopathology is not possible (Friman, Hayes, & Wilson, 1998). Further, as psychiatric symptoms are influenced by one's genetics and biology, as well as social and environmental influences (Rutter, Moffitt, & Caspi, 2006), utilizing a data-driven assessment method to identify the intersection of one's biopsychosocial functioning and their cognitive, emotional, and behavioral symptoms is imperative to ensure that the prescribed intervention is individualized and, in theory, more effective.

The purpose of this chapter is to provide an introduction into the incorporation of functional assessment for psychiatric disorders. An overview of those conditions, or symptom clusters, where the utility of functional assessment has been established will be discussed first, followed by areas where functional assessment has emerging utility. A brief discussion of the symptoms of each condition will be provided, as well as an overview of how functional assessment is specifically used for treatment planning or progress purposes. This chapter is by no means exhaustive. However, the chapter provides context for how identifying environmental relationships to a person's behavioral and emotional functioning leads to effective interventions for a wide variety of mental health symptoms that are pervasive and impairing to the affected individual.

Oppositional Defiant Disorder

An individual with Oppositional Defiant Disorder (ODD) exhibits a frequent and persistent pattern of angry/irritable mood, argumentative/defiant behavior, or vindictiveness. Individuals with ODD may frequently lose their temper, are easily annoyed and deliberately annoy others, argue with and deft authority figures, or blame others for their mistakes. These behaviors must generally occur at least once per week and must cause impairment or distress in the individual or his or her immediate social context (APA, 2013). In children younger than 5 years, behaviors must occur most days for a period of 6 months or more. About 10% of individuals in the United States will be diagnosed with ODD in their lifetime, and prevalence rates are similar for males and females (Nock, Kazdin, Hiripi, & Kessler, 2007). In a national epidemiologic study, median age-of-onset for ODD was found to be age 12 (Nock et al., 2007).

Given its typical age of onset, ODD is commonly conceptualized as a childhood disorder. Therefore, most assessment and treatment research has focused on treatment for ODD in childhood and adolescence. The American Academy of Child and Adolescent Psychiatry practice parameters for ODD recommend multimodal treatment, including parent management training approaches with contingency management (Steiner & Remsing, 2007). A recent review similarly identifies individual and group parent management training as a well-established treatment for ODD in childhood and adolescence (Kaminski & Claussen, 2017).

Before treatment of ODD can begin, the first step is to conduct a functional analysis (or assessment) of the child's problem behaviors (Steiner & Remsing, 2007). This functional assessment is necessary to identify the factors that maintain disruptive behavior, including antecedents, consequences, and setting events. Problem behaviors in children and teens with ODD are the result of youth selecting maladaptive solutions to a challenging environment. As part of the assessment, then, the therapist should focus on environmental factors that may be contributing to the problem behavior. This allows the therapist to work with caregivers to modify the environment to elicit adaptive behaviors and maintain them over time (del Valle, Kelley, & Seoanes, 2001). Caregivers track antecedents and consequences of problem behaviors over a period of 1–2 weeks. The therapist and caregivers then work together to identify possible functions for these behaviors, such as gaining attention, escaping or delaying non-preferred tasks or activities, and gaining access to preferred items or activities.

During treatment, caregivers are encouraged to reduce positive reinforcement of problem behaviors and increase reinforcement for prosocial and compliant behaviors. For example, therapists will recommend that caregivers ignore attention-seeking tantrum behavior and provide positive attention when their child is calm. Similarly, therapists will recommend that caregivers follow through with directions so that noncompliance is not reinforced. When their child complies with directions, caregivers provide praise and/or rewards to reinforce this positive behavior. Additionally, caregivers identify common antecedents or triggers for problem behaviors and use antecedent management strategies to reduce the likelihood of problem behaviors occurring.

Conduct Disorder

Conduct Disorder (CD) is characterized by a pattern of behavior in which the individual violates the basic rights of others or major age-appropriate societal norms. Behaviors can include aggression to people and animals, destruction of property, deceitfulness or theft, or serious violations of rules (e.g., frequent school truancy before age 13 years). The pattern of behavior must be repetitive and persistent (i.e., at least three behaviors in the past 12 months), and must cause clinically significant impairment in functioning (APA, 2013). In diagnosing CD, it is important to determine whether the disorder had childhood onset (before age 10) or adolescent onset (after age 10), as research suggests distinct pathways for antisocial behavior between these groups, with earlier onset predicting worse outcomes (Moffitt, Caspi, Harrington, & Milne, 2002). Additionally, it is important to determine whether individuals with CD also show callous-unemotional symptoms (e.g., lack of guilt, remorse, or empathy; deficient affect), as these individuals tend to have more stable behavior problems and poorer response to treatment (Fairchild et al., 2019). A U.S. national survey estimated the lifetime prevalence of CD is about 12% in males and 7% in females, with median onset at age 11.6 years (Nock, Kazdin, Hiripi, & Kessler, 2006).

In early to middle childhood, the recommended first-line approach for treating CD is parent management training (Fairchild et al., 2019), the same approach described previously for youth with ODD which begins with a functional analysis of the problem behaviors. When children with CD in early to middle childhood also exhibit callous-unemotional symptoms, adding a child-focused empathic-emotion recognition training to parent management training can enhance its effects (Dadds, Cauchi, Wimalaweera, Hawes, & Brennan, 2012). In late childhood and adolescence, Multisystemic Therapy (Henggeler, 2001) and Oregon Multidimensional Treatment Foster Care (Chamberlain, 2003) are recommended treatments. These programs integrate parenting components similar to parent management training, including contingency management, with family-focused strategies, youth skill-building, and cognitive-behavioral therapy (Fairchild et al., 2019). Functional assessment is used in the context of these intensive treatments to identify and modify factors that lead to serious offenses. For example, if a youth committed a sexual offense against a younger child and a driver of their offending behavior was frequent unmonitored babysitting, this access to younger children would be eliminated (Letourneau et al., 2009). Similarly, for youth with substance-use problems, a detailed functional analysis of substance-use related behavior is used as the basis for intervention planning. Youth are encouraged to avoid identified triggers (e.g., spending time with peers who engage in substance use) and caregivers deliver contingent consequences following frequent drug screens (Holth, Torsheim, Sheidow, Ogden, & Henggeler, 2011).

Attention-Deficit/Hyperactivity Disorder

Attention-deficit/hyperactivity disorder (ADHD) is a chronic neurodevelopmental disorder. Individuals with ADHD exhibit impairing patterns of inattentive and/or hyperactive-impulsive symptoms in at least two settings. Inattentive symptoms include difficulty paying attention to details, trouble organizing tasks, being easily distracted, etc. Hyperactive and impulsive symptoms include fidgeting, running about (or feeling restless for adolescents and adults), talking excessively, interrupting, etc. Importantly, several symptoms must be present before age 12 years in order to diagnose ADHD in adolescents and adults. Additionally, there must be clear evidence that these symptoms cause impairment in functioning (APA, 2013). ADHD is one of the most common psychiatric disorders, affecting an estimated 7.2% of children and adolescents (Thomas, Sanders, Doust, Beller, & Glasziou, 2015) and 4.4% of adults (Kessler et al., 2006).

The American Academy of Pediatrics practice guidelines for ADHD in children and adolescents recommend behavior therapy (including parent management training and school-based behavior therapy) as the first line of treatment for preschool-aged children. For children aged 6–11 years, evidence-based behavior therapy and/or FDA-approved medications (e.g., stimulants) can be considered as first line of treatment. For adolescents, FDA-approved medications should be prescribed, and behavior therapy may be added (Wolraich et al., 2011). For adults, combination treatment including psychoeducation, initial medication trial and titration to ideal dose, assessment of residual symptoms, and long-term community follow-up is recommended (Gibbins & Weiss, 2007).

A variety of parent- and/or teacher-administered behavioral strategies has been found to be effective to improve ADHD symptoms in youth. Thus, once the therapist has determined an individual meets diagnostic criteria for ADHD, the next step is to identify target behaviors that should be changed, followed by a functional assessment of these behaviors used to select the most appropriate intervention strategies (Dupaul & Ervin, 1996). For example, if a child exhibits increased inattentive behavior during homework (antecedent) when their caregiver frequently reminds the child to get back on-task, it could be hypothesized that the inattentive behavior is maintained by caregiver attention. An appropriate intervention, then, could be for the caregiver to provide intermittent reinforcement following specified periods of on-task behavior (Dupaul & Ervin, 1996). Overall, meta-analytic research has found larger effects for interventions for youth with ADHD when the intervention was based on functional analysis (Miller & Lee, 2013).

For adults with ADHD, psychosocial treatments typically include organizational and attentional skills training and/or cognitive behavioral therapy derived from a functional assessment of the individual's symptoms. In the cognitive-behavior therapy (CBT) approach, it is hypothesized that maladaptive cognitions reinforce chronic patterns of procrastination and disorganization, leading to avoidance of related tasks and failure to use compensatory strategies (e.g., planning, problem-solving) that could improve ADHD symptoms (Knouse & Safren, 2010; Safren, Sprich, Chulvick, & Otto, 2004). Therapists work with individuals to identify maladaptive cognitions and conduct a functional analysis to identify hypothesized functions. For example, an individual may experience stress when remembering a task is due soon (antecedent), followed by thinking a maladaptive thought (e.g., "I can get it done later."), leading to a feeling of relief (consequence). In this case, the function of the maladaptive thought was removal of stress related to the triggering event (Knouse & Mitchell, 2015). Therapists then help individuals identify their avoidance patterns, including related maladaptive cognitions and their functions, and replace them with alternative coping strategies.

Social Anxiety Disorder

An individual with social anxiety disorder experiences significant fear or anxiety about social situations in which they anticipate scrutiny or judgment from others. The level of anxiety must be clearly out of proportion to the situation. The person fears they will behave in a way that will be embarrassing by either showing anxiety symptoms, such as shaking, perspiring, or speaking in a tremulous voice, or that they will do something else for which they will be negatively judged, such as giving a wrong answer, or saying something that others think is odd (APA, 2013). Antecedents or triggers for anxiety can include activities such as giving a presentation, ordering in a restaurant, meeting new people, or even walking or eating in view of others. The triggering situations are either avoided or endured with intense discomfort perhaps with the aid of safety behaviors that aim to reduce anxiety. Safety behaviors can range from mildly to extremely maladaptive, including actions such as avoiding eye contact, sitting rather than standing at all social events, drinking alcohol or using other substances during or before social events, or perhaps only engaging in such events or activities if accompanied by certain individuals (Buckner & Heimberg, 2010; Spence & Rapee, 2016). Maladaptive safety behaviors are targeted in treatment for elimination or replacement with more adaptive behaviors. There are mixed findings regarding whether all safety behaviors must be eliminated for treatment to be effective (Meulders, Van Daele, Volders, & Vlaeyen, 2016); however, any that are significantly maladaptive will be targeted for elimination. Other individuals may engage in behaviors in response to the person with social anxiety's distress that actually serve to maintain the avoidance such as speaking for them, or making excuses for their absence or departure from events; these behaviors must also be identified and, most likely, targeted for elimination. The 12-month prevalence estimate of Social Anxiety Disorder in the United States is approximately 7% (APA, 2013).

CBT is the treatment of choice for social anxiety with many variants employing gradual exposure to feared situations as a key component of treatment (Kaczkurkin & Foa, 2015; Mayo-Wilson et al., 2014; Rodebaugh, Holaway, & Heimberg, 2004). Avoidance and maladaptive safety behaviors that the person utilizes to reduce distress in feared social situations, and any behaviors performed by others that serve to maintain the person's avoidance, are eliminated in a gradual fashion. The goal is to help the person achieve the goal of distress reduction without engaging in avoidance of necessary or desired social activities and without relying on maladaptive behaviors to tolerate the feared situations. The first step in this process involves identifying the antecedents or triggering situations in the environment as well as accompanying thought patterns that increase anxiety. Examples of anxiety-increasing anxiety include overestimating the chance of bad things happening, overestimating how bad the feared outcome will be if it does happen, and underestimating their ability to cope with a bad outcome. Current strategies the person is using to manage these triggers are also identified, along with any reactions from others that occur in response to their anxiety. Thinking errors that occur during exposure situations, such as inferring negative reactions from others where none may have been present, are identified. In short, any reactions or consequences to the person's behavior in the triggering social situation that appears to be serving to maintain the avoidance or other maladaptive behaviors need to be identified.

During CBT, access to any items in the environment that serve as safety behaviors is reduced, others are instructed to eliminate their own behaviors that facilitate avoidance, such as speaking for the person, or making excuses for the person's absence or departure from events. The person is provided with alternate, more adaptive strategies, such as relaxation techniques and cognitive restructuring that focus on modification of the thought patterns that increase anxiety and/or encourage avoidance. The person will be advised to utilize these more adaptive behaviors before, during, and after engaging in exposure to previously avoided situations. Distress in response to the antecedents or triggers will gradually decrease via desensitization after repeated exposure occurs with no truly bad outcomes. In addition, residual anxiety can be effectively managed via the more adaptive behavioral strategies of relaxation exercises and cognitive restructuring.

Panic Disorder

A person with Panic Disorder experiences recurrent, unexpected panic attacks which are episodes of intense fear that have an abrupt onset and are accompanied by a wide range of physical and cognitive symptoms including, but not limited to, rapid or pounding heartbeat, shortness of breath, a sensation of choking, dizziness, feelings of unreality, or fear of losing control or going "crazy". The person also experiences one or both of the following: (1) Persistent worry about the panic attacks themselves, due to panic being an aversive experience, or worry about consequences of panic, such as worry that panic will lead to a heart attack. (2) Significant behavioral changes that aim to reduce the possibility of panic attacks, such as avoiding certain places, situations, or certain physiological sensations, such as elevated heart rate resulting from exercise. The 12-month prevalence estimate for adolescents and adults in the United States is approximately 2–3% (APA, 2013).

CBT that includes either or both interoceptive exposure, which involves induction of, and graduated desensitization to the physical sensations associated with panic, or exposure to situational triggers is a well-supported treatment for panic disorder (Craske & Barlow, 2007; Kaczkurkin & Foa, 2015; Mitte, 2005). A person with panic disorder can rapidly develop extensive avoidance and other maladaptive behaviors that serve the perceived function of reducing the chance of panic attacks (Craske & Barlow, 2007).

Tracking of antecedents to panic attacks is critical. Common panic attack antecedents can include environmental variables such as being in a crowded room, being somewhere unfamiliar, or being in a hot environment; physical sensations such a rapid heartbeat or dizziness; thought patterns such as anticipating high likelihood of a panic attack in a certain situation or overestimating how bad it would be to have a panic attack in a certain situation. The person is likely to utilize avoidance of situations that they believe will trigger an attack and may also engage in other "safety behaviors" that they believe will reduce the chance of a panic attack but may be maladaptive (Craske & Barlow, 2007). For example, a person may spend a significant amount of time researching escape routes from a school or conference room if they were to need to leave due to a panic attack, or they may leave an event if they cannot ensure that they can be near an exit at all times. They may need to have very particular items or people with them when away from home in order to reduce the chance of panic and to feel they will be safe if they do have a panic attack. In addition, others may engage in behaviors in response to the individual's avoidance and safety behaviors, that may partially maintain the avoidance and safety behaviors (Craske & Barlow, 2007) such as facilitating the safety behaviors or inadvertently removing any negative consequences of avoidance, by doing things such as permitting an adolescent with panic in the school setting to be homeschooled or running an excessive number of errands for an adult. If these behaviors in others are not identified and addressed, it may be challenging for an individual to optimally motivate themselves for treatment.

The functional assessment of panic forms the basis of developing the treatment plan. A hierarchy of antecedents is constructed and the individual will engage in gradual exposure to each item on the hierarchy without engaging in avoidance or safety behaviors. They are instructed in techniques such as deep breathing, progressive muscle relaxation, and cognitive restructuring to facilitate staying in the exposure without experiencing excessive distress or panic. Cognitive restructuring addresses maladaptive beliefs that can drive panic. For example: "my heart is beating fast and I'm short of breath; I must be having a heart attack" can be replaced by "I know that this is what my body does when my fight or flight response is activated, but I'm safe, and I'm fine, I can handle this; my body can handle this." Friends and family members are also instructed to gradually reduce accommodations that remove potential negative consequences of engaging in avoidance. Gradually beginning to permit natural consequences of avoidance can help motivate continued exposure work.

Trichotillomania

An individual with trichotillomania engages in recurrent hair pulling from the scalp or other areas such as eyebrows, eyelashes, or body that results in hair loss. The pulling is not done for cosmetic reasons, and the person struggles to stop the pulling. The 12-month prevalence estimate for trichotillomania in adolescents and adults in the United States is approximately 1–2% (APA, 2013). While typical age of onset is estimated to be between 10 and 13 years of age, estimates of prevalence in childhood are not available; the majority of epidemiological data for this disorder is drawn from college-age populations (Grant & Chamberlain, 2016).

Habit reversal training is the best-supported treatment for trichotillomania (Elliott & Fuqua, 2000; Friman, Finney, & Christophersen, 1984; Morris, Zickgraf, Dingfelder, & Franklin, 2014). Functional assessment is a core component of this treatment; identifying high-risk situations or other antecedents for pulling as well as perceived positive consequences of pulling such as comfort, pleasure, satisfaction, or distress reduction is key to developing the treatment plan.

Antecedent situations for hair pulling can include relaxing activities such as watching television, engaging in pleasure reading or falling asleep, activities the person finds boring such as sitting in a non-engaging lecture, or activities the person finds anxiety provoking, and/or those that require a lot of mental energy and effort such as studying for or taking a test. The function, or desirable consequence, of the hair pulling typically differs depending on the antecedent and so identifying the antecedents correctly is key to developing successful alternative behaviors as well as to determining when and which stimulus control strategies might be most appropriate. For example, if pulling occurs during relaxing activities, such as watching television, and serves a soothing function, the person would be provided with an adaptive alternative soothing behavior that is readily available and incompatible with pulling, such as keeping both hands on a soft blanket or pillow while watching television. If the pulling occurs when the person is going to sleep, stimulus control, such as directing the person to wear a lightweight hat and/or gloves to bed, will be a critical component of treatment.

Tic Disorders

A person with a tic disorder experiences motor and/or vocal tics which are movements or sounds that occur in a sudden, rapid, and nonrhythmic manner. Transient tics are common in childhood with the prevalence of Tourette's Disorder, which includes both motor and vocal tics which are present for a year or more, at 0.3–0.8% in school aged children. Many children continue to experience tics through adolescence and into adulthood (APA, 2013).

Functional assessment and intervention is a core component of Comprehensive Behavioral Intervention for Tourette's (CBIT) which is an evidence-based intervention for Tourette's Disorder and other tic disorders (Piacentini et al., 2010). A structured functional assessment is conducted to determine antecedents and consequences for each target tic (Woods et al., 2008). Antecedents can include situations, behaviors, or emotions and can be fairly general, such as feeling anxious, or quite specific, such as running late for school. Consequences can include social attention that is either positive or negative, being excused from tasks, being punished or excluded from an activity, or being given extra privileges or rewards. Antecedents and consequences of tics are eliminated or reduced if it is realistic to do so, or they are modified if elimination is not realistic. For example, if being in a completely silent room is an antecedent for a burst of vocal tics, a fan, other white noise, or other background noise is introduced. If others provide social attention in response to the tics by either telling the child to stop having the tics, laughing at or comforting the child, they are asked to stop attending to the tics. If the child is permitted to get out of a task, such as homework or chores, due to tics, this consequence is eliminated even if modifications are necessary such as having an assignment read to the child if an eye darting tic is preventing reading.

Depressive Disorders

Depressive disorders such as Major Depressive Disorder, Disruptive Mood Dysregulation Disorder, and Persistent Depressive Disorder (previously termed Dysthymia) share the common feature of sad, empty, or irritable mood with accompanying somatic and cognitive symptoms (APA, 2013).

An individual with Major Depressive Disorder experiences depressed mood most of the day, nearly every day. In children and adolescents, this can present as irritable mood rather than an overtly sad mood state. The person may lose interest or pleasure in activities and hobbies that they previously enjoyed. They may experience feelings of worthlessness, hopelessness, helplessness, or excessive guilt. Thoughts of death and dying, including suicidal thoughts, may also be present. Depressed individuals also often struggle with physical and somatic complaints. They report fatigue, loss of energy, and problems with concentrating (APA, 2013). Major Depression is one of the most common mental disorders in the United States and has a 12-month prevalence estimate of approximately 7% across all ages with the highest rates occurring among 18–29-year olds (APA, 2013).

Disruptive Mood Dysregulation Disorder is a recently recognized psychiatric condition. The disorder is a new diagnostic addition in the DSM-5 to help differentiate children and adolescents who in the past were misdiagnosed and treated for Bipolar Disorder (APA, 2013). Children and adolescents with Disruptive Mood Dysregulation Disorder have persistent severe irritability and/or angry mood state and display frequent episodes of extreme behavior, which may include temper outbursts, verbal and/or physical aggression. This differs from Bipolar Disorder in that the negative mood states persist and are not episodic in nature. Researchers have noted over time that in practice, children and adolescents diagnosed with Bipolar Disorder were comprised of two very distinct and notably different clinical presentations. The addition of Disruptive Mood Dysregulation Disorder is an attempt to separate out children and adolescents with severe, persistent irritability from children and adolescents presenting with classic, episodic bipolar symptoms including mania (APA, 2013). The onset of Disruptive Mood Dysregulation Disorder must occur before the age of 10. The diagnosis age at this time is limited to the age range of 7–18 years of age; adults cannot currently be provided the diagnosis (APA, 2013). Initial prevalence estimates for Disruptive Mood Dysregulation Disorder fall within the 2–5% range of children and adolescents (APA, 2013).

Persistent Depressive Disorder (Dysthymia) is characterized by a chronic depressed or irritable mood lasting for over 2 years for adults or 1 year for children and adolescents. Adults with Persistent Depressive Disorder often report that they have always felt this way. The 12-month prevalence estimate for Persistent Depressive Disorder across all ages in the United States is in the range of 0.5 and 1.5% (APA, 2013).

CBT and Dialectical Behavior Therapy (DBT) are two evidenced-based interventions for the treatment of depression and suicidality (DeCou, Comtois, & Landes, 2019; Hollon & Ponniah, 2010; Tolin, 2010; Turner, Austin, & Chapman,

2014). Similar to CBT descriptions described for other conditions in this chapter, CBT for depression and suicidality focuses on the relationship between cognitions, affect, and behavior (Beck, 1979) and utilizes both cognitive techniques and behavioral strategies. DBT has a significant behavioral focus and is the merging of behavioral change strategies with acceptance-based (focusing on accepting one's emotional experiences rather than labeling as a problem or symptom) techniques (Linehan, 2015; Miller, Rathus, & Linehan, 2007; Rathus & Miller, 2014). Both approaches, thus, incorporate significant behavioral techniques and rely on functional assessment.

CBT and DBT therapists both incorporate functional assessment into their approaches by assessing the relationship between thoughts, feelings, behaviors, and environmental/situational factors. In CBT, this relationship is often taught to patients through the use of the cognitive triangle, thought monitoring, and the use of thought records (McManus, Van Doorn, & Yiend, 2012; Stark, Sander, Yancy, Bronik, & Hoke, 2000). The cognitive triangle looks at the interrelationship between thoughts, feelings, and behaviors in relation to a specific event and how each of these can affect and potentially change the other. For example, an adolescent receiving a bad grade on a test may have the thought, "this is unfair and the teacher is out to get me," which might then correspond with a feeling of anger, and a behavioral action of ripping up the test and yelling at the teacher. Similarly, an adolescent receiving a bad grade may have the thought, "I am stupid and never do well" which could correspond to a feeling of sadness and hopelessness, and a behavioral action of skipping class or decreased academic effort next exam. Each instance had the same triggering event but feelings and behavioral actions varied based on the thought or belief about the event. CBT therapists use thought records to help monitor and identify patterns in automatic thoughts and underlying beliefs that correspond with negative mood states and problem behaviors.

In DBT, the relationship between thoughts, feelings, behaviors, and environmental/situational factors is taught through chain analysis – a technique often viewed as the heart of DBT individual therapy work (Linehan, 2015; Miller et al., 2007; Rathus & Miller, 2014; Rizvi & Ritschel, 2014). DBT chain analysis is an expanded form of functional assessment incorporating the vulnerability factors, thoughts, body sensations, action urges, and feelings leading up to a targeted problematic behavior such as self-harm or non-suicidal self-injury (Linehan, 2015; Miller et al., 2007; Rathus & Miller, 2014; Rizvi & Ritschel, 2014). The therapist works with the patient to identify each of the many links in the chain leading up to the targeted behavior including reinforcement the individual experiences following the targeted behavior. Identifying the factors related to the maintenance of the targeted behavior is an important concept in treatment and acknowledges that the person has perceived benefits or is reinforced by the targeted problem behavior. Non-suicidal self-injury, a common referral reason for DBT which is frequently seen with depressive disorders, often serves many functions and can be positively and negatively reinforced (Walsh, 2006). For example, take the example of the adolescent ("Tom") that received that bad test grade. After receiving the bad grade, Tom went into the school bathroom and cut himself in an episode of non-suicidal self-injury. The first step in the chain analysis for this event would be to identify associated vulnerability factors. Tom notes that he stayed up late the night before and was tired, was hungry, and was stressed due to his parents yelling at him that morning about uncompleted chores. As a result, he was already more vulnerable to experiencing negative mood states and engaging in targeted problem behavior. The next step in the chain analysis is to identify the triggering event that started the chain. In this case, Tom notes that as the teacher passed out the exams, she mentioned she was pleased with how well the class did. Tom identifies that based on the teacher's comment, he expected a high score and was surprised to learn he had scored poorly. Next, in the chain analysis is identifying the different body sensations they experienced when the event occurred: Tom felt his heart racing, pressure in his temples, and was hot all over. Then, the individual must identify their "in the moment "feelings and provide a Subjective Units of Distress rating: Tom identifies he felt angry, foolish, disappointed, embarrassed, and ashamed with a distress level of 60 (moderate distress; on a scale of 0–100). In the next step, action urges corresponding to the "in the moment" feelings are identified. In Tom's case, he notes he had the urge to escape the situation, hide, and avoid others. Next, any thoughts associated with the action step are identified: Tom notes he was stupid, not as good as everyone else, and a complete failure. Tom then points out that he acted on his action urge to escape and left the classroom on a pretext to use the bathroom. The DBT therapist encouraged Tom to look at each new chain link including factors as they occurred in the bathroom. Tom notes that leaving the classroom resulted in an immediate, albeit time-limited, decrease in distress level. He mentions that because he was alone in the bathroom, he started having increased negative thoughts and new body sensations (e.g., pounding/tightening of their chest); he felt hopeless and helpless; his distress level increased to 85 (extremely high distress); and he began thinking he could not tolerate feeling this way much longer. Tom experienced a new action urge to "do something" to make the distress stop. Upon seeing a sharp edge on a paper towel dispenser, he impulsively acted on his urge to self-injure, resulting in an immediate decrease in distress to a 50 (mild–moderate distress). Next, looking at the positive and negative consequences occurring after Tom's self-injury, he notes that he felt immediately relieved from his negative emotional state and high distress, and was relieved to have been able to hide his feelings from peers. However, Tom reports that much later he felt shame and failure because of action on his self-injury urge. After completing each link of the chain, the DBT therapist will determine specific skills and strategies the individual can use that can end with a different, more adaptive outcome. Thus, chain analysis, a form of functional assessment, is an essential component to the treatment of suicidal and self-harm behavior within the DBT framework.

Another essential behavioral change strategy incorporated into both CBT and DBT for the treatment of depressive disorders is Behavioral Activation. Behavioral Activation, first delineated by Lewinsohn (1975), is an important component to CBT and DBT treatment approaches for depression and suicidality (Manos, Kanter, & Busch, 2010). In DBT skills training, for example, this intervention is the focus of the ABC Please skill from the Emotion Regulation module (Linehan, 2015;

Miller et al., 2007; Rathus & Miller, 2014). Patients working on this skill will work on "accumulating positive experiences" and pick from a list of pleasant activities those that they enjoy or currently use and those that may want to try (Rathus & Miller, 2014). The goal of behavioral activation is to reduce symptoms of anhedonia, isolation, and withdrawal, while increasing positive experiences and activity engagement.

Individuals with depressive disorders experience many internal and external barriers to engaging in pleasant activities. Functional assessment can be critical to identifying barriers. A key step in the intervention process is to help eliminate these barriers, such as breaking the activity into smaller more accomplishable tasks. For example, setting a goal to text a friend three times this week could be an initial behavioral goal as opposed to the more advanced goal of leaving the house at least three times per week for a month. Behavioral tracking and monitoring is an important part of this process; patients in both CBT and DBT often keep logs of their efforts. Behavioral activation is an important component to the treatment of depression within both the CBT and DBT frameworks. Additionally, there has been some research supporting the use of Behavioral Activation as a stand-alone treatment for depression for mild-to-moderate depression (Manos et al., 2010; Sturmey, 2009; Tindall et al., 2017).

Another behavioral change strategy incorporated into DBT that relies heavily on functional assessment is the targeting of therapy interfering behaviors. In DBT, therapy interfering behaviors include noncompliance with therapy tasks and completion of therapy homework (i.e., filling out Diary Card, skill practice outside of session), as well as in-session behavior such as nonparticipation or refusing to talk, aggression or self-harm behavior in session, problems with motivation, etc. (Miller et al., 2007). Therapy interfering behaviors are important to address, as they may result in treatment failure or discontinuation of treatment. In DBT, addressing these behaviors is an expected and integral part of treatment. Therapy interfering behaviors can also occur from family members and other collaterals, as well as the therapists themselves.

Chain analysis, a form of functional assessment, is utilized to address therapy interfering behaviors. DBT uses functional assessment to breakdown the antecedents and consequences to therapy interfering behaviors. For example, in the case of therapy homework noncompliance, a DBT therapist will use functional assessment via chain analysis to identify the reasons for lack of compliance (i.e., too hard, overwhelming, too boring, insecurity, etc.) and break down the homework tasks to address these concerns and use reinforcement to shape compliance. For example, an adolescent ("Kate") is asked to complete and bring to session a Diary Card, but has not for several consecutive sessions. The DBT therapist performs a chain analysis in session with Kate and identifies several contributing factors to homework noncompliance. First, the therapist notes that the adolescent plans each day to complete therapy homework after school homework. After school homework, Kate notes she is tired and often frustrated. When attempting to complete her therapy work, she feels stressed as she is unsure what to write and experiences aversive bodily sensations (e.g., abdomen tightening) resulting in the action urge to avoid. Further, not completing homework and not bringing the Diary Card to sessions has also resulted in continuing to work on skill practice during therapy which simultaneously allows Kate to avoid discussing difficult topics that she finds aversive. Based on the outcomes, Kate and her therapist decide that she will complete therapy homework prior to school homework. Future sessions are restructured to focus first on review of Kate's Diary Card, then an in-session reward card game for homework completion, and finally skill practice with any remaining time.

Emerging Areas

While the following conditions affecting one's mental health and wellness may not presently have enough established data supporting the use of functional assessment, it is highly likely that the use of functional assessment could be of some benefit to developing cohesive and effective treatment plans.

Conversion Disorder Conversion Disorder is characterized as an individual having one or more symptoms of altered voluntary motor and sensory function. A medical workup (e.g., imaging, EEG, etc.) and physical exam demonstrate that the symptoms are incompatible with neurological or medical conditions. Symptoms of conversion disorder include the following: weakness or paralysis, abnormal movement, swallowing symptoms, speech symptoms (e.g., dysphonia and slurred speech), seizures, anesthesia or sensory loss, and sensory symptoms (e.g., visual, olfactory, or hearing problems). An individual with Conversion Disorder may have one or more of the symptoms listed above (APA, 2013). Kozlowska, Scher, and Williams (2011) found that 67% of children diagnosed with Conversion Disorder had one or more symptoms. Forty-seven percent had psychogenic nonepileptic seizures, 47% had sensory symptoms (e.g., blindness and visual loss), and 64% had motor symptoms (e.g., gait disturbance, paralysis, weakness of limbs). Though the incident rate of Conversion Disorder is unknown, it is estimated to be 2–5 out of 100,000 per year (APA, 2013).

The empirically supported psychotherapy for Conversion Disorder is CBT as it reduces somatic symptoms and improves physical functioning (Jing, Neeraj, Teodorczuk, Zhan-jiang, & Sun, 2019). A functional assessment is needed with Conversion Disorder to determine factors that are contributing to the development and maintenance of symptoms. Antecedent interventions are essential in the treatment of psychogenic nonepileptic seizures (PNES), a symptom of Conversion Disorder. At the beginning of treatment, patients track their PNES to gain insight into their triggers or antecedents for their episodes. Patients are then taught seizure-control techniques such as relaxation skills to decrease PNES (Goldstein et al., 2015; Lefrance et al., 2009).

In addition to antecedent interventions for PNES, patients are taught techniques to extinguish reinforcement for all symptoms of Conversion Disorder. Children with Conversion Disorder may experience anticipatory anxiety that they may have an onset of symptoms in specific situations. As such, children often avoid situations where they are likely to have a physical response. Continued avoidance of situations further exacerbates their anxiety and somatic symptoms. Use of exposures and cognitive restructuring of the anticipatory anxiety decreases future avoidance. Besides teaching children interventions, parent training is an integral part of treatment of Conversion Disorder. A functional assessment is important to determine how the parent's behavior is maintaining the child's symptoms. Parents often decrease expectations of their children (e.g., fewer chores), significantly change the child's schedule (e.g., later bed and wake times, more screen time), allow the child to stay home from school, permit decreased interactions with family and friends, and give the child more attention for their symptoms further reinforcing their child's symptoms. In treatment, parents are encouraged to limit attention to symptoms; increase the child's involvement in social, family, and extracurricular activities; implement age-appropriate expectations and consequences; and have the child return to school (Williams & Zahka, 2017).

Childhood Obesity While not considered a psychiatric disorder, childhood obesity is a global public health problem that increases the risk of premature death, as well as developing a myriad of medical complications (e.g., diabetes, cancer, asthma, hypertension, and heart disease), physical conditions, and negative social outcomes into adulthood (Barlow & Dietz, 1998; Daniels, 2009; U.S. Department of Health and Human Services, 2012). Being obese as a child (i.e., Body Mass Index [BMI] at or above the 95th percentile for age and gender) is strongly correlated with psychological consequences including anxiety, depression, sleep disorders, compromised perceived quality of life, and low self-esteem affecting the social and educational relationships of children (Rankin et al., 2016). Approximately 18.5% of children aged 2–19 years of age in the United States are considered obese (Hales, Carroll, Fryar, & Ogden, 2017) with prevalence data varying by age group (i.e., those 12–19 years are most at risk), by socioeconomic status (i.e., those of lowest income groups are most at risk), and by ethnic status (i.e., non-Hispanic black and Hispanic children are most at risk) (Ogden, Carroll, Kit, & Flegal, 2012). Of those children considered obese, approximately 70% continue to be obese or overweight as adults (Hales et al., 2017).

Given that childhood obesity is associated with a wide range of negative outcomes, it is imperative to identify and intervene upon factors that may moderate its development and maintenance. At the individual level, obesity is thought to be due to a number of interacting genetic, behavioral, psychological, and environmental factors. Children whose parents are obese are more than 50–60% more likely to also struggle with obesity or other weight-related concerns (Bahreynian et al., 2017; Keane, Layte, Harrington, Kearney, & Perry, 2012). While these outcomes in combination with outcomes from twin studies point to a genetic predisposition for pediatric obesity, external factors also have an impact in the developmental, maintenance, and treatment of obesity and related concerns (Hebebrand & Hinney, 2008). Further, external influences are those that are more amenable to assessment and intervention. For example, data suggest that children whose parents and/or siblings who are obese tend to live in homes where calorie-dense foods are readily available, are more likely to dine out of the home, engage in more sedentary leisure activities, and have lower than average opportunities for physical activity (Pinard et al., 2012) resulting in increased likelihood to become obese than a similar child with fewer risk factors. Researchers also suggest that obese individuals may find food more reinforcing than healthy-weight peers (Epstein, Lin, Carr, & Fletcher, 2012). Further, obese children appear to value energy-dense food more than other potential reinforcers such as spending time with peers, and as a result may need larger portion sizes to feel satiated and have poorer impulse control when it comes to making food choices (French, Epstein, Jeffery, Blundell, & Wardle, 2012; Nederkoorn, Braet, Van Eijs, Tanghe, & Jansen, 2006). Finally, obese children are more likely to experience multiple associated psychosocial problems further affecting their presentation and making treatment more complex.

Treatment for childhood obesity has become a growing field over the past 10 years due to the rising prevalence rates and poor outcomes associated with the condition. Interventions targeting children who are obese primarily focus on modifying caloric consumption or food choices, and increasing physical activity (Luzier, Berlin, & Weeks, 2010; McGovern et al., 2008). Targets for treatment often include limiting nonacademic screen time, reducing inactivity and slowly increasing physical activity to a daily goal of 60 minutes of a moderate to vigorous level, encouraging healthy eating habits in accordance with American Academy of Pediatrics and US Agricultural Department, focusing on a calorie-controlled diet, identify and intervene on maladaptive parent practices regarding diet and exercise, treating co-occurring psychiatric symptoms with evidenced-based psychotherapy or pharmacotherapy, and supporting parenting practices that contribute to child's self-esteem (Rajjo et al., 2017). A family-centered approach to therapy is also recommended, given the high likelihood of childhood obesity occurring in homes where parents and/or siblings also have weight-related issues, and many risk factors for maintenance of obesity (e.g., food availability, eating habits, leisure skill/physical activity choice) may be immediately affected by the home environment (Epstein, Valoski, Wing, & McCurley, 1994; Wilfley & Balantekin, 2018). Bariatric surgery is recommended as a last resort for obese adolescents (Sugerman et al., 2003). However, children and adolescents who fair best (with or without surgery) are those that are involved in a multitiered and multidisciplinary approach to intervention targeting both the individual child and the child's family, and also addresses interfering behaviors, symptoms, events, and family dynamics or the home environment.

Eating Disorders

Eating disorders (i.e., Anorexia Nervosa, Bulimia Nervosa, and Binge Eating Disorder) are abnormalities in eating or eating-related behaviors resulting in changes in the absorption or consumption of food which cause decreased psychosocial functioning or impairs physical health (APA, 2013). Those meeting criteria for anorexia nervosa often have a body weight that is well-below normal level of age, sex, developmental trajectory, and physical health due to food restriction, intense fear of gaining weight or engaging in behaviors the interfere with gaining weight, and abnormal perception of their weight or body shape (APA, 2013). Those with bulimia nervosa and binge eating disorder are often within the normal weight to overweight range as a result of repeatedly eating an excessive amount of food during discrete time periods while experiencing a self-perceived lack of intake control and extreme distress. In those with bulimia nervosa, the binging episode is followed by compensatory behaviors to prevent weight gain (e.g., self-induced vomiting, laxatives or other medications, fasting, or excessive exercise), whereas, those with binge eating disorder do not engage in compensatory behavior. Eating disorders can be severe and even life threatening, with those with anorexia nervosa being 10x more like to die prematurely from symptom complications (e.g., circulatory collapse, organ failure) (Fichter & Quadflieg, 2016). In addition, adolescents and adults are at a heightened risk to engage in self-harm, have suicidal ideation, or attempt suicide than their peers without an eating disorder (Cucchi et al., 2016; Kostro, Lerman, & Attia, 2014).

Present data suggest that approximately 5.2% of females and 1.2% of males aged 8–20 years-old meet criteria for an eating disorder (Smink, Van Hoeken, & Hoek, 2012; Stice, Marti, Shaw, & Jaconis, 2009). While an eating disorder can occur in childhood, the most common age range for onset of symptoms consistent with anorexia nervosa, bulimia nervosa, and binge eating disorder is in adolescence to young adulthood (Swanson, Crow, Le Grange, Swendsen, & Merikangas, 2011). There is a high prevalence of comorbid psychiatric conditions in this population. Over 55%, 88%, and 83% of patients with anorexia nervosa, bulimia nervosa, and binge eating disorder, respectively, have a comorbid psychiatric diagnosis (Swanson et al., 2011). The most common comorbid psychiatric disorders across all eating disorders are mood and anxiety disorders (Herpertz-Dahlmann, 2015).

Given the negative outcomes and poor long-term trajectory for individuals with an eating disorder, there is a growing need to improve response rates to evidence-based treatment. Increasing treatment success is of dire importance, as 25–50% of patients with an eating disorder do not respond to treatment and there is a high likelihood of symptom relapse (Ghaderi, 2007; Redlin, Miltenberger, Crosby, Wolff, & Stickney, 2002). Thus, using functional assessment to improve treatment outcomes is imperative.

Multiple antecedents have been identified in eating disorders. In general, common precipitators include exposure to social values of thinness, having been mocked by peers for weight or other body characteristics, prior sexual or trauma, family history of eating disorders, childhood adversity (i.e., family discord, parent separation, domestic violence, substance use), dissatisfaction with body shape and weight, obesity or family history of obesity, and preoccupation with food. Specific antecedents that can be addressed with functional analysis of anorexia nervosa include comments about weight from family or peers, perfectionistic personality traits, and a history of sexual trauma. Consequences that reinforce behavior in anorexia nervosa include control over an area of life when control is unattainable in other areas, endogenous opioid release obtained with starvation, prevention of

sexual contact, and amenorrhea (Meyer, 2008). For binge eating disorder and bulimia, consequences that reaffirm behavior include attenuation of negative mood after
a binge due to endogenous opioid release (Meyer, 2008). An example of how these
behaviors may be addressed for an individual suffering from binge eating disorder
is an adolescent female who is engaged in restrictive food intake days before social
events to be "thin" and then engaged in binge eating at or after the event, a modification could be to implement three healthy, moderately sized meals per day to reduce
starvation leading to a binge.

Across all eating disorders, CBT is the first-line intervention (Hilbert, Hoek, &
Schmidt, 2017; National Guideline Alliance, 2017). Nutritional counseling is also
recommended. With respect to distinct eating disorders, there are additional recommendations for effective interventions. For anorexia nervosa, family therapy in
combination with CBT is the main component of treatment (Hilbert et al., 2017;
National Guideline Alliance, 2017). An alternative or concurrent therapy with CBT
for bulimia nervosa is interpersonal psychotherapy; however, younger children
highly benefit from family therapy. There is a paucity of research on psychopharma-
cology to treat core symptoms of an eating disorder; however, guidelines recommend antidepressants for co-occurring depressive and obsessive or compulsive
symptoms.

Psychotic Disorders

Psychotic disorders including delusional disorder and schizophrenia spectrum disorders are very rare in childhood and adolescence. Symptoms of psychosis include
hallucinations, delusions, abnormal thoughts, movements, or negative symptoms
(APA, 2013). The estimated prevalence for schizophrenia in prepubertal children is
between 0.04% and 0.1% (Gordon et al., 1994; National Collaborating Centre for
Mental Health (Great Britain), 2013; Ritsner, 2011). The prevalence rate increases
in adolescence to 0.5% of the adolescent population. Age of onset for early-onset
schizophrenia typically occurs between ages 15 and 25 years old (Ritsner, 2011).

A functional assessment can be beneficial in targeting multiple symptom areas
that often accompany psychosis in children and adolescents. In psychotic disorders,
postulated events which may increase the risk that psychotic symptoms emerge
include childhood adversity including sexual trauma, physical abuse, and parental
separation, living in urban environments, and social isolation and defeat (the negative experience of being isolated from a majority group) (Rosenfarb, 2013; Selten,
van der Ven, Rutten, & Cantor-Graae, 2013). Reinforcing consequences for hallucinations include distraction from negative emotions, reduced social isolation, and
increased attention from others (Rosenfarb, 2013). Negative symptoms may emerge
to help cope with positive symptoms. Verbal outbursts of disorganized speech may
be reinforced by escape from unwanted tasks or increased attention (Wilder,
Masuda, O'Connor, & Baham, 2001). For example, if a 17-year-old male is observed
to be talking to a small child that no one else in the room can see, the therapist

would attempt to determine what conditions increased this behavior. If it was determined that when the patient engages in this behavior, staff talk to him more about his hallucinations and engage with him; then, training could occur for both the patient and the staff on how to appropriately engage in conversation and withdrawal attention when the patient is engaging in bizarre speech and giving attention when he is communicating effectively.

Despite the rarity of psychotic illnesses in childhood and adolescence, there are established guidelines for recommendations and treatments. However, more treatment research is needed given the severity of early psychotic symptoms and their impact on long-term prognosis. Referring to a child psychiatrist is the first step of treatment for youth (Abidi et al., 2017). Antipsychotic medications, specifically second-generation neuroleptics, are first line for schizophrenia spectrum disorders in youth (Abidi et al., 2017; McClellan & Stock, 2013). In addition to medication, psychotherapy including family therapy, CBT, education/employment programs has also been shown to be effective (Lecomte et al., 2017). Additionally, there is increasing literature that early intervention with coordinated specialty care, a clinic that provides multidisciplinary services including access to psychotherapy, medication management, family education and support, case management, work or education support is imperative to improve outcomes in this population (Kane et al., 2016).

Habit Disorders

Internet Gaming Disorders

Internet gaming disorder is a proposed condition in the DSM-5 for individuals who exhibit symptoms for at least a year such as preoccupation with games, inability to control amount of time spent gaming, using gaming to escape from reality, loss of prior hobbies, and continuing to game despite social consequences (e.g., loss of work or relationships) (APA, 2013). The age of onset of symptoms consistent with internet gaming disorder typically occurs in adolescence to young adulthood. Prevalence of internet gaming disorder varies in the literature ranging from 1.6% to 8% in those aged 12–20 years old (Feng, Ramo, Chan, & Bourgeois, 2017; Gentile et al., 2017; Paulus, Ohmann, Von Gontard, & Popow, 2018). Males are four times more likely to have symptoms of internet gaming disorder compared to females.

Given the increasing prevalence of this disorder, functional assessment to assist with evidenced-based treatment is imperative to improve outcomes. Scales to assist with functional assessment have been studied and developed in this population (Buono, Upton, Griffiths, Sprong, & Bordieri, 2016; Sprong, Griffiths, Lloyd, Paul, & Buono, 2019). The most significant motivators for pathological video gaming include escape from reality, social outlet, and motivation for in-game rewards. Additionally, biopsychosocial factors increasing risk for gaming disorder include poor family relationship, increased impulsivity, comorbid depression and anxiety, single-parent home, increased level of parent anxiety, decreased parental attachment, and limited parental supervision (Milani et al., 2018; Sugaya, Shirasaka, Takahashi, & Kanda, 2019). In knowing the specific factors that may be maintaining pathological gaming, the therapist and families can develop interventions to mitigate undesirable behavior. For example, if a patient engages in pathological gaming for a social outlet, the therapist and patient could work to develop a behavioral plan that targets alternative social interactions such as board games or sports to engage the patient in other ways.

There is a paucity of literature on evidenced-based treatment for internet gaming disorder. Several studies evaluated antidepressants that target co-occurring mood disorders such as depression and anxiety, have been promising; however, methodology and sample size make it difficult to draw conclusions and make recommendations (King et al., 2017; Zajac, Ginley, Chang, & Petry, 2017). Furthermore, CBT, targeting gaming cravings and reduction in gaming hours, and family therapy, targeting family cohesion, effective communication of the adolescents needs, and increasing shared activities, have shown some efficacy in this population (King et al., 2017; Zajac et al., 2017). More research is needed that include randomized clinical trials with a control group so that conclusions about efficacy may be evaluated for specific interventions. Future studies should also include long-term follow-up and have a structured protocol for interventions.

Substance-Use Disorders

Substance-related and addictive disorders are a set of conditions that impact a person's school, work, and home environment due to an inability to control the use of the substance. Symptoms that are pervasive or impairing include increased tolerance to the substance, withdrawal when the substance is not used, spending time seeking the substance, and continued use of the substance despite difficulties at work, home, or school related to the substance (APA, 2013). While substance classes do have various distinctions in abuse potential, symptoms, and treatment modalities, addictive disorders will be discussed as a category more broadly. Over 40% of youth have tried illicit substances at least once in their life with 13% engaging in binge drinking (Office of Adolescent Health, 2019). Around 7–9% of adolescents between ages 12 and 17 years old meet DSM criteria for substance-use disorder (Mericle et al., 2015). Risk factors for substance-use disorders include other substance-use disorders, Hispanic ethnicity, younger age at first exposure, lack of parental supervision, poverty, involvement in child-welfare system, involvement with legal system, and family history of substance use (Fettes, Aarons, & Green, 2013; Lopez-Quintero et al., 2011; Swendsen et al., 2012). Additionally, the new method of nicotine intake, electronic cigarettes (i.e., vaping), is also being consumed by adolescents with 13% of adolescents reporting smoking e-cigarettes within the past 30 days (Farsalinos, Tomaselli, & Polosa, 2018; Yoong et al., 2018).

Multiple variables have been identified as antecedents substance use in adolescence including increased aggressiveness, impulsivity, involvement with legal system, peer pressure, decreased parental supervision, parent–child relationship dysfunction, and parent substance use (Poikolainen, 2002). While some of anteced-ents for adolescent substance use are genetically influenced (aggressiveness, impul-sivity, parent substance use), many factors exist that can be targeted through treatment, including parent–child relationship and parental supervision. The preva-lence of comorbid psychiatric disorders is high in adolescents with substance use: 61–88% are diagnosed with at least one co-occurring psychiatric diagnosis. Externalizing disorders (e.g., attention-deficit disorder and conduct disorder) co-occur more frequently than internalizing disorders (e.g., anxiety, depression) (Couwenbergh et al., 2006). Additionally, adolescents are highly likely to engage in polysubstance use, and often meet criteria for multiple substance-use disorders. Knowing the individual variables that increase the likelihood of substance use or interfere with treatment can aid into developing a cohesive and effective treatment plan for the adolescent with substance use. For example, Tod, a 16-year-old male is referred to the clinic for alcohol-use disorder. He used to be involved in football but was kicked off the team due to poor academic performance resulting from substance use, change in peer group, and emerging depression. His mother and father recently divorced and now his mother (whom he primarily lives with) works longer hours. As a result of decreased parental supervision, he spends time with friends after school and on the weekend, he engages in drinking and playing pool with his friends. Thus, an intervention could be to increase his participation in alternative social outlets (e.g., other extracurricular activities) that do not involve drinking with his peers and increase adult supervision through utilization of after-school study sessions, working with a tutor, or enlisting assistance from other family members.

By integrating outcomes from the functional assessment into the treatment plan-ning and implementation process, overall behavior will improve, and symptoms related to substance use/abuse will reduce. Current guidelines for adolescents with a substance-use-related disorder recommend the use of family, CBT, motivational interviewing, and contingency management training therapy targeting parental drug use, parent–child relationships, communication, supervision and management of behavior, social skills, anger control, problem-solving, and using incentives to encourage desired behavior (Barnett, Sussman, Smith, Rohrbach, & Spruijt-Metz, 2012; National Institute on Drug Abuse, 2014; Stanger, Lansing, & Budney, 2016). Additionally, pharmacotherapeutics can be utilized as needed to aid with with-drawal and cravings (Bukstein, 2005).

Gambling Disorders

Gambling disorder is a persistent and recurrent uncontrollable urge to gamble resulting in a significant and pervasive negative impact on an individual's life (APA, 2013). While gambling disorder has historically been believed to be a condition that affects adults, recent trend data suggest that adolescents can also display symptoms consistent with gambling disorder. The worldwide prevalence of problematic gam-bling among adolescents ranges between 0.2% and 12.3%, which is substantially higher than the 1–2% prevalence in adults (Floros, 2018). The wide variance in adolescent gambling disorder is thought to be due to inclusion criteria in different studies, methodological differences between country to country, and the candidness of information in various populations.

While the gambling disorder in adolescents is higher than adults, the motivations for gambling are different. Data suggest that adolescents gamble as a social outlet and to dissociate from stressful life events rather than for monetary value (Wilber & Potenza, 2006). Other factors that increase likelihood for adolescent gambling include male gender, parental supervision, impulsivity, poor academic performance, living in a single-parent home, parents with gambling or addiction disorders, and comorbid psychiatric diagnosis (Buth, Wurst, Thon, Lahusen, & Kalke, 2017; Dowling et al., 2017; Floros, 2018). Thus, one approach could be to help identify triggers (e.g., stress) and work to develop alternative coping habits and alternative social outlets.

Literature on treatment for gambling disorder is scant. Studies examining treatment modalities for gambling disorder in adolescents includes motivational interviewing and CBT targeting cognitive distortions surrounding their gambling behavior and challenge underestimated beliefs of their problem behavior (Menchon, Mestre-Bach, Steward, Fernandez-Aranda, & Jimenez-Murcia, 2018). There currently are no randomized trials in children for pharmacotherapy treatment in gambling disorder. However, researchers have noted some efficacy with opioid antagonist and antidepressants for gambling disorders in adulthood (Grant & Potenza, 2010).

Conclusion

Psychiatric disorders and other associated mental health conditions significantly impact an individual's functioning across all environments hindering their ability to lead successful and healthy lives. Finding ways to enhance already established evidenced-based therapies to treat psychiatric symptoms is vital to ensuring individual outcomes are improved and maintaining across time. Although the majority of psychiatric disorders have a genetic or biological component to symptom emergence, environmental and psychosocial variables play a large role in the maintenance and exacerbation of symptoms. The addition of functional assessment strategies to assess the effect of environmental and psychosocial factors on an individual's presentation has a clear role in the treatment planning of psychiatric conditions. However, the use of a functional assessment paradigm has yet to be fully recognized as a useful tool across the broad array of psychopathology.

The first step to utilizing a functional assessment paradigm for psychiatric conditions is to understand the nature, prevalence, and characteristics of the disorder. Without a clear understanding of potential presenting symptoms and their relationship with a person's behavioral, emotional, and social functioning, being able to identify and develop assessment and treatment strategies best suited for the individual may prove difficult. The goal of this chapter was to introduce the reader to how functional assessment can be utilized to offer a viable method for elucidating environmental and other biopsychosocial factors that influence a person's behavioral and emotional health. More research is needed to identify the optimal methodology to integrate a functional assessment paradigm into psychopathology more broadly as well as for specific conditions or symptom clusters. Further, finding additional data-driven methods to assess, modify interventions, and track progress over time for those with psychopathology and other associated conditions will yield increased positive outcomes, thus enabling the individual to achieve a more optimal quality of life.

References

Abidi, S., Mian, I., Garcia-Ortega, I., Lecomte, T., Raedler, T., Jackson, K., … Addington, D. (2017). Canadian guidelines for the pharmacological treatment of schizophrenia spectrum and other psychotic disorders in children and youth. *The Canadian Journal of Psychiatry, 62*(9), 635–647.

American Psychiatric Association. (2013). *Diagnostic and statistical manual of mental disorders* (5th ed.). Washington, DC: American Psychiatric Association.

Bahreynian, M., Qorbani, M., Khaniabadi, B. M., Motlagh, M. E., Safari, O., Asayesh, H., & Kelishadi, R. (2017). Association between obesity and parental weight status in children and adolescents. *Journal of Clinical Research in Pediatric Endocrinology, 9*(2), 111.

Barlow, S. E., & Dietz, W. H. (1998). Obesity evaluation and treatment: Expert committee recommendations. *Pediatrics, 102*(3), e29–e29.

Barnett, E., Sussman, S., Smith, C., Rohrbach, L. A., & Spruijt-Metz, D. (2012). Motivational interviewing for adolescent substance use: A review of the literature. *Addictive Behaviors, 37*(12), 1325–1334.

Beavers, G. A., Iwata, B. A., & Lerman, D. C. (2013). Thirty years of research on the functional analysis of problem behavior. *Journal of Applied Behavior Analysis, 46*(1), 1–21.

Beck, A. T. (Ed.). (1979). *Cognitive therapy of depression*. New York, NY: The Guilford Press.

Buckner, J. D., & Heimberg, R. G. (2010). Drinking behaviors in social situations account for alcohol related problems among socially anxious individuals. *Psychology of Addictive Behaviors, 24*(4), 640–648.

Bukstein, O. G. (2005). Practice parameter for the assessment and treatment of children and adolescents with substance use disorders. *Journal of the American Academy of Child & Adolescent Psychiatry, 44*(6), 609–621.

Buono, F. D., Upton, T. D., Griffiths, M. D., Sprong, M. E., & Bordieri, J. (2016). Demonstrating the validity of the video game functional assessment-revised (VGFA-R). *Computers in Human Behavior, 54*, 501–510.

Buth, S., Wurst, F. M., Thon, N., Lahusen, H., & Kalke, J. (2017). Comparative analysis of potential risk factors for at-risk gambling, problem gambling and gambling disorder among current gamblers—Results of the austrian representative survey 2015. *Frontiers in Psychology, 8*, 2188.

Chamberlain, P. (2003). The Oregon multidimensional treatment foster care model: Features, outcomes, and progress in dissemination. *Cognitive and Behavioral Practice, 10*(4), 303–312.

Couwenbergh, C., van den Brink, W., Zwart, K., Vreugdenhil, C., van Wijngaarden-Cremers, P., & van der Gaag, R. J. (2006). Comorbid psychopathology in adolescents and young adults treated for substance use disorders. *European Child & Adolescent Psychiatry, 15*(6), 319–328.

Craske, M. G., & Barlow, D. H. (2007). *Mastery of your anxiety and panic* (4th ed.). New York, NY: Oxford University Press.

Cucchi, A., Ryan, D., Konstantakopoulos, G., Stroumpa, S., Kaçar, A. Ş., Renshaw, S., … Kravariti, E. (2016). Lifetime prevalence of non-suicidal self-injury in patients with eating disorders: A systematic review and meta-analysis. *Psychological Medicine, 46*(7), 1345–1358.

Dadds, M. R., Cauchi, A. J., Wimalaweera, S., Hawes, D. J., & Brennan, J. (2012). Outcomes, moderators, and mediators of empathic-emotion recognition training for complex conduct problems in childhood. *Psychiatry Research, 199*(3), 201–207.

Daniels, S. R. (2009). Complications of obesity in children and adolescents. *International Journal of Obesity, 33*(1), S60–S65.

DeCou, C., Comtois, K., & Landes, S. (2019). Dialectical behavior therapy is effective for the treatment of suicidal behavior: A meta-anaylsis. *Behavior Therapy, 50*, 60–72.

del Valle, P., Kelley, S. L., & Seoanes, J. E. (2001). The "oppositional defiant" and "conduct disorder" child: A brief review of etiology, assessment, and treatment. *Behavioral Development Bulletin, 10*(1), 36–41.

Dowling, N., Merkouris, S., Greenwood, C., Oldenhof, E., Toumbourou, J., & Youssef, G. (2017). Early risk and protective factors for problem gambling: A systematic review and meta-analysis of longitudinal studies. *Clinical Psychology Review, 51*, 109–124.

Dupaul, G. J., & Ervin, R. A. (1996). Functional assessment of behaviors related to attention-deficit/hyperactivity disorder: Linking assessment to intervention design. *Behavior Therapy, 27*, 601–622.

Elliott, A. J., & Fuqua, A. J. (2000). Trichotillomania: Conceptualization, measurement and treatment. *Behavior Therapy, 31*, 529–545.

Epstein, L. H., Lin, H., Carr, K. A., & Fletcher, K. D. (2012). Food reinforcement and obesity. Psychological moderators. *Appetite, 58*(1), 157–162.

Epstein, L. H., Valoski, A., Wing, R. R., & McCurley, J. (1994). Ten-year outcomes of behavioral family-based treatment for childhood obesity. *Health Psychology, 13*(5), 373.

Fairchild, G., Hawes, D. J., Frick, P. J., Copeland, W. E., Odgers, C. L., Franke, B., … De Brito, S. A. (2019). Conduct disorder. *Nature Reviews Disease Primers, 5*(1), 1–25.

Farsalinos, K., Tomaselli, V., & Polosa, R. (2018). Frequency of use and smoking status of US adolescent e-cigarette users in 2015. *American Journal of Preventive Medicine, 54*(6), 814–820.

Feng, W., Ramo, D. E., Chan, S. R., & Bourgeois, J. A. (2017). Internet gaming disorder: Trends in prevalence 1998-2016. *Addictive Behaviors, 75*, 17–24.

Fettes, D. L., Aarons, G. A., & Green, A. E. (2013). Higher rates of adolescent substance use in child welfare versus community populations in the United States. *Journal of Studies on Alcohol and Drugs, 74*(6), 825–834.

Fichter, M. M., & Quadflieg, N. (2016). Mortality in eating disorders-results of a large prospective clinical longitudinal study. *International Journal of Eating Disorders, 49*(4), 391–401.

Floros, G. D. (2018). Gambling disorder in adolescents: Prevalence, new developments, and treatment challenges. *Adolescent Health, Medicine and Therapeutics, 9*, 43–51.

French, S. A., Epstein, L. H., Jeffery, R. W., Blundell, J. E., & Wardle, J. (2012). Eating behavior dimensions. Associations with energy intake and body weight. A review. *Appetite, 59*(2), 541–549.

Friman, P. C., Finney, J. W., & Christophersen, E. R. (1984). Behavioral treatment of trichotillomania: An evaluative review. *Behavior Therapy, 15*, 249–265.

Friman, P. C., Hayes, S. C., & Wilson, K. G. (1998). Why behavior analysts should study emotion: The example of anxiety. *Journal of Applied Behavior Analysis, 31*(1), 137–156.

Gentile, D. A., Bailey, K., Bavelier, D., Brockmyer, J. F., Cash, H., Coyne, S. M., … Young, K. (2017). Internet gaming disorder in children and adolescents. *Pediatrics, 140*(Suppl 2), S81–S85.

Ghaderi, A. (2007). Logical functional analysis in the assessment and treatment of eating disorders. *Clinical Psychologist, 11*(1), 1–12.

Gibbins, C., & Weiss, M. (2007, October). Clinical recommendations in current practice guidelines for diagnosis and treatment of ADHD in adults. *Current Psychiatry Reports, 9*, 420–426.

Goldstein, L. H., Mellers, J. D. C., Landau, S., Stone, J., Carson, A., Medford, N., & Reuber, M…
Chalder, T. (2015). Cognitive behavioral therapy vs standardized medical care for adults with
dissociative non-epileptic seizures (CODES): A multi-centre randomized controlled trial protocol. *BMC Neurology, 15*(98), 1–13.

Gordon, C. T., Frazier, J. A., McKenna, K., Giedd, J., Zametkin, A., Kaysen, D., … Hong, W.
(1994). Childhood-onset schizophrenia: An NIMH study in progress. *Schizophrenia Bulletin,
20*(4), 697–712.

Grant, J. E., & Chamberlain, S. R. (2016). Trichotillomania. *American Journal of Psychiatry,
173*(9), 868–874.

Grant, J. E., & Potenza, M. N. (2010). Pharmacological treatment of adolescent pathological gambling. *International Journal of Adolescent Medicine and Health, 22*(1), 129–138.

Hales, C. M., Carroll, M. D., Fryar, C. D., & Ogden, C. L. (2017). *Prevalence of obesity among
adults and youth : United States, 2015-2016. NCHS Data Brief, no 288*. Hyattsville, MD:
National Center for Health Statistics.

Hanley, G. P., Iwata, B. A., & McCord, B. E. (2003). Functional analysis of problem behavior: A
review. *Journal of Applied Behavior Analysis, 36*(2), 147–185.

Hebebrand, J., & Hinney, A. (2008). Environmental and genetic risk factors in obesity. *Child &
Adolescent Psychiatric Clinics of North America, 18*, 83–94.

Henggeler, S. W. (2001). Multisystemic therapy. *Residential Treatment for Children and Youth,
18*(3), 75–85.

Herpertz-Dahlmann, B. (2015). Adolescent eating disorders: Update on definitions, symptomatology, epidemiology, and comorbidity. *Child and Adolescent Psychiatric Clinics of North
America, 24*(1), 177–196. https://doi.org/10.1016/j.chc.2014.08.003

Hilbert, A., Hoek, H. W., & Schmidt, R. (2017). Evidence-based clinical guidelines for eating
disorders: International comparison. *Current Opinion in Psychiatry, 30*(6), 423–437.

Hollon, S., & Ponniah, K. (2010). A review of empirically supported psychological therapies for
mood disorders. *Depression & Anxiety, 27*(10), 891–932.

Holth, P., Torsheim, T., Sheidow, A. J., Ogden, T., & Henggeler, S. W. (2011). Intensive quality
assurance of therapist adherence to behavioral interventions for adolescent substance use problems. *Journal of Child and Adolescent Substance Abuse, 20*(4), 289–313.

Jing, L., Neeraj, S. G., Teodorczuk, A., Zhan-jiang, L., & Sun, J. (2019). The efficacy of cognitive
behavioral therapy in somatoform disorders and medically unexplained physical symptoms:
A meta-analysis of randomized controlled trials. *Journal of Affective Disorders, 245*, 98–112.

Kaczkurkin, A. N., & Foa, E. B. (2015). Cognitive behavioral therapy for anxiety disorders: An
update on the empirical evidence. *Dialogues in Clinical Neuroscience, 17*(3), 337–346.

Keane, E., Layte, R., Harrington, J., Kearney, P. M., & Perry, I. J. (2012). Measured parental
weight status and familial socio-economic status correlates with childhood overweight and
obesity at age 9. *PLoS One, 7*(8), e43503.

Kaminski, J. W., & Claussen, A. H. (2017). Evidence base update for psychosocial treatments for
disruptive behaviors in children. *Journal of Clinical Child & Adolescent Psychology, 46*(4),
477–499.

Kane, J. M., Robinson, D. G., Schooler, N. R., Mueser, K. T., Penn, D. L., Rosenheck, R. A., …
Estroff, S. E. (2016). Comprehensive versus usual community care for first-episode psycho-
sis: 2-year outcomes from the NIMH RAISE early treatment program. *American Journal of
Psychiatry, 173*(4), 362–372.

Kessler, R. C., Adler, L., Berkley, R., Biederman, J., Conners, C. K., Demler, O., … Zaslavsky,
A. M. (2006). The prevalence and correlates of adult ADHD in the United States: Results
from the National Comorbidity Survey Replication. *American Journal of Psychiatry, 163*(4),
716–723.

King, D. L., Delfabbro, P. H., Wu, A. M., Doh, Y. Y., Kuss, D. J., Pallesen, S., … Sakuma, H.
(2017). Treatment of internet gaming disorder: An international systematic review and
CONSORT evaluation. *Clinical Psychology Review, 54*, 123–133.

Knouse, L. E., & Mitchell, J. T. (2015). Incautiously optimistic: Positively valenced cognitive avoidance in adult ADHD. *Cognitive and Behavioral Practice, 22*(2), 192–202.

Knouse, L. E., & Safren, S. A. (2010). Current status of cognitive behavioral therapy for adult attention-deficit hyperactivity disorder. *Psychiatric Clinics of North America, 33*, 497–509.

Kozlowska, K., Scher, S., & Williams, L. M. (2011). Patterns of emotional-cognitive functioning in pediatric conversion patients: Implications for the conceptualization of conversion disorder. *Psychosomatic Medicine, 73*(9), 775–788.

Kostro, K., Lerman, J. B., & Attia, E. (2014). The current status of suicide and self-injury in eating disorders: A narrative review. *Journal of Eating Disorders, 2*(1), 19.

Lecomte, T., Abidi, S., Garcia-Ortega, I., Mian, I., Jackson, K., Jackson, K., & Norman, R. (2017). Canadian treatment guidelines on psychosocial treatment of schizophrenia in children and youth. *The Canadian Journal of Psychiatry, 62*(9), 648–655.

Lefrance, W. C., Miller, I. W., Ryan, C. E., Blum, A. S., Solomon, D. A., Kelley, J. E., & Keitner, G. I. (2009). Cognitive behavioral therapy for psychogenic nonepileptic seizures. *Epilepsy & Behavior, 14*, 591–596.

Letourneau, E. J., Henggeler, S. W., Borduin, C. M., Schewe, P. A., McCart, M. R., Chapman, J. E., & Saldana, L. (2009). Multisystemic therapy for juvenile sexual offenders: 1-year results from a randomized effectiveness trial. *Journal of Family Psychology, 23*(1), 89–102.

Lewinsohn, P. M. (1975). The behavioral study and treatment of depression. In M. Hersen, R. M. Eisler, & P. M. Miller (Eds.), *Progress in behavioral modification* (Vol. 1, pp. 19–65). New York, NY: Academic.

Linehan, M. (2015). *DBT skills training manual* (2nd ed.). New York, NY: The Guilford Press.

Lopez-Quintero, C., de los Cobos, J. P., Hasin, D. S., Okuda, M., Wang, S., Grant, B. F., & Blanco, C. (2011). Probability and predictors of transition from first use to dependence on nicotine, alcohol, cannabis, and cocaine: Results of the national epidemiologic survey on alcohol and related conditions (NESARC). *Drug and Alcohol Dependence, 115*(1–2), 120–130.

Luzier, J. L., Berlin, K. S., & Weeks, J. W. (2010). Behavioral treatment of pediatric obesity: Review and future directions. *Children's Health Care, 39*(4), 312–334.

Manos, R., Kanter, J., & Busch, A. (2010). A critical review of assessment strategies to measure the behavioral activation model of depression. *Clinical Psychology Review, 30*, 547–561.

Mayo-Wilson, E., Dias, S., Mavranezouli, I., Kew, K., Clark, D. M., Ades, A. E., & Pilling, S. (2014). Psychological and pharmacological interventions for social anxiety disorder in adults: A systematic review and network meta-analysis. *The Lancet Psychiatry, 1*(5), 368–376.

McClellan, J., & Stock, S. (2013). Practice parameter for the assessment and treatment of children and adolescents with schizophrenia. *Journal of the American Academy of Child & Adolescent Psychiatry, 52*(9), 976–990.

McGovern, L., Johnson, J. N., Paulo, R., Hettinger, A., Singhal, V., Kamath, C., … Montori, V. M. (2008). Treatment of pediatric obesity: A systematic review and meta-analysis of randomized trials. *The Journal of Clinical Endocrinology & Metabolism, 93*(12), 4600–4605.

McManus, F., Van Doorn, K., & Yiend, J. (2012). Examining the effects of thought records and behavioral experiments in instigating belief change. *Journal of Behavior Therapy and Experimental Psychiatry, 43*(1), 540–547.

Menchon, J. M., Mestre-Bach, G., Steward, T., Fernandez-Aranda, F., & Jimenez-Murcia, S. (2018). An overview of gambling disorder: From treatment approaches to risk factors. *F1000Research, 7*, 434.

Mericle, A. A., Arria, A. M., Meyers, K., Cacciola, J., Winters, K. C., & Kirby, K. (2015). National trends in adolescent substance use disorders and treatment availability: 2003–2010. *Journal of Child & Adolescent Substance Abuse, 24*(5), 255–263.

Meulders, A., Van Daele, T., Volders, S., & Vlaeyen, J. W. S. (2016). The use of safety-seeking behavior in exposure-based treatments for fear and anxiety: Benefit or burden? A meta-analytic review. *Clinical Psychology Review, 45*, 144–156.

Meyer, S. B. (2008). Functional analysis of eating disorders. *Journal of Behavior Analysis in Health, Sports, Fitness and Medicine, 1*(1), 26.

Milani, L., La Torre, G., Fiore, M., Grumi, S., Gentile, D. A., Ferrante, M., … Di Blasio, P. (2018). Internet gaming addiction in adolescence: Risk factors and maladjustment correlates. *International Journal of Mental Health and Addiction, 16*(4), 888–904.

Miller, F. G., & Lee, D. L. (2013). Do functional behavioral assessments improve intervention effectiveness for students diagnosed with ADHD? A single-subject meta-analysis. *Journal of Behavioral Education, 22*(3), 253–282.

Miller, A., Rathus, J., & Linehan, M. (2007). *Dialectical behavior therapy with suicidal adolescents*. New York, NY: The Guilford Press.

Mitte, K. (2005). A meta-analysis of the efficacy of psycho- and pharmaco-therapy in panic disorder with and without agoraphobia. *Journal of Affective Disorders, 88*, 27–45.

Moffitt, T. E., Caspi, A., Harrington, H., & Milne, B. J. (2002). Males on the life-course-persistent and adolescence-limited antisocial pathways: Follow-up at age 26 years. *Development and Psychopathology, 14*(1), 179–207.

Morris, S. H., Zickgraf, H. F., Dingfelder, H. E., & Franklin, M. E. (2014). Habit reversal training in trichotillomania: Guide for the clinician. *Expert Review of Neurotherapeutics, 13*(9), 1067–1077.

National Collaborating Centre for Mental Health (Great Britain). (2013). *Psychosis and schizophrenia in children and young people: Recognition and management*. RCPysch Publications.

National Guideline Alliance. (2017). Eating disorders: Recognition and treatment. Retrieved from https://www.nice.org.uk/guidance/NG69

National Institute on Drug Abuse. (2014). Principles of adolescent substance use disorder treatment: A research-based guide, 2014. Retrieved from https://www.drugabuse.gov/publications/principles-adolescent-substance-use-disorder-treatment-research-based-guide/acknowledgements

Nederkoorn, C., Braet, C., Van Eijs, Y., Tanghe, A., & Jansen, A. (2006). Why obese children cannot resist food: The role of impulsivity. *Eating Behaviors, 7*(4), 315–322.

Nock, M. K., Kazdin, A. E., Hiripi, E., & Kessler, R. C. (2006). Prevalence, subtypes, and correlates of DSM-IV conduct disorder in the National Comorbidity Survey Replication. *Psychological Medicine, 36*(5), 699–710.

Nock, M. K., Kazdin, A. E., Hiripi, E., & Kessler, R. C. (2007). Lifetime prevalence, correlates, and persistence of oppositional defiant disorder: Results from the National Comorbidity Survey Replication. *Journal of Child Psychology and Psychiatry, 48*(7), 703–713.

Office of Adolescent Health. (2019). United states adolescent substance abuse facts. Retrieved from https://www.hhs.gov/ash/oah/facts-and-stats/national-and-state-data-sheets/adolescents-and-substance-abuse/united-states/index.html

Ogden, C. L., Carroll, M. D., Kit, B. K., & Flegal, K. M. (2012). Prevalence of obesity and trends in body mass index among US children and adolescents, 1999-2010. *Journal of the American Medical Association, 307*(5), 483–490.

O'Neill, R. E., Albin, R. W., Storey, K., Horner, R. H., & Sprague, J. R. (2014). *Functional assessment and program development*. Toronto, ON, Canada: Nelson Education.

Paulus, F. W., Ohmann, S., Von Gontard, A., & Popow, C. (2018). Internet gaming disorder in children and adolescents: A systematic review. *Developmental Medicine & Child Neurology, 60*(7), 645–659.

Piacentini, J., Woods, D. W., Scahill, L., Wilhelm, S., Peterson, A. L., Chang, S., … Walkup, J. T. (2010). Behavior therapy for children with Tourette disorder: A randomized controlled trial. *Journal of the American Medical Association, 303*(19), 1929–1937.

Pinard, C. A., Yaroch, A. L., Hart, M. H., Serrano, E. L., McFerren, M. M., & Estabrooks, P. A. (2012). Measures of the home environment related to childhood obesity: A systematic review. *Public Health Nutrition, 15*(1), 97–109.

Poikolainen, K. (2002). Antecedents of substance use in adolescence. *Current Opinion in Psychiatry, 15*(3), 241–245.

Rajjo, T., Mohammed, K., Alsawas, M., Ahmed, A. T., Farah, W., Asi, N., … Murad, M. H. (2017). Treatment of pediatric obesity: An umbrella systematic review. *The Journal of Clinical Endocrinology & Metabolism, 102*(3), 763–775.

Rankin, J., Matthews, L., Cobley, S., Han, A., Sanders, R., Wiltshire, H. D., & Baker, J. S. (2016). Psychological consequences of childhood obesity: Psychiatric comorbidity and prevention. *Adolescent Health, Medicine and Therapeutics, 7*, 125.

Rathus, J., & Miller, A. (2014). *DBT skills manual for adolescents*. New York, NY: Guilford Publications.

Redlin, J., Miltenberger, R., Crosby, R., Wolff, G., & Stickney, M. (2002). Functional assessment of binge eating in a clinical sample of obese binge eaters. *Eating and Weight Disorders-Studies on Anorexia, Bulimia and Obesity, 7*(2), 106–115.

Ritsner, M. S. (2011). *Handbook of schizophrenia spectrum disorders, volume III: Therapeutic approaches, comorbidity, and outcomes*. New York, NY: Springer.

Rizvi, S., & Ritschel, L. (2014). Mastering the art of chain analysis in dialectical behavior therapy. *Cognitive and Behavioral Practice, 21*(3), 335–349.

Rodebaugh, T. L., Holaway, R. M., & Heimberg, R. G. (2004). The treatment of social anxiety disorder. *Clinical Psychology Review, 24*, 883–908.

Rosenfarb, I. S. (2013). A functional analysis of schizophrenia. *The Psychological Record, 63*(4), 929–946.

Rutter, M., Moffitt, T. E., & Caspi, A. (2006). Gene–environment interplay and psychopathology: Multiple varieties but real effects. *Journal of Child Psychology and Psychiatry, 47*(3–4), 226–261.

Safren, S. A., Sprich, S., Chulvick, S., & Otto, M. W. (2004, June). Psychosocial treatments for adults with attention-deficit/hyperactivity disorder. *Psychiatric Clinics of North America, 27*, 349–360.

Selten, J., van der Ven, E., Rutten, B. P., & Cantor-Graae, E. (2013). The social defeat hypothesis of schizophrenia: An update. *Schizophrenia Bulletin, 39*(6), 1180–1186.

Smink, F. R., Van Hoeken, D., & Hoek, H. W. (2012). Epidemiology of eating disorders: Incidence, prevalence and mortality rates. *Current Psychiatry Reports, 14*(4), 406–414.

Spence, S. H., & Rapee, R. M. (2016). The etiology of social anxiety disorder: An evidence-based model. *Behavior Research and Therapy, 86*, 50–67.

Sprong, M. E., Griffiths, M. D., Lloyd, D. P., Paul, E., & Buono, F. D. (2019). Comparison of the video game functional assessment-revised (VGFA-R) and internet gaming disorder test (IGD-20). *Frontiers in Psychology, 10*, 310.

Stark, K., Sander, J., Yancy, M., Bronik, M., & Hoke, J. (2000). Treatment of depression in childhood and adolescence: Cognitive-behavioral procedures for the individual and the family. In *Child and adolescent therapy: Cognitive-behavioral procedures*. New York, NY: The Guilford Press.

Steiner, H., & Remsing, L. (2007). Practice parameter for the assessment and treatment of children and adolescents with oppositional defiant disorder. *Journal of the American Academy of Child & Adolescent Psychiatry, 46*(1), 126–141.

Stice, E., Marti, C. N., Shaw, H., & Jaconis, M. (2009). An 8-year longitudinal study of the natural history of threshold, subthreshold, and partial eating disorders from a community sample of adolescents. *Journal of Abnormal Psychology, 118*(3), 587.

Stanger, C., Lansing, A. H., & Budney, A. J. (2016). Advances in research on contingency management for adolescent substance use. *Child and Adolescent Psychiatric Clinics of North America, 25*(4), 645–659.

Sturmey, P. (2009). Behavioral activation is an evidenced based treatment for depression. *Behavior Modification, 33*(6), 818–829.

Sugaya, N., Shirasaka, T., Takahashi, K., & Kanda, H. (2019). Bio-psychosocial factors of children and adolescents with internet gaming disorder: A systematic review. *BioPsychoSocial Medicine, 13*(1), 3.

Sugerman, H. J., Sugerman, E. L., DeMaria, E. J., Kellum, J. M., Kennedy, C., Mowery, Y., & Wolfe, L. G. (2003). Bariatric surgery for severely obese adolescents. *Journal of Gastrointestinal Surgery, 7*(1), 102–108.

Swanson, S. A., Crow, S. J., Le Grange, D., Swendsen, J., & Merikangas, K. R. (2011). Prevalence and correlates of eating disorders in adolescents: Results from the national comorbidity survey replication adolescent supplement. *Archives of General Psychiatry, 68*(7), 714–723.

Swendsen, J., Burstein, M., Case, B., Conway, K. P., Dierker, L., He, J., & Merikangas, K. R. (2012). Use and abuse of alcohol and illicit drugs in US adolescents: Results of the national comorbidity survey–adolescent supplement. *Archives of General Psychiatry, 69*(4), 390–398.

Tindall, L., Mikocka-Walus, A., McMillan, D., Wright, B., Hewitt, C., & Gascoyne, S. (2017). Is behavioral activation effective in the treatment of depression in young people? A systematic review and meta-analysis. *Psychology and Psychotherapy, 90*(4), 770–796.

Thomas, R., Sanders, S., Doust, J., Beller, E., & Glasziou, P. (2015, April 1). Prevalence of attention-deficit/hyperactivity disorder: A systematic review and meta-analysis. *Pediatrics, 135*, e994–e1001.

Tolin, D. (2010). Is cognitive-behavioral therapy more effective than other therapies? A meta-analytic review. *Clinical Psychology Review, 30*, 710–720.

Turner, B., Austin, S., & Chapman, A. (2014). Treating non-suicidal self-injury: A systematic review of the psychological and pharmacological interventions. *Canadian Journal of Psychiatry, 59*(11), 576–585.

U.S. Department of Health and Human Services. (2012). *The surgeon general's vision for a healthy and fit nation*. Rockville, MD: U.S. Department of Health and Human Services.

Walsh, B. (2006). *Treating self-injury: A practical guide*. New York, NY: The Guilford Press.

Wilber, M. K., & Potenza, M. N. (2006). Adolescent gambling: Research and clinical implications. *Psychiatry (Edgmont), 3*(10), 40.

Wilder, D. A., Masuda, A., O'Connor, C., & Baham, M. (2001). Brief functional analysis and treatment of bizarre vocalizations in an adult with schizophrenia. *Journal of Applied Behavior Analysis, 34*(1), 65–68.

Wilfley, D. E., & Balantekin, K. N. (2018). Family-based behavioral interventions for childhood obesity. In *Pediatric obesity* (pp. 555–567). Cham, Switzerland: Humana press.

Williams, S. E., & Zahka, N. E. (2017). *Treating somatic symptoms in children and adolescents*. New York, NY: The Guilford Press.

Wolraich, M., Brown, L., Brown, R. T., DuPaul, G., Earls, M., Feldman, H. M., … Davidson, C. (2011, November). ADHD: Clinical practice guideline for the diagnosis, evaluation, and treatment of attention-deficit/ hyperactivity disorder in children and adolescents. *Pediatrics, 128*, 1007–1022.

Woods, D. W., Piacentini, J. C., Chang, S. W., Deckersbach, T., Ginsburg, G. S., Peterson, A. L., … Wilhem, S. (2008). *Managing Tourette syndrome: A behavioral intervention for children and adults*. New York, NY: Oxford University Press.

Yoong, S. L., Stockings, E., Chai, L. K., Tzelepis, F., Wiggers, J., Oldmeadow, C., … Attia, J. (2018). Prevalence of electronic nicotine delivery systems (ENDS) use among youth globally: A systematic review and meta-analysis of country level data. *Australian and New Zealand Journal of Public Health, 42*(3), 303–308.

Zajac, K., Ginley, M. K., Chang, R., & Petry, N. M. (2017). Treatments for internet gaming disorder and internet addiction: A systematic review. *Psychology of Addictive Behaviors, 31*(8), 979.

Chapter 8
Observing Behaviors in Functional Assessment

Steven G. Little, Margaret Gopaul, and Angeleque Akin-Little

Observing Behaviors in Functional Assessment

Many of the principles developed under the theories of operant conditioning and eventually applied behavior analyses were later applied to functional assessment. This chapter covers: Operational definitions, behavioral observations including their principles and behavioral observation methods, the reliability of behavioral observations, and factors affecting behavioral observations.

Operational Definitions

An operational definition of behavior presents a clear (i.e., provides unambiguous descriptions), concise (i.e., free of extraneous detail), objective (i.e., refers to only observable features of responding), and detailed (i.e., differentiate between responses that should and should not be considered an occurrence definition of the behavior or behaviors of interest) definition of behavior (Cooper, Heron, & Heward, 2007, 2020; Lerman et al., 2010). The definition is provided in a way that is observable, measurable, and repeatable and provides complete information about a behavior's occurrence. An operational definition should include a description of the particular action that can be seen or heard using precise language that can be replicated by a stranger. In other words, if an individual unfamiliar with the client, one who had never observed the client before, could read the operational definition and be relatively clear on

S. G. Little (✉) · A. Akin-Little
Walden University, Minneapolis, MN, USA

M. Gopaul
Liberty University, Lynchburg, VA, USA

© Springer Nature Switzerland AG 2021
J. L. Matson (ed.), *Functional Assessment for Challenging Behaviors and Mental Health Disorders*, Autism and Child Psychopathology Series,
https://doi.org/10.1007/978-3-030-66270-7_8

instances of the defined behavior. For example, Harry pointed his middle finger in the direction of the teacher, rather than Harry made inappropriate gestures towards the teacher. Also, it is best to define behaviors with an observable beginning and end and/ or the time/duration or frequency count. For example, Harry pointed his middle finger three times in one hour at his teacher, rather than Harry often used inappropriate gestures towards his teacher. A similar example would be Harry was out of his seat for 17.5 minutes during a 30-minute class instead of Harry was out of his seat for most of the class. Generating this type of operational definition means that two or more individuals could independently observe that behavior and agree when the behavior is occurring and is not occurring (Cooper et al., 2007).

Why Operational Definitions Are Important?

The need for operational definitions is fundamental. When behavior is operationally defined, these clear and concise target behavior definitions enable clinicians and researchers to accurately and consistently measure the same behavior within and across studies, settings, or time (Cooper et al., 2020). It is essential that everyone has the same understanding and collects data in a standardized manner. Operational definitions should therefore be completed before any data collection begins. It can be very difficult to describe a behavior without being influenced by subjective or personal factors. Teachers and parents have their own perspectives and expectations which can, even inadvertently, become part of their understanding of the behavior. For example, they may think the child chooses to engage in a specific behavior, especially misbehavior. Lerman et al. (2010) evaluated the feasibility and utility of a laboratory model for examining observer accuracy within the framework of signal-detection theory (SDT). They illustrated that bias may be reduced by providing observers with a more complete and detailed definition of behavior, in this case aggression, resulted in a reduction in the likelihood and amount of response bias, as well as a decrease in the incidence of false alarms.

How to Write an Operational Definition?

An operational definition of behavior demonstrates validity if it facilitates observers to accurately identify every feature of the behavior of concern that is distinguishable from other behaviors (Cooper et al., 2007). There are four basics to operationally defining a behavior. These include a label, definition, examples, and nonexamples. For example, if an off-task behavior is selected as the target behavior; this might be operationally defined as doing various tasks in class besides those which were assigned. Examples might include texting or talking to classmates, looking out window, and scribbling on paper. Nonexamples might include attending to assignment, following teacher's instructions, and accessing materials related to the assignment.

Remember, a behavior is operationally defined when it provides an opportunity to obtain complete information about a behavior's occurrence (Cooper et al., 2007). One way to help evaluate completeness of an operational definition is the dead man's test for deciding if something is a behavior. The Dead Man's Test is a simple procedure developed by Ogden Lindsley in 1965 (Lindsley, 1991). Ask "can a dead man do it?" If a dead man can do it, it is not a behavior; and if a dead man cannot do it, then it is a behavior. For example, can a dead man be quiet? Yes, he can, therefore it would not be considered a behavior for an operational definition. Similarly, can a dead man talk? No, he cannot, therefore it would be considered a behavior for an operational definition.

Examples of NonOperational and Operational Definitions

- Nonoperational (subjective) Definition: Matt blurts out questions in class. You need to know: which class? What does blurt mean? How often does he blurt? Is he asking questions that relate to the class? (Webster, 2019).
- Operational Definition: Matt shouts out relevant questions without raising his hand 3–5 times during each Language Arts class (Webster, 2019).
- Nonoperational (subjective) Definition: Karen throws temper tantrums during recess (Webster, 2019). You need to know: What behaviors constitute a tantrum? How often do these "tantrums" occur? Are there any specific conditions (antecedents) to the tantrums?
- Operational Definition: Karen shouts, cries, or throws objects each time she participates in group activities during recess (3–5 times per week) (Webster, 2019).

Types of Target Behavior Definitions

When accessing a target behavior, it can be defined either functionally or topographically (Cooper et al., 2020). Function-based definitions are recommended as the first choice when possible since it covers all applicable forms of the response group. Whereas, target behaviors based on a list of topographies could overlook applicable response groups or provide irrelevant response topographies (Cooper et al., 2020).

Function-Based Definitions A function-based definition encompasses all relevant forms of the response class. Below are examples of function-based definitions of various target behaviors:

Elopement: "Any part of the participant's body passing through the doorway and moving or attempting to move 3 m (or more) away from the therapist" (Piazza et al., 1999, p. 65).

Hand Mouthing: "Placement of the hand past the plane of the lips or repetitive contact between the hand and mouth or tongue" (Roscoe, Iwata, & Zhou, 2013, p. 183).

Aggression: "Hitting, throwing items at people, kicking, and pushing" (Wacker et al., 2013, p. 35).

Property destruction: "Throwing, banging, or ripping objects" (Greer et al., 2013, p. 290).

Head hitting: "Forceful contact against the head or face by hand or fist" (Vollmer, Marcus, & Ringdahl, 1995, p. 18).

Topographically Based Definitions Topographically based definitions identify the behavior by its shape or form (Cooper et al., 2020) and are used when you do not have easy access to the functional outcome of the behavior, or the function of the behavior varies by the environment. Below are examples of topographically based definitions of various target behaviors:

Tantrum: "The child threw herself on the floor and kicked and screamed in a high-pitched voice." (Webster, 2020).

Golf Swing: Because even a bad golf swing may result in a good outcome (e.g., ball on the green) describing the position of the feet, hands, head, etc. may be preferred (Cooper et al., 2020).

Slouching: The student lowers his upper torso and places hands and lower arms on desk.

Operation Definitions in the Literature

A review of the literature found reference to the importance of operational definitions as early as 1935 (Stevens, 1935) and anecdotally the first author remembers professors stressing the importance of operationally defining behavior in the 1970s. However, comprehensive reviews of the literature indicate that published research does not always provide operational definitions of treatments in psychology in general and behavior analysis specifically, although it has been improving during the past 20 years. Peterson, Homer, and Wonderlich (1982), were the first to investigate operationalization of treatments in a review of articles published in the *Journal of Applied Behavior Analysis* from 1968 to 1980. They reported only that less than 80% of articles provided an operational of treatment. Kazdin (1990) reviewed articles investigating child and adolescent psychotherapy from 1970 to 1988 and found that 55.6% reported treatment operationalization. Gresham, Gansle, and Noell (1993) reviewed research in applied behavior analysis with children and Gresham, Gansle, Noell, Cohen, and Rosenblum (1993) reviewed school-based behavioral intervention studies. While there was overlap in these two data sets, only 34.2% and 35%, respectively, reported an operationalization of treatment. More recently Borrelli et al. (2005), in a review of major journals in health behavior change research similarly found only 35% of studies reporting an operational definition of treatment. Finally, a review by McIntyre, Gresham, DiGennaro, and Reed (2007) reviewed school-based intervention studies published in the *Journal of Applied Behavior Analysis* from 1991 to 2005. They found that 95% of studies reported an operational definition of treatment, providing a much more optimistic view of operational definitions in research

Behavioral Observation

There are a number of reliable and valid behavioral assessment methods available and the most highly utilized is direct behavior observation (Watson & Watson, 2009). Behavioral observation includes watching and recording the behavior of an individual within their regular environment or an analog setting (Watson & Steege, 2003). Briefly, direct behavior observation refers to observing, monitoring, and recording a behavior as it actually occurs in real time. Prior to actually observing behavior, one must first operationally define the target behavior, determine when and where observation will occur, choose a method for recording behavior (i.e., frequency, duration, interval recording, time sampling), and choose a recording instrument (e.g., paper/pencil, tablet, or other electronic device). For example, a child may be observed within their classroom, on the playground, at home, etc. Observers most commonly focus on how often a behavior occurs (frequency), but other characteristics may be focused on, such as how intense a behavior is (magnitude) and how long a behavior lasts (duration). The goal is that the data collected will be based on objective findings as opposed to perceptions of that behavior/individual (Watson & Steege, 2003).

It is, however, not always possible to directly observe behavior as it occurs, as may be the case with low frequency, high-intensity behaviors (e.g., aggressive outbursts). It may become necessary to use indirect methods, such as interviews, to obtain information from those in the student's environment who have had the opportunity to observe the behavior. The focus of this chapter is not on interviews but recognizes that they may be necessary in the case of the low- frequency behaviors mentioned above or in cases when there are multiple behaviors of concern and the practitioner would like to narrow down the behaviors in order to target one or more for intervention. Questionnaires and/or interviews could be general (e.g., the *Achenbach System of Empirically Based Assessment*, Achenbach & Rescorla, 2001) or related to discerning the function of a particular behavior (e.g., *Functional Assessment Informant Record-Teacher; FAIR-T*, Edwards, 2002). Regardless of the format, the main goals in a behavioral assessment are to identify: (1) under what conditions the behavior occurs, (2) the contextual factors that may contribute to the problem, (3) extra-environmental variables, (4) the peer's and teacher's responses to the behavior, (5) related skill and/or performance deficits, and (6) previous and/or ongoing interventions (Watson & Watson, 2009).

Principles of and Approaches to Behavioral Observation

Verner, Wichnick, and Poulson (2017) and Watson and Watson (2009) identify some general principles and approaches to behavioral observation. These include direct observation. Observation in the naturalistic environment, analog observations, role-play, self-monitoring, and functional behavior assessment.

Direct Observation of Behavior Direct observation of behavior refers to observing, monitoring, and recording a behavior as it actually occurs in real time. It is one of the fundamentals of behavioral assessment and is considered to be a low-inference methodology (Watson & Watson, 2009). Before observing behavior, it is important to operationally define the target behavior (see above), determine when and where observation will occur, choose a method for recording behavior (e.g.,, frequency, duration, interval recording, time sampling), and choose a recording instrument (e.g., paper/pencil, electronic).

Natural Environment It is ideal, when possible to measure the behavior of the individual in their naturalistic environment as opposed a contrived setting. These observations can be structured using a reliable method to sample the individual (e.g., time sampling, momentary time-sampling) or unstructured. The latter, identified in behavior analysis as naturalistic-free operant observation (Cooper et al., 2020) involves observing the individual in their everyday environment (e.g., classroom, playground, home) and recording how the individual allocates their time and the number of minutes devoted to each activity. Using either approach, the observer should be as unobtrusive as possible.

Analog Observations As opposed to natural settings, observations are sometimes conducted in an environment where the conditions can be more closely controlled (Alberto & Troutman, 2013). This is especially true when conducting a functional behavior assessment (FBA) or with behaviors that are of low frequency so that a naturalistic environment is not possible. In an analog observation, the setting, antecedents, and consequent stimuli can be controlled to maximize the likelihood of the target behavior and/or more clearly identify functions of the behavior.

Role-Play Role-play is a specific type of analog setting in which the two or more individuals are presented with a sample situation and told to act as if it were actually occurring (Verner et al., 2017). While usually used as a therapeutic technique, it can also be used to identify behavioral responses to specific stimuli. It is primarily used when evaluating social interactional variables. While not used as an assessment technique, Jafer, Tayyebeh, Reza, Mansoureh, and Zahra (2014) evaluated the efficacy of role-playing along with applied behavioral analysis (ABA) on social behavior of children with autism. They found that role-play along with ABA interventions can increase social behaviors of children with autism more than either intervention alone. This suggests that role-play could validly be used as an assessment technique also.

Self-Monitoring Cooper et al. (2020) define self-monitoring as "a procedure whereby a person systematically observes his behavior and records the occurrence or nonoccurrence of the target behavior" (p. 692). While self-monitoring may have reactive effects, that is, the measurement procedure may itself produce a change in the individual's behavior; the outcome may have a positive clinical effect (e.g., increase incidence of a desirable behavior or decrease incidence of an undesirable behavior). Self-monitoring has also been shown to have positive effects by allowing data recording of nonovert events such as thoughts or physiological changes (Verner et al., 2017). Xu, Wang, Lee, and Luke (2017) investigated self-monitoring with guided goal setting to increase academic engagement for a 9-year-old boy on the autism spectrum (IQ = 69), displaying disruptive behaviors in an inclusive classroom in China. Not only was this boy able to be taught to accurately record his own behavior, but also results of the intervention were very positive with academic engagement increasing from a mean of 10.6% of intervals in baseline to a terminal criterion of 80% over five phases (27 days) using a changing criterion design.

Methods of Behavioral Observation

There are different methods of behavioral observation which strive to deliver objective and quantitative data. Those objective and quantitative data can then be used by teachers/practitioners to establish current levels of target behavior(s), customize goals for behavioral improvement, and revise intervention plans (Watson & Steege, 2003). Dimensions of behavior refer to the frequency or rate of behavior, the duration of a behavior, the relative intensity/magnitude with which a behavior occurs, and the latency of a behavior (Watson & Watson, 2009).

Frequency refers to the absolute number of times that an event occurs, or how often a behavior occurs (Cooper et al., 2020). To best use a frequency measure, the target behavior should have a discrete beginning and end (i.e., clear starts and stops). Rate refers to the number of times the behavior occurs per specific period of time (e.g., minute, 30-minute class, etc.). For example, if the target behavior occurred 14 times in a 10-minute observation session, the rate would be 1.4 occurrences per minute. Rate measures are particularly useful because they allow for comparisons across observations of unequal lengths and are considered a direct measure of behavior (Watson & Watson, 2009).

Duration is simply the amount of time the behavior occurred from onset to cessation. The most accurate method to record duration is via real-time recording (Watson & Watson, 2009). In real-time recording, a sample of time is selected (e.g., 30 minutes) and the observer uses a stopwatch to record the actual amount of time the student engages in the target behavior and then converts the resulting amount to a percentage of time. For example, a student who is observed to be academically engaged for 33 minutes of a 50-minute class would have been academically engaged

66% of the time. As simple as it is, it can be time-intensive and requires considerable effort by the observer.

Intensity, or magnitude, is frequently difficult to operationalize and measure. For example, how does one rate the intensity of a tantrum? You could measure the level of sound using an electronic measuring device, but such devices may be expensive or not readily available. For this reason, intensity is often measured via a subjective rating scale (e.g., a 1–10 scale, where one is the least intense and 10 which is the most intense). These types of subjective scales have been shown to be useful and valid for rating the intensity of pain behaviors (Allen & Matthews, 1998) as well as behaviors that occur in a classroom setting (Watson & Watson, 2009).

Latency is best defined as the elapsed time from the onset of a stimulus to the initiation of a response (Cooper et al., 2020). Although latency is an important behavioral dimension, it is probably not often assessed (Watson & Watson, 2009). A disadvantage of measuring latency is that it is time-consuming and the observer may take 10–15 minutes to adequately observe and record the behaviors. The primary advantage is by identifying problems in latency and addressing those concerns may also reduce or eliminate irritating behaviors that may occur during the latency period.

Analysis of Antecedent Events

Antecedent events are stimuli that occur immediately before an identified target behavior occurs. Functionally, they can be thought of as "triggers" or "cues" for a behavior. The main advantage of identifying and measuring antecedents is that one can manipulate them as an intervention to facilitate behavior change (Watson & Watson, 2009). Analysis of antecedent events can be incorporated into behavioral observation and interviews. When conducting an observation, one can note the stimuli that are temporally related to the target behavior. Although one cannot make causal statements about the relationship between the stimulus event and interfering behavior based on such an observation, the information can be used when conducting an FBA to allow one to begin formulating hypotheses about the conditions that prompt the target behavior.

Anecdotal (A-B-C) Recording

The direct observation method is often used when first collecting data on a targeted behavior (Neitzel & Bogin, 2008). This direct method, which is also called anecdotal observation, typically includes the use of an antecedent-behavior-consequence (A-B-C) data chart. This method is one exception to collect objective and quantifiable information since it involves recording and interpreting a narrative of behavior. The narrative is recorded during an observation period using an A-B-C chart for interpreting the target behavior (Neitzel & Bogin, 2008). The A-B-C data chart allows the teacher/practitioner to:

(a) Record what happened immediately preceding the target behavior(s) (*antecedent*).
(b) Observe and record occurrences of the target behavior(s). (*behavior*)
(c) Record what happened immediately following the target behavior(s) (*consequence*).

Below is an example of an A-B-C data collection chart.

A (Antecedent)	B (Behavior)	C (Consequence)
Provide a descriptive account of activities and specific events that occur prior to the behavior.	*Provide a descriptive account of what the behavior looked like when it occurred.*	*Provide a descriptive account of the events that followed or the consequence(s) of the behavior.*
Example: 10:30 am. The teacher asks students (including Jane) to form a circle and hold hands.	*Example*: 10:32 am. Jane shoved a peer in the circle.	*Example*: 10:34 am. Jane was made to sit out the activity.

These data can provide valuable information into the learner/client's behavior which can be used to identify target behaviors (Cooper et al., 2007; Neitzel & Bogin, 2008). According to Sugai, Sprague, Horner, and Walker (2000), "if we can identify the conditions under which problem behavior is likely to occur (triggering antecedents and maintaining consequences), we can arrange environments in ways that reduce occurrences of problem behavior and teach and encourage positive behaviors that can replace problem behaviors" (p. 137). The goal is to identify and catch patterns within the learner's behavior to identify the function of behavior.

Behavior Sampling (Event Recording)

Behavioral sampling or event recoding is a good choice for recording the frequency of a behavior, assuming that the behavioral definitions are written to distinguish between instances of a behavior (Cooper et al., 2020). There are some drawbacks to using event recording. For instance, it requires accurate behavioral definitions; it is not useful for behaviors that are challenging to observe and record (e.g., inattentiveness), and those behaviors that occur infrequently. The two types of behavioral sampling are frequency measures and discrete categorization (Cooper et al., 2020).

Frequency measures This method requires simply tallying the number of times the behavior occurs in a given period (Cooper et al., 2007). This is best for discrete responses (having a clear beginning and end) so that separate instances can be counted. These data can be interpreted as the number of times the behavior occurred. For example, saying hello or punching are both behaviors where there is a discrete beginning and ending. However, this is less applicable for ongoing behaviors such as smiling, talking, or behaviors with long duration (Cooper et al., 2007). Data can be recorded as rate, if the data comparisons are done across observations of different lengths. For example, if five behaviors occurred during a 5-minute observation, the rate would be 1 behavior per minute. Hence, a rate of response can be obtained by dividing the frequency by number of minutes observed

Discrete categorization This is a useful method to classify behaviors into discrete categories, such as in seat - out of seat, and appropriate – inappropriate. Discrete categorization is similar to frequency measures but it provides a broader category (Cooper et al., 2007).

Time Sampling

Time sampling uses various methods to record target behavior(s) at specific instants. The observer typically divides the observation period into intervals, after which, the observer records the occurrence or lack of occurrence of a behavior within that interval or at the end of the interval (Tieghi-Benet et al., 2003). The advantages of time sampling include:

(a) Its utility for high-rate behaviors that are difficult to count.
(b) Its utility for behaviors with no clear beginning or end.
(c) Allow for brief (10 minutes plus) observations or extended periods of time.
(d) Data can be converted to percentages allowing for the use of a plotted graph to monitor behavioral changes over time (Tieghi-Benet et al., 2003).

On the other hand, the disadvantages of time sampling include:

(a) Its limitation of only providing an approximation of the behavior(s).
(b) The sample produced may not be representative.
(c) Typically, it requires the observer's full attention and alternative observer(s) may be required.
(d) Tools are needed, such as a timekeeping device (Tieghi-Benet et al., 2003).

Interval recording methods These methods provide data to document the number of intervals during which there is the presence or absence of targeted behavior(s) (Cooper et al., 2020). Interval recording consists of three basic variations, namely, partial-interval recording, whole-interval recording, and momentary time sampling.

Partial-interval recording Here, the observer is focused on if the behavior(s) occurs or does not occur within the duration of that interval and to ensure that the particular behavior is not present for the entire interval (Alberto & Troutman, 2013). Discrete behaviors that are observable using partial-interval recording may include participation in a class activity, punching a peer, complimenting a peer, or cursing.

After the recording is finished, the observer tallies the number of intervals that included the observed behavior (Cooper et al., 2020). Multiple occurrences are scored as one occurrence. The observer then records these data as percentage of intervals for when the behavior occurred. The partial interval recording method provides an estimation of frequency and duration of a behavior. It can also help the observer recognize where behaviors are occurring throughout the observational period. On the other hand, a drawback to using partial-interval recording is that it requires an observer's full attention and it may overestimate behaviors (Cooper et al., 2020; Tieghi-Benet et al., 2003).

Whole-interval recording This type of interval recording is similar to partial-interval recording in all aspects except it is best used to measure more continuous or long-lasting behaviors (Cooper et al., 2007). For example, if inattention is the target behavior, at the end of the interval it will only be recorded if inattentive behavior occurred throughout the entire interval. Data are totaled by adding the number of intervals in which the behavior occurred and dividing the sum by the number of observed intervals multiplied by 100. The result reflects the percentage of intervals in which the observed behavior occurred. If the target behavior occurs at a constant but moderate rate, whole-interval recording is typically recommended (Cooper et al., 2007). However, since whole-interval recording requires that the behavior must occur during the entire interval, there is a tendency for this method to underestimate behavior.

Momentary time-sampling In momentary time-sampling, behaviors are recorded at specified time intervals. For example, the observer defines the interval of time, say 1 minute, and look up at the end of that interval. The observer records whether the behavior is occurring or is not occurring at that particular point in time. In practice, the observer creates a grid, with each box representing each interval. Using a timer, the observer momentarily observes the individual for the target behavior at the end of the interval. If the behavior was observed at that moment, then it is recorded in the box. For instance, a 30-minute observation may be constructed in 1-minute intervals whereby the observer will have 30 moments to observe the behavior. Momentary time-sampling is beneficial since it does not require the observer's undivided attention and it is an excellent choice for continuous or high-frequency behaviors. An advantage to momentary time-sampling is that it provides observers with the option of observing multiple behaviors or individuals at the same time (Cooper et al., 2007). Momentary time-sampling has some drawbacks in that it can underestimate the rate of occurrence of the behavior (Cooper et al., 2007). For example, it is possible that the behavior occurs during the interval but stops just prior to the "moment" of observation at the end of the interval. Therefore, this behavior would be missed and as such behaviors that could be recorded during that interval time may not be recorded unless they happen to be occurring at the end of the interval (Cooper et al., 2007).

Duration recording This type of recording allows the observer to report the percentage of time at which the individual engaged in the target behavior (Cooper et al., 2007; Tieghi-Benet et al., 2003). Essentially, duration recording provides a report of the length of the behavior by allowing the observer to record the time when the behavior begins to when it ceases. Duration data are aggregated by calculating of the totals of all the durations then divided by the number of occurrences. For example, John engaged in three incidences (125 seconds, 365 seconds, and 45 seconds) of talking to peers during 15-minute recess resulting in an average of 3 minutes per talking to peers during recess (Tieghi-Benet et al., 2003).

Duration recording is most useful when the main concern is the length or duration of the behavior (Cooper et al., 2007; Tieghi-Benet et al., 2003). For example, this measurement may not be suitable for behaviors such as hitting or smoking since greater concern would be the frequency and not so much the length of these behaviors. However, there are instances where duration recording may be appropriate such as daydreaming or tantrums as well as behaviors that occur frequently or those that are harder to measure as discrete entities, such as talking to peers or pencil tapping. On the other hand, a drawback of duration recording is that it can be challenging to obtain an accurate report if the observer is not exclusively assigned to this task for the entire observation period (Cooper et al., 2007; Tieghi-Benet et al., 2003).

Latency recording As mentioned previously, latency recording is defined as the elapsed time from the onset of a stimulus to the initiation of a response (Cooper et al., 2020). It is frequently helpful to assess the amount of time it takes an individual to perform or complete a target behavior once a verbal cue or demand is received. For example, how long it takes for a kindergartner to join circle time or put toys away once he/she is prompted. This method of assessment can be conducted when a specific verbal instruction or an event can be identified that precedes the target behavior. It can also be used when there is a need to assess the time it takes for a student to respond/comply, or when interested in when to prompt a communication skill. Latency recording is beneficial in that it allows the observer to record ongoing progress in responding to verbal cues (Cooper et al., 2007). On the other hand, a drawback of latency recording is the time it takes to accurately conduct the observation.

Permanent products This type of measurement is used when occurrence of the target behavior(s) produces a relatively permanent product (Cooper et al., 2020). Common examples of permanent products recording are the number of pieces of litter deposited in an area, number of words spelled correctly, number of completed homework assignments, etc. Permanent products are beneficial in that it is less time-consuming for practitioners and few adjustments are needed to their routine/schedule (Cooper et al., 2020). Also, this type of measurement is not only deemed convenient but also effective since the data can be securely stored away for later verification or review. A drawback of permanent products is that the data recorded may not provide details of how the student participated in the behavior. For example, a student may have failed to complete some of the short essays questions in class on a particular day. However, the permanent product report may not be able to inform that the student was interrupted by a peer on serval occasions. Hence, this method may be more effective when used along with direct observation methods (Cooper et al., 2007).

Reliability of Behavioral Observation

Reliability is the consistency of the assessment's data reported which is valuable to the purposes of behavioral observation. Types of reliability are consistency, test-retest, and inter-rater reliability. Of these three types of reliability, inter-rater reliability is the most relevant to behavioral observation (Cooper et al., 2020). It involves having two individuals observing the student at the same time and the degree to which they agree about the occurrence or nonoccurrence of the behavior. Having accurate and precise behavioral definitions and establishing skilled training for behavioral observers are two factors needed when expecting inter-rater reliability. Generally, when inter-rate agreement is less than 100%, data need to be checked for accuracy (Cooper et al., 2020).

Factors Affecting Behavioral Observation

While observation is the primary manner of data collection in applied behavior analysis, there are a number of threats to the accuracy of measurement. According to Repp, Nieminen, Olinger, and Brusca (1988), there are multiple major factors that may potentially affect accuracy of observational data including: (a) reactivity, (b) observer drift, (c) the recording procedure, (d) location of the observation, (e) reliability, and (f) expectancy.

Reactivity

This is an occurrence whereby the participant or person being observed changes their behavior due to the awareness that they are being observed (Cooper et al., 2020). It would be faulty to presume that an individual's behavior is the same as it would be if the observer was not present. However, reactivity surely occurs in some of these cases, as subjects respond to the presence of observers by changing their behaviors (Repp et al., 1988). There may also be observer reactivity in which the observer changes his/her behavior is changed by the knowledge that others will be evaluating the data (Cooper et al., 2020). Observers can reduce reactivity by being as unobtrusive as possible, repeating observations after reactivity subsides, or taking reactivity into account when interpreting the data (Cooper et al., 2020). Monitoring observers as unobtrusively as possible on an unpredictable schedule should help reduce the observer reactivity (Cooper et al., 2020).

Observer Drift

This is a cognitive phenomenon that involves a gradual shift by the observer from the original response definition that results in behavior being inconsistently recorded (Cooper et al., 2007). When drift occurs, the data collected are no longer directly comparable across conditions, because they no longer quantify the same precise response. In addition, the amount of drift may vary from observer to observer. Cooper et al. (2020) recommend providing observers with occasional training sessions throughout the investigation to minimize observer drift.

Recording Procedure

In general, the more complicated the recording system, the more likely there will be error(s) (Cooper et al., 2020). In addition, the method of sampling behavior may itself lead to error. According to Repp et al. (1988), studies have found that (a) partial-interval overestimates, (b) whole-interval underestimates, (c) momentary time-sampling is preferred, because it randomly overestimates and underestimates and thus produces a fairly accurate average, and (d) shorter observation intervals produce far more accurate data than do longer intervals.

Location of the Observation

Most of the data from direct observation are collected in the naturalistic environment with the observer present. However, it is also possible to collect behavioral data via electronic recording equipment in an effort to reduce the obtrusiveness of observations. While electronic recording devices may cause some reactivity initially, studies have suggested that this effect is at most short-lived (Repp et al., 1988). With advances in the miniaturization of cameras, they may be virtually impossible to detect, thus reducing reactivity even further.

Reliability

Reliability in this context refers to interobserver agreement, or the degree to which two observers agree that responding has occurred. One of the simplest ways to increase reliability is to ensure that all observers have consistent and adequate training. In addition, research has suggested that observers who know that reliability checks are being conducted tend to be more accurate (Repp et al., 1988).

Expectancy

Observers may be biased through expectations of subject performance that are based on factors such as gender, the behavior of peers, or the purpose of the intervention (Repp et al. (1988). Research has suggested that the best way to minimize these effects is through comprehensive training of the observers. Experimenter feedback may also affect the behavior of observers.

Conclusion

Before any valid and reliable functional behavior assessment (FBA) can be conducted, it is important that there is a clear and unambiguous definition of the target behavior. Therefore, developing an operational definition of the target behavior is essential and the first step in an FBA. This chapter discussed operational definition in detail, their rationale, and provided examples and suggestions on writing an operational definition.

Once a behavior has been defined, it is important that observations be conducted to assess it in a manner that will allow an understanding of the function of the behavior as well as its rate of occurrence and other factors that may be important. Therefore, this chapter discussed behavioral observations, the principles undergirding behavioral observations, behavioral observation methods, the reliability of behavioral observations, and factors affecting behavioral observations. Regardless of the type, typography, or frequency of the target behavior, defining it and reliably measuring it are essential in the development of any intervention. Albert Einstein once said: "If I had only one hour to save the world, I would spend 55 minutes defining the problem, and only 5 minutes finding the solution." The same applies to behavior analysis, spend your time defining and understanding the behavior, the intervention will become obvious.

References

Achenbach, T. M., & Rescorla, L. A. (2001). *Manual for the ASEBA school-age forms & profiles*. Burlington, VT: University of Vermont, Research Center for Children, Youth, & Families.

Alberto, P. C., & Troutman, A. C. (2013). *Applied behavior analysis for teachers* (9th ed.). Columbus, OH: Merrill.

Allen, K. D., & Matthews, J. R. (1998). Behavior management of recurrent pain in children. In T. S. Watson & F. M. Gresham (Eds.), *Handbook of child behavior therapy* (pp. 263–286). New York, NY: Plenum Press.

Borrelli, B., Sepinwall, D., Ernst, D., Bellg, A. J., Czajkowski, S., Breger, R., ... Orwig, D. (2005). A new tool to assess treatment fidelity and evaluation of treatment fidelity across 10 years of health behavior research. *Journal of Consulting and Clinical Psychology, 73*, 852–860. https://doi.org/10.1037/0022-006X.73.5.852

Cooper, J. O., Heron, T. E., & Heward, W. L. (2007). *Applied behavior analysis* (2nd ed.). Upper Saddle River, NJ: Pearson Education, Inc..

Cooper, J. O., Heron, T. E., & Heward, W. L. (2020). *Applied behavior analysis* (3rd ed.). Upper Saddle River, NJ: Pearson Education, Inc..

Edwards, R. P. (2002). A tutorial for using the Functional Assessment Informant Record-Teachers (FAIR-T). *Proven Practice: Prevention and Remediation Solutions for Schools, 4,* 31–38.

Greer, B. D., Neidert, P. L., Dozier, C. L., Payne, S. W., Zonneveld, K. L., & Harper, A. M. (2013). Functional analysis and treatment of problem behavior in early education classrooms. *Journal of Applied Behavior Analysis, 46,* 289–295. https://doi.org/10.1002/jaba.10

Gresham, F. M., Gansle, K. A., & Noell, G. H. (1993). Treatment integrity in applied behavior analysis with children. *Journal of Applied Behavior Analysis, 26,* 257–263. https://doi.org/10.1901/jaba.1993.26-257

Gresham, F. M., Gansle, K. A., Noell, G. H., Cohen, S., & Rosenblum, S. (1993). Treatment integrity of school-based behavioral intervention studies: 1980–1990. *School Psychology Review, 22,* 254–272.

Jafer, A. S., Tayyebeh, S., Reza, A. B. H., Mansoureh, H., & Zahra, K. (2014). Effectiveness of role-playing and applied behavior analysis: Increases in social behavior in children with autism. *Journal of Research in Behavioural Sciences, 12,* 351–359.

Kazdin, A. E. (1990). Psychotherapy for children and adolescents. *Annual Review of Psychology, 41,* 21–54. https://doi.org/10.1146/annurev.ps.41.020190.000321

Lerman, D. C., Tetreault, A., Hovanetz, A., Bellaci, E., Miller, J., Karp, H., … Toupard, A. (2010). Applying signal-detection theory to the study of observer accuracy and bias in behavioral assessment. *Journal of Applied Behavior Analysis, 43,* 195–213. https://doi.org/10.1901/jaba.2010.43-195

Lindsley, O. R. (1991). From technical jargon to plain English for application. *Journal of Applied Behavior Analysis, 24,* 449–458. https://doi.org/10.1901/jaba.1991.24-449

McIntyre, L. L., Gresham, F. M., DiGennaro, F. D., & Reed, D. D. (2007). Treatment integrity of school-based interventions with children in the Journal of Applied Behavior Analysis 1991–2005. *Journal of Applied Behavior Analysis, 40,* 659–672. https://doi.org/10.1901/jaba.2007.659-672

Neitzel, J., & Bogin, J. (2008). *Steps for implementation: Functional behavior assessment.* Chapel Hill, NC: The National Professional Development Center on Autism Spectrum Disorders, Frank Porter Graham Child Development Institute, The University of North Carolina.

Peterson, L., Homer, A. L., & Wonderlich, S. A. (1982). The integrity of independent variables in behavior analysis. *Journal of Applied Behavior Analysis, 15,* 477–492. https://doi.org/10.1901/jaba.1982.15-477

Piazza, C. C., Bowman, L. G., Contrucci, S. A., Delia, M. D., Adelinis, J. D., & Goh, H. L. (1999). An evaluation of the properties of attention as reinforcement for destructive and appropriate behavior. *Journal of Applied Behavior Analysis, 32,* 437–449. https://doi.org/10.1901/jaba.1999.32-437

Repp, A. C., Nieminen, G. S., Olinger, E., & Brusca, R. (1988). Direct observation: Factors affecting the accuracy of observers. *Exceptional Children, 55,* 29–36. https://doi.org/10.1177/001440298805500103

Roscoe, E. M., Iwata, B. A., & Zhou, L. (2013). Assessment and treatment of chronic hand mouthing. *Journal of Applied Behavior Analysis, 46,* 181–198. https://doi.org/10.1002/jaba.14

Stevens, S. S. (1935). The operational definition of psychological concepts. *Psychological Review, 42,* 517–527.

Sugai, G., Sprague, J. R., Horner, R. H., & Walker, H. M. (2000). Preventing school violence: The use of office discipline referrals to assess and monitor school-wide discipline interventions. *Journal of Emotional and Behavioral Disorders, 8,* 94–101. https://doi.org/10.1177/106342660000800205

Tieghi-Benet, M. C., Miller, K., Reiners, J., Robinett, B. E., Freeman, R. L., Smith, C. L., ... Palmer, A. (2003). *Encouraging Student Progress (ESP), student/team book.* Lawrence, KS: University of Kansas.

Verner, S. M., Wichnick, A. M., & Poulson, C. L. (2017). Observation methods. In J. L. Matson (Ed.), *Handbook of social behavior and skills in children* (pp. 83–100). Cham, Switzerland: Springer International Publishing.

Vollmer, T. R., Marcus, B. A., & Ringdahl, J. E. (1995). Noncontingent escape as treatment for self-injurious behavior maintained by negative reinforcement. *Journal of Applied Behavior Analysis, 28,* 15–26. https://doi.org/10.1901/jaba.1995.28-15

Wacker, D. P., Lee, J. F., Dalmau, Y. C. P., Kopelman, T. G., Lindgren, S. D., Kuhle, J., ... Waldron, D. B. (2013). Conducting functional communication training via telehealth to reduce the problem behavior of young children with autism. *Journal of Developmental and Physical Disabilities, 25,* 35–48. https://doi.org/10.1007/s10882-012-9314-0

Watson, T. S., & Steege, M. W. (2003). *Conducting school-based functional behavioral assessments: A practitioner's guide.* New York, NY: Guilford Press.

Watson, T. S., & Watson, T. S. (2009). Behavioral assessment in the schools. In A. Akin-Little, S. G. Little, M. Bray, & T. Kehle (Eds.), (pp. 27–41). Washington, DC: APA Books.

Webster, J. (2019). *Operational definition of behavior in a school setting.* Retrieved from https://www.thoughtco.com/operational-definition-of-behavior-3110867

Webster, J. (2020). *The topography of behavior.* Retrieved from https://www.thoughtco.com/topography-of-behavior-3110854

Xu, S., Wang, J., Lee, G. T., & Luke, N. (2017). Using self-monitoring with guided goal setting to increase academic engagement for a student with autism in an inclusive classroom in China. *The Journal of Special Education, 51,* 106–114. https://doi.org/10.1177/0022466916679980

Chapter 9
Interviews and Report Writing in the Context of Functional Assessment

Michael P. Kranak, Meagan K. Gregory, and Griffin W. Rooker

Individuals with intellectual and developmental disabilities (IDD) commonly engage in forms of challenging behavior such as aggression, property destruction, elopement, yelling, and screaming, or self-injurious behavior (SIB; Crocker et al., 2006), with some prevalence estimates indicating SIB occurs in more than 30% of individuals with autism spectrum disorder (Soke et al., 2016). These individuals can exhibit challenging behavior across various settings including their homes, schools, clinics, and the community (Falligant et al., 2020; Muething et al., 2020; Podlesnik et al., 2017). Because treatment of these behaviors has been demonstrated to be more effective when the reasons why challenging behavior occurs are known (Didden et al., 2006), the first step in designing behavioral treatments for challenging behaviors is to conduct a functional assessment to identify the variables that occasion and maintain challenging behavior. Functional assessment is not simply the implementation of a single instrument, tool, or test, but rather refers to the process of determining variables that impact the occurrence of problem behavior (cf. Neef & Peterson, 2007). Functional assessments can include any combination of three components: (a) indirect assessments, (b) direct and descriptive assessments, and (c) experimental functional analyses[1] (FAs). One type of indirect assessment is an interview (Floyd et al., 2005). In this chapter, we describe and focus specifically on interviews as an aspect of indirect assessment, the various published methods of

---

[1] Experimental, in this sense, means the manipulation of consequences (i.e., independent variables) not that the analysis and assessment itself is untested or exploratory.

M. P. Kranak (✉)
Oakland University, Rochester, MI, USA
e-mail: kranak@oakland.edu

M. K. Gregory · G. W. Rooker
Kennedy Krieger Institute, Baltimore, MD, USA

Johns Hopkins University School of Medicine, Baltimore, MD, USA

© Springer Nature Switzerland AG 2021
J. L. Matson (ed.), *Functional Assessment for Challenging Behaviors and Mental Health Disorders*, Autism and Child Psychopathology Series,
https://doi.org/10.1007/978-3-030-66270-7_9

interviews related to challenging behavior, and how information garnered from the interview may be included in final reports.

Interviews Within the Functional Assessment Process

Indirect assessments are often the first part of the overall functional assessment process. Interviews are an important part of this process, as information obtained through interview can: (a) enable clinicians to identify potential target or interfering behaviors, (b) enable clinicians to identify potential evocative antecedents and maintaining consequences, (c) generate operational definitions, and (d) generate testable hypotheses regarding behavior function. It is important to note that interviews are not a means of determining behavioral function. In fact, conducting only an interview will not produce results that are valid and is therefore not recommended (Roscoe et al., 2009; Verriden & Roscoe, 2018). Rather, these tools are designed and validated as first steps in the process of determining behavioral function. Additionally, interviews present clinicians with an opportunity to build rapport or improve upon existing relationships with clients and their families. Table 9.1 depicts examples of rapport building statements and topics. Rapport building is integral to effectively building trust between clinicians and the clients and families with whom they are working, therefore making informants more likely to share pertinent information (Andzik & Kranak, 2020; Bailey & Burch, 2013).

Potential Interview Candidates

Clients undergoing functional assessments or receiving (or preparing to receive) behavioral services are likely to have many potential informants involved their lives. These informants can include family members and/or caretakers, as well as other professionals that may be providing various therapeutic services

Table 9.1 Potential rapport building statements

Potential Topic	Statements
Recent weather	"Glad we have had a break in the humidity. Do you prefer hot or colder weather? "That storm last night was enjoyable. Were things calm in your neck of the woods?
Community events	"Have you had a chance to visit the local farmer's market?" "Does [client's name] partake in any sports or clubs?"
Informant/familial interests	"That's a cool [sports related name/theme] jacket you wore today. Have you always been a fan of/liked [team/sport]?"

(LaFrance et al., 2019). As such, each individual may provide a unique perspective, insight, or experience regarding the client. As an illustrative example, consider a client who may be receiving services from a speech-language pathologist (SLP) to improve some aspects of swallowing and articulation. In this situation, it is likely that the SLP would be more equipped to provide detailed and nuanced information regarding swallowing and communication in comparison to a family member (e.g., Gerber, 2013). On the other hand, it is unlikely that the SLP (or any other professional) is with the client at all times and the duration of their relationship with the client may vary. Thus, parents or primary caregivers are likely the best interview candidates to speak towards day-to-day activities, transitions, and sleep time routines (Vladescu et al., 2020) as well as the client's behavior over a longer period of time.

It is unlikely that it will be possible to interview every individual who interacts with the client. Thus, it may be advantageous to prioritize those that spend the most time with the client (i.e., parents or primary caregivers) or professionals that have worked with the client for an extended amount of time. Said another way, one ought to choose interview informants wisely (Borgmeier & Horner, 2006). Table 9.2 depicts a list of potential interview candidates and information that could be obtained from each candidate, respectively. Although each can provide insights specifically related to their roles in the client's life, it is also important to consider if certain informants or candidates can speak to multiple areas (e.g., parents and teachers both able to speak about daily routines). Moreover, interviewing multiple people can allow interviewers to get a "second opinion" on why behavior may be occurring in certain contexts and not others. Said another way, it is not about tattling on another party, but rather getting a more nuanced look at why behaviors may or may not be occurring. This way, interviewers are maximizing the allotted, available interview time.

Table 9.2 Individuals with whom to potentially conduct interviews

Person/Relation to Client	Potential Information
Parent or primary caregiver	Topographies of challenging behavior. Other individuals in the household. Potential triggers and variables surrounding challenging behavior. Patterns of behavior over a longer time period.
Teacher	Tasks that may be aversive. Tasks in which client may enjoy engaging. Determine if challenging behavior occurs across settings (e.g., home and school).
Other family member (e.g., grandparent)	Determine if challenging behavior occurs across settings *or* family members.
Other professionals (e.g., speech-language pathologists, physical therapist)	Identify areas of strength, if challenging behavior is displayed across various therapy sessions.

Interview Structure and Procedures for Incorporating Methods into Interview

The type, standard, and quality of information obtained from interviews can vary widely due to a number of factors. First, interviews rely primarily on subjective recall on the part of the informant rather than direct behavioral observations (Rooker et al., 2015). Second, when the interview is more open-ended and informal, there is some evidence to suggest that interpersonal variables (interviewer skills and personality) can influence the quality of information obtained (Jäckle et al., 2011). Third, experience of the interviewer can certainly play a role in the outcome of an interview, as more experienced interviewers are likely to obtain better information than interviewers with minimal experience (LeBlanc & Luiselli, 2016). Because of this, structured interviews methods have been developed to guide interviewers to prompt informants to provide pertinent information they may not have shared otherwise (Table 9.3).

Structured Interview Tools

One commonly used and well-supported interview tool is the Questions About Behavioral Function, or QABF (Matson & Vollmer, 1995). The QABF is a 25-item rating scale designed to aid in identifying the function of a challenging behavior. Every item requires the informant to respond on a Likert-style rating scale rather than in an open-ended fashion. Based on responses to these 25 items, the QABF then produces a score in five function categories: attention, escape, tangible, physical, and nonsocial (automatic). Scores in those categories can help clinicians in developing hypothesis to test in the experimental FA.

A second interview tool is the Motivation Assessment Scale (MAS; Durand & Crimmins, 1988). The MAS is a 16-item questionnaire that aims to identify situations and settings in which clients may engage in challenging behaviors. Similar to

Table 9.3 Standardized interview aids

Interview Aid	Description
Questions About Behavioral Function (QABF)	Brief Likert-scale styled structured aid. Produces score indicating potential function.
Motivation Assessment Scale (MAS)	Brief Likert-scale styled structured aid. Produces score indicating potential function.
Functional Assessment Screening Tool (FAST)	Brief yes/no question structured aid. Produces score indicating potential function.
Functional Assessment Interview (FAI) Interview-Informed Synthesized Contingency Analysis (IISCA, interview portion only)	Long form, fully structured interview comprised of open-ended questions. Permits more flexibility in the overall interview process. Interview supplement used to design a specific experimental analysis. Interview is open-ended to permit as much flexibility as possible.

the QABF, the MAS presents all items in the form of a Likert-scale regarding the frequency with which behaviors occur in certain settings. The MAS also produces scores in four function categories: sensory, escape, attention, and tangible. Like the QABF, these results and scores can guide clinicians' decisions regarding additional assessments.

A third form of a structured interview aid is the Functional Analysis Screening Tool (FAST; Iwata et al., 2013). In contrast to the QABF and MAS, the FAST does not include Likert-scale questions. Rather, the FAST utilizes 16 yes/no questions in conjunction with additional questions regarding demographics and topographies. Based on the scores from the yes/no questions, a potential source of reinforcement is identified as either: social positive (attention/preferred items), social negative (escape from tasks/activities), automatic positive (sensory stimulation), or automatic negative (pain attenuation). Although shorter and stylistically different than the previous two aids, the FAST also provides information that clinicians can use to develop hypotheses regarding the function(s) of challenging behavior.

Open-Ended Interview Aids

Although structured aids can provide more continuity throughout the interview process with various informants and may make the ability to gather important information more reliable, it is possible that the close-ended format of the questions may not capture all of the variables related to challenging behavior. That is, by providing a set list of questions, the information gathered is necessarily circumscribed. As such, open-ended aids provide a format for the overall interview, aimed at obtaining pertinent information regarding challenging behavior(s), but permit more flexibility than the QABF, MAS, and FAST.

Similar to other structured interview aids, these open-ended interview aids help clinicians determine what questions to ask and how to phrase them in a way that encourages informants to provide more accurate and complete information. However, unlike the aids in the previous section, these aids neither use ranking or rating scales nor produce scores that indicate potential functions of behavior. Instead, these aids are comprised of open-ended questions to which informants are able to provide as much information as possible, and this information can be used to determine when to conduct direct observations so as to maximize the likelihood of observing problem behavior and to design conditions in a functional analysis to test possible functions.

Two notable open-ended aids are the Functional Assessment Interview (FAI; cf. O'Neill et al., 1997) and the interview portion of the interview-informed synthesized contingency analysis (that is, the II portion of the IISCA; Hanley, 2012; Hanley et al., 2014). For both aids, questions are broken down into nine sections. In the first section, informant's answer questions regarding what challenging behaviors occur, what they look like, how often they occur, and how intense they can be. This is an important first step in identifying the potential target behaviors for further assessment. This is especially true in the case when both very severe and mild challenging behaviors are exhibited (e.g., SIB and stereotypy). In this scenario, SIB would certainly be prioritized, with clinicians triaging SIB before moving to stereotypy. The second section focuses on daily routines and other ecological variables (e.g., medications, eating habits) that can potentially impact the challenging behaviors. Additionally, informants are provided an opportunity to describe daily activities and client's reactions to those activities, which can indicate potential preferred and nonpreferred activities. Third, informants are asked about very specific events that can trigger or occasion challenging behaviors. For example, informants are asked about what one event they could do in order to ensure the behavior happens and what they could do to ensure it does *not* occur.

The fourth and fifth sections focus on potential strengths and weakness (or, rather, adaptive abilities and deficits) and typical consequences of certain client behaviors. These two sections can help determine not only potential setting events and establishing operations, but also potential replacement or alternative behaviors that may already be in the client's repertoire. Similarly, the sixth, seventh, and eighth sections focus on the client's communication skills. In particular, when moving through these sections, the interviewer is able to ask about specific communication modalities that may be best suited for the client, based on skill level or situations that are the most difficult in terms of communication. Finally, in the ninth section, the interviewer is able to briefly summarize the information and hypothesize what functions certain behaviors may serve.

It is important to note that every interview session should be designed on a case-by-case basis. No two informants are the same, and no two clients are the same. As such, it is important to rely on clinical expertise, as well as input from colleagues and other clinical team members regarding how to best structure interviews to make sure all relevant information is obtained. If the interviewing clinician is working as part of an interdisciplinary team, this may also impact the structure and content of the interview. Multi or interdisciplinary teams may have guidelines and clearly delineated boundaries regarding the types of questions asked by each member of the team. For example, behavior analysts may ask strictly about behavior, whereas pediatricians are responsible for asking about medications, allergies, and other health issues. On the other hand, transdisciplinary teams incorporate role release, in which members of the team may ask about areas that are not strictly within their discipline based on the ebbs and flows of the interview (e.g., King et al., 2009). For example, if a pediatrician were to ask a question about how well a client walks and the informant were to bring up how it seems the client cannot hear well while walking or engaging in another physical activity, the physical therapist might naturally ask about the client's hearing or other situations in which they do not seem to hear well. This question may seem better suited for an audiologist, but given the nature of transdisciplinary teams, it is actually encouraged for members to ask questions about other areas and disciplines. Lastly, the structure of an interview should still have some element of fluidity and flexibility. Said another way, just because the interview starts out moving through all portions of the QABF, there may be areas that the informant really wants to expand upon in detail. Thus, clinicians ought to be able to switch gears between structured interview aids and guidelines, as well as more informal narrative interviewing.

Comparing and Contrasting Structured and Open-Ended Interview Aids

Both structured and open-ended interviews have strengths and limitations. For example, structured interview aids can limit biases related to informant traits but may produce other sorts of biases. For example, the order in which Likert-style questions are presented in structured aids can result in biased answers on the part of the informant (Chan, 1991). Informants are also likely to respond to Likert-style questions in extreme fashions. That is, they are likely to indicate behaviors as occurring more frequently and intensely than they otherwise would have stated in response to an open-ended question. In addition, although structured interviews may be simpler for a less-experienced clinician to implement and may produce more easily digestible results (i.e., they may suggest a possible function), they also may not capture as much information as open-ended aids. This applies both to variables that may impact the challenging behavior directly as well as potential replacement behaviors (e.g., questions related to replacement behaviors already in the client's repertoire are only posed in open-ended aids). There are additional biases that exist that go beyond the scope of this chapter, thus, we encourage readers to keep strengths and limitations of each method in mind when utilizing them in clinical practice.

Report Writing in the Context of Functional Assessment

Following completion of the functional assessment (including interviews), results should be summarized. This report will include not only those results from interviews as discussed in the current chapter, but also results from other assessment methods. Depending on the type and number of team members that will be contributing to the report, it can be difficult to determine what to include or exclude and how to write results in a manner consumable to many audiences. To that end, we discuss specifically how to incorporate information obtained in an interview into a final report (see Fig. 9.1 for an illustrative example).

Informant Interview
    Format: Functional Assessment Interview (FAI)
    Interviewer: Shawn; 3/18/20
    Who was interviewed: Nancy (relation to client: mother)
    Summary of Results: During interview (according to the FAI sheet), Mom primarily focused on the aggression and elopement. Aggression was listed as highest priority. Behaviors are likely to occur with mom, any family member in home, and BCBA at center. The most troublesome times are when they are out in community, which is not often *because* they currently cannot safely handle elopement, and at school. Mom noted aggression was more likely to happen when: access to food was denied, preferred activity was interrupted, or when a demand was placed on him (in particular, at the center). Mom is unsure how they handle issues at school. Mom has tried time out; BCBA is currently providing attention when he elopes. Neither procedure has been effective at decreasing the behavior. Based on the information provided in the FAI, the hypothesized functions of aggression and elopement are denied access to tangibles and escape from demands.

Fig. 9.1 Example of interview write-up in final report

What to Incorporate and How to Incorporate It?

Depending on how many people were interviewed and what (if any) structured interviews were completed, it can seem daunting to have to summarize every individual interview. However, there are a few items that ought to be present in any interview summary contained in a report. First, the format or type of interview should be specified. This can include any of the structured formats discussed herein (e.g., FAI, QABF), or if the interview was informal and no aid was used, clinicians should consider indicating "Informal" as the interview type. Second, logistical details of the interview should be noted. These details include who was interviewed and their relation to the client, who conducted the interview, the date and time, and the setting in which it took place. Third, the results of the interview should be briefly discussed. The description of the results will differ depending upon the type of interview conducted and the topics of discussion. In short, any summary of results should include the details about what happened and what was discussed during the interview, and what those findings indicated with respect to the challenging behavior.

Speaking to Multiple Audiences

In terms of how to incorporate all of the above discussed components, first and foremost, all information must be presented accurately. This is especially true in terms of summarizing interviews, as one does not want to mischaracterize informants' responses or to suggest that the results of an interview definitively indicate the consequences (i.e., payoffs) that maintain the occurrence of the challenging behavior. One challenge with presenting information accurately may be how to present it without using technical jargon—especially in terms of adhering to the professional and ethical compliance code behavior analysts must follow (Behavior Analyst Certification Board, 2014). Thus, it is critical to consider who will be reading the report (and, if those reading the report will have a team member present to assist them with interpretation). For example, parents and/or caregivers will certainly have an opportunity to read and review the report. Consider the likelihood parents and caregivers are familiar with phrases such as behavior maintained by access to positive reinforcement (e.g., behavior maintained by access to adult attention or by access to specific tangible items) and results of a FAST. In this case, it may be more appropriate to not only use the technical terms, but also brief definitions (e.g., writing that behaviors occur to get adult to pay attention to them) that can make the findings included in the report more palatable. The same can be said if the report will be read by other professionals with minimal experience or exposure to behavior analysis.

Focusing on the Referral Issue

In any case, no matter the intended audience, it is important to focus on and prioritize the issue for which the client was referred (Janney & Snell, 2000). For example, the client may have been referred for engaging in aggression and elopement. However, in the course of the interviews (and overall assessment process), some academic issues may have been brought up. In this scenario, it can be easy to make recommendations regarding curriculum revision or additional classroom supports. However, clinicians need to prioritize the issue for which services were sought (i.e., aggression and elopement) and continue to act within their clinical scope of competence (Janney & Snell, 2000; Brodhead et al., 2018). Depending upon the makeup of the team and individuals writing the report, it may be possible that there will be an opportunity to comment on other issues that arose during the assessment. But, overall, the majority of the report ought to be reflective of the primary issue for which the client was referred.

Hypothesized Functions and Evidence-Based Recommendations

Following indirect assessments (including interviews described herein), clinicians will be able to generate hypotheses regarding functions of nominated challenging behaviors. In addition, clinicians will be able to make potential treatment recommendations based upon those hypotheses. However, as previously discussed, indirect assessments are not an end to themselves; they are the first steps in the assessment process. Additional assessments must be conducted prior to treatment. Indirect assessments are meant to supplement and guide direct observation and experimental assessments in order to identify the functions of challenging behaviors (Roscoe et al., 2015). Roscoe et al. evaluated FAs modified specifically from information garnered through indirect assessments (i.e., interviews) and found that FAs modified based on informant information resulted in differentiation of responding during test conditions otherwise undifferentiated in previous FAs. Indeed, these results further support the use of interviews and other indirect assessments to guide additional assessments.

Conclusions

In this chapter, we described various methods of how to structure interviews during the functional assessment process, how to incorporate interview results into final reports, and considerations with writing final reports. It is important to note that the guidelines presented in the current chapter are not hard rules, but rather recommendations and thoughts to consider when conducting functional assessments. It is likely that every team and/or agency has its own standards, protocols, or guidelines regarding the assessment and interview process. As such, one must be cognizant of immediate rules, contingencies, and guidelines that need to be followed under those certain contexts. Interviews are critical components to the overall functional assessment process. They can guide decisions for future descriptive or experimental assessments and enable clinicians to generate hypotheses regarding behavioral functions. Reports serve as both legal and ethical documentation of client needs and proposed actionable and tenable steps towards meeting and addressing those needs. Interviews are but one of the assessment measures included in the report, and are not a sufficient means to conclude behavioral function or develop a treatment plan. Thus, we encourage readers to consume the remaining chapters on descriptive and experimental assessments.

Author Note The authors wish to thank Elissa Spinks for her assistance in compiling resources and references.

References

Andzik, N. R., &Kranak, M. P. (2020). The softer side of supervision: Recommendations when teaching and evaluating behavior-analytic professionalism. *Behavior Analysis: Research and Practice*. Advance online publication. https://doi.org/10.1037/bar0000194.

Bailey, J. S., & Burch, M. R. (2013). *How to think like a behavior analyst: Understanding the science that can change your life*. Taylor & Francis.

Behavior Analyst Certification Board. (2014). *Professional and ethical compliance code for behavior analysts*. Littleton, CO: Author.

Borgmeier, C., & Horner, R. H. (2006). An evaluation of the predictive validity of confidence ratings in identifying functional behavior assessment hypothesis statements. *Journal of Positive Behavior Interventions, 8*(2), 100–105. https://doi.org/10.1177/10983007060080020101

Brodhead, M. T., Quigley, S. P., & Wilczynski, S. M. (2018). A call for discussion about scope of competence in behavior analysis. *Behavior Analysis in Practice, 11*(4), 424–435. https://doi.org/10.1007/s40617-018-00303-8

Chan, J. C. (1991). Response-order effects in Likert-type scales. *Education and Psychological Measurement, 51*, 531–540.

Crocker, A. G., Mercier, C., Lachapelle, Y., Brunet, A., Morin, D., & Roy, M. E. (2006). Prevalence and types of aggressive behaviour among adults with intellectual disabilities. *Journal of Intellectual Disability Research, 50*, 652–661.

Durand, V. M., & Crimmins, D. B. (1988). Identifying the variables maintaining self-injurious behavior. *Journal of Autism and Developmental Disorders, 18*(1), 99–117. https://doi.org/10.1007/BF02211821

Didden, R., Korzilius, K., van Oorsouw, W., & Sturmey, P. (2006). Behavioral treatment of challenging behaviors in individuals with mild mental retardation: Meta-analysis of single-subject research. *American Journal on Mental Retardation, 111*(4). https://doi.org/10.1352/0895-8017(2006)111[290:BTOCBI]2.0CO;2

Falligant, J. M., Kranak, M. P., McNulty, M. K., Schmidt, J. D., Hausman, N. L., &Rooker, G. W. (2020). Prevalence of renewal of problem behavior: Replication and extension to an inpatient setting. *Journal of Applied Behavior Analysis*. Advance online publication.https://doi.org/10.1002/jaba.740.

Floyd, R. G., Phaneuf, R. L., & Wilczynksi, S. M. (2005). Measurement properties of indirect assessment methods for functional behavioral assessment: A review of research. *School Psychology Review, 34*, 58–73.

Gerber, S. (2013). A developmental perspective on language assessment and intervention for children on the autistic spectrum. *Topics in Language Disorders, 23*(2), 74–94. https://doi.org/10.1097/00011363-200304000-00003

Hanley, G. P. (2012). Functional assessment of problem behavior: Dispelling myths, overcoming implementation obstacles, and developing new lore. *Behavior Analysis in Practice, 5*(1), 54–72. https://doi.org/10.1007/BF03391818

Hanley, G. P., Jin, C. S., Vanselow, N. R., & Hanratty, L. A. (2014). Producing meaningful improvements in problem behavior of children with autism via synthesized analyse and treatments. *Journal of Applied Behavior Analysis, 47*(1), 16–36. https://doi.org/10.1002/jaba.106

Iwata, B. A., DeLeon, I. G., & Roscoe, E. M. (2013). Reliability and validity of the functional analysis screening tool. *Journal of Applied Behavior Analysis, 46*(1), 271–284. https://doi.org/10.1002/jaba.31

Jäckle, A., Lynn, P., Sinibaldi, J., &Tipping, S. (2011). *The effect of interviewer personality, skills and attitudes on respondent co-operation with face-to-face surveys* (No. 2011–14). ISER Working PaperSeries.

Janney, R., & Snell, M. E. (2000). *Behavioral support*. Baltimore, MD: Paul H. Brookes.

King, G., Strachan, D., Tucker, M., Duwyn, B., Desserud, S., & Shillington, M. (2009). The application of transdisciplinary model for early intervention services. *Infants & Young Children, 22*(3), 211–223.

LaFrance, D. L., Weiss, M. J., Kazemi, E., Gerenser, J., & Dobres, J. (2019). Multidisciplinary teaming: Enhancing collaboration through increased understanding. *Behavior Analysis in Practice, 12*(3), 709–726. https://doi.org/10.1007/s40617-019-00331-y

LeBlanc, L. A., & Luiselli, J. K. (2016). Refining supervisory practices in the field of behavior analysis: Introduction to the special section on supervisor. *Behavior Analysis in Practice, 9*(4), 271–273. https://doi.org/10.1007/s40617-016-0156-6

Matson, J. L., & Vollmer, T. R. (1995). *Questions about behavioral function (QABF)*. Baton Rouge, LA: Disability Consultants.

Muething, C., Call, N., Pavlov, A., Ringdahl, J., Gillespie, S., Clark, S., & Mevers, J. L. (2020). Prevalence of renewal of problem behavior during context changes. *Journal of Applied Behavior Analysis, 53*(3), 1485–1493. https://doi.org/10.1002/jaba.672

Neef, N. A., & Peterson, S. M. (2007). Functional behavior assessment. In J. O. Cooper, T. E. Heron, & W. E. Heward (Eds.), *Applied behavior analysis* (pp. 500–524). Upper Saddle River, NJ: Pearson/Merrill-Prentice Hall.

O'Neill, R. H., Albin, R. W., Sprague, J. R., Storey, K., & Newton, J. S. (1997). *Functional assessment and program development for problem behavior*. Pacific Grove, CA: Brooks/Cole Publishing.

Podlesnik, C. A., Kelley, M. E., Jimenez-Gomez, C., & Bouton, M. E. (2017). Renewed behavior produced by context change and its implications for treatment maintenance: A review. *Journal of Applied Behavior Analysis, 50*, 675–697.

Roscoe, E. M., Rooker, G. W., Pence, S. T., & Longworth, L. J. (2009). Assessing the utility of a demand assessment for functional analysis. *Journal of Applied Behavior Analysis, 42*(4), 819–825. https://doi.org/10.1901/jaba.2009.42-819

Roscoe, E. M., Schlichenmeyer, K. J., & Dube, W. V. (2015). Functional analysis of problem behavior: A systematic approach for identifying idiosyncratic variables. *Journal of Applied Behavior Analysis, 48*(2), 289–314. https://doi.org/10.1002/jaba.201

Rooker, G. W., DeLeon, I. G., Borrero, C. S. W., Frank-Crawford, M. A., & Roscoe, E. M. (2015). Reducing ambiguity in the functional assessment of problem behavior. *Behavioral Interventions, 30*(1), 1–35. https://doi.org/10.1002/bin.1400

Soke, G. N., Rosenberg, S. A., Hamman, R. F., Fingerlin, T., Robinson, C., Carpenter, L., … DiGiuseppi, C. (2016). Brief report: Prevalence of self-injurious behaviors among children with autism spectrum disorder–a population-based study. *Journal of Autism and Developmental Disorders, 46*(11), 3607–3614. https://doi.org/10.1007/s10803-016-2879-1

Verriden, A. L., & Roscoe, E. M. (2018). An evaluation of a punisher assessment for decreasing automatically reinforced problem behavior. *Journal of Applied Behavior Analysis, 52*(1), 205–226. https://doi.org/10.1002/jaba.509

Vladescu, J. C., Schnell, L. K., & Day-Watkins, J. (2020). Infant positioning: A brief review. *Journal of Applied Behavior Analysis, 53*(3), 1237–1241.

Chapter 10
The Evolution of Functional Analysis

Allie E. Rader, Justin B. Leaf, and Joseph H. Cihon

The Evolution of Functional Analysis

Interventionists providing treatment for individuals diagnosed with developmental and/or intellectual disabilities (e.g., behavior analysts, teachers, paraprofessionals) have the unique opportunity to improve the quality of the lives of their clients. This often means improving or developing prosocial behaviors (e.g., social, language, academics) and ameliorating aberrant behavior (e.g., self-injurious behavior, stereotypic behaviors). Aberrant behaviors commonly demonstrated by individuals diagnosed with autism spectrum disorder (ASD), intellectual disabilities (ID), and other developmental disabilities (DD) can create a major barrier to this goal (Blacher & McIntyre, 2006). In some cases, these behaviors are part of a diagnostic criteria that characterizes a disability (e.g., stereotypic behaviors related to ASD). In other cases, aberrant behaviors might develop because of limited communication skills (Kaiser & Roberts, 2011), reduced independence, or other impairments resulting from the primary diagnosis (Dominick, Davis, Lainhart, Tager-Flusberg, & Folstein, 2007; Nagai, Hinobayashi, & Kanazawa, 2017).

The prevalence and impact of aberrant behaviors varies greatly from individual to individual. Aberrant behaviors range from minor interferences with learning, such as hand-flapping, tapping materials, and other stereotypical behaviors to dangerous behaviors such as self-injury and aggression. For instance, one survey of

A. E. Rader
Endicott College, Beverly, MA, USA

May Institute, Randolph, MA, USA

J. B. Leaf (✉) · J. H. Cihon
Endicott College, Beverly, MA, USA

Autism Partnership Foundation, Seal Beach, CA, USA

© Springer Nature Switzerland AG 2021
J. L. Matson (ed.), *Functional Assessment for Challenging Behaviors and Mental Health Disorders*, Autism and Child Psychopathology Series,
https://doi.org/10.1007/978-3-030-66270-7_10

over 8000 children diagnosed with ASD found that 27.7% engaged in self-injurious behavior (Soke et al., 2016). Another indicated the prevalence of self-injury was somewhere between 4% to 12% and 33% to 71% for individuals diagnosed with ID with individuals diagnosed with ASD, respectively (Richards, Oliver, Nelson, & Moss, 2012). Furthermore, rates of aggressive behaviors toward others has been documented to be anywhere from 7% to 56% in children with ASD (Kanne & Mazurek, 2011).

Severe topographies of aberrant behavior, such as self-injury and aggression, may pose serious risks of harm to the impacted individuals as well as their families, caregivers, and society (Pelios, Morren, Tesch, & Axelrod, 1999). Beyond the risk of bodily harm, aberrant behaviors can have profound effects on the overall well-being of families (Blacher & McIntyre, 2006). Chronic engagement in dangerous behaviors may result in institutionalization and seclusion of individuals from their families and society (Pelios et al., 1999). Additionally, parents of individuals that engage in chronic dangerous behaviors are more likely to suffer from low personal morale, stress, and depression (Blacher & McIntyre, 2006).

Because of the detrimental effects aberrant behaviors have on the lives of individuals and their families, reliance on evidence-based practice to safely and effectively ameliorate these behaviors is imperative. One field dedicated to evidenced-based interventions and a focus on function (the conditions under which behavior occurs) is applied behavior analysis (ABA). ABA is a systematic approach to understanding behaviors of social interest (Baer, Wolf, & Risley, 1968). As a field of scientific investigation, ABA currently provides the most reliable empirical support for effective treatments of aberrant behaviors associated with developmental disabilities (Reichow, 2012).

Research within the field of ABA indicates interventions for reducing aberrant behavior are most effective when they are function-based (Vollmer, Iwata, Zarcone, Smith, & Mazaleski, 1993); in other words, when interventions are developed using the reinforcing consequences previously available for aberrant behavior. Subsequent function-based treatments typically involve teaching the individual how to access that consequence in more socially preferred ways. For example, an individual may engage in aggression to escape or delay academic tasks. The interventionist will first assess the aggression to determine whether it is, in fact, functioning to escape or delay academic tasks. Following this assessment, the interventionist will identify a way that the individual can escape or delay academic tasks that is more socially preferred (e.g., asking for a break when an academic task is presented).

To prescribe function-based treatments, it is essential to accurately identify the variables maintaining the behavior. One method of identifying function is to assess these variables as part of a functional behavioral assessment (FBA). FBAs are assessments that investigate environmental variables that might influence behavior such as providing demands, withholding attention, or terminating access to preferred items (Oliver, Pratt, & Normand, 2015). These variables are identified for the purpose of determining potential functional relationships between aspects of the environment and the behavior of interest.

FBAs often include an indirect assessment that involves interviewing people in the individual's environment (Oliver et al., 2015). These interviews may include interviewing caregivers and family members or having them complete assessments and/or rating scales (Zaja, Moore, Van Ingen, & Rojahn, 2011). Some popular rating scales include the Motivational Assessment Scale (MAS; Durand & Crimmins, 1988), the Functional Analysis Screening Tool (FAST; Iwata, DeLeon, & Roscoe, 2013), and the Questions About Behavioral Function (QABF; Matson & Vollmer, 1995). While commonly used, some studies have indicated that the reliability and validity of these questionnaires are not adequate for treatment development without supplemental assessment (Iwata et al., 2013). Further analysis is recommended to develop effective treatment.

An additional component common to the FBA that might supplement the use of questionnaires and interview is a descriptive assessment (Hanley, 2012). A descriptive assessment involves observing and documenting the environmental conditions that tend to surround the behavior of interest (Sloman, 2010). One of the most common descriptive assessments is known as A-B-C data collection (Sloman, 2010), which was first described by Bijou, Peterson, and Ault (1968). This method involves observing the target behavior in the natural setting and recording the events that happen directly before and after its occurrence. Like interviews and questionnaires, no experimental manipulation is included in this method of evaluation, and results have been shown to be inconsistent with more rigorous methods of assessment (Hall, 2005; Sloman, 2010; Thompson & Iwata, 2007).

A final component of an FBA may be the interventionist implementing a functional analysis (Iwata et al., 1982), although a functional analysis is not always implemented as part of an FBA and functional analysis might also be conducted as an isolated or stand-alone procedure. The term *functional analysis* (FA) has been used to describe empirical demonstrations of cause-effect relationships (see, however, Hanley, Iwata, & McCord, 2003, for an extended discussion of the term). It is the only commonly used method for evaluating function that demonstrates a functional relation (Oliver et al., 2015). The FA evaluates behavioral function through direct manipulation of environmental variables that are hypothesized to maintain a behavior. Typically, several conditions are designed to arrange the conditions under which the behavior of interest is likely to occur. If the target behavior occurs, then the putative reinforcer specific to that condition is provided. The specific methods and nuances of FA are numerous, and best practices are often debated by researchers and interventionists (Hanley, 2012). The continued refinement and discussion regarding FA has led to one of the most robust literatures in the field of ABA (Beavers, Iwata, & Lerman, 2013; Hanley et al., 2003).

Given the central role the development and implementation of FA plays in the treatment of aberrant behavior, it is important to understand the historical underpinnings and current applications of this methodology. Therefore, the purpose of this chapter is to provide an overview of the history of functional analysis, discuss various types of functional analyses and how these types address barriers to the implementation of functional analysis, and suggest future directions for research related to FA.

History of Functional Analysis

Skinner (1953) described the term *functional relation* for use in behavior analysis as a replacement for the typical use of cause-and-effect (p. 23). He was careful, however, to note that while "a 'cause' becomes a 'change in an independent variable' and an 'effect' a 'change in a dependent variable'" (Skinner, 1953, p. 23), a *functional relation* does not suggest how a cause causes its effect. Notably, Skinner's (1953) use of the term described a functional relationship in which objective variables affecting behavior may be analyzed. Skinner (1953) went on to introduce the term *functional analysis* when stating, "The external variables of which behavior is a function provide for what may be called a causal or functional analysis. We undertake to predict and control the behavior of the individual organism" (p. 35). In *Verbal Behavior*, Skinner (1957) elaborated on this premise. Specifically, Skinner (1957) provided a context for how such a functional analysis might apply to human behavior in a description of the maintaining variables of verbal behavior when stating:

> The probability that a verbal response of given form will occur at a given time is the basic datum to be predicted and controlled. It is the 'dependent variable' in a *functional analysis*. The conditions and events to which we turn in order to achieve prediction or control—the 'independent variables'—must now be considered. (pp. 28–29)

Here, Skinner (1957) provided the theoretical framework for the prediction and control of topographies of behavior beyond verbal responses. For instance, the adjective "verbal" may be replaced with "aberrant." Thus, the interventionist might conduct a functional analysis to consider which independent variables might be manipulated to predict and control the aberrant response.

While focus on function was implicit in Skinner's work, early applications seldom emphasized identification of a function to inform treatment (Dixon, Vogel, & Tarbox, 2012). Aberrant behavior was typically treated using arbitrary but powerful reinforcement and punishment contingencies (Iwata & Bailey, 1974; Lovaas & Simmons, 1969; Zeilberger, Sampen, & Sloane, 1968). These contingencies were arbitrary in that they held no specific relevance to the maintaining variables of the aberrant behavior in question. Without considering the function of behavior in development of an intervention, punishment was found to be more effective (Pelios et al., 1999). However, the use of punishment had undesirable side effects and raised ethical concerns (Sidman & Center, 1991).

Despite widespread use of arbitrary contingencies and punishment, some early research did consider functional relationships with respect to aberrant behavior. This early work set the stage for the formal development of a methodology to evaluate the function of aberrant behavior. For example, one early researcher who emphasized the importance of function in the treatment of aberrant behavior was Ferster (1964). Ferster advocated for the adaptation of experimental methods used for control of nonhuman participants in the lab for application to human participants. Importantly, Ferster recognized the essential role of social contingencies (the behavior of others) in the shaping and maintenance of aberrant behaviors in humans.

Ferster referred to social reinforcement as "reinforcements of the world" and proposed that individuals who engage in aberrant behaviors might do so because of an inability to engage in behaviors that contact such reinforcement. Ferster wrote a "characterization of the behavior of the psychiatric patient in terms of a functional analysis," in which he proposed three explanations for why an individual might engage in aberrant behaviors. These included (1) an inadequate reinforcement history, (2) an inadequate schedule of reinforcement, or (3) excessive punishment that produces excess avoidant behavior.

Lovaas was another researcher that recognized the influence of social contingencies on the maintenance of aberrant behavior and was one of the first to adapt this knowledge for what might be considered an early functional analysis. Lovaas identified social reinforcers that were effective in teaching new behaviors to children who demonstrate self-injurious behaviors. He hypothesized that if social reinforcers might be used to teach and maintain new behaviors, they might also be involved in the maintenance of aberrant behaviors (Lovaas, Freitag, Gold, & Kassorla, 1965).

To test this hypothesis, Lovaas et al. (1965) developed a series of unique experimental manipulations. Social reinforcement was used to teach new behaviors, and then the new behavior was placed on extinction by abruptly ceasing delivery of contingent reinforcement. Lovaas and colleagues found that the frequency of the new skill quickly decreased and that there was a reciprocal increase in what was termed *self-destructive behavior* (i.e., self-injury). This inverse relationship led to the researchers' conclusion that these behaviors might share a common reinforcer, that is, the new behavior and the aberrant behavior might belong to the same response class. The final phase of the study experimentally demonstrated that social reinforcement did, in fact, maintain self-destructive behavior for the participant. In this final phase, Lovaas and colleagues conducted numerous, alternating sessions in which all social reinforcement was either absent or delivered contingent upon emission of self-destructive behavior. Results showed that the rate of self-destructive behavior was much higher during contingent delivery of social reinforcement than in its absence.

Carr, Newsom, and Binkoff (1976) expanded upon the work of Lovaas et al. (1965). Like Lovaas' work, Carr et al. evaluated self-injury but evaluated the manipulation of environmental changes that occurred before self-injury (i.e., antecedent conditions) rather than manipulating the consequence. Carr et al. identified a participant for whom known treatments for self-injurious behavior involving manipulation of consequences had been unsuccessful. They observed that self-injury was more likely to occur during situations when demands were placed frequently. To test the hypothesis that self-injury was evoked by demands and reinforced by the subsequent removal of those demands, an assessment was designed with three conditions: (1) mands, (2) tacts, and (3) free time. The results of Carr et al. (1976) indicated that self-injury occurred more often during the mand condition and almost never in the tact and free-time conditions. Carr, Newsom, and Binkoff (1980) would later go on to describe the application of the same assessment toward the identification of maintaining variables of aggressive behavior.

The early research on behavioral function by researchers such as Ferster, Lovaas, Carr, and others led to a call for interventionists to develop a broad evaluative tool for identifying the function(s) of aberrant behavior (Dixon et al., 2012). The term "functional analysis" was formally adopted by Iwata, Dorsey, Slifer, Bauman, and Richman (1982) to describe such a methodology. In this seminal paper, the authors presented methods for directly assessing the function of self-injurious behavior. This methodology has been referred to as the standard FA (SFA; Ala'i-Rosales et al., 2019).

Iwata et al. (1982) evaluated the self-injury of nine individuals under four distinct conditions using a multielement experimental design. These conditions were designed to test the sensitivity of self-injury to isolated contingencies. The first two conditions were designed to evaluate the effects of socially mediated contingencies: (1) a *social disapproval condition* and (2) an *academic demand condition*. The third condition was an *unstructured play condition*, and the fourth was an *alone condition*. After 15 min of a condition, the next condition was implemented in an order that was predetermined and randomly assigned.

Each condition was designed so the individual was deprived of the relevant putative reinforcer until an instance of self-injury occurred. During the *social disapproval* (attention) *condition*, the participant was instructed to play with toys while the experimenter worked. All social attention was withheld until an occurrence of self-injury, at which time the interventionist provided statements of disapproval such as "don't do that, you're going to hurt yourself." While attention was only delivered contingent upon self-injury, the participant had free access to toys throughout the condition. The *academic demand condition* comprised of educational tasks the participants were likely to encounter in a special education setting. The tasks were presented, and the interventionist provided prompts until the participant complied or engaged in self-injury. Following any instance of self-injury, the experimenter ended the task and turned away from the participant for 30 s. Following task completion, the experimenter provided praise.

An *unstructured play condition* was conducted as a control and an enriched environment. No tasks or demands were presented, and toys were freely available. Attention was provided in the form of social praise and brief touch for appropriate behavior at least every 30 s. There were no programmed consequences provided for self-injury. Finally, the *alone condition* was conducted to evaluate if self-injury occured in the absence of another person in an impoverished environment. There were no toys, materials, or other people present in the room. Although the SFA is often associated with a third socially mediated condition, tangible, this was not described in the literature until Mace and West (1986). Furthermore, it was not a separate condition as part of the SFA until 1995 (Vollmer, Marcus, Ringdahl, & Roane, 1995).

Iwata and colleagues' (1982) results indicated the maintaining variables of self-injury were differentiated for most of the participants. In other words, the rate of self-injury was consistently higher in one condition than any other. Four participants engaged in higher rates of self-injury during the alone condition, indicating self-injury was maintained through contingencies that did not require social mediation (e.g., automatic reinforcement). Two participants showed markedly higher rates of self-injury during the demand condition, indicating that self-injury was maintained by escape from demands. One participant engaged in more self-injury when attention was provided contingent upon its occurrence. Finally, three participants' results were either unclear or the occurrence of self-injury was equally frequent across conditions. These results demonstrated a reliable methodology for identifying a functional relationship between aberrant behavior and environmental variables.

The publication of Iwata and colleagues' (1982) seminal study was particularly impactful on the field of ABA (Beavers et al., 2013; Hanley, 2012; Hanley et al., 2003) and was subsequently republished in 1994 in a special edition of the *Journal of Applied Behavior Analysis* (JABA) dedicated to the current use and influence of functional analysis. There were additional seminal studies such as Carr and Durand (1985). In this seminal study, Carr and Durand hypothesized that aberrant behavior and verbal behavior could be functionally equivalent. Carr and Durand developed an assessment in which they systematically varied difficulty of demands as well as frequency of teacher attention to identify the function of aberrant behavior. This assessment was followed by treatment using differential reinforcement of functional communication.

The effect of these seminal studies on practice is apparent by the rapid adoption of the core features of the SFA in research on functional analysis published after 1994 (Jessel, Hanley, & Ghaemmaghami, 2019). These core features included (a) multiple test conditions, (b) uniform test conditions, (c) isolated test components, and (d) a play control condition (Jessel, Hanley, & Ghaemmaghami, 2016). Following the publication of Iwata et al. (1982), there have been hundreds of published studies on the effectiveness of functional analysis (Beavers et al., 2013; Hanley, 2012; Hanley et al., 2003) and the methodology has been adopted into clinical practice (Oliver et al., 2015) and has been part of US Law (i.e., Individuals with Disabilities Education Act, 1990).

As more implementation of SFAs by interventionist began to increase, practical concerns with the methodology outlined by Iwata et al. (1982/1994) arose. One concern was the time and resources required for implementation of functional analysis (Wacker et al., 1994). Furthermore, ethical and safety concerns arose regarding the reinforcement of aberrant behavior (Thomason-Sassi, Iwata, Neidert, & Roscoe, 2011). The applicability of experimental functional analysis was questioned in settings outside of highly controlled, laboratory settings (Ruiz & Kubina, 2017). These concerns and others were likely antecedents to the development of alterations of the SFA.

Variations to the Standard Functional Analysis

Variations of the SFA have been studied extensively (Beavers et al., 2013; Hanley et al., 2003). Among the most common variations are the brief FA, trial-based FA, latency-based FA, and precursor FA. More recently, research has explored alternatives to the SFA such as the interview-informed synthesized contingency analysis (IISCA; Hanley, Jin, Vanselow, & Hanratty, 2014) and preventative approaches to aberrant behavior (Ala'i-Rosales et al., 2019).

Brief Functional Analysis

The brief FA addressed one of the most commonly cited concerns regarding the SFA, its duration (Wacker et al., 1994). A single condition of an SFA, as described in the seminal study by Iwata et al. (1982/1994), required 15 min to complete. Thus, to conduct one SFA session consisting of four conditions, a interventionist must invest at least 60 min. Furthermore, numerous sessions were usually required to complete a thorough and accurate SFA in which clear differentiation was demonstrated (Wallace & Iwata, 1999). In contrast, conditions in the brief FA last 5–10 min, substantially decreasing the time required to conduct an FA (Northup et al., 1991). Another modification commonly implemented in a brief FA is decreased iterations (only one or two) of conditions before development of an intervention (Northup et al., 1991). Using this variation the entire assessment could be conducted in 90 min, which allows for the assessment to be completed in settings that could not accommodate repeated testing such as outpatient psychological services (Wacker et al., 1994).

One of the first publications of a brief FA was conducted by Northup et al. (1991). In this study, the researchers shortened the duration of test conditions and used paired control conditions that matched each test condition rather than a single play control condition. Furthermore, the authors were able to identify a functionally equivalent alternative behavior for treatment during the abbreviated assessment. Subsequent treatment used differential reinforcement of a functionally equivalent mand. Shortened condition length was further investigated by Wallace and Iwata (1999), who retrospectively analyzed results of SFAs from 46 individuals and evaluated whether shortening condition lengths would affect the ultimate conclusion of function. Results indicated the conclusion would have remained identical for all FAs if only the first 10 min had been conducted. Indeed, conventional use of SFA methodology often includes 10 min conditions rather than the 15 min sessions first described by Iwata et al. (1982/1994). Wallace and Iwata and other replications indicate the brief FA is a viable alternative to the SFA (Derby et al., 1992; Wacker et al., 1994; Wallace & Knights, 2003).

Trial-Based Functional Analysis

A second variation is the trial-based FA. Similar to the brief FA, a trial-based FA often begins each condition with a matched control (Rispoli, Ninci, Neely, & Zaini, 2014). For example, before running an attention condition in which attention is withheld until the occurrence of aberrant behavior, an attention control is conducted in which attention is continuously delivered. Test and control condition lengths are typically short (e.g., 2 min) making this another variation that is time-efficient (Ruiz & Kubina, 2017). Another unique feature of trial-based FAs is only requiring one instance of aberrant behavior during each test condition. Furthermore, trial-based FAs are conducted using discrete trials within the individual's natural environment (Rispoli et al., 2014).

Trial-based FAs also address concerns with repeatedly evoking and reinforcing aberrant behavior (Thomason-Sassi et al., 2011). It is an alternative that provides fewer exposures to conditions in which aberrant behavior will intentionally contact reinforcement (Thomason-Sassi et al., 2011). Furthermore, trial-based FAs are conducted in the individual's natural environment, as opposed to a decontextualized, analogue setting common in SFAs (Ruiz & Kubina, 2017). By conducting the assessment in the natural environment, this method ensures results are ecologically valid for the setting or context in which treatment will be conducted.

Modifications to the SFA characteristic of trial-based FAs were first described by Sigafoos and Saggers (1995). The purpose of Sigafoos and Saggers was to demonstrate an effective alternative to SFA for use within a special education classroom in which SFAs may be less feasible. In this study, FA conditions began with a 1 min test condition in which the putative reinforcer was only delivered contingent upon emission of the target aberrant response (e.g., attention was withheld until self-injury occurred). This was followed by a 1 min control condition in which the putative reinforcer was delivered noncontingently. Several replications and extensions of this methodology have shown that trial-based FAs successfully indicated a function of aberrant behavior, supporting the conclusion that the variation is a reasonable alternative to SFA (Rispoli et al., 2014). However, studies comparing the SFA and the trial-based variation indicated that results between the two methods did not always agree (Ruiz & Kubina, 2017).

Latency-Based Functional Analysis

A third variation is the latency-based FA. The latency-based FA is a method that, like the SFA, uses the four standard test conditions (i.e., attention, demand, tangible, alone) and a play control condition (Neidert, Iwata, Dempsey, & Thomason-Sassi, 2013). This methodology relies on the assumption that a shorter latency to aberrant behavior during a given condition correlates with the strength of the response (Call, Pabico, & Lomas, 2009). As soon as each condition begins, a timer is started and the latency to the first occurrence of aberrant behavior is measured (Neidert et al., 2013). After one occurrence of the aberrant behavior, the condition is ended (Neidert et al., 2013). This shares similarities to the trial-based approach, in which only one instance of aberrant behavior is necessary in each test condition.

This modification provides an alternative to the concern of repeatedly reinforcing aberrant behavior in an SFA (Thomason-Sassi et al., 2011). Latency-based FAs also provide a potential solution to another notable barrier. In some idiosyncratic scenarios, responses may not feasibly occur more than once in a given time frame (Neidert et al., 2013). Examples of such responses include vomiting, eloping, or disrobing. By using latency as a measure of response strength rather than repeated occurrences, these unique behaviors can be evaluated using FA methodology.

Call et al. (2009) created a hierarchy of demand aversiveness based upon the latency from a demand to aberrant behavior. This hierarchy was used to inform the development of a functional analysis in which latency to aberrant behavior was the unit of analysis. Test conditions included traditional attention, tangible, ignore, and toy play. However, the demand condition was unique in that it tested a *highly aversive* and *less aversive* demand situation. Thomason-Sassi et al. (2011) further evaluated the use of latency as a measure of response strength by analyzing data from existing functional analyses. Thomason-Sassi et al. found an inverse relationship between response rate and latency (i.e., high rates of aberrant behaviors corresponded to short latencies to the first instance of aberrant behavior). They found that latency data accurately predicted the outcomes of SFAs in most cases. These results indicated that latency is a viable measure of response strength for use in functional analysis. Neidert et al. (2013) then applied these findings to successfully conduct latency-based FAs of elopement for two individuals. They tested ignore, attention, and demand conditions and utilized multielement and reversal designs. They found that, while elopement was maintained by multiple variables, latency to elopement was consistently much longer during the control (toy play) condition than any other condition. Despite evidence that makes latency-based FAs theoretically compelling, Beavers et al. (2013) indicated that less than 10% of articles reviewed utilized latency as a variation to the SFA.

Precursor Functional Analysis

A fourth variation is a precursor FA. This variation relies on knowledge derived from research on response classes and hierarchical responding in which one behavior predictably precedes another (Heath & Smith, 2019). In an attempt to minimize risks associated with the SFA, the precursor FA replaces the aberrant, potentially dangerous behavior with a less dangerous behavior that has been demonstrated to reliably occur prior to the aberrant behavior. In this manipulation, the behavior is observed and analyzed to identify precursors that might be reinforced in the assessment in lieu of reinforcing dangerous behaviors.

Smith and Churchill (2002) investigated the effects of delivering reinforcement associated with severe topographies of behavior for precursory responses. They evaluated whether this would lead to the safer assessments while maintaining reliable identification of function for the more severe topography. Precursors were identified through caregiver report and direct observation. The FA was then conducted in a similar fashion to the Iwata et al. (1982/1994) but by replacing the target response with the identified precursor. Smith and Churchill compared these results to results of a traditional SFA. They found that standard models and precursor models resulted in the same conclusion, while the SFA evoked far more severe aberrant behavior than the precursor FA. This finding is consistent with other studies in which precursor FA and SFA results were compared (Heath & Smith, 2019). Further research has explored the best methods to identify reliable precursor behaviors. While some studies used indirect measures such as interviews (Smith & Churchill, 2002), others have used direct observation and conditional probability assessments (Borrero & Borrero, 2008; Langdon, Carr, & Owen-Deschryver, 2008).

Informed Synthesized Contingency Analysis (Practical Functional Assessment)

A fifth variation, and perhaps the methodology that most markedly departs from the core features of the SFA, is the IISCA (Hanley et al., 2014) or practical functional assessment (Practical Functional Assessment, 2015). This methodology begins with an open-ended interview in which information is gathered from caregivers to identify circumstances that commonly occasion the behavior of interest. This information is then used to design a single test condition that replicates the antecedent and consequent conditions hypothesized to maintain the behavior. The test is juxtaposed with a control condition that matches the test in every way except that it is devoid of the relevant reinforcing contingency (Hanley et al., 2014). Fewer replications of conditions are necessary than in more traditional methods, and condition lengths are relatively short (i.e., 5 or 10 min). Like other modifications of the SFA, the IISCA places an emphasis on efficiency. However, the IISCA presents a unique departure from the SFA in several ways.

First, as indicated in the title, a hallmark of IISCA is the use of an open-ended interview to design the conditions. This, in turn, informs treatment once the assessment is complete. Treatment based on an IISCA is typically in the form of an omnibus functional communication response such as "my way" (Coffey et al., 2019). While an open-ended interview is the approach that was originally used by Iwata et al. (1982/1994) to inform their assessment, this style of interview has largely been replaced by closed-ended methods (Hanley, 2012). Use of the open-ended interview process allows the interventionist to avoid the pitfalls associated with other indirect measures that are notoriously unreliable and lead to narrow hypotheses of generic functions (Hanley, 2012). Likewise, it avoids reliance on descriptive analyses with similar drawbacks (Hanley, 2012). The open-ended interview allows the interventionist to capture nuances that might not be captured by testing isolated attention, escape, and tangible conditions. This results in an assessment that is highly flexible and individualized.

Second, the IISCA uses a single test condition rather than multiple conditions. The single condition is markedly distinct from those in other FA methodologies in that it synthesizes all hypothesized contingencies into one test condition (e.g., escape to attention). This synthesis is intended to more closely align with natural contexts identified in the interview process. Such a personalized test condition is a notable departure from the uniform test conditions of the SFA. While the SFA tests isolated test contingencies, the control condition in the SFA is a synthesis of all of the possible reinforcers with access provided noncontingently. In the IISCA, the synthesized test condition is compared to a control condition that matches the test condition. This means the only reinforcers provided noncontingently in the control condition are those hypothesized to maintain aberrant behavior and also evaluated in the test condition.

Another unique feature of the IISCA is the broad response class that is reinforced during the test condition. Rather than providing the relevant reinforcer for a specific response of concern, the IISCA test condition includes delivery of reinforcement for engagement in any behaviors that have been reported to frequently co-occur or precede the behavior of interest. Like the precursor FA, this makes the IISCA a safer alternative to the standard model. It also improves efficiency because interventionists do not have to continue to run multiple conditions when a specific target response does not occur. That is, the IISCA is more likely to evoke behavior in the response class and is therefore less likely to lead to tests in which the behavior cannot be evaluated because of nonoccurrence.

Despite being a relatively recent addition to the FA literature, the IISCA has a growing literature base (Coffey et al., 2019). Importantly, the research on the IISCA has emphasized the subsequent treatment effects of the analysis. Results of studies using a treatment informed from an IISCA have demonstrated highly effective treatments (Coffey et al., 2019). Coffey et al. (2019) reported that all the studies reviewed using IISCA-informed treatment resulted in at least a 90% reduction in aberrant behavior and half of the studies reported a 100% reduction.

Preventative and Progressive Model

The final variation discussed in this chapter represents a progression from current conventions with respect to aberrant behavior. It has recently been proposed that interventionists should focus efforts on the prevention of aberrant behaviors (Ala'i-Rosales et al., 2019). One preventative strategy is called the "Big Four" which represents a progressive approach to aberrant behavior. If aberrant behaviors can be precluded from becoming part of an individual's repertoire through early intervention, fewer resources will be needed in treatment. Extensive research on FAs has demonstrated that aberrant behaviors are more likely to occur in one or a combination of four conditions (i.e., attention, escape, tangible, or automatic). This makes it possible to preemptively treat individuals at risk for developing aberrant behaviors by developing repertoires that permit individuals to safely navigate these conditions. While the Big Four is a theoretical model, it builds upon and is informed by decades of empirical literature.

One premise is that aberrant behaviors are often reinforced by a combination of the four standard categories (synthesized) and that they should be preemptively treated as such. Ala'i-Rosales et al. (2019) proposed that research in SFA can directly inform treatment of aberrant behavior of at-risk individuals before aberrant behaviors arise. This research informed the conceptualization of four focus areas of skills to teach all at-risk children at an early age. These may be summarized as (a) communicating wants and needs, (b) gaining attention, (c) independent leisure skills, and (d) tolerating adversity. These skills, when taught, permit individuals to safely and socially appropriately navigate their environments in ways that continue contact reinforcement and build repertoires (i.e., behavioral cusps).

Furthermore, Ala'i-Rosales et al. (2019) discussed that there may be other variables that occasion aberrant behavior that are not encompassed by the conditions typically addressed in the SFA. These include control as a function (also described by Bowman, Fisher, Thompson, & Piazza, 1997) and antecedent control (i.e., respondent behavior). Although, not described by Ala'i-Rosales and colleagues, another component of a progressive approach to aberrant behavior is conducting in-the-moment assessment of function as opposed to an SFA or modified FA. In-the-moment assessment of function consists of the interventionist observing and assessing the variables occurring in the present environment (e.g., behavior, antecedent, consequence, nonverbal behavior, attention) and considering all previous, similar occurrences (e.g., past antecedents, past consequences, sleep behavior, medical issues). This allows an interventionist to determine the function of the behavior and "on the fly" to enhance and modify intervention as needed in a structured, yet flexible manner (Leaf et al., 2016). Finally, if aberrant behavior is already being displayed, then it would be still beneficial to teach all of the functions to the learner.

Other Functional Analysis Methodologies

It is important to note that other, less commonly implemented modifications to the SFA as well as combinations of methods and experimental designs have been developed and evaluated (Hanley et al., 2003). For example, one method derived from the early analyses by Carr et al. (1976, 1980) is an antecedent-only FA, in which relevant evocative contexts are simulated without reinforcement of aberrant behavior. Despite the importance of this method to the formulation of SFA methodology, Hanley et al. (2003) found that only 20% of published studies on functional analysis followed an antecedent-only approach. Another example is the extended FA in which conditions can last hours to capture low-frequency, high-magnitude behavior (Dixon et al., 2012). Furthermore, the experimental design used in FAs has not been historically constrained to multielement designs, although this design is the most common (Hanley et al., 2003). Other designs have included the pairwise and reversal designs (Hanley et al., 2003).

Future Research

While FA is one of the most researched topics within behavior analysis (Matson & Williams, 2014), several topics within the FA methodology and literature require further investigation. These include testing functions outside of the standard four functions (i.e., attention, escape, tangible, and automatic), further analysis of synthesized contingencies, the role of respondent behavior in functional analysis, in-the-moment assessment of function, and the role of choice in assessing aberrant behavior.

Explore Additional Sources of Control

Research examining functions of behavior originated with investigation of SIB and was solidified by Carr (1977) in a paper describing the four hypothesized maintaining variables (i.e., attention, tangible, escape, automatic reinforcement). Since then, research has shown that these hypothesized functions can also maintain other response topographies beyond self-injury (Beavers et al., 2013). These four functions of behavior are often conceived as fitting broadly into the categories of positive or negative reinforcement and encompassing all other nuanced forms of reinforcement. However, there could be additional functions (e.g., control or antecedent control as in the case with respondent behavior) that are the cause of aberrant behavior. The limited research on these functions does not provide interventionists with methods to properly treat aberrant behavior, and as such more research is needed.

Continue Examining Synthesized Contingencies

Second, further analysis of synthesized contingencies could help guide interventionists in selecting the most appropriate and effective method for implementing FAs. There has been an increase in the research demonstrating that the IISCA (practical functional assessment) can identify the conditions under which aberrant behavior occurs and, more importantly, decrease the probability of aberrant behavior (Jessel et al., 2016). However, there have been several professionals who have raised doubts about the use of the IISCA (e.g., Fisher, Greer, Romani, Zangrillo, & Owen, 2016). As such, more research is needed on the IISCA across topographies of aberrant behavior, research groups, and various participant demographics.

Explore the Use of Concurrent Operant Assessments

Third, some research has avoided evoking aberrant behavior altogether. In one example, a functional relation between an aberrant behavior and its maintaining variables is demonstrated by making reinforcement available for engaging in an alternative response and demonstrating that responses are reallocated from aberrant behavior to the alternative response when a putative reinforcer is made available for that response (Finkel, Derby, Weber, & McLaughlin, 2003). This is done using a concurrent operant assessment in which participants are provided the choice between two and more concurrently available schedules of reinforcement (e.g., Hood, Rodriguez, Luczynski, & Fisher, 2019). For example, a room may be divided in half with each half of the room associated with a specific schedule or reinforcement (Harding et al., 1999). When predictable and orderly patterns of response allocation result, experimental control is demonstrated. Large gaps exist in the limited body of research using concurrent operant assessments to identify functions of aberrant behavior. These studies lack replication, and there has not been a comparison of results of such concurrent operant assessments with results of SFA. The reliability and validity of this method, though theoretically compelling, requires further replication and exploration.

Expand FA Methodology to More Populations

Fourth, while research on FA has shown that the methods are widely applicable to different topographies of behaviors, it has yet to be shown how broadly applicable FA methods are across a variety of populations. Research has largely focused on individuals diagnosed with developmental disabilities (Dixon et al., 2012). Some have indicated that research with typically developing populations would expand our knowledge base of the efficacy of FA (Dixon et al., 2012). Applying FA methodology with populations with mental health concerns (e.g., obsessive-compulsive disorder, depression) or behavior concerns common to typically developing youth or an aging population can further demonstrate the generality of this practice (Beavers et al., 2013).

Examine Barriers Impeding FAs in Practice

Fifth, the SFA has been described as a flexible methodology that is adaptable and can be individualized for clinical practice (Hanley, 2012; Iwata & Dozier, 2008). Despite the extensive research on modifications to the SFA to increase efficiency and practical implementation, a survey of the Board Certified Behavior Analysts (BCBAs) found that over half (63%) of behavior analysts reported they "never or almost never" conduct functional analyses (Oliver et al., 2015). Given that FA has a large evidence base supporting its use, research should emphasize identification and removal of barriers to implementation in practice.

Oliver et al. (2015) suggested that one barrier to implementation of FAs in practice might be lack of training for interventionists. They suggested that graduate studies should go beyond teaching FA philosophy and logic and should focus on teaching the implementation of FA. Some research has focused on training teachers how to implement FAs (Rispoli et al., 2015; Rispoli, Neely, Healy, & Gregori, 2016). However, little research has focused on training BCBAs, who are most likely to be responsible for conducting FAs. This research and training should teach BCBAs how to implement all functional analysis procedures (e.g., SFA, IISCA, and in-the-moment assessment of function). Investigation might also be conducted on the scope of FA training that is currently offered or required in graduate programs and ensure that all graduate students have knowledge and can implement the continuum of FAs.

Experimentally Evaluate the Big Four

Finally, future researchers should empirically evaluate the "Big Four" proposed by Ala'i-Rosales et al. (2019). Although Ala'i-Rosales and colleagues laid out a compelling case for a preventative approach to aberrant behavior, it has yet to be evaluated empirically. As such, future researchers should evaluate if proactively establishing the repertoires required to successfully navigate the four conditions within SFAs prevents the onset of aberrant behavior. One potential method to evaluate the "Big Four" could be similar to evaluations of Preschool Life Skills (for a detailed description, see Hanley, Heal, Tiger, & Ingvarsson, 2007), which was designed as a preventative approach to prevent the development of aberrant behavior for young children. The methods employed in this research could also be informed by recent evaluations of preventative approaches within the laboratory (e.g., Fahmie, Macaskill, Kazemi, & Elmer, 2018). Regardless of the methods, it is clear our field is beginning to progress from a reactive to a preventative approach to aberrant behavior, and our research should continue to reflect that progression.

Conclusion

FA has a robust literature base with some modifications and progressions only beginning to be explored (e.g., IISCA, the Big Four). Continued progression and cutting-edge research can provide conceptually systematic and technological methodologies to expand our breadth and depth of knowledge without sacrificing rigor.

Researchers continue to explore relationships between aberrant behaviors and their contextual variables through variations and modifications to the SFA. Some variations have been extensively studied and provide a myriad of methodologies from which a professional might choose when conducting an FA as part of an FBA or in isolation. Many of these variations have permitted researchers to effectively address concerns regarding efficiency, safety, and ethics.

The SFA and FA variations also contribute to the rich history of research and focus on function-based treatment of aberrant behavior as discussed by Skinner and promulgated by researchers such as Lovaas, Carr, and Iwata. The emphasis on function-based treatment continues to be impactful in remediating the detrimental effects aberrant behaviors have on the lives of individuals and their families. Continued use of FA as an evidence-based practice to safely and effectively reduce aberrant behaviors remains paramount, especially given findings of idiosyncrasies and nuances of maintaining variables of aberrant behaviors for individuals with disabilities. Interventionists who provide intervention for individuals who engage in aberrant behaviors can fulfill their obligation to improve lives by reliance on extant literature regarding FA.

References

Ala'i-Rosales, S., Cihon, J. H., Currier, T. D. R., Ferguson, J. L., Leaf, J. B., Leaf, R., … Weinkauf, S. M. (2019). The big four: Functional assessment research informs preventative behavior analysis. *Behavior Analysis in Practice, 12*(1), 222–234. https://doi.org/10.1007/s40617-018-00291-9

Baer, D. M., Wolf, M. M., & Risley, T. R. (1968). Some current dimensions of applied behavior analysis. *Journal of Applied Behavior Analysis, 1*(1), 91–97. https://doi.org/10.1901/jaba.1968.1-91

Beavers, G. A., Iwata, B. A., & Lerman, D. C. (2013). Thirty years of research on the functional analysis of problem behavior: Thirty years of functional analysis. *Journal of Applied Behavior Analysis, 46*(1), 1–21. https://doi.org/10.1002/jaba.30

Bijou, S. W., Peterson, R. F., & Ault, M. H. (1968). A method to integrate descriptive and experimental field studies at the level of data and empirical concepts. *Journal of Applied Behavior Analysis, 1*(2), 175–191. https://doi.org/10.1901/jaba.1968.1-175

Blacher, J., & McIntyre, L. L. (2006). Syndrome specificity and behavioural disorders in young adults with intellectual disability: Cultural differences in family impact. *Journal of Intellectual Disability Research, 50*(3), 184–198. https://doi.org/10.1111/j.1365-2788.2005.00768.x

Borrero, C. S., & Borrero, J. C. (2008). Descriptive and experimental analyses of potential precursors to problem behavior. *Journal of Applied Behavior Analysis, 41*, 83–96. https://doi.org/10.1901/jaba.2008.41-83

Bowman, L. G., Fisher, W. W., Thompson, R. H., & Piazza, C. C. (1997). On the relation of mands and the function of destructive behavior. *Journal of Applied Behavior Analysis, 30*(2), 251–265. https://doi.org/10.1901/jaba.1997.30-251

Call, N. A., Pabico, R. S., & Lomas, J. E. (2009). Use of latency to problem behavior to evaluate demands for inclusion in functional analyses. *Journal of Applied Behavior Analysis, 42*(3), 723–728. https://doi.org/10.1901/jaba.2009.42-723

Carr, E. G. (1977). The motivation of self-injurious behavior: A review of some hypotheses. *Psychological Bulletin, 84*(4), 800–816. https://doi.org/10.1037/0033-2909.84.4.800

Carr, E. G., & Durand, V. M. (1985). Reducing behavior problems through functional communication training. *Journal of Applied Behavior Analysis, 18*(2), 111–126. https://doi.org/10.1901/jaba.1985.18-111

Carr, E. G., Newsom, C. D., & Binkoff, J. A. (1976). Stimulus control of self-destructive behavior in a psychotic child. *Journal of Abnormal Child Psychology, 4*(2), 139–153. https://doi.org/10.1007/BF00916518

Carr, E. G., Newsom, C. D., & Binkoff, J. A. (1980). Escape as a factor in the aggressive behavior of two retarded children. *Journal of Applied Behavior Analysis, 13*(1), 101–117. https://doi.org/10.1901/jaba.1980.13-101

Coffey, A., Shawler, L., Jessel, J., Nye, M., Bain, T., & Dorsey, M. (2019). Interview-informed synthesized contingency analysis (IISCA): Novel interpretations and future directions. *Behavior Analysis in Practice*. https://doi.org/10.1007/s40617-019-00348-3

Derby, K. M., Wacker, D. P., Sasso, G., Steege, M., Northup, J., Cigrand, K., & Asmus, J. (1992). Brief functional assessment techniques to evaluate aberrant behavior in an outpatient setting: A summary of 79 cases. *Journal of Applied Behavior Analysis, 25*(3), 713–721. https://doi.org/10.1901/jaba.1992.25-713

Dixon, D. R., Vogel, T., & Tarbox, J. (2012). History of functional analysis and applied behavior analysis.

Dominick, K. C., Davis, N. O., Lainhart, J., Tager-Flusberg, H., & Folstein, S. (2007). Atypical behaviors in children with autism and children with a history of language impairment. *Research in Developmental Disabilities, 28*(2), 145–162. https://doi.org/10.1016/j.ridd.2006.02.003

Durand, V. M., & Crimmins, D. B. (1988). The motivation assessment scale. In *Dictionary of behavioral assessment techniques* (pp. 309–310).

Fahmie, T. A., Macaskill, A. C., Kazemi, E., & Elmer, U. C. (2018). Prevention of the development of problem behavior: A laboratory model. *Journal of Applied Behavior Analysis, 51*(1), 25–39. https://doi.org/10.1002/jaba.426

Ferster, C. B. (1964). Reinforcement and punishment in the control of human behavior by social agencies. In *Experiments in behaviour therapy* (pp. 189–206). New York, NY: Macmillan Co..

Finkel, A. S., Derby, K. M., Weber, K. P., & McLaughlin, T. F. (2003). Use of choice to identify Behavioral function following an inconclusive brief functional analysis. *Journal of Positive Behavior Interventions, 5*(2), 112–121. https://doi.org/10.1177/10983007030050020601

Fisher, W. W., Greer, B. D., Romani, P. W., Zangrillo, A. N., & Owen, T. M. (2016). Comparisons of synthesized and individual reinforcement contingencies during functional analysis. *Journal of Applied Behavior Analysis, 49*(3), 596–616. https://doi.org/10.1002/jaba.314

Hall, S. S. (2005). Comparing descriptive, experimental and informant-based assessments of problem behaviors. *Research in Developmental Disabilities, 26*(6), 514–526. https://doi.org/10.1016/j.ridd.2004.11.004

Hanley, G. P. (2012). Functional assessment of problem behavior: Dispelling myths, overcoming implementation obstacles, and developing new Lore. *Behavior Analysis in Practice, 5*(1), 54–72. https://doi.org/10.1007/BF03391818

Hanley, G. P., Heal, N. A., Tiger, J. H., & Ingvarsson, E. T. (2007). Evaluation of a class wide teaching program for developing preschool life skills. *Journal of Applied Behavior Analysis, 40*(2), 277–300. https://doi.org/10.1901/jaba.2007.57-06

Hanley, G. P., Iwata, B. A., & McCord, B. E. (2003). Functional analysis of problem behavior: A review. *Journal of Applied Behavior Analysis, 36*(2), 147–185. https://doi.org/10.1901/jaba.2003.36-147

Hanley, G. P., Jin, C. S., Vanselow, N. R., & Hanratty, L. A. (2014). Producing meaningful improvements in problem behavior of children with autism via synthesized analyses and treatments: Severe problem behavior. *Journal of Applied Behavior Analysis, 47*(1), 16–36. https://doi.org/10.1002/jaba.106

Harding, J. W., Wacker, D. P., Berg, W. K., Cooper, L. J., Asmus, J., Mlela, K., & Muller, J. (1999). An analysis of choice making in the assessment of young children with severe behavior problems. *Journal of Applied Behavior Analysis, 32*(1), 63–82. https://doi.org/10.1901/jaba.1999.32-63

Heath, H., & Smith, R. G. (2019). Precursor behavior and functional analysis: A brief review. *Journal of Applied Behavior Analysis, 52*(3), 804–810. https://doi.org/10.1002/jaba.571

Hood, S. A., Rodriguez, N. M., Luczynski, K. C., & Fisher, W. W. (2019). Evaluating the effects of physical reactions on aggression via concurrent-operant analyses. *Journal of Applied Behavior Analysis, 52*(3), 642–651. https://doi.org/10.1002/jaba.555

Individuals with Disabilities Education Act of 1990, 20 U.S.C. § 1400 *et seq.* (1990) (amended 1997, 2004).

Iwata, B. A., & Bailey, J. S. (1974). Reward versus cost token systems: An analysis of the effects on students and teacher. *Journal of Applied Behavior Analysis, 7*(4), 567–576. https://doi.org/10.1901/jaba.1974.7-567

Iwata, B. A., DeLeon, I. G., & Roscoe, E. M. (2013). Reliability and validity of the functional analysis screening tool: Functional analysis screening tool. *Journal of Applied Behavior Analysis, 46*(1), 271–284. https://doi.org/10.1002/jaba.31

Iwata, B. A., Dorsey, M. F., Slifer, K. J., Bauman, K. E., & Richman, G. S. (1982/1994). Toward a functional analysis of self-injury. *Journal of Applied Behavior Analysis, 27*(2), 197–209. https://doi.org/10.1901/jaba.1994.27-197

Iwata, B. A., & Dozier, C. L. (2008). Clinical application of functional analysis methodology. *Behavior Analysis in Practice, 1*(1), 3–9. https://doi.org/10.1007/BF03391714

Jessel, J., Hanley, G. P., & Ghaemmaghami, M. (2016). Interview-informed synthesized contingency analyses: Thirty replications and reanalysis. *Journal of Applied Behavior Analysis, 49*(3), 576–595. https://doi.org/10.1002/jaba.316

Jessel, J., Hanley, G. P., & Ghaemmaghami, M. (2019). On the standardization of the functional analysis. *Behavior Analysis in Practice.* https://doi.org/10.1007/s40617-019-00366-1

Kaiser, A. P., & Roberts, M. Y. (2011). Advances in early communication and language intervention. *Journal of Early Intervention, 33*, 298–309. https://doi.org/10.1177/1053815111429968

Kanne, S. M., & Mazurek, M. O. (2011). Aggression in children and adolescents with ASD: Prevalence and risk factors. *Journal of Autism and Developmental Disorders, 41*(7), 926–937. https://doi.org/10.1007/s10803-010-1118-4

Langdon, N., Carr, E., & Owen-DeSchryver, J. (2008). Functional analysis of precursors for serious problem behavior and related intervention. *Behavior Modification, 32*, 804–827. https://doi.org/10.1177/0145445508317943

Leaf, J. B., Leaf, R., McEachin, J., Taubman, M., Ala'i-Rosales, S., Ross, R. K., … Weiss, M. J. (2016). Applied Behavior Analysis is a Science and, Therefore, Progressive. Journal of Autism and Developmental Disorders, 46(2), 720–731. https://doi.org/10.1007/s10803-015-2591-6.

Lovaas, O. I., Freitag, G., Gold, V. J., & Kassorla, I. C. (1965). Experimental studies in childhood schizophrenia: Analysis of self-destructive behavior. *Journal of Experimental Child Psychology, 2*(1), 67–84. https://doi.org/10.1016/0022-0965(65)90016-0

Lovaas, O. I., & Simmons, J. Q. (1969). Manipulation of self-destruction in three retarded children. *Journal of Applied Behavior Analysis, 2*(3), 143–157. https://doi.org/10.1901/jaba.1969.2-143

Mace, F. C., & West, B. J. (1986). Analysis of demand conditions associated with reluctant speech. *Journal of Behavior Therapy and Experimental Psychiatry, 17*, 285–294.

Matson, J. L., & Vollmer, T. R. (1995). *User's guide: Questions about behavioral function (QABF).* Baton Rouge, LA: Scientific Publishers.

Matson, J. L., & Williams, L. W. (2014). Functional assessment of challenging behavior. *Current Developmental Disorders Reports, 1*(2), 58–66. https://doi.org/10.1007/s40474-013-0006-y

Nagai, Y., Hinobayashi, T., & Kanazawa, T. (2017). Influence of early social-communication Behaviors on maladaptive behaviors in children with autism spectrum disorders and intellectual disability. *Journal of Special Education Research, 6*(1), 1–9. https://doi.org/10.6033/specialeducation.6.1

Neidert, P. L., Iwata, B. A., Dempsey, C. M., & Thomason-Sassi, J. L. (2013). Latency of response during the functional analysis of elopement: Elopement. *Journal of Applied Behavior Analysis, 46*(1), 312–316. https://doi.org/10.1002/jaba.11

Northup, J., Wacker, D., Sasso, G., Steege, M., Cigrand, K., Cook, J., & DeRaad, A. (1991). A brief functional analysis of aggressive and alternative behavior in an outclinic setting. *Journal of Applied Behavior Analysis, 24*(3), 509–522. https://doi.org/10.1901/jaba.1991.24-509

Oliver, A. C., Pratt, L. A., & Normand, M. P. (2015). A survey of functional behavior assessment methods used by behavior analysts in practice: Functional behavior assessment survey. *Journal of Applied Behavior Analysis, 48*(4), 817–829. https://doi.org/10.1002/jaba.256

Pelios, L., Morren, J., Tesch, D., & Axelrod, S. (1999). The impact of functional analysis methodology on treatment choice for self-injurious and aggressive behavior. *Journal of Applied Behavior Analysis, 32*(2), 185–195. https://doi.org/10.1901/jaba.1999.32-185

Practical Functional Assessment. (2015). Retrieved December 2, 2019, from Practical Functional Assessment website: https://practicalfunctionalassessment.com/

Reichow, B. (2012). Overview of meta-analyses on early intensive Behavioral intervention for young children with autism spectrum disorders. *Journal of Autism and Developmental Disorders, 42*(4), 512–520. https://doi.org/10.1007/s10803-011-1218-9

Richards, C., Oliver, C., Nelson, L., & Moss, J. (2012). Self-injurious behaviour in individuals with autism spectrum disorder and intellectual disability: Self-injury in autism spectrum disorder. *Journal of Intellectual Disability Research, 56*(5), 476–489. https://doi.org/10.1111/j.1365-2788.2012.01537.x

Rispoli, M., Burke, M. D., Hatton, H., Ninci, J., Zaini, S., & Sanchez, L. (2015). Training head start teachers to conduct trial-based functional analysis of challenging behavior. *Journal of Positive Behavior Interventions, 17*(4), 235–244. https://doi.org/10.1177/1098300715577428

Rispoli, M., Neely, L., Healy, O., & Gregori, E. (2016). Training public school special educators to implement two functional analysis models. *Journal of Behavioral Education, 25*(3), 249–274. https://doi.org/10.1007/s10864-016-9247-2

Rispoli, M., Ninci, J., Neely, L., & Zaini, S. (2014). A systematic review of trial-based functional analysis of challenging behavior. *Journal of Developmental and Physical Disabilities, 26*(3), 271–283.

Ruiz, S., & Kubina, R. M. (2017). Impact of trial-based functional analysis on challenging behavior and training: A review of the literature. *Behavior Analysis: Research and Practice, 17*(4), 347–356. https://doi.org/10.1037/bar0000079

Sidman, M., & Center, D. B. (1991). Coercion and its fallout. *Behavioral Disorders, 16*(4), 315–317. https://doi.org/10.1177/019874299101600403

Sigafoos, J., & Saggers, E. (1995). A discrete-trial approach to the functional analysis of aggressive behaviour in two boys with autism. *Australia and New Zealand Journal of Developmental Disabilities, 20*(4), 287–297.

Skinner, B. F. (1953). *Science and human behavior.* New York, NY: Free Press.

Skinner, B. F.(1957). Verbal behavior (B. F. Skinner reprint series; edited by Julie S. Vargas book 1) (pp. 28-29). B. F. Skinner foundation. Kindle edition.

Sloman, K. N. (2010). Research trends in descriptive analysis. *The Behavior Analyst Today, 11*(1), 20. https://doi.org/10.1037/h0100686

Smith, R. G., & Churchill, R. M. (2002). Identification of environmental determinants of behavior disorders through functional analysis of precursor behaviors. *Journal of Applied Behavior Analysis, 35,* 125–136. https://doi.org/10.1901/jaba.2002.35-125

Soke, G. N., Rosenberg, S. A., Hamman, R. F., Fingerlin, T., Robinson, C., Carpenter, L., … DiGuiseppi, C. (2016). Brief report: Prevalence of self-injurious Behaviors among children with autism Spectrum disorder—A population-based study. *Journal of Autism and Developmental Disorders, 46*(11), 3607–3614. https://doi.org/10.1007/s10803-016-2879-1

Thomason-Sassi, J. L., Iwata, B. A., Neidert, P. L., & Roscoe, E. M. (2011). Response latency as an index of response strength during functional analyses of problem behavior. *Journal of Applied Behavior Analysis, 44*(1), 51–67. https://doi.org/10.1901/jaba.2011.44-51

Thompson, R. H., & Iwata, B. A. (2007). A comparison of outcomes from descriptive and functional analyses of problem behavior. *Journal of Applied Behavior Analysis, 40*(2), 333–338. https://doi.org/10.1901/jaba.2007.56-06

Vollmer, T. R., Iwata, B. A., Zarcone, J. R., Smith, R. G., & Mazaleski, J. L. (1993). The role of attention in the treatment of attention-maintained self-injurious behavior: Noncontingent reinforcement and differential reinforcement of other behavior. *Journal of Applied Behavior Analysis, 26*(1), 9–21. https://doi.org/10.1901/jaba.1993.26-9

Vollmer, T. R., Marcus, B. A., Ringdahl, J. E., & Roane, H. S. (1995). Progressing from brief assessments to extended experimental analyses in the evaluation of aberrant behavior. *Journal of Applied Behavior Analysis, 28*(4), 561–576. https://doi.org/10.1901/jaba.1995.28-561

Wacker, D. P., Berg, W. K., Cooper, L. J., Derby, K. M., Steege, M. W., Northup, J., & Sasso, G. (1994). The impact of functional analysis methodology on outpatient clinic services. *Journal of Applied Behavior Analysis, 27*(2), 405–407. https://doi.org/10.1901/jaba.1994.27-405

Wallace, M. D., & Iwata, B. A. (1999). Effects of session duration on functional analysis outcomes. *Journal of Applied Behavior Analysis, 32*(2), 175–183. https://doi.org/10.1901/jaba.1999.32-175

Wallace, M. D., & Knights, D. J. (2003). An evaluation of a brief functional analysis format within a vocational setting. *Journal of Applied Behavior Analysis, 36*(1), 125–128. https://doi.org/10.1901/jaba.2003.36-125

Zaja, R. H., Moore, L., Van Ingen, D. J., & Rojahn, J. (2011). Psychometric comparison of the functional assessment instruments QABF, FACT and FAST for self-injurious, stereotypic and aggressive/destructive behaviour. *Journal of Applied Research in Intellectual Disabilities, 24*(1), 18–28. https://doi.org/10.1111/j.1468-3148.2010.00569.x

Zeilberger, J., Sampen, S. E., & Sloane, H. N. (1968). Modification of a child's problem behaviors in the home with the mother as therapist. *Journal of Applied Behavior Analysis, 1*(1), 47–53. https://doi.org/10.1901/jaba.1968.1-47

Chapter 11
Scaling Methods in Functional Assessment

Paige A. Weir, Johnny L. Matson, and Joshua Montrenes

Introduction

Several types of function-based assessments exist to identify the maintaining factors of challenging behaviors exhibited by individuals with developmental disabilities. Challenging behaviors often include self-injurious behavior (SIB), aggression, stereotypic or repetitive behavior, and property destruction. Identifying the primary function of challenging behavior helps inform treatment planning that minimizes maladaptive behavior and increases prosocial behavior. In order to develop an effective treatment plan, environmental variables that inform the clinician of the antecedents and the reinforcing consequences or functions of the behavior must be identified.

Iwata, Dorsey, Slifer, Bauman, and Richman (1982, 1994) originally proposed a behavioral assessment model using operant methodology to identify functional relationships between environmental events and self-injurious behavior of individuals with developmental disabilities. A substantial amount of literature has replicated, expanded, and discussed this assessment model (Beavers, Iwata, & Lerman, 2013). Today, functional assessment (FA) represents an overarching category of behavioral methods used to identify environmental variables that cause behaviors to occur and become reinforced (Ellingson, Miltenberger, & Long, 1999; Iwata, Vollmer, & Zarcone, 1990; Lennox & Miltenberger, 1989).

Several FA methods are used to develop effective treatment for challenging behaviors (Ellingson et al., 1999). Ellingson et al. (1999) surveyed 36 behavioral programming agencies that specialize in treatment for individuals with developmental disabilities. The survey collected information regarding FA strategies used to inform treatment plans for the clients with challenging behaviors (e.g., indirect, direct, and functional analysis). The most common use of indirect methods were

P. A. Weir (✉) · J. L. Matson · J. Montrenes
Department of Psychology, Louisiana State University, Baton Rouge, LA, USA
e-mail: pweir1@lsu.edu

© Springer Nature Switzerland AG 2021

J. L. Matson (ed.), *Functional Assessment for Challenging Behaviors and Mental Health Disorders*, Autism and Child Psychopathology Series,
https://doi.org/10.1007/978-3-030-66270-7_11

scaling tools such as the Functional Analysis Screening Tool (FAST) (Ellingson et al., 1999). The direct method most reported among participants was the Antecedent-Behavior-Consequence (ABC) assessment. Experimental Functional Analysis (EFA) was most commonly used in natural settings. Additionally, the indirect tools (e.g., behavior checklists and rating scales) were endorsed as the easiest to use, while direct observation methods were perceived to be the most effective when identifying the function of behavior. However, when additional information was needed, EFA was perceived as the most useful method when creating effective treatment (Ellingson et al., 1999).

While this study demonstrated the pros and cons of using certain functional strategies, indirect observation assessments, direct observation assessments, and EFAs are the most used methods when conducting FAs. Each of these methods aim to identify the primary factor that maintains a challenging behavior; however, they differ in the time it takes to collect data, the ease of use, and the level of experimental manipulation involved (Ellingson et al., 1999; Iwata et al., 1994). Therefore, it is essential to note that there is not a single gold standard procedure used to conduct an FA (Sasso, Conroy, Stichter, & Fox, 2001). Fortunately, literature has produced a tiered behavioral assessment model when addressing challenging behavior.

This behavioral assessment model contains a three-tiered functional analysis paradigm, designed to help family and practitioners remediate and prevent challenging behaviors in young children (Conroy, Davis, Fox, & Brown, 2002). It was developed to not only reduce the intensity and frequency of the maladaptive behaviors, but it also provided a model for intervention to prevent the behaviors from reoccurring. The model begins by focusing on preventing challenging behaviors from occurring in a global environment (Conroy et al., 2002).

The first tier starts with an assessment of challenging behaviors that occur in global or group settings (e.g., classrooms). Intervention then takes place through the manipulation of variables in the group environment; variables may include physical environment changes and/or instructional adjustments. The second tier then targets challenging behaviors that occur in children who are unresponsive to environmental interventions of the first level and are therefore at a higher risk for developing more severe behaviors. This second tiered assessment procedure implements the use of direct observation and/or caregiver interviews in order to gain additional information about the targeted challenging behaviors. Lastly, the third tier targets children who were unresponsive to the first two tiers. This tier implements assessment and intervention that are individualized to a particular child. Some methods used to implement FA for this tier are EFA and scaling methods. Both of these methods target the challenging behavior of a child and identify specific maintaining factors while gaining detailed information regarding antecedents and reinforcing consequences (Conroy et al., 2002).

While scaling methods of FA are the primary focus of this chapter, the most common methods of FA will be briefly discussed. In addition, the benefits and limitations to choosing each method will also be mentioned. Following, popular indirect scaling methods will be discussed and reviewed in detail.

Functional Assessment Methods

As previously mentioned, direct observational methods, indirect observation methods, and EFAs are the most common techniques used to identify the function of challenging behavior (Ellingson et al., 1999). Each method aims to gain topographic information of the target behavior and identify environmental variables that may be motivating and reinforcing the individual's maladaptive behavior. The following section briefly describes each method, instances in which the methods may or may not be appropriate, and common tools that are used to implement each technique.

Direct Observation

Direct FA methods use observations of environmental events, such as variables/factors that are present before and after a behavior occurs. These direct observations allow the opportunity to identify behavioral patterns and relationships between the antecedent, the behavior, and the reinforcing consequences. Common strategies used to collect observational data are ABC descriptive/checklists and/or scatter plots (Ellingson et al., 1999; Iwata, Pace, et al., 1994; Miltenberger, 1997). Direct observation methods focus on challenging behavior as it occurs in a natural environment. The collection of observational data can be beneficial as the recording takes place in a natural environment setting and adds ecological validity. Additionally, the findings better generalize to real-world scenarios, and the methods do not require information from a secondary source. While these direct methods can be advantageous, variables are not manipulated or changed in a controlled environment; therefore, the data is strictly correlational, and causation cannot be applied to determine the function of the behavior (Hall, 2005).

ABC Data

ABC descriptive data and checklists specify environmental events that occur before and after a behavior takes place. The goal of ABC data is to identify the maintaining factor or function of a behavior. While the collection of descriptive ABC data includes writing one's observations of the antecedent, behavior, and consequence, an ABC checklist is a more simplified version for a behavior that has already been observed for possible antecedents and consequences. The observer simply checks off the corresponding antecedents and consequences that take place each time the behavior occurs (Ellingson et al., 1999). Although ABC descriptive data can be time-consuming, ABC checklists allow for a simpler alternative for applied settings. Additionally, the descriptive data obtained may offer more detailed information and prove to be helpful when identifying the function of the behavior. However, it is important to note that the detail and accuracy of ABC data recorded by the observer is subjective (Joyce, 2006; Sulzer-Azaroff & Mayer, 1977).

Scatterplots

Scatterplots create a visual representation of the frequency and duration in which a challenging behavior occurs over time. The scatterplot aims to correlate behavioral events with a specific time of day. Once an interval of time is determined as the *y*-axis (e.g., 30 minutes), the observer records the frequency and duration the behavior occurs during the interval. Then, with the *x*-axis representing days of the week, the data is plotted and becomes a visual representation of the time of day behavior is most likely to occur (Ellingson et al., 1999; Touchette, MacDonald, & Langer, 1985). This method allows a clinician or provider to analyze and interpret behavior patterns from a visual display. Scatterplots can be simple to collect, leading to higher use in applied settings. However, the antecedents and consequences of a behavior can be difficult to collect when using this method, and little research examining the psychometric properties of scatterplots as an FA method exist (Bosma & Mulick, 1990; Matson & Minshawi, 2007).

Indirect Observation

Indirect FA methods rely on the responses of an informant. In order to qualify as a reliable informant, the informant must have frequent experience interacting with the individual and observing their challenging behavior. Informants may be relatives, caregivers, teachers, or staff of the individual (Ellingson et al., 1999). Common indirect methods include interviews and rating scales (Lennox & Miltenberger, 1989). While each indirect method aims to gain information about the time in which the challenging behavior occurs and antecedents and consequences related to the behavior through different methods, research surrounding the reliability and validity of indirect measures are limited and exhibit mixed findings (Ellingson et al., 1999). For example, an informant must be reliable when participating in an indirect functional assessment. However, over-reporting and under-reporting still may occur and affect the accuracy of the information obtained (Vincent Mark Durand & Crimmins, 1990). In addition, similarly to direct observation methods, providers must note that indirect measures only obtain correlational information regarding the cause and function of a behavior (Hall, 2005).

While there are several limitations that a clinician and researcher must consider when utilizing indirect methods of FA, a number of benefits exist as well. For instance, indirect methodology can be less intrusive than direct contact methods (Floyd, Phaneuf, & Wilczynski, 2005). Indirect methods do not require the behavior to be exhibited during the time of assessment as it relies on the participation of a third party that has observed the behavior in question. Additionally, indirect methods allow the informants to reflect on the entire history in which they've observed behaviors occurring (O'Neill et al., 1997). Therefore, indirect methods may capture behaviors that occur less frequently. It is also advantageous to note that some behaviors may be dangerous or unethical to evoke for a direct assessment (e.g., self-injurious behaviors); therefore, indirect methods provide an alternative strategy for the clinician to form hypotheses and identify the motivating operations of behavior (O'Neill et al., 1997). Lastly, indirect methods can be used to inform direct observation methods by identifying the primary conditions in which a behavior occurs prior to an EFA. A clinician can then use the conditions identified by the indirect measure to create an EFA that is efficient at identifying the function of a behavior (Floyd et al., 2005).

Behavioral Interviews

Interviews that aim to identify the function of behavior include questions aimed to identify variables contributing to behavior occurring. The interview questions are often answered by an informant that knows the individual and has observed the behavior being targeted. Interview questions collect information regarding the topography of the behavior, the setting(s) in which the behavior occurs, events that often take place prior to and after the behavior takes place, any prior treatment attempts, and information about potential related factors/events (Ellingson et al., 1999; Floyd et al., 2005). The most commonly used behavioral interview is the Functional Assessment Interview (FAI; O'Neill et al., 1997). The FAI is a comprehensive interview that consists of open-ended questions that target challenging behaviors and can be administered in 45–90 minutes (Cunningham & O'Neill, 2000). Behavioral interviews like the FAI are flexible and allow for additional probing when necessary. However, research that uses interview methods or studies that investigate their psychometric properties are limited (Ellingson et al., 1999; Floyd et al., 2005).

Informant-Based Rating Scales

Informant-based rating scales/measures aim to identify the function of behavior by asking a respondent to answer questions regarding a challenging behavior that takes place by using a Likert-type scale. Informant-based scales are often administered in a paper-pencil format or administered to the respondent by the clinician. The rating scales should be administered to or completed by respondents who know the individual well and have directly observed the challenging behavior being targeted (e.g., parents and teachers). When the informant completes a scaling measure, each item should be answered with the setting in which the informant has observed the challenging behavior or the setting in which the informant knows the individual best (e.g., classroom, home). The question is then answered using the respective Likert-type scale, and based on the subscales or factors for each measure, a score is quantified and a rating is calculated to help determine the function or motivating factor of the behavior.

Informant-based rating scales typically have a short administration time compared to behavioral interviews and other functional assessment methods. Rating scales are used among many professionals as they are easily administered, scored, and interpreted. Additionally, informant-based rating scales can easily be administered at regular intervals if the function of behavior needs to be monitored or if the function is suspected to have changed. Similar to behavioral interviews, scaling methods rely on third-party reports and recollection of when behavior takes place. Therefore, the potential of inaccurate reports is high and the reliability and validity of informant-based rating scales are questionable (Crawford, Brockel, Schauss, & Miltenberger, 1992; Ellingson et al., 1999; Zarcone, Rodgers, Iwata, Rourke, & Dorsey, 1991). The most commonly used scales are the Motivation Assessment Scale (MAS; Durand & Crimmins, 1988) and the Questions About Behavior Function (QABF; Matson & Vollmer, 1995).

Experimental Functional Analysis (EFA)

An EFA is a functional assessment method that includes the manipulation of antecedents and/or consequences to demonstrate the effects of these variables on a targeted challenging behavior (Ellingson et al., 1999). EFAs are conducted by a clinician or provider and require the individual to participate and evoke the targeted challenging behavior. EFAs are conducted in controlled environment settings (e.g., clinics, observation rooms, offices) or in natural environment settings where the challenging behavior typically occurs (e.g., group home, classroom, or work). The results of an EFA demonstrate a functional relationship between the antecedents and consequences surrounding a challenging behavior (Ellingson et al., 1999). However, EFAs should be used with caution, as they can create unnecessary stress for an individual, and ethical considerations should be a priority. Unfortunately, EFAs are often time-consuming (Lennox & Miltenberger, 1989), can be rigorous and complex when developed and administered (Durand & Crimmins, 1988), and are not an ideal method of assessment for infrequent challenging behavior (Ellingson et al., 1999). In contrast, EFAs can be beneficial in limiting confounding variables to best identify the primary function of a behavior and, in turn, allow for the development of a comprehensive and effective treatment plan (Iwata, Vollmer, Zarcone, & Rodgers, 1993; Lennox & Miltenberger, 1989). Lastly, an EFA can be used in the event that previous functional assessment methods have unsuccessfully informed treatment plans to reduce challenging behavior (Conroy et al., 2002).

Scaling Methods

As mentioned previously in this chapter, there is not a single gold standard procedure used to implement functional assessment (Sasso et al., 2001). However, EFAs and scaling methods are used as the most individualized functional analysis methodology of the three-tiered functional analysis paradigm. The implementation of EFAs and scaling methods target challenging behavior on the individual level. These methods identify the function(s) of challenging behavior while obtaining detailed information regarding antecedents and reinforcing consequences in the individuals environment (Conroy et al., 2002). Gaining specific information about an individual's challenging behaviors aids practitioners in creating individualized treatment plans that are more likely to be effective when implemented. In particular, scaling methods are frequently used in applied settings and are often preferred by clinicians and providers, prior to implementing an EFA. Scaling methods appeal to practitioners as they do not require the behavior to be exhibited in the moment, do not risk evoking challenging behavior using aversive environment, and can usually be administered, scored, and interpreted in an acceptable amount of time (Bodfish, 2004; Guess & Carr, 1991; O'Neill et al., 1997). Additionally, scaling methods traditionally follow a set of established psychometric rules. For instance, scaling measures set a standard in which each client's behavior can be judged. Creating a standard scaling method typically includes a normed group, scores that denote severity, and demonstrates reliability and validity to ensure consistency in measuring the targeted behavior. Also, factor analysis is often used to establish subscales. This psychometric approach has been influential in developing functional assessment measures.

Over the decades, several informant-based scaling methods have been developed, discussed in literature, and applied in clinical settings. Although there are several functional assessment scaling methods, the most studied scales are the Questions About Behavioral Function (QABF), Motivation Assessment Scale (MAS), the Functional Assessment for Multiple Causality (FACT), the Motivation Analysis Rating Scale (MARS), and the Functional Analysis Screening Tool (FAST) (Matson & Williams, 2014).

The remainder of this chapter will review popular scaling methods for identifying the function challenging behaviors exhibited by individuals with developmental disabilities. The review of each scale will include a detailed description of the measure, including its development, administration, scoring and interpretation. The most updated review of literature regarding the scale's reliability and validity and the benefits and limitations of each measure will also be discussed. The scales that are most commonly used will be reviewed first, followed by other popular measures.

Motivation Assessment Scales (MAS)

Description

One of the most clinically used and researched indirect FA scales is the Motivation Assessment Scale (Durand & Crimmins, 1988; Sigafoos, Kerr, & Roberts, 1994; Toogood & Timlin, 1996). The MAS has been clinically used to decrease challenging behaviors among individuals with developmental disabilities by identifying motivating factors that may be maintaining those behaviors (Ray-Subramanian, 2013). The MAS is an informant-based measure composed of 16 items. The items are individually rated on a seven-point Likert-type scale ranging from "0 (never)" to "6 (always)". Example items are "Does this behavior occur when you are talking to other persons in the room?" and "Does the behavior occur whenever you stop attending to the person?". The measure has four subscales, measured by four items each. Each subscale represents a function that may motivate the individual to engage in the targeted challenging behavior. The four subscales include (1) escape from aversive events, (2) gaining access to social attention, (3) gaining access to tangibles, and (4) sensory reinforcement (Boothroyd, 2001; Durand & Crimmins, 1988).

Scale Development

The MAS was originally developed to identify the motivating factor of self-injurious behavior in individuals with developmental disabilities (Durand & Crimmins, 1988). While the MAS administration manual does not give a thorough description of the scale's development (Boothroyd, 2001), the administration guide does specify that the MAS was developed over a 4-year period (Durand & Crimmins, 1988). Four subscales were created based on common functions of self-injurious behavior identified in previous literature (i.e., social attention, tangible consequences, escape from unpleasant situations, and sensory consequences). The items were derived from interviews with teachers, clinicians, and parents who had direct contact with individuals with autism and developmental disabilities. In addition, questions were added and removed to gain interrater reliability across a variety of settings (Boothroyd, 2001; Durand & Crimmins, 1988; Ray-Subramanian, 2013).

Administration

Prior to administering the MAS, the developers require a detailed description of the challenging behavior being assessed as well as the setting in which the behavior occurs. Raters should also be familiar with each item, for which an explanation of the intended meaning of each item and guidelines for rating each item are provided in the administration guide. In addition, the scale was designed to be completed by various raters such as caregivers, teachers, and service providers. However, the developers emphasize that only raters who have experienced direct contact or observation of the individual for several weeks should complete the MAS (Boothroyd, 2001; Durand & Crimmins, 1992). The MAS should be administered to an informant that has directly observed the challenging behavior and knows the individual well. The scale can be completed by paper and pencil or as an interview. While the developers did not specify an administration length of time, the administration guide states that the scale should not be administered for an entire day (Boothroyd, 2001; Durand & Crimmins, 1992).

Scoring and Interpretation

The MAS items are recorded on a scoring sheet, and the measure is scored by hand. After an informant completes all 16 items, the individual items are then transferred to a scoring grid. Total scores are obtained for each subcategory by obtaining the sum of the rating for each of the four motivations. Mean scores are then calculated by dividing each of the total subscale scores by 4. A ranking of 1, 2, 3, or 4 is given to each subscale based on the mean score of each subscale category. The ranking of "1" is assigned to the category with the highest mean, indicating the most likely motivation for the challenging behavior. The subscale with the second highest mean is assigned a ranking of "2," indicating the second most likely motivation and so on, until the ranking of "4" indicates the lowest motivation (Boothroyd, 2001; Durand & Crimmins, 1992).

When interpreting scores of the MAS, those who administer the scale should rely on the rankings of the motivation categories rather than the total subscale scores or means (Boothroyd, 2001; Durand & Crimmins, 1992). While the administration manual does not specify what is considered to be a high score, high scores suggest that the subscale's function may be maintaining the individual's problem behavior (Durand & Crimmins, 1992; Ray-Subramanian, 2013). In the event that two or more categories receive high scores, the authors recommend that the administrator revisit the behavior definition as well as the setting that is defined. Lastly, when two subscales receive equal mean scores or the difference between two mean scores are 0.5 or less, this indicates that both motivation categories may be responsible for maintaining the challenging behavior (Durand & Crimmins, 1988; Durand & Crimmins, 1992; Ray-Subramanian, 2013). Once a motivating function is identified, the results can then be used to develop an intervention to decrease the challenging behavior and reinforce replacement behaviors (Ray-Subramanian, 2013).

Reliability

The interrater reliability of the MAS was originally assessed by comparing the ratings of teachers and assistant teachers of 50 children with developmental disabilities that engaged in self-injurious behavior. Both interrater reliability and test-retest reliability were found to be high. Pearson correlations between raters ranged between 0.80 and 0.95 (Durand & Crimmins, 1992; Ray-Subramanian, 2013). The test-retest reliability after 30 days ranged from 0.89 to 0.98. The developers did not provide individual test-retest or internal consistency reliability estimates for the four motivational categories or subscales (Ray-Subramanian, 2013). Therefore, some critics have argued that the MAS should be used with direct observation methods as its psychometric properties have demonstrated limitations (Duker & Sigafoos, 1998; Ray-Subramanian, 2013; Spreat & Connelly, 1996).

Although initial studies described the MAS to be psychometrically sound, additional studies have not been able to replicate similar findings. Newton and Sturmey (1991) found an interrater reliability ranging from 0.20 to 0.70 and poor internal consistency; two other studies have found similar results (Goza & Ricketts, 1993; Zarcone et al., 1991). Although the MAS was initially promising and has been considered to be unprecedented in quality, other instruments have psychometrically surpassed the scale (Belva, Hattier, & Matson, 2013).

Validity

The developers of the MAS were also the first to examine the validity of the scale. The authors compared the MAS to the results of an EFA of eight children and identified high agreement between the two measures; therefore, demonstrating results with good validity relative to analogue assessments (Durand & Crimmins, 1992). Additionally, convergent validity of the MAS compared to EFAs demonstrated a 43.8% agreement, while the agreement between the MAS and the QABF was 61.5% (Paclawskyj, Matson, Rush, Smalls, & Vollmer, 2001).

The creators of the MAS provided additional support for validity of the MAS scale. A factor analytic study conducted by Bihm, Kienlen, Ness, and Poindexter (1991) provided support for the validity of the four MAS subscales that were found by Durand and Crimmins (1992). The validity of the MAS used the teachers MAS rating to predict how individuals would behave in the administration of an EFA, and results demonstrated good validity relative to analogue assessments (Durand & Crimmins, 1992)

Questions About Behavior Function (QABF)

Description

The Questions About Behavior Function (QABF) is a 25-item indirect informant-based measure of behavioral function designed for individuals with developmental disabilities evincing challenging behaviors such as aggression and self-injury. Each item is scored by a four-point Likert-type scale representing the frequency in which the target behavior occurs in the listed setting. The response options are never, rarely, some, and often. The scale has five items that represent each of the five categories or subscales of behavioral functions. Some example questions include "engages in the behavior because he/she is in pain" and "engages in the behavior to try to get a reaction from you." The five-factor measure includes the subscale categories of attention, escape, physical, tangible, and nonsocial (Matson & Vollmer, 1995). The results of a QABF provide the clinician with information that is helpful in creating hypotheses of behavior functions to treat various challenging behaviors. The QABF is a scale that can be quickly administered and easily interpreted and includes a graph to demonstrate the primary function of the target behavior (Sturmey, 1996).

Compared to EFAs, the QABF does not require the behavior to be evinced, thus avoiding potential reinforcement of maintaining factors or the introduction/reinforcement of maladaptive behaviors (Matson & Minshawi, 2007). In addition, the measure requires less training and resources than an EFA when used in applied settings (Matson & Vollmer, 1995; Sturmey, 1995). The QABF can also be used to assess high-impact, low-frequency behaviors (Matson & Vollmer, 1995). Lastly, the QABF is helpful in aiding a clinician in the formation and implementation of functionally based treatment plans. In particular, the scale is useful for a large number of persons evincing a wide range of behavior problems (Matson & Vollmer, 1995) and for functionally based clinical research using large group designs (Applegate, Matson, & Cherry, 1999; Matson & Vollmer, 1995).

Scale Development

Studies have been conducted supporting the factor structure of the QABF, indicating statistical rationale for scale's implementation in applied settings for individuals with developmental disabilities. Matson and Vollmer (1995), the developers of the QABF, conducted an exploratory factor analysis that used a sample of 462 individuals with intellectual disability (ID), who were between the ages of 13 and 86 years old and exhibited the challenging behaviors of self-injurious behavior (SIB), aggression, or property destruction. The factor analysis results explained 74.5% of the variance and supported the following five factors including attention, escape, physical, tangible, and nonsocial functions of behavior. A replication of the factor analysis on the severity scores of the QABF included 40 younger individuals with ID who collectively evinced a total of 118 challenging behaviors (Nicholson, Konstantinidi, & Furniss, 2006). The results support the original five factors, explaining 73% of the variance. Although the QABF has been shown to identify at least one primary behavioral function in 84% of cases (Matson, Bamburg, Cherry, & Paclawskyj, 1999), some challenging behaviors are maintained by more than one function (Matson & Boisjoli, 2007; Matson & Vollmer, 1995).

Administration

The QABF can typically be administered in approximately 30 minutes. The test is administered in an interview format with a respondent who is familiar with the person being assessed and the problem behavior being examined. Although the QABF may be used for more than one behavior, each behavior should be assessed separately (Matson & Vollmer, 1995). According to the administration manual, the QABF requires the target behavior to first be operationally defined (Matson & Vollmer, 1995). Administrators must also implement inclusion criteria in order for a behavior to be scored, and exclusion criteria may be included as well. Next, the clinician should choose an informant that has known or worked with the individual for at least 6 months and is familiar with the behavior being targeted. When administering the scale, the clinician should read the instruction and explain the Likert-scale options to the informant. The items are then read verbatim to the informant, and their answer is recorded on the protocol sheet (Matson & Vollmer, 1995).

Scoring and Interpretation

When scoring the QABF, columns of each category are scored using a scoring sheet. The first column of each category includes items that are endorsed in each category. The first column represents frequency and receives an endorsement score of "1" for each item listened that was originally endorsed and "0" if it was not endorsed. The number of items that were endorsed for each category, the number (0–5), should be circled for the corresponding category on the scoring graph. The second column represents severity, and each item should be scored for each function category by recording the number endorsed for each item (i.e., 0, never; 1, rarely; 2, some; and 3, often). The summed total for each of the subscale's five items (0–5) is then circled on the scoring graph for each function category. Lastly, the frequency scores and severity scores should be connected by two separate lines. The lines represent a visualization of the frequency and severity of the target behavior among different functional categories (Matson & Vollmer, 1995).

When interpreting the QABF, a clear function is considered an endorsement when there is a frequency score of four or five and no other categories are significantly endorsed. Two or more elevated scales may indicate multiple functions of a behavior and should be interpreted accordingly. The most elevated should be considered the most prominent function, though categories that have equal scores are a possibility. The developers suggest that an EFA should be conducive if the function of a behavior is unclear or the individual's response to the treatment is unsatisfactory (Matson & Vollmer, 1995).

Reliability

The QABF has been found to have good test-retest reliability and interrater reliability (Belva et al., 2013; Leader & Mannion, 2016; Matson et al., 1999; Paclawskyj, Matson, Rush, Smalls, & Vollmer, 2000). The test-retest reliability and interrater reliability were examined with a sample of 57 individuals with profound or severe ID (Paclawskyj et al., 2000). Test-retest reliability was high and the interrater reliability was good, with total agreement ranging from 69.67% to 95.65% (Paclawskyj et al., 2000).

Interrater agreement was explored in a sample of 40 individuals with autism and/or severe learning difficulties and severe challenging behavior. Results demonstrated an interrater agreement of a primary function for 59% of the QABFs, for which interrater agreement was higher for higher-rate behaviors and lower for lower-rate behaviors. Internal consistency was also found to be high (Nicholson et al., 2006).

Validity

The QABF demonstrated predictive validity when targeting challenging behaviors of 398 individuals with developmental disabilities. SIB, aggression, and stereotypy significantly decreased after the implementation of a QABF-informed treatment plan. The treatment outcomes of individuals who were administered the QABF were more successful than the treatment outcomes of controls receiving standard treatments not based on functional analysis. These findings validated the utility of the QABF, particularly in applied settings (Matson et al., 1999).

When the convergent validity of the QABF compared to EFA was examined, the QABF and EFA method showed a 56.3% agreement on the maintaining function, slightly higher than when the MAS was compared to EFA. Additionally, the MAS and QABF were in agreement 61% of the time, which was an improvement when the scales were compared with the EFA method (Paclawskyj et al., 2001). Overall, the QABF has been shown to have good stability and validity, therefore establishing the measure as a sound scale to assess for behavioral functions (Leader & Mannion, 2016).

Functional Assessment for Multiple Causality (FACT)

Description

When determining the function of a challenging behavior using indirect measures, difficulties arise when multiple maintaining functions are identified. According to research, nearly half of challenging behaviors are found to serve multiple functions (Matson & Boisjoli, 2007). Although a challenging behavior may have multiple maintaining factors, identifying the primary function aids in developing an effective treatment plan. The FACT is an informant-based measure that is used to identify the most prominent function of a challenging behavior. The FACT is a 35-item forced-choice measure and requires the informant to choose between two possible functions in order to identify the primary behavioral function (Matson et al., 2003). According to a study that examined the usefulness of a force-choice measure when a clear behavioral function is not identified, the developers suggest that the FACT be administered as a second-tier scaling method for behavioral function (Matson et al., 2003).

Scale Development

The FACT was developed to identify a hierarchy of functions for challenging behavior exhibited by individuals with developmental disabilities. This forced-choice scale was designed for informants to choose between two behavioral function options that vary in validity, so a clear behavioral function may be identified. The frequency in which option is endorsed indicates the overall validity of each function. Therefore, the frequency that an option is endorsed may indicate the treatment priority of the corresponding behavioral function (Matson et al., 2003).

The original version of the scale included 50 items with three possible response options for each. However, due to the length of time it took to administer the measure, some items were eliminated, resulting in a 35-item informant-based measure with only two response options. An example item from the FACT is "engages in the behavior more (A) to get attention or more (S) as a form of "self-stimulation" or (N) neither?" A factor analysis was conducted with a five factor model. The five factors found were consistent with the five subscales of the QABF: tangible, physical, attention, escape, and nonsocial (Matson et al., 2003).

Administration

According to the administration manual, the FACT should be administered by a clinician or practitioner that has a degree in a mental health-related field. Similar to previously mentioned scales, the FACT should be administered to an informant that has known the individual at least 6 months. The interviewer then reads each item verbatim, providing explanations as needed. The chosen option for each item is then recorded (Matson et al., 2003).

Scoring and Interpretation

Once all the informant's answers are recorded, the clinician then uses the scoring sheet to total the number of each letter. Next, the frequency of each letter is graphed under the corresponding behavioral function subscale. Each behavioral function subscale then has a corresponding column that indicates the percentage in which the function was endorsed. The higher the percentage, the higher the likelihood that the corresponding subscale is the maintaining factor of the target behavior (Matson et al., 2003).

Reliability

A sample of 297 individuals with intellectual disabilities ranging from 9 to 85 years was utilized to test the internal consistency across subscales, which was found to be excellent. Another study was then conducted with 197 individuals with intellectual disabilities, ranging from 16 to 85 years of age, and all subscales demonstrated good to high estimates of reliability (0.88–0.92). However, more research is needed to determine the validity and general utility of the FACT (Matson et al., 2003).

Validity

While the FACT demonstrated good to excellent reliability and may not be first used or identify behavioral functions, more research to demonstrate the validity and utility of the FACT are warranted (Matson et al., 2003). In addition, although the scale may be useful in determining which behavior could be initially targeted in a treatment plan, limited research supports the utility of the scale (Belva et al., 2013).

Motivation Analysis Rating Scale (MARS)

Description

The Motivation Analysis Rating Scale (MARS) was one of the first functional assessment scales developed. The scale consists of six items that are rated on a five-point Likert-type frequency scale ranging from "0, never" to "4, almost always." An example item is "when ___ behavior occurs, the resident is trying to acquire something he wants" (Sturmey, 1994; Wieseler, Hanson, Chamberlain, & Thompson, 1985). While this scale was one of the first to be created, research examining its psychometric properties is limited; therefore, limiting the utility of the measure (Belva et al., 2013; Sturmey, 1994).

Development

The MARS was originally developed to identify the function of challenging behaviors, particularly stereotypy and self-injury. The informants were originally intended to be staff members of a residential hospital for individuals with developmental disabilities, explaining the terminology of the word "resident" that refers to the individual exhibiting the target behavior (Wieseler et al., 1985).

Administration

The MARS can be administered to an informant that knows the individual and is familiar with the challenging behavior being targeted. Each item is read to or read by the informant, and a frequency option is then selected. When considering the best frequency option to select, the measure provides percentage equivalents for some options of the Likert-type scale such as (1) almost never, (2) less than 50% of the time, (3) more than 50% of the time, and (4) almost always (Wieseler et al., 1985).

Scoring and Interpretation

When scoring the MARS, three pairs of items are summed to represent each of the following subscales: positive environmental consequences, task escape/avoidance, and self-stimulation. The subscale with the highest summed frequency endorsement is considered the primary function of the behavior (Wieseler et al., 1985).

Reliability

The psychometrics of the scale were assessed using 96 staff ratings of 60 individuals with self-injurious behavior and stereotypy. The interrater reliability was evaluated only for the primary motivating function and was found to be in the lower range of 73% (Wieseler et al., 1985). Some limitations regarding the psychometrics of this scale exist. For instance, it is important to note that no data was originally published regarding the internal consistency of the measure (Sturmey, 1994). Additionally, questions arise regarding the length of the measure as six-item functional assessments are rare unless the short scales have a strong empirical foundation. Additionally, no reliability data has been provided for individual items or scale totals (Belva et al., 2013; Sturmey, 1994).

Validity

Compared to the lower reliability, the validity of the scale was found to be high (95%). The validity of the scale was assessed by comparing the MARS with ABC data of the target behavior. Only the validity of the primary motivating function was evaluated and was found to be 95% between the two methods (Wieseler et al., 1985). The high validity in relation to the lower reliability is unusual and raises questions among critics. The difference may be explained by the method in which validity was determined as the validity was calculated only when two raters agreed on the same primary function, therefore potentially biasing and inflating the validity results (Sturmey, 1994).

Functional Assessment Screening Tool (FAST)

Description

The Functional Analysis Screening Tool (FAST) is a 16-item informant-based functional assessment measure and is used to determine factors that may be influencing challenging behaviors. The scale is recommended to be used as a screener for behavioral functionality prior to conducting a comprehensive functional analysis. There are four behavioral functions that the scale measures including social (attention/preferred items), social (escape from tasks/activities), automatic (sensory stimulation), and automatic (pain attenuation). An example item is "Does the problem behavior occur even when no one is nearby or watching?", and each item is rated "Yes", "No," or "N/A" (Iwata, DeLeon, & Roscoe, 2013). In an effort to improve the consistency of verbal report, the developers derived items from environmental conditions identified in FA research (Beavers et al., 2013; Iwata et al., 2013).

Scale Development

The FAST was originally developed to identify the contingencies that maintain challenging behavior in individuals with developmental disabilities, particularly the contingencies of positive and negative reinforcement. At the beginning of development, the scale consisted of 32 items. However, during continued development, the scale was modified through an evaluation process. For a 4-month trial period, members of a psychology department at a residential facility for individuals with disabilities used the scale during their assessment of challenging behaviors. Written feedback regarding scale content and format were obtained, and revisions were made to modify wording and formatting of items. The scale was then administered to informants of 182 individuals where reliability scores were calculated and items were reworded or deleted based on the lowest reliabilities. The final scale consisted of 16 items (Iwata et al., 2013).

Administration

The developers recommend the scale be administered to several staff or caregivers that interact with the individual. Prior to administering the items to the informant, the Informant-Client Relationship and Problem Behavior Information sections should be completed. These sections collect qualitative information such as how long the informant has known the individual and the capacity in which they interact with them. When administering the items, each item is read verbatim to the informant, and an answer is selected (Iwata et al., 2013).

Scoring and Interpretation

After the administration of the FAST is complete, items that have a rating of "Yes" are circled in the scoring summary. Then, the number of items that are circled are transferred to the respective subscale column totals. The totals for each subscale are then summed, and the subscale that has the highest number of "Yes" answers is determined as the primary reinforcing factor of the target behavior (Iwata et al., 2013; Leader & Mannion, 2016).

Reliability

Data was collected for 151 individuals with ID or ASD that exhibited challenging behavior. Overall interrater agreement for the FAST was found to be moderate at best (71.5%), similar to that of previously studied instruments (Beavers et al., 2013; Iwata et al., 2013). Agreement for individual items ranged from 53.3% to 84.5%, and outcome agreement in which two informants' most frequent "Yes" answers were for the same function was 64.8%.

Validity

The FAST was also compared to the outcomes of 59 EFAs to test validity and utility of the measure. The FAST was found to predict that the highest rate of problem behavior was only 63.8% of the time, which was inadequate when compared to the results of EFAs (Iwata et al., 2013; Wieseler et al., 1985). Overall, research of the FAST's psychometric properties is limited, and more literature regarding the utility of this measure is still needed (Beavers et al., 2013; Iwata et al., 2013; Matson & Williams, 2014).

Conclusion

In summary, extensive literature has established that challenging behavior is maintained by environmental conditions, and FA is an essential technique in identifying environmental contingencies (Bachman, 1972; Carr, 1977; Iwata et al., 1982; Iwata, Dorsey, Slifer, Bauman, & Richman, 1994). Several methods have been used to assess for maintaining functions of behavior. In particular, direct and indirect methods are valuable in identifying functions of behavior and informing individualized treatment plans (Leader & Mannion, 2016; Matson et al., 2003). Traditionally, FA has relied primarily on the direct method of EFA to identify maintaining factors of behavior, requiring the replication of environmental conditions to identify those causal variables. Although EFA is supported by substantial research and determined to be the most effective in identifying the function of challenging behaviors (Iwata, Dorsey, et al., 1994; Leader & Mannion, 2016; Northup et al., 1991), EFAs can be time-consuming and resource intensive, therefore making its use impractical in many applied settings (Matson et al., 2003). In order to address these limitations, indirect scaling methods are often used to supplement or at times replace EFAs (Beavers et al., 2013). Scaling methods provide a supplemental alternative that is often more realistic for applied settings and can be used prior to EFAs and inform the development of individual treatment plans (Paclawskyj et al., 2000). While the use of indirect scaling methods are often brief and economical and can often be more sensitive to certain behaviors than direct methods, the function of some behaviors can still remain undetermined, in which case a comprehensive EFA may be warranted to inform an effective treatment plan (Matson et al., 2003; Paclawskyj et al., 2001).

References

Applegate, H., Matson, J. L., & Cherry, K. E. (1999). An evaluation of functional variables affecting severe problem behaviors in adults with mental retardation by using the questions about behavioral function scale (QABF). *Research in Developmental Disabilities, 20*, 229–237.

Bachman, J. A. (1972). Self-injurious behavior: A behavioral analysis. *Journal of Abnormal Psychology, 80*, 211–224.

Beavers, G. A., Iwata, B. A., & Lerman, D. C. (2013). Thirty years of research on the functional analysis of problem behavior. *Journal of Applied Behavior Analysis, 46*, 1–21.

Belva, B. C., Hattier, M. A., & Matson, J. L. (2013). Assessment of problem behavior. In D. D. Reed, F. D. DiGennaro Reed, & J. K. Luiselli (Eds.), *Handbook of crisis intervention and developmental disabilities* (pp. 123–146). New York, NY: Springer.

Bihm, E. M., Kienlen, T. L., Ness, M. E., & Poindexter, A. R. (1991). Factor structure of the motivation assessment scale for persons with mental retardation. *Psychological Reports, 68*(Suppl 3), 1235–1238.

Bodfish, J. W. (2004). Treating the core features of autism: Are we there yet? *Mental Retardation and Developmental Disabilities Research Reviews, 10*(4), 318–326.

Boothroyd, R. A. (2001). Review of the motivation assessment scale. In *The fourteenth mental measurements yearbook*. Lincoln, NE: Buros Institute of Mental Measurements.

Bosma, A., & Mulick, J. A. (1990). Brief report: Ecobehavioral assessment using transparent scatter plots. *Behavioral Interventions, 5*(2), 137–140.

Carr, E. G. (1977). The motivation of self-injurious behavior: A review of some hypotheses. *Psychological Bulletin, 84*(4), 800–816.

Conroy, M. A., Davis, C. A., Fox, J. J., & Brown, W. H. (2002). Functional assessment of behavior and effective supports for young children with challenging behaviors. *Assessment for Effective Intervention, 27*(4), 35–47.

Crawford, J., Brockel, B., Schauss, S., & Miltenberger, R. G. (1992). A comparison of methods for the functional assessment of stereotypic behavior. *Journal of the Association for Persons with Severe Handicaps, 17*(2), 77–86.

Cunningham, E., & O'Neill, R. E. (2000). Comparison of results of functional assessment and analysis methods with young children with autism. *Education and Training in Mental Retardation and Developmental Disabilities, 35*(4), 406–414.

Duker, P. C., & Sigafoos, J. (1998). The motivation assessment scale: Reliability and construct validity across three topographies of behavior. *Research in Developmental Disabilities, 19*(2), 131–141.

Durand, V., & Crimmins, D. (1992). *The motivation assessment scale (MAS) administration guide*. Topeka, KS: Monaco.

Durand, V. M., & Crimmins, D. B. (1988). Identifying the variables maintaining self-injurious behavior. *Journal of Autism and Developmental Disorders, 18*(1), 99–117.

Durand, V. M., & Crimmins, D. B. (1990). Chapter 3: Assessment. In *Severe behavior problems: A functional communication training approach*. New York, NY: Guilford Press.

Ellingson, S. A., Miltenberger, R. G., & Long, E. S. (1999). A survey of the use of functional assessment procedures in agencies serving individuals with developmental disabilities. *Behavioral Interventions, 14*(4), 187–198.

Floyd, R. G., Phaneuf, R. L., & Wilczynski, S. M. (2005). Measurement properties of indirect assessment methods for functional behavioral assessment: A review of research. *School Psychology Review, 34*(1), 58–73.

Goza, A. B., & Ricketts, R. W. (1993). The motivation assessment scale: Analysis of inter-rater and test-retest reliability. In *Annual meeting of the Association for Behavior Analysis-International*. Chicago, IL.

Guess, D., & Carr, E. (1991). Emergence and maintenance of stereotypy and self-injury. *American Journal of Mental Retardation, 96*(3), 299–319.

Hall, S. S. (2005). Comparing descriptive, experimental and informant-based assessments of problem behaviors. *Research in Developmental Disabilities, 26*(6), 514–526.

Iwata, B. A., DeLeon, I. G., & Roscoe, E. M. (2013). Reliability and validity of the functional analysis screening tool. *Journal of Applied Behavior Analysis, 46*(1), 271–284.

Iwata, B. A., Dorsey, M. F., Slifer, K. J., Bauman, K. E., & Richman, G. S. (1982). Toward a functional analysis of self-injury. *Analysis and Intervention in Developmental Disabilities, 2*(1), 3–20.

Iwata, B. A., Dorsey, M. F., Slifer, K. J., Bauman, K. E., & Richman, G. S. (1994). Toward a functional analysis of self-injury. *Journal of Applied Behavior Analysis, 27*(2), 197–209.

Iwata, B. A., Pace, G. M., Dorsey, M. F., Zarcone, J. R., Vollmer, T. R., Smith, R. G., ... Willis, K. D. (1994). The functions of self-injurious behavior: An experimental-epidemiological analysis. *Journal of Applied Behavior Analysis, 27*(2), 215–240.

Iwata, B. A., Vollmer, T. R., & Zarcone, J. R. (1990). The experimental (functional) analysis of behavior disorders: Methodology, applications, and limitations. In *Perspectives on the use of nonaversive and aversive interventions for persons with developmental disabilities* (pp. 301–330). Sycamore, IL: Sycamore Publishing Company.

Iwata, B. A., Vollmer, T. R., Zarcone, J. R., & Rodgers, T. A. (1993). Treatment classification and selection based on behavioral function. In R. Van Houten & S. Axelrod (Eds.), *Behavior analysis and treatment* (pp. 101–125). Boston, MA: Springer.

Joyce, T. (2006). Functional analysis and challenging behaviour. *Psychiatry, 5*(9), 312–315.

Leader, G., & Mannion, A. (2016). Challenging behaviors. In J. L. Matson (Ed.), *Handbook of assessment and diagnosis of autism spectrum disorder* (pp. 209–232). Cham, Switzerland: Springer International Publishing.

Lennox, D. B., & Miltenberger, R. G. (1989). Conducting a functional assessment of problem behavior in applied settings. *Research and Practice for Persons with Severe Disabilities, 14*(4), 304–311.

Matson, J. L., Bamburg, J. W., Cherry, K. E., & Paclawskyj, T. R. (1999). A validity study on the questions about behavioral function (QABF) scale: Predicting treatment success for self-injury, aggression, and stereotypies. *Research in Developmental Disabilities, 20*(2), 163–175.

Matson, J. L., & Boisjoli, J. A. (2007). Multiple versus single maintaining factors of challenging behaviours as assessed by the QABF for adults with intellectual disabilities. *Journal of Intellectual and Developmental Disability, 32*(1), 39–44.

Matson, J. L., Kuhn, D. E., Dixon, D. R., Mayville, S. B., Laud, R. B., Cooper, C. L., ... Matson, M. L. (2003). The development and factor structure of the Functional Assessment for multiple causaliTy (FACT). *Research in Developmental Disabilities, 24*(6), 485–495.

Matson, J. L., & Minshawi, N. F. (2007). Functional assessment of challenging behavior: Toward a strategy for applied settings. *Research in Developmental Disabilities, 28*(4), 353–361.

Matson, J. L., & Vollmer, T. R. (1995). *Questions about behavioral function (QABF)*. Baton Rouge, LA: Disability Consultants, LLC.

Matson, J. L., & Williams, L. W. (2014). Functional assessment of challenging behavior. *Current Developmental Disorders Reports, 1*(2), 58–66.

Miltenberger, R. G. (1997). *Behavior modification: Principles and procedures*. Pacific Grove, CA: Brooks/Cole : ITP.

Newton, J. T., & Sturmey, P. (1991). The motivation assessment scale: Inter-rater reliability and internal consistency in a British sample. *Journal of Intellectual Disability Research, 35*(5), 472–474.

Nicholson, J., Konstantinidi, E., & Furniss, F. (2006). On some psychometric properties of the questions about behavioral function (QABF) scale. *Research in Developmental Disabilities, 27*(3), 337–352.

Northup, J., Wacker, D., Sasso, G., Steege, M., Cigrand, K., Cook, J., & DeRaad, A. (1991). A brief functional analysis of aggressive and alternative behavior in an out clinic setting. *Journal of Applied Behavior Analysis, 24*(3), 509–522.

O'Neill, R. E., Horner, R. H., Albin, R. W., Sprague, J. R., Storey, K., & Newton, J. S. (1997). *Functional assessment and program development for problem behavior: A practical handbook*. New York, NY: Cole Publishing.

Paclawskyj, T. R., Matson, J. L., Rush, K. S., Smalls, Y., & Vollmer, T. R. (2000). Questions about behavioral function (QABF): A behavioral checklist for functional assessment of aberrant behavior. *Research in Developmental Disabilities, 21*(3), 223–229.

Paclawskyj, T. R., Matson, J. L., Rush, K. S., Smalls, Y., & Vollmer, T. R. (2001). Assessment of the convergent validity of the Questions About Behavioral Function scale with analogue functional analysis and the Motivation Assessment Scale. *Journal of Intellectual Disability Research, 45*(Pt 6), 484–494.

Ray-Subramanian, C. (2013). Motivation assessment scale. In *Encyclopedia of autism spectrum disorders*. New York, NY: Springer.

Sasso, G. M., Conroy, M. A., Stichter, J. P., & Fox, J. J. (2001). Slowing down the bandwagon: The misapplication of functional assessment for students with emotional or behavioral disorders. *Behavioral Disorders, 26*(4), 282.

Sigafoos, J., Kerr, M., & Roberts, D. (1994). Interrater reliability of the motivation assessment scale: Failure to replicate with aggressive behavior. *Research in Developmental Disabilities, 15*(5), 333–342.

Spreat, S., & Connelly, L. (1996). Reliability analysis of the motivation assessment scale. *American Journal of Mental Retardation, 100*(5), 528–532.

Sturmey, P. (1994). Assessing the functions of aberrant behaviors: A review of psychometric instruments. *Journal of Autism and Developmental Disorders, 24*(3), 293–304.

Sturmey, P. (1995). Analog baselines: A critical review of the methodology. *Research in Developmental Disabilities, 16*(4), 269–284.

Sturmey, P. (1996). *Functional analysis in clinical psychology*. New York, NY: Wiley.

Sulzer-Azaroff, B., & Mayer, G. R. (1977). *Applying behavior-analysis procedures with children and youth*. New York, NY: Holt, Rinehart, Winston.

Toogood, S., & Timlin, K. (1996). The functional assessment of challenging behaviour: A comparison of informant-based, experimental and descriptive methods. *Journal of Applied Research in Intellectual Disabilities, 9*(3), 206–222.

Touchette, P. E., MacDonald, R. F., & Langer, S. N. (1985). A scatter plot for identifying stimulus control of problem behavior. *Journal of Applied Behavior Analysis, 18*(4), 343–351.

Wieseler, N. A., Hanson, R. H., Chamberlain, T. P., & Thompson, T. (1985). Functional taxonomy of stereotypic and self-injurious behavior. *Mental Retardation, 23*(5), 230.

Zarcone, J. R., Rodgers, T. A., Iwata, B. A., Rourke, D. A., & Dorsey, M. F. (1991). Reliability analysis of the motivation assessment scale: A failure to replicate. *Research in Developmental Disabilities, 12*(4), 349–360.

Part III
Treatment

Chapter 12
Function-Based Treatments for Severe Problem Behavior

Sarah K. Slocum and Nathan A. Call

Overview

As described in previous chapters, best practices for behavioral interventions begin by isolating the reason for (i.e., the function of) a particular problem behavior using a functional behavioral assessment (Hagopian, Dozier, Rooker, & Jones, 2013). Although there are a wide range of functional assessment methodologies, the gold-standard approach is an experimental or functional analysis (Iwata, Dorsey, Slifer, Bauman, & Richman, 1982). The existing evidence strongly indicates that behavioral treatments selected based upon the results of an assessment are more effective than those that are not (Heyvaert, Saenen, Campbell, Maes, & Onghena, 2014; Ingram, Lewis-Palmer, & Sugai, 2005). Function-based treatments have been demonstrated to be effective for individuals who are typically developing (Gardner, Spencer, Boelter, Dubard, & Jennett, 2012; Grandy & Peck, 1997; Woods et al., 2001) as well as those diagnosed with dementia (Baker, Hanley, & Mathews, 2006), traumatic brain injuries (Dixon et al., 2004), schizophrenia (Wilder, Masuda, O'Connor, & Baham, 2012), among other diagnoses. These approaches have even been applied successfully to nonhuman animal populations (Dorey, Rosales-Ruiz, Smith, & Lovelace, 2009; Feuerbacher & Wynne, 2016; Hall, Protopopova, & Wynne, 2015; Martin, Bloomsmith, Kelley, Marr, & Maple, 2011; Morris & Slocum, 2019). Although function-based interventions have been implemented with individuals from a wide range of populations, the vast majority of research evaluating the use of functional assessments and function-based treatments has been conducted

S. K. Slocum (✉) · N. A. Call
Severe Behavior Department, Marcus Autism Center, Atlanta, GA, USA

Division of Autism & Related Disorders, Department of Pediatrics, Emory University School of Medicine, Atlanta, GA, USA
e-mail: sarah.slocum.freeman@choa.org

© Springer Nature Switzerland AG 2021
J. L. Matson (ed.), *Functional Assessment for Challenging Behaviors and Mental Health Disorders*, Autism and Child Psychopathology Series,
https://doi.org/10.1007/978-3-030-66270-7_12

with individuals with intellectual or development disabilities (IDD; Beavers, Iwata, & Lerman, 2013).

Individuals with IDD have likely become the primary recipients of behavioral interventions for several reasons: First, problem behavior is more prevalent among individuals with IDD than their neurotypical peers (Emerson, 2001). As a result, they are in greater need for interventions to address problem behavior. Second, the reinforcers used in the assessment and treatment process have historically been under the control of interventionists of individuals with IDD to a greater degree than for those working with other populations. That is, typically developing individuals may have control over these variables themselves; the stimuli that function as reinforcers for typically developing individuals may be more difficult to manipulate (e.g., one's paycheck).

Finally, there has been a societal shift more broadly towards the inclusion of individuals with IDD with their typically developing peers, with the most recent data indicating a decrease in individuals with IDD residing in institutions from almost 200,000 in 1967 to 33,000 in 2009 (National Council on Disability, 2009). Subsequently, legislation (e.g., Individuals with Disabilities Education Act, 2004) and the formation of organizations that represent their interests (e.g., Autism Speaks) have raised even greater awareness of the treatment needs of the IDD population. This shift has likely produced an increase in both clinical services for and research with those with IDD. More individuals are receiving treatment for problem behavior because of insurance mandates for behavior analytic services (Johnson, Danis, & Hafner-Eaton, 2014). Furthermore, the focus on individuals with IDD such as autism spectrum disorder (ASD) in the research literature has been driven in part by an increase in research funding related to treatments for these individuals (Singh, Illes, Lazzeroni, & Hallmayer, 2009). As a result of all of these factors, the focus of the current chapter on individuals with IDD will mirror the emphasis of research on function-based treatments with this population.

Topography Versus Function

Prior to the advent of formal assessment methods for identifying the function of a targeted problem behavior, behavioral interventions were often selected based on the physical presentation or *topography* of the problem behavior in question. Clearly, the topography of problem behavior is an important factor when it comes to treatment. For example, it is necessary to have a clear operational definition of the problem behavior to measure and observe changes during the treatment process. The topography also plays a role in selecting the appropriate setting and implementing safety measures. For example, clinicians may need to include specific items in treatment sessions when pica is the topography of the targeted problem behavior. Studies of behavioral treatments of pica have used rooms baited with items that resemble the inedible items that the individual regularly ingests when engaging in pica, but that are safe to consume (Piazza, Hanley, & Fisher, 1996). In contrast, treating elopement requires a space from which an individual can run or wander safely while the interventionist is still able to monitor and retrieve the individual (Piazza et al., 1997). However, although the topography of the problem behavior plays a role in the treatment process, research shows that selecting treatments based on topography is less likely to result in positive outcomes compared to those that are function-based (Heyvaert et al., 2014).

When based upon topography rather than function, treatment strategies must rely upon arbitrarily selected interventions rather than functional reinforcers, a treatment approach dubbed "behavior modification" by Mace (1994). These interventions have the potential to be successful, but they typically require a trial-and-error approach that is generally inconsistently effective. That is, an interventionist may be able to develop an effective behavior modification strategy if he or she is able to identify powerful arbitrary reinforcers or to select the functional reinforcer through chance. However, sufficiently powerful reinforcers do not always exist nor can they always be identified on the first attempt. As a result, several unsuccessful treatments may be attempted before an effective one can be identified. Perhaps even more problematic, such trial-and-error approaches to treatment selection sometimes lead to deploying counter-therapeutic interventions. For example, an interventionist without the benefit of a functional assessment may select time-out as an intervention to treat escape-maintained problem behavior. Such time-out procedures often involve moving an individual away from a situation contingent on a targeted problem behavior. Thus, rather than being an effective treatment, it is likely to instead function as a reinforcer for escape-maintained problem behavior by removing the individual from an aversive situation. As a result, arbitrarily selecting time-out has the potential to exacerbate rather than ameliorate problem behavior of this type. The fact that arbitrarily selected interventions are not matched to the function therefore increases the likelihood that punishment may be necessary to produce clinically significant reductions in problem behavior.

Punishment-based treatments for problem behavior were not uncommon in the period leading up to the development of functional assessment methods (Birnbrauer, 1968; Corte, Wolf, & Locke, 1971; Sajwaj, Libet, & Agras, 1974; Tanner & Zeiler, 1975). Punishment procedures, including the application of electric shock (Birnbrauer, 1968), aromatic ammonia (Tanner & Zeiler, 1975), restraint (Favell, McGimsey, & Jones, 1978), exercise or work (Luce, Delquadri, & Hall, 1980), and the oral administration of lemon juice (Sajwaj et al., 1974), have all been employed in the past as a means of reducing problem behavior. Although these punishers are all capable of producing intended reductions in problem behavior, the ethics of applying an aversive stimulus to individuals with IDD is at best considered debatable and is generally considered unacceptable except under dire circumstances (Behavior Analyst Certification Board, 2014; Vollmer et al., 2011). Yet, when the function of a problem behavior is unknown, punishment may be the only treatment capable of producing a clinically significant improvement because no arbitrary reinforcers are more powerful than the functional one(s). For example, Corte et al. (1971) compared reinforcement and punishment strategies to treat self-injurious behavior with four subjects. Punishment was more effective than the reinforcement-based interventions, likely because the authors did not first identify the function of self-injurious behavior. There is some evidence that the formalization of functional assessment methodology has corresponded with a reduction in the use of punishment-based treatments for problem behavior (Pelios, Morren, Tesch, & Axelrod, 1999).

Extinction

In a seminal paper, Carr (1977) reviewed several studies that employed a behavior modification approach and suggested the inconsistent findings regarding treatment effectiveness may be due to misunderstanding the variables that maintain problem behavior. Rather, he suggested that the most parsimonious explanation for the etiology of problem behavior such as self-injurious behavior is that it is maintained by a contingency of reinforcement. As such, the most straightforward function-based treatment is to disrupt that contingency, a procedure referred to as *extinction*. Implementing extinction typically involves the discontinuation of the reinforcer(s) maintaining a behavior (Iwata, Pace, Cowdery, & Miltenberger, 1994). Because extinction is defined in terms of the relationship between the behavior and the consequence that maintains it, the procedure for implementing extinction differs significantly depending on the function of the problem behavior.

Extinction of problem behavior maintained by socially mediated positive reinforcers (e.g., attention or tangible items) consists of preventing the delivery of the relevant positive reinforcer when problem behavior occurs (e.g., Mazaleski, Iwata, Vollmer, Zarcone, & Smith, 1993). For example, consider disruptive behavior such as throwing academic materials in a classroom setting. It is possible this behavior is maintained by adult attention, and in that case, extinction would consist of ignoring or otherwise not attending to the student when disruptive behavior occurs. It is also possible this behavior is maintained by access to a preferred item in the classroom such as a soothing toy or snack. In this case, extinction would consist of not allowing the student access to the preferred items when disruptive behavior occurs. Of course, these exact procedures may not be feasible (i.e., a teacher may not be able to allow the individual to disrupt an entire classroom or destroy expensive equipment while ignoring problem behavior), but these forms of extinction can effectively reduce problem behavior if they are matched to its function and can be implemented.

Extinction of problem behavior maintained by socially mediated negative reinforcers (e.g., demands or social interaction) differs substantially from extinction of problem behavior maintained by positive reinforcement. For this class of behavior, extinction involves the continuation of the condition that evoked the problem behavior (e.g., Iwata, Pace, Kalsher, Cowdery, & Cataldo, 1990). In other words, escape from or discontinuation of the aversive situation is prevented. Consider the above example of a student engaging in disruptive behavior in a classroom. It is also possible this behavior is maintained by the teacher sending the student to the principal's office, a form of escape from the class and any aversive tasks or stimuli. In this case, extinction would consist of requiring the student to remain in the academic setting even if disruptive behavior occurs. As outlined above, these exact procedures may not be feasible (i.e., a teacher may not be able to follow through with a demand to complete a math problem if the student throws the academic materials across the room), but these forms of extinction can effectively reduce problem behavior if they are matched to its function and can be implemented.

For problem behavior maintained by automatic reinforcement, extinction can be challenging to implement because the person implementing the intervention generally does not have control over the functional reinforcer. In fact, a lack of control over the functional reinforcer is viewed as the main reason automatically reinforced problem behavior is more difficult to treat than problem behavior maintained by social reinforcers (Vollmer, Peters, & Slocum, 2015). However, the principles of extinction remain the same. Research has found that in some cases it is possible to conduct assessments to identify the source of automatic reinforcement maintaining a targeted problem behavior, such as the specific form of sensory stimulation it produces (e.g., Kennedy & Souza, 1995; Moore, Fisher, & Pennington, 2004). When the specific maintaining reinforcer produced by the problem behavior can be identified, it is sometimes possible to control it. When such is the case, problem behavior could be placed on extinction, such as through the use of protective equipment that prevents sensory input resulting from head-banging (Rincover, 1978; Rincover, Cook, Peoples, & Packard, 1979; Rincover, Newsom, & Carr, 1979). Similarly, Kennedy and Souza (1995) used goggles to eliminate the physical sensation produced by eye poking, and Moore et al. (2004) evaluated the use of a helmet and splints to reduce self-injurious body hitting maintained by automatic reinforcement. In both evaluations, experimenters alternated between times in which subjects wore and did not wear protective equipment, demonstrating the protective equipment's suppressive effects on problem behavior.

Researchers have also examined the utility of response blocking as another form of extinction for problem behavior maintained by automatic reinforcement (Reid, Parsons, Phillips, & Green, 1993). Response blocking involves physically preventing an individual from contacting the source of automatic reinforcement maintaining a behavior. For example, Reid et al. (1993) blocked hand mouthing for two subjects. The experimenters blocked subjects' attempts to insert their hands into their mouths (but still allowed the individuals to move their hands, even up to their mouths), resulting in reductions in mouthing for both subjects. In addition to hand mouthing, response blocking has been used to successfully treat property destruction (Fisher, Lindauer, Alterson, & Thompson, 1998), pica (McCord, Grosser, Iwata, & Powers, 2005), and self-injurious behavior (Smith, Russo, & Le, 1999).

Response interruption and redirection (RIRD) is similar to response blocking in that the interventionist prevents problem behavior from occurring, but it includes an added component of redirecting the individual to engage in an incompatible or more appropriate behavior. For example, Ahearn, Clark, MacDonald, and Chung (2007) treated vocal stereotypy using this approach. When vocal stereotypy occurred, the authors interrupted the subject by stating his or her name and subsequently asked questions that required a vocal response. Response interruption and redirection has been effective in treating self-injurious behavior maintained by automatic reinforcement as well (Jennett, Jann, & Hagopian, 2011). Jennett et al. (2011) first conducted a competing stimulus assessment to empirically identify an activity to which they would redirect subjects who engaged in self-injurious behavior maintained by automatic reinforcement. Subjects' interaction with these competing stimuli was initially quite limited. However, after adding a prompt to engage with items appropriately, the experimenters observed a reduction in self-injurious behavior and a concomitant increase in item interaction.

The effects of extinction are not always immediate (Goh & Iwata, 1994). Rather, interventionists should be aware that extinction frequently produces a delayed or gradual reduction in problem behavior. In addition, extinction can also have some negative side effects (Lerman & Iwata, 1996; Lerman, Iwata, & Wallace, 1999; Lovaas, Freitag, Gold, & Kassorla, 1965; Piazza, Patel, Gulotta, Sevin, & Layer, 2003). For example, extinction can produce a temporary increase in problem behavior before a subsequent reduction is observed. These extinction bursts occur in about 39% of cases and can be ameliorated by the addition of reinforcement procedures (Lerman et al., 1999). Individuals experiencing extinction may also engage in emotional responding or engage in novel forms of problem behavior. This extinction induced variability has been shown to occur in about 22% of cases (Lerman et al., 1999). One commonly reported challenge to using extinction as a treatment component is that caregivers may begin implementing it but discontinue extinction when they experience an extinction burst or new and unexpected forms of problem behavior. It is imperative for caregivers to persist with extinction in these situations to avoid (a) differentially reinforcing the now more-intense topography of problem behavior and (b) reinforcing problem behavior on an intermittent schedule of reinforcement (Arkoosh et al., 2007), which has the potential to produce behavior more resistant to subsequent attempts at extinction (Bijou, 1957). Concern regarding these side effects of extinction should not necessarily dissuade interventionists from using it, as extinction is a core component of most behavioral treatments and can be highly effective while not always producing these side effects.

Several studies have shown that reinforcement-based interventions may not be effective without the inclusion of extinction (Hagopian, Fisher, Sullivan, Acquisto, & LeBlanc, 1998; Mazaleski et al., 1993). Although the long-term effects of extinction are not fully known, some research suggests that extinction may produce long-lasting improvements. For example, Fisher, Piazza, Cataldo, and Harrell (1993) found that after exposing subjects to extinction and then removing extinction, reductions in problem behavior persisted. However, interventions consisting solely of extinction are not recommended because they do not provide individuals with the opportunity to access the functional reinforcer. In many instances, access to the functional reinforcer is appropriate or even desirable. Rather, the issue is that the individual is using problem behavior to do so. Thus, differential reinforcement strategies that make access to the functional reinforcer contingent upon an appropriate alternative behavior should almost always be employed alongside extinction. Arranging for an alternative means by which an individual can access the functional reinforcer can also attenuate the side effects of extinction (Lerman et al., 1999).

Differential Reinforcement

Treatments that adopt an approach of including both extinction and ensuring an alternative means to contact the functional reinforcer are referred to as *differential reinforcement*. As with extinction, the implementation of differential reinforcement varies according to the function of the targeted problem behavior. Although there are several specific forms of differential reinforcement, two main types are most commonly used (Vollmer & Iwata, 1992): differential reinforcement of other behavior (DRO) and differential reinforcement of alternative behavior (DRA).

Differential Reinforcement as a Treatment for Problem Behavior Maintained By Social Reinforcement

Conceptually, *differential reinforcement of other behavior* (DRO) consists of reinforcing any behavior other than the targeted problem behavior. However, procedurally DRO entails delivery of the functional reinforcer following an interval in which problem behavior does not occur (Allen & Harris, 1966). Vollmer, Iwata, Zarcone, Smith, and Mazaleski (1993) successfully treated attention-maintained self-injurious behavior with three subjects using DRO. The experimenters delivered attention following intervals without problem behavior, and problem behavior did not produce attention (i.e., they included extinction). If the subjects refrained from engaging in problem behavior for the duration of that interval, then the experimenters provided the functional reinforcer. However, if problem behavior occurred, they reset the DRO interval. The DRO procedure effectively reduced the self-injurious behavior of all three subjects. DROs have also been found to be effective in treating vocal stereotypy, motor stereotypy, aggression, property destruction, and tantrums (Weston, Hodges, & Davis, 2018).

Many procedural variations of DRO interventions have appeared in the literature, including (a) basing the initial reinforcement schedule on the rate of the targeted problem behavior during baseline (e.g., Lindberg, Iwata, Kahng, & DeLeon, 1999); (b) deciding to either reset or not reset the DRO interval contingent on problem behavior (e.g., Gehrman, Wilder, Forton, & Albert, 2017); and (c) methods for gradually increasing the DRO schedule over time (e.g., Rozenblat, Brown, Brown, Reeve, & Reeve, 2009). Further, research has examined (d) the use of an *interval* DRO in which the functional reinforcer is delivered when problem behavior does not occur for the entirety of a fixed interval duration (e.g., Azrin, Basalel, Jamner, & Caputo, 1988) or an interval of varying duration (e.g., Della Rosa, Fellman, DeBiase, DeQuinzio, & Taylor, 2015); as well as (e) the use of a *momentary* DRO in which reinforcement is delivered so long as the problem behavior is not occurring at the precise moment the interval ends (Heffernan & Lyons, 2016). Each of these several variations has been used successfully. Thus, selecting the specific DRO procedure for any given application can be challenging. Fortunately, several useful guidelines on the use of DRO exist (e.g., Jessel & Ingvarsson, 2016; Vollmer & Iwata, 1992; Weston et al., 2018), so readers seeking greater depth on the use of DRO for a specific scenario are referred there.

Unlike DRO, in which any topography other than the targeted problem behavior can result in reinforcement, in *differential reinforcement of alternative behavior (DRA)*, the functional reinforcer is delivered contingent upon the individual engaging in a specified alternative behavior (Petscher, Rey, & Bailey, 2009). When using DRA, the results of a functional assessment can inform not only which reinforcer to deliver and how to implement extinction, but also the specific topography of the alternative behavior. That is, some behaviors are more appropriate alternatives for specific functional reinforcers than others. For example, compliance is often the most appropriate alternative behavior to problem behavior maintained by escape from demands (Marcus & Vollmer, 1995). Thus, when selecting an alternative behavior for use in a DRA-based treatment, it can be helpful to consider how others typically access the specific functional reinforcer in a socially appropriate manner.

One of the most common types of DRA is *functional communication training* (FCT), in which the alternative appropriate behavior consists of a communication response such as a request (Carr & Durand, 1985). Similar to DRO interventions, several factors should be considered when implementing FCT, beginning with which modality of communication to select. A variety of modalities have been used in FCT, including vocal speech (Carr & Durand, 1985), card exchange (Anderson, Barretto, McLaughlin, & McQuaid, 2016), manual sign (Falcomata, Wacker, Ringdahl, Vinquist, & Dutt, 2013), or activation of an augmentative communication device (Durand, 1999), among others. However, when selecting a specific communication response, it is important to prioritize those that are (a) already in the individual's repertoire, (b) of low response effort compared to the targeted problem behavior (Richman, Wacker, & Winborn, 2001), (c) preferred by the individual (Falcomata, Ringdahl, Christensen, & Boelter, 2010; Torelli et al., 2016; Winborn-Kemmerer, Ringdahl, Wacker, & Kitsukawa, 2009), (d) recognized by the individual's community of listeners, and (e) likely to be reinforced every time it occurs (at least initially). As with DRO, the selection of a communicative alternative behavior that addresses each of these priorities for any given application can be challenging. Fortunately, Tiger, Hanley, and Bruzek (2008) have provided a helpful tutorial.

Differential Reinforcement as a Treatment for Problem Behavior Maintained By Automatic Reinforcement

As discussed above, the treatment of problem behavior maintained by automatic reinforcement usually requires a different approach than interventions targeting problem behavior maintained by socially mediated reinforcers. Consider an individual who engages in self-injurious behavior in the form of eye poking. This behavior could serve any of several functions, including social positive reinforcement (e.g., attention), automatic positive reinforcement (e.g., visual stimulation), or automatic negative reinforcement (e.g., alleviation of the pain produced by an ocular migraine). If an individual's eye poking is attention-maintained, it may be appropriate to block eye poking while minimizing attention and deliver high-quality attention contingent on refraining from eye poking for set intervals (DRO) or the individual saying "play with me" (DRA/FCT). However, if eye poking is maintained by automatic positive reinforcement in the form of the visual stimulation it produces, then problem behavior may be reduced through the use of a DRO or DRA arrangement that includes the delivery of a competing or even more preferred source of visual stimulation, such as a toy with flickering lights. Conversely, if eye poking is maintained by automatic negative reinforcement in the form of alleviation of pain from a headache, the functional reinforcer may be outside of an interventionist's control. In such a situation, it may be necessary to augment medical interventions to address the headache with behavior modification approaches such as the delivery of a highly preferred leisure item, edible item, or attention contingent on the individual not engaging in problem behavior (DRO). Further evaluation on these types of interventions is discussed below.

Function-Based Interventions in the Absence of Extinction

Differential reinforcement is the gold-standard behavioral treatment for problem behavior (Cooper, Heron, & Heward, 2007). As described above, these procedures typically include the use of extinction to reduce the likelihood of problem behavior in the future paired with reinforcement of an appropriate alternative response. Although the superiority of this strategy over nonfunction-based ones has been empirically demonstrated, it is not always practical for interventionists to implement with high fidelity. As an example, a caregiver of a large individual with escape-maintained problem behavior may not be able to implement escape extinction using hand-over-hand guidance because the individual is physically stronger than the caregiver. Similarly, a teacher may not be able to ignore a student engaging in attention-maintained problem behavior in the form of throwing a computer towards a peer in the classroom because of the risk of injury to the peer and the cost of the resulting property damage. Thus, when developing an intervention strategy, it is necessary to consider a range of factors to arrive at an effective but also feasible function-based intervention.

When extinction is impossible or unlikely to be implemented with fidelity, manipulating various parameters of the relevant reinforcers can still produce significant improvements (Athens & Vollmer, 2010; Hoch, McComas, Thompson, & Paone, 2002; Kelley, Lerman, & Van Camp, 2002; Piazza et al., 1997). Such parameters include the quality and magnitude of the reinforcers provided contingent upon problem or appropriate behavior. Hoch et al. (2002) evaluated qualitatively different reinforcers for compliance and escape-maintained problem behavior. In their evaluation, problem behavior still produced a break from instructions (i.e., extinction was not used). However, compliance with an instruction produced a break that included access to preferred activities. This difference in the quality of reinforcement for both responses produced an increase in compliance and a reduction in problem behavior.

Athens and Vollmer (2010) conducted an experiment in which they delivered attention for both problem behavior and appropriate behavior for seven subjects. Under these initial conditions, problem behavior occurred at higher rates compared to appropriate behavior. However, when the authors manipulated the quality of attention such that high-quality attention was provided for appropriate behavior and low-quality attention was provided for problem behavior, the balance shifted such that they observed more appropriate behavior and less problem behavior. The authors found that they could also bias responding away from problem behavior and towards appropriate behavior by manipulating the magnitude of reinforcement available for each response. That is, when problem behavior produced a 10-s break from instruction, but appropriate behavior produced a 30-s break, subjects allocated more responding towards appropriate behavior than problem behavior.

It can be worthwhile to consider the benefits of manipulating other parameters of the contingency between behavior and reinforcement. These include the delay to reinforcement following appropriate or problem behavior and the effort required to produce reinforcement. With regards to the former, all else being equal, a shorter delay to reinforcement following appropriate behavior compared to problem behavior will result in more favorable outcomes (Athens & Vollmer, 2010). With respect to response effort, the effect of different schedules of reinforcement for problem behavior and appropriate behavior has been evaluated as a potential form of treatment that does not require extinction. For example, Kelley et al. (2002) found that delivering reinforcement for problem behavior on a lean intermittent schedule of reinforcement compared to delivering reinforcement for appropriate behavior every time it occurred produced more appropriate behavior and reduced problem behavior.

The degree to which an individual engages in problem or appropriate behavior that produces different consequences can be conceptualized as a concurrent operants arrangement, or choice paradigm, and modeled using the matching law (Baum, 1974; Herrnstein, 1970). Research on this model with problem behavior has demonstrated that responding towards two concurrently available choices tends to occur in proportion to the relative amount of reinforcement available for each (Borrero et al., 2010; Borrero & Vollmer, 2013). Consider an example similar to those described above in which problem behavior produces 30 s of attention, whereas appropriate behavior produces 5 min of attention (i.e., 10 times more attention for appropriate behavior). The matching law predicts that in this situation an individual who engages in attention-maintained problem behavior will be 10 times more likely to engage in appropriate behavior than problem behavior.

Antecedent Interventions

To this point, the function-based treatments discussed have been consequence-based strategies in that they manipulate what happens after problem behavior and/or an appropriate alternative behavior. However, it is also possible to produce reductions in problem behavior by changing the environment prior to its occurrence to alter the motivating operation responsible for evoking problem behavior (see Carr, Severtson, & Lepper, 2009 for a review). Common antecedent interventions include noncontingent reinforcement (NCR; Vollmer, Ringdahl, Roane, & Marcus, 1997), the use of cues or signals (Cote, Thompson, & Mckerchar, 2005; Gouboth, Wilder, & Booher, 2007; Mace, Shapiro, & Mace, 1998), the high-probability instructional sequence (Lipschultz & Wilder, 2017), and incorporating choice (Shogren, Faggella-Luby, Bae, & Wehmeyer, 2004), among others.

Noncontingent reinforcement (NCR) is an intervention that includes the delivery of the functional reinforcer, but it is not provided contingent on the occurrence of any specific behavior (Carr et al., 2009). Noncontingent reinforcement is often implemfvented alongside extinction, similar to the differential reinforcement interventions described in the previous section. Vollmer et al. (1997) began treating aggression maintained by access to leisure items by providing subjects with continuous access to those preferred items. This initial continuous access diminished the motivating operation such that there was no reason to engage in problem behavior. However, over time the experimenters incorporated longer intervals in which the items were unavailable. Slocum, Grauerholz-Fisher, Peters, and Vollmer (2018) applied the same technique with one subject who engaged in attention-maintained problem behavior, starting with continuous access to attention and gradually decreasing the amount of attention over time. Both of these studies found that continuous access to the functional reinforcer reduced or eliminated problem behavior. Although providing such dense access to the functional reinforcer may not be feasible over the long term, this type of NCR can be worthwhile for situations in which it is too dangerous to allow problem behavior to occur (e.g., when a larger student with IDD who engages in severe aggression towards peers is in the lunchroom at school).

In the examples above, NCR was provided in the form of continuous access to the functional reinforcer. However, noncontingent delivery of a functional reinforcer can also be intermittent (Van Camp, Lerman, Kelley, Contricci, & Vorndran, 2000). For example, reinforcer delivery can occur based on a fixed-time or variable-time schedule of reinforcement, but still be delivered independent of the individual's behavior. Although there is evidence that this approach can produce a reduction in problem behavior (Carr et al., 2009), multiple mechanisms have been theorized as being responsible for its effect. One such hypothesis is that time-based reinforcement produces a change in the motivating operation through satiation (Slocum et al., 2018; Vollmer et al., 1997). This phenomenon is especially likely with dense schedules of NCR. Alternatively, some researchers have suggested that under lean schedules of NCR, extinction is likely the mechanism responsible for reductions in problem behavior (Hagopian, Fisher, & Legacy, 1994; Wallace, Iwata, Hanley, Thompson, & Roscoe, 2012). Like extinction, NCR, or time-based delivery of a reinforcer, is another way of disrupting the relationship between behavior and reinforcement. Thus, the reductions in problem behavior produced by lean schedules of NCR may be due to such an effect.

Noncontingent reinforcement for problem behavior maintained by automatic reinforcement typically includes the use of competing or matched stimuli (Piazza, Adelinis, Hanley, Goh, & Delia, 2000; Rapp, 2007). Matched stimuli are those that produce the same or a similar form of sensory input as that which maintains the problem behavior. Consider the earlier example of eye poking; a toy with flickering lights may match the type of automatically reinforcing visual stimulation that is produced by eye poking. Thus, free access to such a toy could reduce the establishing operation to engage in that form of problem behavior. Piazza et al. (2000) compared the availability of functionally matched and arbitrarily selected stimuli on the rate of three subjects' problem behavior in the form of hand mouthing, saliva play, and dangerous jumping and climbing. Matched stimuli were those that the authors hypothesized generated similar sensory stimulation as the problem behavior (e.g., shaving cream on a mirror as a matched stimulus for saliva play). For all three subjects, matched stimuli produced greater reductions in problem behavior compared to arbitrary stimuli. Overall, noncontingent access to items that produce matched forms of sensory stimulation is a promising approach to reducing problem behavior maintained by automatic reinforcement.

Signals are another common antecedent strategy that can produce a reduction in problem behavior (Cote, Thompson, & Mckerchar, 2005; Gouboth et al., 2007; Mace et al., 1998). In one arrangement, Gouboth et al. (2007) compared NCR without signals to NCR that included signals prior to the removal of an item in the form of a statement explaining the contingencies (e.g., "I am taking the toy. When the timer rings, I will give it back to you."). Noncontingent reinforcement reduced problem behavior, but the addition of the signal produced even greater reductions: For one subject, NCR produced a 35% reduction in problem behavior, whereas the inclusion of the signal produced an 83% reduction. Signals are particularly useful in situations in which a behavior is sometimes permissible rather than problematic in all situations or at all times. For example, Conroy, Asmus, Sellers, and Ladwig (2005) used signals to indicate times during which a student was and was not allowed to engage in motor stereotypy. In this case, because the topography of problem behavior was hand flapping and mild in nature, it was considered acceptable to allow the individual to hand flap outside of instructional time. In the presence of the signal indicating that hand flapping was unavailable, the experimenters verbally reminded the individual not to engage in the behavior contingent on hand flapping. This treatment reduced hand flapping during times in which problem behavior was signaled as unavailable.

Another common antecedent-based treatment is the *high-probability instructional sequence*, which is often used with escape-maintained problem behavior. This strategy involves the presentation of demands that are highly likely to result in and build a recent history of compliance before presenting a demand unlikely to result in compliance (Mace et al., 1998). This procedure has been shown to be effective with individuals across a range of different ages, populations, and in various settings (Lipschultz & Wilder, 2017). Another antecedent strategy that can improve problem behavior is presentation of *choices*. Several studies have demonstrated the potential benefits of the fact that choice can function as a reinforcer in and of itself (Tiger, Hanley, & Hernandez, 2006). A meta-analysis conducted by Shogren et al. (2004) concluded that embedding choices into an individual's daily routine can reduce problem behavior. Choice was evaluated differently across studies, but generally fell into two categories: subjects that could either make choices concerning the order in which tasks were completed or could make choices between two or more activities. Choice is a relatively simple intervention for situations in which any of several options are acceptable. For example, it may not matter if someone brushes their teeth before or after using the bathroom in a bedtime routine. However, it may not be good to incorporate a choice between these two tasks, as both are necessary.

This chapter has highlighted only a few of the wide array of antecedent strategies for reducing problem behavior. Others include prompts (Sprague & Horner, 1992; Wilder, Allison, Nicholson, Abellon, & Saulnier, 2010), adding routines and structure (Bohn, Roehrig, & Pressley, 2004), decreasing task difficulty (Pace, Iwata, Cowdery, Andree, & McIntyre, 1993), and interspersing easy and difficult tasks (Ebanks & Fisher, 2003). Several review chapters have been written on these types of antecedent-based strategies (e.g., Kern & Chen, 2019), and readers interested in a more in-depth review are encouraged to seek them out.

Function-Based Treatments Using Arbitrary Reinforcers

This chapter focuses on function-based treatments for problem behavior. Indeed, the literature cited above clearly indicates interventions that incorporate the findings of a functional assessment have better outcomes than those that do not (Ingram et al., 2005). However, the use of arbitrary reinforcers may still be necessary in some cases. Arbitrary reinforcers may be necessary when interventionists lack control over the functional reinforcer, such as in the treatment of problem behavior maintained by automatic reinforcement (e.g., Toussaint & Tiger, 2012), or when the functional reinforcer cannot be identified. Alternatively, arbitrary reinforcers may be added to function-based treatments to produce even greater reductions in problem behavior (e.g., Zangrillo, Fisher, Greer, Owen, & DeSouza, 2016).

Although interventionists relied more heavily upon arbitrary reinforcers prior to the advent of functional assessment methods, these procedures continue to be implemented with some success under certain situations. For example, Toussaint and Tiger (2012) used a DRO intervention to reduce skin picking. The presumed functional automatic reinforcer (i.e., the sensory stimulation produced by skin picking) could not be replicated by the interventionists. The experimenters instead delivered praise and a token contingent on intervals elapsing without skin picking. The subject was subsequently allowed to exchange tokens for access to a video after each session. Although this DRO arrangement effectively reduced skin picking, it likely would not have been effective if the automatic reinforcer produced by skin picking was more powerful than access to the video. Furthermore, although the intervention did not manipulate the functional reinforcer, the results of the functional assessment could still be considered useful in that the experimenters were aware of the fact that the problem behavior was maintained by automatic reinforcement, and therefore were able to avoid mistakenly implementing counter-therapeutic interventions.

Lustig et al. (2014) and Scalzo, Forwell, and Suto (2016) similarly implemented DRO procedures with arbitrary reinforcers to reduce stereotypy maintained by automatic reinforcement. Lustig et al. delivered computer time, and Scalzo et al. delivered a hand towel (both found to be preferred items) within DRO arrangements. It is difficult to isolate the mechanism responsible for the reduction of problem behavior in these situations because functional assessments can produce a false-positive determination of an automatic function when the maintaining social variable cannot be controlled. Generally, it is assumed that these procedures will produce a reduction in problem behavior if the consequence is powerful enough to overpower reinforcement provided by the problem behavior itself (Vollmer & Iwata, 1992).

The inclusion of arbitrary reinforcers to enhance the effectiveness of function-based treatments has also been demonstrated to be effective across a wide range of applications. Slocum et al. (2018) provided free access to a nonfunctional reinforcer in the form of attention or preferred items when the functional reinforcer in the form of preferred items or attention was not available. This approach successfully reduced problem behavior even when the functional reinforcer was only available under lean schedules. Enhancing the potency of the functional reinforcer has also been applied to the treatment of escape-maintained problem behavior by providing items during breaks from demands as mentioned before (Zangrillo et al., 2016) as well as throughout demand contexts to make them less aversive (Cote et al., 2005; Park & Scott, 2009).

Interestingly, examples exist suggesting that treatments using arbitrary reinforcers can be effective even when the functional reinforcer has been identified and can be controlled. Fischer, Iwata, and Mazaleski (1997) delivered arbitrary reinforcers in an NCR arrangement and successfully reduced self-injurious behavior maintained by positive reinforcement. Similarly, the delivery of edible items either noncontingently within an NCR arrangement (Lomas, Fisher, & Kelley, 2010) or contingent on an appropriate behavior such as compliance in a DRA (Lalli et al., 1999; Piazza et al., 1997; Slocum & Vollmer, 2015) has been shown to reduce problem behavior maintained by escape, even when problem behavior continues to produce the functional reinforcer (i.e., without extinction).

In many studies evaluating the inclusion of positive reinforcers in the treatment of escape behavior, some of the subjects engaged in problem behavior maintained by negative *and* positive reinforcement (e.g., Slocum & Vollmer, 2015). Thus, it is possible the delivery of edible items could have actually been considered a function-based intervention in those cases. Further, there is a lack of understanding regarding the mechanism by which these interventions reduce problem behavior. One possibility is that edible items and breaks are asymmetrical with respect to their availability outside of the contingency for problem behavior. For example, edible items are commonly restricted for individuals with IDD for lengthy intervals. Other than mealtimes, an individual may only obtain edible items controlled by caregivers contingent upon specific behavior. That is, edible items likely operate within a relatively *closed economy*. In contrast, attention and breaks from demands are typically provided freely throughout the day – a relatively *open economy*. Roane, Falcomata, and Call (2005) showed that reinforcers in a closed economy are more powerful for individuals with IDD than those in an open economy. Thus, the degree to which an arbitrary reinforcer is available within an open or closed economy may need to be equated across breaks and edible items to truly compare function-based interventions and those that use arbitrary reinforcers. Unfortunately, this comparison would be quite challenging from a research design perspective, particularly with respect to arranging a closed economy. That is, although edible items or other positive reinforcers can be restricted to evaluate the effect of a closed economy, restriction of breaks would require arranging for the continuous presentation of some aversive stimulus (such as demands).

Although treatments using arbitrary reinforcers do not reduce problem behavior through the same mechanism as those that alter the contingencies of the functional reinforcer, functional assessment still guides the selection of treatments that rely upon arbitrary reinforcers. We are not suggesting that treatments can be selected randomly or without a functional assessment. In many of the studies described above, the function of problem behavior was known and contributed to intervention selection. Additional research on the efficacy of interventions using arbitrary reinforcers is necessary to draw more thorough conclusions, including work focused on the relative long-term outcomes of function-based treatments and those employing arbitrary reinforcers.

Programming for Maintenance of Function-Based Treatment Effects

The literature presented thus far has included several strategies shown to effectively reduce problem behavior, but many of these strategies are not feasible over the long term. For instance, delivering an edible item for every instance of compliance will likely lead to a reduction in escape-maintained problem behavior. However, if the individual becomes satiated on the edible item, that intervention may cease to be effective. Furthermore, over time there are likely to be substantial health concerns given the high caloric intake of an individual receiving such an intervention. Similarly, teaching an individual with a history of engaging in problem behavior maintained by attention to instead say, "Talk to me please," may be effective. However, without additional steps the individual is likely to continuously request attention, which is unlikely to be possible for most caregivers to reinforce. Thus, it is critical to reduce the rate of the alternative response or to bring it under the control of some stimulus or schedule controlled by a caregiver (Hagopian, Boelter, & Jarmolowicz, 2011). There are several such ways to extend behavioral interventions to increase their social validity (i.e., interventions with goals of social significance, procedures of social appropriateness, and effects of social importance; Wolf, 1978) and ecological validity (i.e., interventions designed to fit within the real-world setting; Schmuckler, 2010).

Delaying Reinforcement

Following training of a functional communication response, a delay to the delivery of the functional reinforcer can be incorporated (see Hagopian et al., 1998 for a review). Grey, Healy, Leader, and Hayes (2009) evaluated the utility of graduated delayed reinforcement procedures to increase the social validity of FCT. After teaching a communication response to replace problem behavior maintained by access to preferred items and activities, the authors gradually increased a delay between the request and access to the functional reinforcer. Grey et al. were able to reach a 10-min delay to reinforcement following a request. When providing a delay to reinforcement, it is common to use a stimulus to signal the delay such as stating "wait" before the delay begins (Hagopian et al., 2011). Graduated delayed reinforcement can be successful for many cases such as in Grey et al. However, delayed reinforcement signaled by a vocal statement may only be effective for briefer delays (Hagopian et al., 2011).

Thinning Reinforcement

Functional communication training has been successfully used to treat problem behavior maintained by escape from demands by replacing that problem behavior with requests for a break. However, in this situation, many individuals will request breaks so frequently that they comply very little with the task, or not at all (Marcus & Vollmer, 1995). Therefore, it is more common to use a DRA procedure in which the alternative response is compliance rather than communication (Geiger, Carr, & LeBlanc, 2010). The social validity of this intervention can be further enhanced by gradually increasing the response requirement (Pace et al., 1993; Ringdahl et al., 2002). Pace et al. (1993) demonstrated that starting with no demands and gradually adding them across consecutive sessions were successful at maintaining reductions in problem behavior while simultaneously increasing compliance. However, although potentially successful, the slow introduction of demands may not be optimal if it is just as efficient to start with the terminal work goal and persist through any problem behavior that occurs. To evaluate this question, Ringdahl et al. (2002) found that slowly increasing the number of demands until a terminal goal was reached did in fact produce less overall problem behavior than beginning with a requirement to complete the number of demands that constituted the terminal goal. Therefore, it may be easier to gradually increase the response requirement over time rather than working through extinction. Researchers have found a similar methodology can be effective in cases that have incorporated FCT or reinforcing requests for a break. Lalli, Casey, and Kates (1995) taught individuals with escape-maintained problem behavior to request a break. They subsequently required compliance with a portion of a task following the request before actually providing the break. Over time, Lalli et al. were able to increase the work requirement until the individual was reliably completing the entire task.

Another approach to increasing the feasibility of DRA interventions is to thin reinforcement for communication responses during FCT (Borrero & Vollmer, 2006). That is, rather than reinforcing every instance of the alternative behavior, the interventionist reinforces some, but not all of them, while gradually thinning the proportion of responses that result in reinforcement. When FCT incorporates certain functional communication responses, such as a picture exchange, another option for thinning the schedule of reinforcement is to briefly restrict access to the materials required to emit that alternative response and gradually increase the interval of restriction (Roane, Fisher, Sgro, Falcomata, & Pabico, 2004). Roane et al. (2004) taught subjects to use a picture exchange to access preferred items. At first, the picture card was available continuously, but over time, the authors made the card unavailable for longer intervals. Although this procedure has been replicated successfully several times (e.g., Fisher, Greer, Querim, & DeRosa, 2014; Hagopian et al., 2011; Roane et al., 2004), there may be some ethical concerns regarding the restriction of an individual's ability to communicate. That is, many individuals with whom these interventions are implemented are not capable of communicating effectively via vocal speech or manual sign. Thus, picture exchange or augmentative communication devices are their primary means of indicating their needs. Restricting access to the stimuli involved in communicating makes these individuals functionally mute rather than teaching them that there are times during which the functional reinforcer is unavailable. For this reason, multiple schedules constitute an appealing strategy for indicating when requests will or will not be reinforced.

Multiple Schedules

A multiple schedule consists of two or more schedules of reinforcement that alternate, with a discriminative stimulus that indicates when each schedule is operative (Herrick, Myers, & Korotkin, 1959). These complex schedules are commonly implemented to teach individuals when an alternative response will be reinforced (an interval denoted as S^D) and when it will not (denoted as S^Δ; e.g., Jarmolowicz, DeLeon, & Kuhn, 2009). It is important to note that problem behavior remains on extinction throughout both phases of a multiple schedule that is employed for this purpose. Several studies have demonstrated that the alternative response can come under the control of the signals associated with each condition, as individuals continue to emit the alternative response in the presence of the S^D, but not in the presence of the S^Δ (Call et al., 2018). Hanley, Iwata, and Thompson (2001) compared the use of a multiple schedule to a mixed schedule that was identical to the multiple schedule but did not include signals. The authors found that including signals produced greater reductions in problem behavior compared to the mixed schedule. As is true when thinning other schedules of reinforcement as described above, the duration of the S^Δ interval of a multiple schedule typically begins as a brief interval that gradually increases (Fisher, Greer, Fuhrman, & Querim, 2015). A key advantage of this approach is that the signals are typically under the control of an interventionist so that he or she is eventually able to deny access to the functional reinforcer at times that it is inconvenient or impossible to deliver.

Reemergence of Problem Behavior

The procedures described above are necessary to increase the practicality of function-based treatments for caregivers of individuals who exhibit problem behavior. It is important to note, however, that problem behavior frequently reemerges after treatments establish reductions, including during schedule thinning (Volkert, Lerman, Call, & Trosclair-Lasserre, 2013) or when an intervention is introduced into a new context (Saini, Sullivan, Baxter, DeRosa, & Roane, 2018). When a previously suppressed behavior reemerges as a result of the alternative response not being reinforced, whether during schedule thinning or a lapse in treatment fidelity, it is called *resurgence* (Greer & Shahan, 2019). In one review, Briggs, Fisher, Greer, and Kimball (2018) found that resurgence occurred for 76% of individuals experiencing scheduling thinning following FCT. Although the magnitude of the resurgence effect (i.e., how much problem behavior was observed) differed across subjects, it is important for interventionists to proactively plan for the possibility that problem behavior may resurge.

Similar to resurgence, renewal occurs in about 42% of cases (Muething et al., 2020). Clinical examples have demonstrated renewal when an individual's problem behavior is reinforced at home (Context A), then placed on extinction in the clinic (Context B), and then the individual transitions back into the home (Context A; Podlesnik, Kelley, Jimenez-Gomez, & Bouton, 2017), where extinction persists. Under this arrangement, it is common to see a relapse in problem behavior, even though extinction continues in the new setting. Just as with resurgence, interventionists should be aware that there is a likelihood renewal could occur when treating problem behavior.

Future Research

Function-based interventions have been shown to be highly effective with individuals of different ages and with different disabilities, in a number of settings, and with several types of interventionists (Beavers et al., 2013). Still, additional research is warranted. The treatment literature for the past several decades has understandably focused primarily upon development of function-based treatments. However, given that certain treatments using arbitrary reinforcers may be more feasible for interventionists to implement with fidelity, it may be time for the field to explore the conditions under which they are most effectively deployed. As described previously, there are situations in which interventions using arbitrary reinforcers can effectively reduce problem behavior (e.g., Lalli et al., 1999; Toussaint & Tiger, 2012). However, the mechanisms responsible for these effects are not always well understood and should be evaluated. For example, as discussed in the preceding section, it may be that the delivery of edible items is more effective at reducing escape-maintained problem behavior than breaks because edibles are less freely available. Alternatively, it may be the case that arbitrary positive reinforcers are simply more preferred than functional reinforcers. Finally, it is important for future research to examine the durability of function-based treatments and treatments using arbitrary reinforcers.

The function-based treatments discussed to this point operate primarily through operant conditioning or contact with reinforcing or punishing consequences (Skinner, 1938). However, the role of respondent conditioning in the treatment of problem behavior is in need of additional research. Respondent behavior is elicited by a stimulus and therefore not dependent on consequences (Cooper et al., 2007). For example, the bottom panel of Fig. 12.1 depicts the results of a treatment for problem behavior maintained by social avoidance or social-negative reinforcement that incorporates two respondent conditioning approaches. First, after establishing a hierarchy of aversiveness for various types of social interaction based upon latency to problem behavior (data not shown), the interventionist implemented the least-aversive form of social interaction. This approach is different from the typical application of a demand latency assessment prior to treating problem behavior maintained by social-negative reinforcement (Call, Pabico, & Lomas, 2009). Demand latency assessments are typically implemented to identify the *most* aversive form of social interaction. Instead, the experimenters first introduced a form of social interaction they had identified as not being aversive. As problem behavior remained low, they gradually progressed through the introduction of increasingly aversive types of social interaction. Second, they paired access to preferred edible and leisure items with social interaction. Both components (fading in more aversive forms of social interaction and access to preferred items) occurred across baseline and FCT conditions (see bottom panel of Fig. 12.1). These approaches were evaluated after operant conditioning alone had been attempted unsuccessfully (top panel of Fig. 12.1). In spite of this successful application of respondent conditioning, more research is necessary to further evaluate its role within behavioral interventions.

Finally, the vast majority of research on behavior analytic treatments of problem behavior has used single-subject research methods. This approach is appropriate because it shows the types of treatment effects that are possible and allows researchers to demonstrate strong relationships between specific behavioral mechanisms and subjects' problem behavior. However, research relying on single-subject methods is less likely to be disseminated to certain key audiences. To reach these audiences, it may be necessary to adopt methods from group designs, including larger sample sizes, randomized controlled trials (RCTs), and effect size calculations (e.g., Lindgren et al., 2016). These methods are also best equipped to address different research questions, including demonstrating which interventions are more or less likely to be effective for certain categories of individuals. Figure 12.2 depicts preliminary data from an example of this type of study, which will include a larger sample size than is typically employed in research on behavioral interventions to evaluate commonly implemented treatments for escape-maintained problem behav-

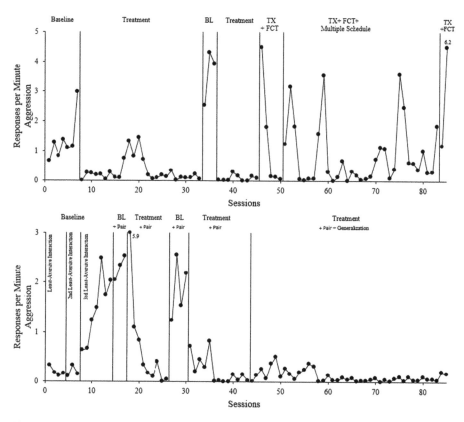

Fig. 12.1 Clinical data for a patient receiving treatment services in the severe behavior intensive outpatient program at the Marcus Autism Center. This individual had problem behavior maintained by social avoidance which was treated through FCT and other antecedent strategies

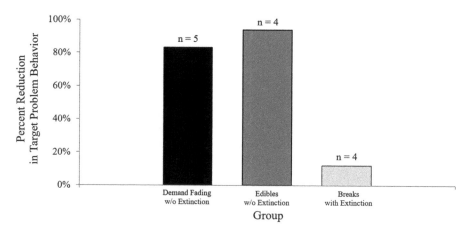

Fig. 12.2 Data obtained across sites on the assessment and treatment of escape-maintained problem behavior. Average percent reduction in problem behavior for the first 10, 5-min treatment sessions is plotted across groups of subjects who received one of three commonly implemented treatments

ior. Specifically, the bars represent average levels of problem behavior during the first 10, 5-min sessions of three interventions: delivering edible items for compliance, delivering breaks for compliance with extinction, and using instructional fading. These data may speak to the broader impact of these interventions such as the likelihood that these treatments will work in the short term for individuals with escape-maintained problem behavior. Although these results are preliminary, there are clear differences in the average percent reduction in problem behavior across the different interventions.

Conclusions

Functional assessments, in their best-known form, first appeared in the literature four decades ago (Iwata et al., 1982). Since then, function-based treatments have been refined such that many procedures have been successfully used to treat a variety of topographies and functions of problem behavior. These include extinction, differential reinforcement, antecedent manipulations, and many more. Understanding the contingencies that maintain problem behavior is integral to treatment effectiveness. Although the treatments discussed above may seem simple, interventionists must consider several variables simultaneously when selecting or implementing them. One such factor that has not always been considered sufficiently in the literature is ecological validity. If interventionists develop a strategy that a caregiver cannot or will not implement with fidelity, then the outcomes of that treatment are null. Therefore, in addition to considering treatment efficacy, interventionists should also devote careful planning to anticipating potential side effects (e.g., extinction bursts) and considering stakeholder buy-in (e.g., caregiver preferences) when selecting a behavioral intervention for problem behavior.

References

Ahearn, W. H., Clark, K. M., MacDonald, R. P. F., & Chung, B. I. (2007). Assessing and treating vocal stereotypy in children with autism. *Journal of Applied Behavior Analysis, 40*, 263–275. https://doi.org/10.1901/jaba.2007.30-06

Allen, K. E., & Harris, F. R. (1966). Elimination of a child's scratching by training the mother in reinforcement procedures. *Behaviour Research and Therapy, 4*, 79–84. https://doi.org/10.1016/0005-7967(66)90046-5

Anderson, E., Barretto, A., McLaughlin, T. F., & McQuaid, T. (2016). Case report: Effects of functional communication training with and without delays to decrease aberrant behavior in a child with autism spectrum disorder. *Journal on Developmental Disabilities, 22*, 101–110.

Arkoosh, M. K., Derby, K. M., Wacker, D. P., Berg, W., McLaughlin, T. F., & Barretto, A. (2007). A descriptive evaluation of long-term treatment integrity. *Behavior Modification, 31*, 880–895. https://doi.org/10.1177/0145445507302254

Athens, E. S., & Vollmer, T. R. (2010). An investigation of differential reinforcement of alternative behavior without extinction. *Journal of Applied Behavior Analysis, 43*, 569–589. https://doi.org/10.1901/jaba.2010.43-569

Azrin, N. H., Basalel, V. A., Jamner, J. P., & Caputo, J. N. (1988). Comparative study of behavioral methods of treating severe self-injury. *Behavioral Interventions, 3*, 119–152. https://doi.org/10.1002/bin.2360030204

Baker, J. C., Hanley, G. P., & Mathews, R. M. (2006). Staff-administered functional analysis and treatment of aggression by an elder with dementia. *Journal of Applied Behavior Analysis, 39*, 469–474. https://doi.org/10.1901/jaba.2006.80-05

Baum, W. M. (1974). On two types of deviation from the matching law: Bias and undermatching. *Journal of the Experimental Analysis of Behavior, 22*, 231–242. https://doi.org/10.1901/jeab.1974.22-231

Beavers, G. A., Iwata, B. A., & Lerman, D. C. (2013). Thirty years of research on the functional analysis of problem behavior. *Journal of Applied Behavior Analysis, 46*, 1–21. https://doi.org/10.1002/jaba.30

Behavior Analyst Certification Board. (2014). *Professional and ethical compliance code for behavior analysts*. Littleton, CO: Author.

Bijou, S. W. (1957). Patterns of reinforcement and resistance to extinction in young children. *Child Development, 28*, 47–54. https://doi.org/10.1111/j.1467-8624.1957.tb04830.x

Birnbrauer, J. (1968). Generalization of punishment effects: A case study. *Journal of Applied Behavior Analysis, 1*, 201–211. https://doi.org/10.1901/jaba.1968.1-201

Bohn, C. M., Roehrig, A. D., & Pressley, M. (2004). The first days of school in the classrooms of two more effective and four less effective primary-grades teachers. *The Elementary School Journal, 104*, 269–287. https://doi.org/10.1086/499753

Borrero, C. S. W., & Vollmer, T. R. (2006). Experimental analysis and treatment of multiply controlled problem behavior: A systematic replication and extension. *Journal of Applied Behavior Analysis, 39*, 375–379. https://doi.org/10.1901/jaba.2006.170-04

Borrero, C. S. W., Vollmer, T. R., Borrero, J. C., Bourret, J. C., Sloman, K. N., Samaha, A. L., & Dallery, J. (2010). Concurrent reinforcement schedules for problem behavior and appropriate behavior: Experimental applications of the matching law. *Journal of the Experimental Analysis of Behavior, 93*, 455–469. https://doi.org/10.1901/jeab.2010.93-455

Borrero, J. C., & Vollmer, T. R. (2013). An application of the matching law to severe problem behavior. *Journal of Applied Behavior Analysis, 35*, 13. https://doi.org/10.1901/jaba.2002.35-13

Briggs, A. M., Fisher, W. W., Greer, B. D., & Kimball, R. T. (2018). Prevalence of resurgence of destructive behavior when thinning reinforcement schedules during functional communication training. *Journal of Applied Behavior Analysis, 51*, 620–633. https://doi.org/10.1002/jaba.472

Call, N. A., Clark, S. B., Lomas Mevers, J., Parks, N. A., Volkert, V. M., & Scheithauer, M. C. (2018). An individualized method for establishing and thinning multiple schedules of reinforcement following functional communication training. *Learning and Motivation, 62*, 91–102. https://doi.org/10.1016/j.lmot.2017.03.006

Call, N. A., Pabico, R. S., & Lomas, J. E. (2009). Use of latency to problem behavior to evaluate demands for inclusion in functional analyses. *Journal of Applied Behavior Analysis, 42*, 723–728. https://doi.org/10.1901/jaba.2009.42-723

Carr, E. G. (1977). The motivation of self-injurious behavior: A review of some hypotheses. *Psychological Bulletin, 84*, 800–816. https://doi.org/10.1037/0033-2909.84.4.800

Carr, E. G., & Durand, V. M. (1985). Reducing behavior problems through functional communication training. *Journal of Applied Behavior Analysis, 18*, 111–126. https://doi.org/10.1901/jaba.1985.18-111

Carr, J. E., Severtson, J. M., & Lepper, T. L. (2009). Noncontingent reinforcement is an empirically supported treatment for problem behavior exhibited by individuals with developmental disabilities. *Research in Developmental Disabilities, 30*, 44–57. https://doi.org/10.1016/j.ridd.2008.03.002

Conroy, M. A, Asmus, J. M, Sellers, J. A, & Ladwig, C. N. (2005). The use of an antecedent-based intervention to decrease stereotypic behavior in a general education classroom: A case study. *Focus on Autism and Other Developmental Disabilities, 20*(4), 223–230.https://doi.org/10.1177/10883576050200040401

Cooper, J. O., Heron, T. E., & Heward, W. L. (2007). *Applied behavior analysis* (2nd ed.). Upper Saddle River, NJ: Pearson.

Corte, H. E., Wolf, M. M., & Locke, B. J. (1971). A comparison of procedures for eliminating self-injurious behavior of retarded adolescents. *Journal of Applied Behavior Analysis, 4*, 201–213. https://doi.org/10.1901/jaba.1971.4-201

Cote, C. A., Thompson, R. H., & McKerchar, P. M. (2005). The effects of antecedent interventions and extinction on toddlers' compliance during transitions. *Journal of Applied Behavior Analysis, 38*, 235–238. https://doi.org/10.1901/jaba.2005.143-04

Della Rosa, K. A., Fellman, D., DeBiase, C., DeQuinzio, J. A., & Taylor, B. A. (2015). The effects of using a conditioned stimulus to cue DRO schedules. *Behavioral Interventions, 30*, 219–230. https://doi.org/10.1002/bin.1409

Dixon, M. R., Guercio, J., Falcomata, T., Horner, M. J., Root, S., Newell, C., & Zlomke, K. (2004). Exploring the utility of functional analysis methodology to assess and treat problematic verbal behavior in persons with acquired brain injury. *Behavioral Interventions, 19*, 91–102. https://doi.org/10.1002/bin.155

Dorey, N. R., Rosales-Ruiz, J., Smith, R., & Lovelace, B. (2009). Functional analysis and treatment of self-injury in a captive olive baboon. *Journal of Applied Behavior Analysis, 42*, 785–794. https://doi.org/10.1901/jaba.2009.42-785

Durand, V. (1999). Functional communication training using assistive devices: Recruiting natural communities of reinforcement. *Journal of Applied Behavior Analysis, 32*, 247–267. https://doi.org/10.1901/jaba.1999.32-247

Ebanks, M. E., & Fisher, W. W. (2003). Altering the timing of academic prompts to treat destructive behavior maintained by escape. *Journal of Applied Behavior Analysis, 36*, 355–359. https://doi.org/10.1901/jaba.2003.36-355

Emerson, E. (2001). *Challenging behaviour. Analysis and intervention in people with severe intellectual disabilities* (2nd ed.). Cambridge, UK: Cambridge University Press.

Falcomata, T. S., Ringdahl, J. E., Christensen, T. J., & Boelter, E. W. (2010). An evaluation of prompt schedules and mand preference during functional communication training. *The Behavior Analyst Today, 11*, 77–84. https://doi.org/10.1037/h0100690

Falcomata, T. S., Wacker, D. P., Ringdahl, J. E., Vinquist, K., & Dutt, A. (2013). An evaluation of generalization of mands during functional communication training. *Journal of Applied Behavior Analysis, 46*, 444–454. https://doi.org/10.1002/jaba.37

Favell, J. E., McGimsey, J. F., & Jones, M. L. (1978). The use of physical restraint in the treatment of self-injury and as positive reinforcement. *Journal of Applied Behavior Analysis, 11*, 225–241. https://doi.org/10.1901/jaba.1978.11-225

Feuerbacher, E. N., & Wynne, C. D. L. (2016). Application of functional analysis methods to assess human–dog interactions. *Journal of Applied Behavior Analysis, 49*, 970–974. https://doi.org/10.1002/jaba.318

Fischer, S. M., Iwata, B. A., & Mazaleski, J. L. (1997). Noncontingent delivery of arbitrary reinforcers as treatment for self-injurious behavior. *Journal of Applied Behavior Analysis, 30*, 239–249. https://doi.org/10.1901/jaba.1997.30-239

Fisher, W. W., Greer, B. D., Fuhrman, A. M., & Querim, A. C. (2015). Using multiple schedules during functional communication training to promote rapid transfer of treatment effects. *Journal of Applied Behavior Analysis, 48*, 713–733. https://doi.org/10.1002/jaba.254

Fisher, W. W., Greer, B. D., Querim, A. C., & DeRosa, N. (2014). Decreasing excessive functional communication responses while treating destructive behavior using response restriction. *Research in Developmental Disabilities, 35*, 2614–2623. https://doi.org/10.1016/j.ridd.2014.06.024

Fisher, W. W., Lindauer, S. E., Alterson, C. J., & Thompson, R. H. (1998). Assessment and treatment of destructive behavior maintained by stereotypic object manipulation. *Journal of Applied Behavior Analysis, 31*, 513–527. https://doi.org/10.1901/jaba.1998.31-513.

Fisher, W. W., Piazza, C., Cataldo, M., & Harrell, R. (1993). Functional communication training with and without extinction and punishment. *Journal of Applied Behavior Analysis, 26*, 23–36. https://doi.org/10.1901/jaba.1993.26-23

Gardner, A. W., Spencer, T. D., Boelter, E. W., Dubard, M., & Jennett, H. K. (2012). A systematic review of brief functional analysis methodology with typically developing children. *Education and Treatment of Children, 35*, 313–332. https://doi.org/10.1353/etc.2012.0014

Gehrman, G., Wilder, D. A., Forton, A. P., & Albert, K. (2017). Comparing resetting to non-resetting DRO procedures to reduce stereotypy in a child with autism. *Behavioral Interventions, 32*, 242–247. https://doi.org/10.1002/bin.1486

Geiger, K. B., Carr, J. E., & LeBlanc, L. A. (2010). Function-based treatments for escape-maintained problem behavior: A treatment-selection model for practicing behavior analysts. *Behavior Analysis in Practice, 3*, 22–32. https://doi.org/10.1007/BF03391755

Goh, H., & Iwata, B. A. (1994). Behavioral persistence and variability during extinction of self-injury maintained by escape. *Journal of Applied Behavior Analysis, 27*, 173–174. https://doi.org/10.1901/jaba.1994.27-173.

Gouboth, D., Wilder, D. A., & Booher, J. (2007). The effects of signaling stimulus presentation during noncontingent reinforcement. *Journal of Applied Behavior Analysis, 40*, 25–30. https://doi.org/10.1901/jaba.2007.725-730.

Grandy, S. E., & Peck, S. M. (1997). The use of functional assessment and self-management with a first grader. *Child and Family Behavior Therapy, 19*, 29–43. https://doi.org/10.1300/J019v19n02_03

Greer, B. D., & Shahan, T. A. (2019). Resurgence as choice: Implications for promoting durable behavior change. *Journal of Applied Behavior Analysis, 52*, 816–846. https://doi.org/10.1002/jaba.573

Grey, I., Healy, O., Leader, G., & Hayes, D. (2009). Using a TimeTimer ™ to increase appropriate waiting behavior in a child with developmental disabilities. *Research in Developmental Disabilities, 30*, 359–366. https://doi.org/10.1016/j.ridd.2008.07.001

Hagopian, L. P., Fisher, W. W., & Legacy, S. M. (1994). Schedule effects of noncontingent reinforcement on attention-maintained destructive behavior in identical quadruplets. *Journal of applied behavior analysis, 27*(2), 317–325. https://doi.org/10.1901/jaba.1994.27-317

Hagopian, L. P., Boelter, E. W., & Jarmolowicz, D. P. (2011). Reinforcement schedule thinning following functional communication training: Review and recommendations. *Behavior Analysis in Practice, 4*, 4–16. https://doi.org/10.1007/BF03391770

Hagopian, L. P., Dozier, C. L., Rooker, G. W., & Jones, B. A. (2013). Assessment and treatment of severe problem behavior. In G. J. Madden (Ed.), *APA handbook of behavior analysis: Vol. 2. Translating principles into practice* (pp. 353–386). Washington, DC: APA.

Hagopian, L. P., Fisher, W. W., Sullivan, M. T., Acquisto, J., & LeBlanc, L. A. (1998). Effectiveness of functional communication training with and without extinction and punishment: A summary of 21 inpatient cases. *Journal of Applied Behavior Analysis, 31*, 211–235. https://doi.org/10.1901/jaba.1998.31-211

Hall, N. J., Protopopova, A., & Wynne, C. D. L. (2015). The role of environmental and owner-provided consequences in canine stereotypy and compulsive behavior. *Journal of Veterinary Behavior, 10*, 24–35. https://doi.org/10.1016/j.jveb.2014.10.005

Hanley, G. P., Iwata, B. A., & Thompson, R. H. (2001). Reinforcement schedule thinning following treatment with functional communication training. *Journal of Applied Behavior Analysis, 34*, 17–38. https://doi.org/10.1901/jaba.2001.34-17

Heffernan, L., & Lyons, D. (2016). Differential reinforcement of other behavior for the reduction of severe nail biting. *Behavior Analysis in Practice, 9*, 253–256. https://doi.org/10.1007/s40617-016-0106-3

Herrick, R. M., Myers, J. L., & Korotkin, A. L. (1959). Changes in Sd and in Sdelta rates during the development of an operant discrimination. *Journal of Comparative Psychology, 52*, 359–363. https://doi.org/10.1037/h0044283

Herrnstein, R. J. (1970). On the law of effect. *Journal of the Experimental Analysis of Behavior, 13*, 243–266. https://doi.org/10.1901/jeab.1970.13-243

Heyvaert, M., Saenen, L., Campbell, J. M., Maes, B., & Onghena, P. (2014). Efficacy of behavioral interventions for reducing problem behavior in persons with autism: An updated quantitative synthesis of single-subject research. *Research in Developmental Disabilities, 35*, 2463–2476. https://doi.org/10.1016/j.ridd.2014.06.017

Hoch, H., McComas, J. J., Thompson, A. L., & Paone, D. (2002). Concurrent reinforcement schedules: Behavior change and maintenance without extinction. *Journal of Applied Behavior Analysis, 35*, 155–169. https://doi.org/10.1901/jaba.2002.35-155.

Individuals with Disabilities Education Act, 20 U.S.C. § 1400 (2004).

Ingram, K., Lewis-Palmer, T., & Sugai, G. M. (2005). Function-based intervention planning: Comparing the effectiveness of FBA function-based and non-function-based intervention plans. *Journal of Positive Behavior Interventions, 7*, 224–236. https://doi.org/10.1177/109.830.0705007.004.0401

Iwata, B. A., Dorsey, M. F., Slifer, K. J., Bauman, K. E., & Richman, G. S. (1982). Toward a functional analysis of self-injury. *Analysis and Intervention in Developmental Disabilities, 2*, 3–20. https://doi.org/10.1016/0270-4684(82)90003-9

Iwata, B. A., Pace, G. M., Cowdery, G. E., & Miltenberger, R. G. (1994). What makes extinction work: An analysis of procedural form and function. *Journal of Applied Behavior Analysis, 27*, 131–144. https://doi.org/10.1901/jaba.1994.27-131

Iwata, B. A., Pace, G. M., Kalsher, M. J., Cowdery, G. E., & Cataldo, M. F. (1990). Experimental analysis and extinction of self-injurious escape behavior. *Journal of Applied Behavior Analysis, 23*, 11–27. https://doi.org/10.1901/jaba.1990.23-11

Jarmolowicz, D., DeLeon, I., & Kuhn, S. (2009). Functional communication during signaled reinforcement and/or extinction. *Behavioral Interventions, 24*, 265–273. https://doi.org/10.1002/bin.288

Jennett, H., Jann, K., & Hagopian, L. P. (2011). Evaluation of response blocking and re-presentation in a competing stimulus assessment. *Journal of Applied Behavior Analysis, 44*, 925–929. https://doi.org/10.1901/jaba.2011.44-925

Jessel, J., & Ingvarsson, E. T. (2016). Recent advances in applied research on DRO procedures. *Journal of Applied Behavior Analysis, 49*, 991–995. https://doi.org/10.1002/jaba.323

Johnson, R. A., Danis, M., & Hafner-Eaton, C. (2014). US state variation in autism insurance mandates: Balancing access and fairness. *Autism, 18*, 803–814. https://doi.org/10.1177/1362361314529191

Kelley, M. E., Lerman, D. C., & Van Camp, C. M. (2002). The effects of competing reinforcement schedules on the acquisition of functional communication. *Journal of Applied Behavior Analysis, 35*, 59–63. https://doi.org/10.1901/jaba.2002.35-59

Kennedy, C. H., & Souza, G. (1995). Functional analysis and treatment of eye poking. *Journal of Applied Behavior Analysis, 28*, 27–37. https://doi.org/10.1901/jaba.1995.28-27

Kern, L., & Chen, R. (2019). Antecedent interventions. In K. C. Radley & E. H. Dart (Eds.), *Handbook of behavioral interventions in schools: Multi-tiered systems of support*. New York, NY: Oxford University Press.

Lalli, J. S., Casey, S., & Kates, K. (1995). Reducing escape behavior and increasing task completion with functional communication training, extinction, and response chaining. *Journal of Applied Behavior Analysis, 28*, 261–268. https://doi.org/10.1901/jaba.1995.28-261

Lalli, J. S., Vollmer, T. R., Progar, P. R., Wright, C., Borrero, J., Daniel, D., … May, W. (1999). Competition between positive and negative reinforcement in the treatment of escape behavior. *Journal of Applied Behavior Analysis, 32*, 285–296. https://doi.org/10.1901/jaba.1999.32-285

Lerman, D. C., & Iwata, B. A. (1996). A methodology for distinguishing between extinction and punishment effects associated with response blocking. *Journal of Applied Behavior Analysis, 29*, 231–233. https://doi.org/10.1901/jaba.1996.29-231

Lerman, D. C., Iwata, B. A., & Wallace, M. D. (1999). Side effects of extinction: Prevalence of bursting and aggression during the treatment of self-injurious behavior. *Journal of Applied Behavior Analysis, 32*, 1–8. https://doi.org/10.1901/jaba.1999.32-1

Lindberg, J. S., Iwata, B. A., Kahng, S., & DeLeon, I. G. (1999). DRO contingencies: An analysis of variable-momentary schedules. *Journal of Applied Behavior Analysis, 32*, 123–126. https://doi.org/10.1901/jaba.1999.32-123.

Lindgren, S., Wacker, D., Suess, A., Schieltz, K., Pelzel, K., Kopelman, T., … Waldron, D. (2016). Telehealth and autism: Treating challenging behavior at lower cost. *Pediatrics, 137*, 167–175. https://doi.org/10.1542/peds.2015-2851O

Lipschultz, J., & Wilder, D. A. (2017). Recent research on the high-probability instructional sequence: A brief review. *Journal of Applied Behavior Analysis, 50*, 424–428. https://doi.org/10.1002/jaba.378

Lomas, J. E., Fisher, W. W., & Kelley, M. E. (2010). The effects of variable-time delivery of food items and praise on problem behavior reinforced by escape. *Journal of Applied Behavior Analysis, 43*, 425–435. https://doi.org/10.1901/jaba.2010.43-425

Lovaas, O. I., Freitag, G., Gold, V. J., & Kassorla, I. C. (1965). Experimental studies in childhood schizophrenia: Analysis of self-destructive behavior. *Journal of Experimental Child Psychology, 2*, 67–84. https://doi.org/10.1016/0022-0965(65)90016-0

Luce, S. C., Delquadri, J., & Hall, R. V. (1980). Contingent exercise: A mild but powerful procedure for suppressing inappropriate verbal and aggressive behavior. *Journal of Applied Behavior Analysis, 13*, 583–594. https://doi.org/10.1901/jaba.1980.13-583

Lustig, N., Ringdahl, J., Breznican, G., Romani, P., Scheib, M., & Vinquist, K. (2014). Evaluation and treatment of socially inappropriate stereotypy. *Journal of Developmental and Physical Disabilities, 26*. https://doi.org/10.1007/s10882-013-9357-x.

Mace, A. B., Shapiro, E. S., & Mace, F. C. (1998). Effects of warning stimuli for reinforcer withdrawal and task onset on self-injury. *Journal of Applied Behavior Analysis, 31*, 679–682. https://doi.org/10.1901/jaba.1998.31-679.

Mace, F. C. (1994). The significance and future of functional analysis methodologies. *Journal of Applied Behavior Analysis, 27*, 385–392. https://doi.org/10.1901/jaba.1994.27-385

Marcus, B. A., & Vollmer, T. R. (1995). Effects of differential negative reinforcement on disruption and compliance. *Journal of Applied Behavior Analysis, 28*, 229–230. https://doi.org/10.1901/jaba.1995.28-229

Martin, A. L., Bloomsmith, M. A., Kelley, M. E., Marr, M. J., & Maple, T. L. (2011). Functional analysis and treatment of human-directed undesirable behavior exhibited by a captive chimpanzee. *Journal of Applied Behavior Analysis, 44*, 139–143. https://doi.org/10.1901/jaba.2011.44-134

Mazaleski, J. L., Iwata, B. A., Vollmer, T. R., Zarcone, J. R., & Smith, R. G. (1993). Analysis of the reinforcement and extinction components in DRO contingencies with self-injury. *Journal of Applied Behavior Analysis, 26*, 143–156. https://doi.org/10.1901/jaba.1993.26-143

McCord, B. E., Grosser, J. W., Iwata, B. A., & Powers, L. J. (2005). An analysis of response-blocking parameters in the prevention of pica. *Journal of Applied Behavior Analysis, 38*, 391–394. https://doi.org/10.1901/jaba.2005.92-04

Moore, J. W., Fisher, W. W., & Pennington, A. (2004). Systematic application and removal of protective equipment in the assessment of multiple topographies of self-injury. *Journal of Applied Behavior Analysis, 37*, 73–77. https://doi.org/10.1901/jaba.2004.37-73

Morris, K. L., & Slocum, S. K. (2019). Functional analysis and treatment of self-injurious feather plucking in a black vulture (Coragyps atratus). *Journal of Applied Behavior Analysis, 52*, 918–927. https://doi.org/10.1002/jaba.639

Muething, C., Call, N., Pavlov, A., Ringdahl, J., Gillespie, S., Clark, S. & Mevers, J. L. (2020). Prevalence of renewal of problem behavior during context changes. *Journal of Applied Behavior Analysis*. https://doi.org/10.1002/jaba.672.

National Council for Disability. (2009). (Retrieved December 4, 2019). Institutions: Definitions, populations, and trends. https://ncd.gov/publications/2012/Sept192012/Institutions

Pace, G. M., Iwata, B. A., Cowdery, G. E., Andree, P. J., & McIntyre, T. (1993). Stimulus (instructional) fading during extinction of self-injurious escape behavior. *Journal of Applied Behavior Analysis, 26*, 205–212. https://doi.org/10.1901/jaba.1993.26-205.

Park, K. L., & Scott, T. M. (2009). Antecedent-based interventions for young children at risk for emotional and behavioral disorders. *Behavioral Disorders, 34*, 196–211. https://doi.org/10.1177/019874290903400402

Pelios, L., Morren, J., Tesch, D., & Axelrod, S. (1999). The impact of functional analysis methodology on treatment choice for self-injurious and aggressive behavior. *Journal of Applied Behavior Analysis, 32*, 185–195. https://doi.org/10.1901/jaba.1999.32-185

Petscher, E. S., Rey, C., & Bailey, J. S. (2009). A review of empirical support for differential reinforcement of alternative behavior. *Research in Developmental Disabilities, 30*, 409–425. https://doi.org/10.1016/j.ridd.2008.08.008

Piazza, C. C., Adelinis, J. D., Hanley, G. P., Goh, H., & Delia, M. D. (2000). An evaluation of the effects of matched stimuli on behaviors maintained by automatic reinforcement. *Journal of Applied Behavior Analysis, 33*, 13–27. https://doi.org/10.1901/jaba.2000.33-13.

Piazza, C. C., Hanley, G. P., Bowman, L. G., Ruyter, J. M., Lindauer, S. E., & Saiontz, D. M. (1997). Functional analysis and treatment of elopement. *Journal of Applied Behavior Analysis, 30*(4), 653–672. https://doi.org/10.1901/jaba.1997.30-653

Piazza, C. C., Hanley, G. P., & Fisher, W. W. (1996). Functional analysis and treatment of cigarette pica. *Journal of Applied Behavior Analysis, 29*, 437–450. https://doi.org/10.1901/jaba.1996.29-437

Piazza, C. C., Patel, M. R., Gulotta, C. S., Sevin, B. M., & Layer, S. A. (2003). On the relative contributions of positive reinforcement and escape extinction in the treatment of food refusal. *Journal of Applied Behavior Analysis, 36*, 309–324. https://doi.org/10.1901/jaba.2003.36-309

Podlesnik, C. A., Kelley, M. E., Jimenez-Gomez, C., & Bouton, M. E. (2017). Renewed behavior produced by context change and its implications for treatment maintenance: A review. *Journal of Applied Behavior Analysis, 50*, 675–697. https://doi.org/10.1002/jaba.400

Rapp J. T. (2007). Further evaluation of methods to identify matched stimulation. *Journal of applied behavior analysis, 40*(1), 73–88. https://doi.org/10.1901/jaba.2007.142-05

Reid, D. H., Parsons, M. B., Phillips, J. F., & Green, C. W. (1993). Reduction of self-injurious hand mouthing using response blocking. *Journal of Applied Behavior Analysis, 26*, 139–140. https://doi.org/10.1901/jaba.1993.26-139

Richman, D. M., Wacker, D. P., & Winborn, L. (2001). Response efficiency during functional communication training: Effects of effort on response allocation. *Journal of Applied Behavior Analysis, 34*, 73–76. https://doi.org/10.1901/jaba.2001.34-73

Rincover, A. (1978). Sensory extinction: A procedure for eliminating self-stimulatory behavior in developmentally disabled children. *Journal of Abnormal Psychology, 6*, 299–310. https://doi.org/10.1007/BF00924733

Rincover, A., Cook, R., Peoples, A., & Packard, D. (1979). Sensory extinction and sensory reinforcement principles for programming multiple adaptive behavior changes. *Journal of Applied Behavior Analysis, 12*, 221–233. https://doi.org/10.1901/jaba.1979.12-221

Rincover, A., Newsom, C. D., & Carr, E. G. (1979). Using sensory extinction procedures in the treatment of compulsive-like behavior of developmentally disabled children. *Journal of Consulting and Clinical Psychology, 4*, 695–701. https://doi.org/10.1037/0022-006X.47.4.695

Ringdahl, J. E., Kitsukawa, K., Andelman, M. S., Call, N., Winborn, L., Barretto, A., & Reed, G. K. (2002). Differential reinforcement with and without instructional fading. *Journal of Applied Behavior Analysis, 35*, 291–294. https://doi.org/10.1901/jaba.2002.35-291

Roane, H. S., Call, N. A., & Falcomata, T. S. (2005). A preliminary analysis of adaptive responding under open and closed economies. *Journal of Applied Behavior Analysis, 38*, 335–348. https://doi.org/10.1901/jaba.2005.85-04.

Roane, H. S., Fisher, W. W., Sgro, G. M., Falcomata, T. S., & Pabico, R. R. (2004). An alternative method of thinning reinforce delivery during differential reinforcement. *Journal of Applied Behavior Analysis, 37*, 213–218. https://doi.org/10.1901/jaba.2004.37-213

Rozenblat, E., Brown, J. L., Brown, A. K., Reeve, S. A., & Reeve, K. F. (2009). Effects of adjusting DRO schedules on the reduction of stereotypic vocalizations in children with autism. *Behavioral Interventions, 24*, 1–15. https://doi.org/10.1002/bin.270

Saini, V., Sullivan, W. E., Baxter, E. L., DeRosa, N. M., & Roane, H. S. (2018). Renewal during functional communication training. *Journal of Applied Behavior Analysis, 51*, 603–619. https://doi.org/10.1002/jaba.471

Sajwaj, T., Libet, J., & Agras, S. (1974). Lemon-juice therapy: The control of life-threatening rumination in a six-month-old infant. *Journal of Applied Behavior Analysis, 7*, 557–563. https://doi.org/10.1901/jaba.1974.7-557

Scalzo, K., Forwell, S., & Suto, M. (2016). An integrative review exploring transition following an unexpected health-related trauma. *Journal of Occupational Science, 23*, 1–20. https://doi.org/10.1080/14427591.2016.1223742

Schmuckler, M. A. (2010). What is ecological validity? A dimensional analysis. *Infancy, 2*, 419–436. https://doi.org/10.1207/S15327072IN0204_02

Shogren, K. A., Faggella-Luby, M. N., Bae, S. J., & Wehmeyer, M. L. (2004). The effect of choice-making as an intervention for problem behavior: A meta-analysis. *Journal of Positive Behavior Interventions, 6*, 228–237. https://doi.org/10.1177/10983007040060040401

Singh, J., Illes, J., Lazzeroni, L., & Hallmayer, J. (2009). Trends in US autism research funding. *Journal of Autism and Developmental Disorders, 39*, 788–795. https://doi.org/10.1007/s10803-008-0685-0

Skinner, B. F. (1938). *The behavior of organisms: An experimental analysis*. New York, NY: Appleton-Century.

Slocum, S. K., Grauerholz-Fisher, E., Peters, K. P. & Vollmer, T. R. (2018). A multicomponent approach to thinning reinforcer delivery during noncontingent reinforcement schedules. *Journal of Applied Behavior Analysis, 51*, 61–69. https://doi.org/10.1002/jaba.427

Slocum, S. K., & Vollmer, T. R. (2015). A comparison of positive and negative reinforcement for compliance to treat problem behavior maintained by escape. *Journal of Applied Behavior Analysis, 48*, 563–574. https://doi.org/10.1002/jaba.216

Smith, R. G., Russo, L., & Le, D. D. (1999). Distinguishing between extinction and punishment effects of response blocking: A replication. *Journal of Applied Behavior Analysis, 32*, 367–370. https://doi.org/10.1901/jaba.1999.32-367

Sprague, J. R., & Horner, R. H. (1992). Covariation within functional response classes: Implications for treatment of severe problem behavior. *Journal of Applied Behavior Analysis, 25*, 735–745. https://doi.org/10.1901/jaba.1992.25-735

Tanner, B. A., & Zeiler, M. (1975). Punishment of self-injurious behavior using aromatic ammonia as the aversive stimulus. *Journal of Applied Behavior Analysis, 8*, 53–57. https://doi.org/10.1901/jaba.1975.8-53

Tiger, J. H., Hanley, G. P., & Bruzek, J. (2008). Functional communication training: A review and practical guide. *Behavior Analysis in Practice, 1*, 16–23. https://doi.org/10.1007/BF03391716

Tiger, J. H., Hanley, G. P., & Hernandez, E. (2006). An evaluation of the value of choice with preschool children. *Journal of Applied Behavior Analysis, 39*, 1–16. https://doi.org/10.1901/jaba.2006.158-04

Torelli, J. N., Lambert, J. M., Da Fonte, M. A., Denham, K. N., Jedrzynski, T. M., & Houchins-Juarez, N. J. (2016). Assessing acquisition of and preference for mand topographies during functional communication training. *Behavior Analysis in Practice, 9*, 165–168. https://doi.org/10.1007/s40617-015-0083-y

Toussaint, K. A., & Tiger, J. H. (2012). Reducing covert self-injurious behavior maintained by automatic reinforcement through a variable momentary DRO procedure. *Journal of Applied Behavior Analysis, 45*, 179–184. https://doi.org/10.1901/jaba.2012.45-179

Van Camp C, M., Lerman D. C., Kelley M. E., Roane H. S., Contrucci S. A., Vorndran C. M. (2000). Further analysis of idiosyncratic antecedent influences during the assessment and treatment of problem behavior. *Journal of Applied Behavior Analysis 33*(2):207–221. https://doi.org/10.1901/jaba.2000.33-207. PMID: 10885528; PMCID: PMC1284239.

Volkert, V. M., Lerman, D. C., Call, N. A., & Trosclair-Lasserre, N. (2013). An evaluation of resurgence during treatment with functional communication training. *Journal of Applied Behavior Analysis, 42*, 145–160. https://doi.org/10.1901/jaba.2009.42-145

Vollmer, T. R., Hagopian, L. P., Bailey, J. S., Dorsey, M. F., Hanley, G. P., Lennox, D., ... Spreat, S. (2011). The association for behavior analysis international position statement on restraint and seclusion. *The Behavior Analyst, 34*, 103–110. https://doi.org/10.1007/bf03392238

Vollmer, T. R., & Iwata, B. A. (1992). Differential reinforcement as treatment for behavior disorders: Procedural and functional variations. *Research in Developmental Disabilities, 13*, 393–417. https://doi.org/10.1016/0891-4222(92)90013-V

Vollmer, T. R., Iwata, B. A., Zarcone, J. R., Smith, R. G., & Mazaleski, J. L. (1993). The role of attention in the treatment of attention-maintained self-injurious behavior: Noncontingent reinforcement and differential reinforcement of other behavior. *Journal of Applied Behavior Analysis, 26*, 9–21. https://doi.org/10.1901/jaba.1993.26-9

Vollmer, T. R., Peters, K. P., & Slocum, S. K. (2015). Treatment of severe behavior disorders. In *Clinical and organizational applications of applied behavior analysis* (pp. 47–67). Waltham, MA: Elsevier.

Vollmer, T. R., Ringdahl, J. E., Roane, H. S., & Marcus, B. A. (1997). Negative side effects of noncontingent reinforcement. *Journal of Applied Behavior Analysis, 30*, 161–164. https://doi.org/10.1901/jaba.1997.30-161

Wallace, M. D., Iwata, B. A., Hanley, G. P., Thompson, R. H., & Roscoe, E. M. (2012). Noncontingent reinforcement: a further examination of schedule effects during treatment. *Journal of applied behavior analysis , 45*(4), 709–719. https://doi.org/10.1901/jaba.2012.45-709

Weston, R., Hodges, A., & Davis, T. N. (2018). Differential reinforcement of other behaviors to treat challenging behaviors among children with autism: A systematic and quality review. *Behavior Modification, 42*, 584–609. https://doi.org/10.1177/0145445517743487

Wilder, D. A., Allison, J., Nicholson, K., Abellon, O. E., & Saulnier, R. (2010). Further evaluation of antecedent interventions on compliance: The effects of rationales to increase compliance among preschoolers. *Journal of Applied Behavior Analysis, 43*, 601–613. https://doi.org/10.1901/jaba.2010.43-601

Wilder, D. A., Masuda, A., O'Connor, C., & Baham, M. (2012). Brief functional analysis and treatment of bizarre vocalizations in an adult with schizophrenia. *Journal of Applied Behavior Analysis, 34*, 65–68. https://doi.org/10.1901/jaba.2001.34-65

Winborn-Kemmerer, L., Ringdahl, J. E., Wacker, D. P., & Kitsukawa, K. (2009). A demonstration of individual preference for novel mands during functional communication training. *Journal of Applied Behavior Analysis, 42*, 185–189. https://doi.org/10.1901/jaba.2009.42-185

Wolf, M. M. (1978). Social validity: The case for subjective measurement or how applied behavior analysis is finding its heart. *Journal of Applied Behavior Analysis, 11*, 203–214. https://doi.org/10.1901/jaba.1978.11-203

Woods, D. W., Fuqua, W., Siah, A., Murray, L. K., Welch, E. B., & Seif, T. (2001). Understanding habits: A preliminary investigation of nail biting function in children. *Education and Treatment of Children, 24*, 199–216. https://www.jstor.org/stable/42899654.

Zangrillo, A. N., Fisher, W. W., Greer, B. D., Owen, T. M., & DeSouza, A. A. (2016). Treatment of escape-maintained challenging behavior using chained schedules: An evaluation of the effects of thinning positive plus negative reinforcement during functional communication training. *International Journal of Developmental Disabilities, 62*, 147–156. https://doi.org/10.1080/20473869.2016.1176308

Chapter 13
The Role of Functional Assessment in Treatment Planning for Challenging Behavior

Kelly M. Schieltz and Wendy K. Berg

Introduction

Functional assessments of severe challenging behavior have become an integral part of developing behavioral treatments to reduce the occurrence of challenging behavior and increase adaptive responses. When the results of a functional analysis (FA; Iwata, Dorsey, Slifer, Bauman, & Richman, 1982/1994) show consistent patterns of challenging behavior within each test condition, and differentiation in behavior between test conditions, identifying the function(s) of the behavior is fairly straightforward. In many cases, knowing the function of a target behavior is sufficient to identify an effective reinforcer-based treatment approach to (a) reduce challenging behavior (e.g., by withholding the identified functional reinforcer via extinction) and (b) increase a desired alternative response (e.g., by providing the same functional reinforcer contingent on an alternative response that serves the same function as challenging behavior) (Beavers, Iwata, & Lerman, 2013; Lerman, 2013).

Once we know the reinforcers maintaining challenging behavior, at least two classes of treatment can be developed, with the first class involving primarily a consequence-based approach to treatment and the second class involving an antecedent-based approach. In both the consequence and antecedent classes of treatment, the active variable in treatment is the functional reinforcer identified via

K. M. Schieltz (✉)
Stead Family Department of Pediatrics, The University of Iowa Carver College of Medicine, The University of Iowa Stead Family Children's Hospital, Iowa City, IA, USA

Center for Disabilities and Development, The University of Iowa Stead Family Children's Hospital, Iowa City, IA, USA
e-mail: kelly-schieltz@uiowa.edu

W. K. Berg
Center for Disabilities and Development, The University of Iowa Stead Family Children's Hospital, Iowa City, IA, USA

© Springer Nature Switzerland AG 2021
J. L. Matson (ed.), *Functional Assessment for Challenging Behaviors and Mental Health Disorders*, Autism and Child Psychopathology Series,
https://doi.org/10.1007/978-3-030-66270-7_13

the FA. The first class of treatment, consequence-based, provides the identified functional reinforcers contingently for appropriate behavior and withholds those same reinforcers for challenging behavior. This approach to treatment has proven to be highly successful, as shown by the large-scale applications of functional communication training (FCT; Carr & Durand, 1985; Kurtz, Boelter, Jarmolowicz, Chin, & Hagopian, 2011; Tiger, Hanley, & Bruzek, 2008). In FCT, we provide the functional reinforcer identified in the FA as maintaining challenging behavior contingently for appropriate communication (Carr & Durand, 1985). Equally important, we make every attempt to withhold the functional reinforcer for challenging behavior. In this case, we are attempting to substitute appropriate behavior for challenging behavior within a differential reinforcement of alternative behavior (DRA) treatment program (Reichle & Wacker, 2017).

The second class of treatment, antecedent-based, involves alterations to the environment prior to the occurrence of challenging behavior. For example, we might provide the functional reinforcer in a time-based treatment, meaning that the reinforcer identified in the FA is now delivered based on the passage of time (e.g., Lalli, Casey, & Kates, 1997; Reed, Ringdahl, Wacker, Barretto, & Andelman, 2005; Vollmer, Iwata, Zarcone, Smith, & Mazaleski, 1993). If we are able to determine that challenging behavior is occurring at a particular rate (e.g., every 60 seconds), then providing the functional reinforcer every 45 seconds should reduce or eliminate the occurrence of challenging behavior. In this case, we are attempting to prevent challenging behavior, or alter its probability of occurrence, by providing the reinforcer "freely" on a schedule that is sufficient to reduce the establishing operation (Laraway, Snycerski, Michael, & Poling, 2003; Michael, 1982) for challenging behavior.

Reinforcement-based treatment, then, can be determined directly from the results of a FA and can focus on antecedent, consequence, or both classes of treatment. If treatments based exclusively on the results of an FA are sufficient for reducing challenging behavior to acceptable levels, then no further assessment is needed, which is often the case in the FCT literature (e.g., Durand & Carr, 1991; Hagopian, Fisher, Thibault Sullivan, Acquisto, & LeBlanc, 1998; Wacker et al., 2013). However, in other cases, more information may be needed, or would be beneficial, in developing an effective treatment. This may especially be the case if the results of the original treatment that was based on the FA suggest that the treatment is not working, or not working as well as we would have preferred. Thus, subsequent assessment is used to improve the effects of treatment, even if the treatment is working well. In these cases, there may be a need to fade some of the treatment components to, for example, reduce the time taken to implement the procedure, the complexity of the treatment, or planning for the long-term maintenance of the results of treatment.

In applied settings, treatment packages often involve more than a specific DRA component, meaning that they are a bit more complex and involve many components comprised of both antecedent and consequence variables. Although the FA is an important initial step in developing an effective treatment for challenging behavior, subsequent consequence and antecedent assessments may be required for further identifying the variables that are related to both the ongoing occurrence of challenging behavior and the display of desired adaptive behavior.

Relative to consequences, the results of a FA identify the response-reinforcer relation between challenging behavior and the reinforcers maintaining that behavior. Subsequent assessments of consequences can provide information that supplement the results of FAs in the following ways. First, identifying other, arbitrary reinforcers for behaviors other than the challenging behavior may provide critical information for developing the treatment (e.g., Fischer, Iwata, & Mazaleski, 1997; Fisher, DeLeon, Rodriguez-Catter, & Keeney, 2004; Fuhrman, Greer, Zangrillo, & Fisher, 2018; Payne & Dozier, 2013). For example, if the individual engages in challenging behavior to escape demands, a preference assessment may reveal what preferred toys should be available during breaks from demands that occur because of compliant behavior. Second, identifying specific qualities or types of reinforcement that are more or less potent for the individual may be useful for treatment planning (e.g., Sumter, Gifford, Tiger, Effertz, & Fulton, 2020). For example, identifying whether attention from another adult (or tangible items) is substitutable for mom's attention (functional reinforcer) may show variations in how adult attention can be provided at home. Third, identifying the schedule of reinforcement that is needed to maintain appropriate responding in the absence of challenging behavior, such as the maximum length of time that occurs between the removal of tangibles or attention and the first occurrence of challenging behavior, would suggest how long treatment sessions should occur and would be important for developing fading plans (e.g., Wacker et al., 2011). Fourth, reinforcer assessments might identify both the reinforcers and the contingencies that maintain appropriate responding versus the occurrence of challenging behavior that is maintained by automatic reinforcement (e.g., Berg et al., 2016).

One advantage of FAs over other functional assessment procedures is that the results identify the motivating operations (MOs) and other specific antecedent stimuli associated with the occurrence of challenging behavior in addition to the reinforcers maintaining challenging behavior. These antecedent conditions are known as MOs, which refer to the events that temporarily alter the value of a reinforcer and thereby alter the occurrence of responses associated with gaining access to the reinforcer in the past (Michael, 1982). MOs are events and other stimuli that temporarily decrease the value of a reinforcer (i.e., abolishing operations; AOs) or increase the value of a reinforcer (i.e., establishing operations; EOs) that maintains a response. These MOs, then, subsequently (but temporarily) decrease or increase, respectively, the likelihood of the future occurrence of the targeted response (Laraway et al., 2003).

For treatment planning purposes, antecedent assessments can supplement FA results, in the following ways. First, identifying conditions that establish the value of the functional reinforcer for appropriate behaviors may provide options for preventing the occurrence of challenging behavior (e.g., Berg et al., 2000; Schieltz, Wacker, & Romani, 2017). For example, providing noncontingent access to preferred toys when parent attention is removed may be an effective approach to prevent challenging behavior maintained by attention. Similarly, signaling the availability of an arbitrary (but potent) positive reinforcer for task completion may be an effective treatment for escape-maintained challenging behavior. Second, identifying conditions that abolish the value of the functional reinforcer for challenging behavior may result in the reduction of challenging behavior (e.g., Gardner, Wacker, & Boelter, 2009). For example, providing noncontingent access to high-quality attention during the presentation of demands may abolish the MO to escape the demand. Similarly, signaling the availability of high preferred tangibles prior to the removal of attention may function as an AO.

The response-reinforcer and stimulus-response relations identified by the results of a FA translate to two classes of treatment, consequence-based and antecedent-based, that can be implemented within each identified function of challenging behavior. The consequence component of a treatment plan for challenging behavior that is maintained by negative reinforcement may include a break from the task, and we may need to enrich those breaks by incorporating highly preferred tangible items into the break. The antecedent components may include a reduction in task amount or difficulty. Relative to challenging behavior maintained by positive reinforcement, consequence treatment components may include adjustments in the qualities or preferences for the functional reinforcers and/or adjustments in the schedule of reinforcement. Relative to antecedent treatment components for challenging behavior maintained by positive reinforcement, components may include providing access to alternative reinforcers during the delay periods to the functional reinforcer or providing noncontingent access to the functional reinforcer as a means for abolishing its value for a period of time. For challenging behavior that is maintained by automatic reinforcement, consequence and antecedent treatment components may include providing contingent or noncontingent access to preferred items that compete with the reinforcers maintaining challenging behavior.

In the following sections, we describe examples of these supplemental consequence and antecedent assessments conducted to inform treatment packages for each identified behavioral function.

Negative Reinforcement

Escape from demands (i.e., negative reinforcement) is the most common function identified for challenging behavior (Beavers et al., 2013; Iwata et al., 1994). This function is identified when challenging behavior occurs following the presentation of a demand and results in the contingent removal of that demand. Demands that have resulted in the occurrence of challenging behavior have ranged from tasks of daily living such as picking up toys and brushing teeth (e.g., Harding, Wacker, Berg, Lee, & Dolezal, 2009; Steege et al., 1990) to academic tasks such as completing math or reading (e.g., McComas, Hoch, Paone, & El-Roy, 2000; Schieltz et al., 2020). With the diverse range and characteristics of demands that result in challenging behavior, further information on the variables associated with demands that occasion or prevent challenging behavior, and the specific consequences that reinforce both problem and compliant behavior, are often needed to prescribe specific treatment plans. For example, evaluations of the effects of potential consequences that can be used in treatment programs to reduce challenging behavior may include manipulations to the response-reinforcer contingencies associated with specific tasks or types of demands (e.g., Richman et al., 2001) and the types of activities that are provided during breaks from the task (e.g., Golonka et al., 2000; Zarcone, Fisher, & Piazza, 1996). Assessments of antecedent variables might involve manipulations of the events prior to the demand (e.g., Lalli et al., 1999; Schieltz et al., 2017) or dimensions of the demand itself (e.g., Boelter et al., 2007; Dunlap, Kern-Dunlap, Clarke, & Robbins, 1991; McComas et al., 2000) to determine if these variables establish or abolish the value of negative reinforcement. Again, we often initiate treatment, such as FCT, immediately following the completion of the FA. If treatment is successful, then no further assessment may be needed, at least until we begin to fade the treatment to promote maintenance. However, if treatment is not successful, or for some reason requires alteration (e.g., the care provider does not find the initial treatment to be acceptable), then the following assessment procedures might be considered. Selected examples of these procedures are provided in Table 13.1 and are briefly described below.

Consequence Assessments   Within the demand condition of the FA, consequences are arranged such that when challenging behavior occurs in response to the presentation of a demand, the demand is removed. When the demand is removed, the individual most commonly receives a brief break from the demand (with the break often not involving anything preferred to the individual). Thus, when planning for treatment to address challenging behavior maintained by negative reinforcement, arrangement of the contingencies for compliance with the demand needs to be considered, as do the variables that are in place during the break. Some options to evaluate include comparisons between breaks alone and enriched breaks (Golonka et al., 2000; Zarcone et al., 1996) and/or distributed and accumulated breaks (Bukala, Hu, Lee, Ward-Horner, & Fienup, 2015; DeLeon et al., 2014; Fulton, Tiger, Meitzen, & Effertz, 2020).

Relative to breaks alone versus enriched breaks, previous studies have demonstrated that enriched breaks were more effective at increasing compliance and decreasing the occurrence of challenging behavior than breaks alone (Golonka et al., 2000; Zarcone et al., 1996). For example, Zarcone et al. (1996) compared the effects of breaks alone and enriched breaks on the rate of task completion displayed by a 10-year-old boy with autism spectrum disorder and profound intellectual disabilities. During the break alone condition, the child received a 20 s break which included the availability to leave the work area and wander around the room. However, no interactions with others or leisure items were available. During the enriched break condition, the child received a 20 s break which included the availability to leave the work area to engage with others and leisure items. Across both conditions, breaks were provided following task completion. Using a combined reversal-multielement design, results showed that task completion occurred at higher rates during the enriched breaks condition, which continued across different

Table 13.1 Summary of selected assessment procedures, rationales, and implications for treatment planning for challenging behavior maintained by negative reinforcement

Assessment procedure	Procedural steps	Rationale	Implications for treatment planning
Consequence assessments			
Reinforcer type assessment	Compare levels of challenging behavior when reinforcers for task completion include access to (a) an enriched break versus (b) a break with nothing	Determine if differentiated responding occurs between types of breaks	Type of negative reinforcement may be helpful in determining whether to enrich the break for task completion
Reinforcer timing assessment	1. Compare levels of challenging behavior when reinforcers for task completion are (a) distributed for completion of portions of the tasks and (b) accumulated throughout the task, but provided at the end of the task 2. Evaluate preference for reinforcer timing arrangement	Determine if differentiated responding occurs between the timing of the reinforcement delivery	Timing of the reinforcer delivery may be helpful in determining whether to intersperse reinforcement for completion of smaller or shorter work requirements
Contingency analysis	Compare levels of challenging behavior and compliance when reinforcers are provided contingent on (a) accurate responding and (b) attempted responding	Determine if differentiated responding occurs between contingencies for accuracy versus attempts	Contingent reinforcers may be more effective when based on the skills of the individual (i.e., reinforcers for accuracy when requesting completion of an independent skill versus reinforcers for attempts when requesting completion of an emerging or difficult skill)
Antecedent assessments			
Reinforcer presentation assessment	Compare levels of task completion and challenging behavior when reinforcers for task completion are (a) signaled vs. unsignaled or (b) contingent vs. noncontingent	Determine if differentiated responding occurs between the presentation of reinforcers	Signaling contingent access to reinforcers for task completion may be an important treatment component for increasing the motivation to engage in desired behaviors

(continued)

Table 13.1 (continued)

Assessment procedure	Procedural steps	Rationale	Implications for treatment planning
Assessment of demand dimensions	Compare levels of task engagement and challenging behavior during various conditions such as (a) preferred vs. non-preferred tasks, (b) choice vs. no choice of tasks, (c) person presenting the demand, (d) type of demand, (e) difficulty level of the demand, (f) amount of the demand, and (g) instructional strategies to assist with the demand	Determine if differentiated responding occurs between antecedent variables that alter various dimensions of the demand	Altering dimensions of the demand may be effective at decreasing the motivation to engage in challenging behavior to obtain escape as a reinforcer

tasks and increased work requirements. Golonka et al. showed similar results for task completion, as well as decreased occurrences of challenging behavior.

Another assessment option to consider related to consequences entails the timing of the reinforcement provision. Some individuals may prefer to receive reinforcers more frequently (distributed reinforcement) whereas others may prefer to receive reinforcers all at once (accumulated reinforcement). For example, Fulton et al. (2020) evaluated the effects of these contingency arrangements on the challenging behavior and compliance of three children, aged 8–11 years old, with diagnoses of autism spectrum disorder and attention deficit hyperactivity disorder. All children engaged in challenging behavior that was maintained by negative reinforcement. During the distributed reinforcement condition, a 30 s enriched break (access to a high preferred leisure item) was provided contingent on compliance on a fixed ratio (FR) 1 schedule. During the accumulated reinforcement condition, praise for compliance was delivered on a FR1 schedule until 15 praise statements had been delivered, wherein the enriched break was provided for 7.5 min. Results of this evaluation, which was conducted within a multielement design, showed different patterns of responding across children. Specifically, for one child, challenging behavior did not occur, and compliance remained high across both conditions. In contrast, for the other two children, challenging behavior continued to occur with varying levels of compliance during the distributed reinforcement condition, whereas challenging behavior decreased to near zero levels with compliance increasing and remaining relatively more stable in the accumulated reinforcement condition. Following the condition comparisons, a preference assessment was conducted to determine each child's relative preference for the distribution timing of the reinforcers for compliance. Results of the preference assessment showed that two of the children exclusively preferred the distributed and accumulated arrangements, respectively, whereas the results for the third child varied across conditions.

In addition to the quality and timing of the reinforcers, the specific reinforcement contingency can also be considered, and especially in relation to demands that interact with skill issues. One example of this type of assessment was provided by Richman et al. (2001) who further showed how antecedent variables can interact with consequence variables. Specifically, Richman et al. evaluated the effects of manipulating the contingencies for receiving reinforcement on task completion and challenging behavior maintained by escape from demands. The effects of providing reinforcement (i.e., praise and a 10–15-sec break from the task) contingent on attempts to complete a task and completing the task accurately were compared with a young girl with challenging behavior maintained by escape from demands. Prior to comparing the effects of different response contingencies for reinforcement, the effects of different types of prompts on the participant's accuracy in completing academic tasks were identified and used to identify a prompt that consistently resulted in accurate responding (one-step verbal prompts) and a prompt that typically resulted in inaccurate responding (three-step verbal prompts). During the response contingency comparison, the investigators used a reversal design to alternate the type of prompt provided (effective versus ineffective) across sessions while comparing the effects of providing reinforcement (i.e., praise and a 10–15 sec break from the task) contingent on attempting the work task or completing the work task accurately. Results showed that the participant responded accurately and without challenging behavior across both reinforcement contingencies (attempts versus accuracy) when effective prompts (one-step instructions) were used to present the task. For three-step instructions, challenging behavior only occurred when reinforcement was contingent on accurate responding. Thus, displays of challenging behavior were related to both the prompts and reinforcement contingencies provided.

As summarized in Table 13.1, reinforcer assessments may identify what reinforcers to include for adaptive/compliant behavior, when to distribute those reinforcers following task completion, and how those reinforcement contingencies may vary across antecedent variables. In addition, if skill issues are interfering with an individual's compliant behavior, altering the dependent variable (the target response) that is reinforced may have the immediate effect of reducing challenging behavior. This may be especially important to care providers who are dealing with very severe challenging behavior or for clients who are displaying severe emotional responding in the presence of some demands but not other demands.

Antecedent Assessments One goal for antecedent assessments associated with negative reinforcement is to identify the specific events that establish or abolish escape as a reinforcer in a specific context, such as with specific tasks. Numerous studies (e.g., Call, Wacker, Ringdahl, Cooper-Brown, & Boelter, 2004; Dunlap et al., 1991; Horner, Day, Sprague, O'Brien, & Heathfield, 1991; Smith, Iwata, Goh, & Shore, 1995) have demonstrated that manipulations to specific independent variables associated with a demand can influence the likelihood that the demand will occasion target behavior. Changes in target behavior associated with these manipulations are used to identify EOs and/or AOs for challenging behavior with specific tasks or in specific contexts. There are so many antecedent variables that can alter

MOs, that we attempt, at least initially, to base the manipulations during assessment on those variables that we hypothesize to be related to challenging behavior. We then use the assessment procedures to vary their presentation systematically, in order to identify the variables that establish or abolish escape as a reinforcer.

Variables related to task demands that have been evaluated include the effects of task preference (e.g., Dunlap et al., 1991; Killu, Clare, & Im, 1999; May, 2019), task choice (e.g., Dunlap et al., 1994; Romaniuk et al., 2002), person presenting the demand (Boelter et al., 2007; Ringdahl & Sellers, 2000), type of demand (e.g., Roscoe, Rooker, Pence, Longworth, & Zarcone, 2009), difficulty level of the demand (e.g., Boelter et al., 2007; Richman et al., 2001), presentation of the demand (e.g., Cengher et al., 2016; Horner et al., 1991; Mace et al., 1988; Richman et al., 2001; Schnell et al., 2020; Seaver & Bourret, 2014), availability of adult attention or other preferred stimuli during the demand (e.g., Call et al., 2004; Gardner et al., 2009; Kettering, Fisher, Kelley, & LaRue, 2018), and use of instructional strategies to support completion of the academic task as the demand (e.g., McComas et al., 1996; McComas et al., 2000; McComas, Wacker, & Cooper, 1996; Schieltz et al., 2020). In the following paragraphs, we briefly highlight preference and choice for the task, difficulty level of the task, and instructional strategies to support completion of the task.

Relative to task preference and task choice, Killu et al. (1999) evaluated the effects of task preference and the opportunity to choose between tasks on task completion with two 12-year-old boys diagnosed with learning disabilities and a 13-year-old boy with developmental delays. Each of the participants showed high levels of off-task behavior during academic tasks. Following preference assessments to identify preferred and non-preferred academic tasks for each participant, the authors compared the levels of task engagement when task preference and task choice varied (i.e., preferred and non-preferred tasks without choice, preferred and non-preferred tasks with choice). Using a case study design, each participant showed greater task completion with preferred tasks than non-preferred tasks, whereas the opportunity to choose between tasks provided no additional effects beyond those of task preference. Although choice of tasks did not result in better outcomes for this study, a review of 38 studies conducted by Howell, Dounavi, and Storey (2019) showed that choice has resulted in better outcomes for 45% of the participants when the variable of choice was evaluated.

Relative to task difficulty, Boelter et al. (2007) demonstrated that challenging behavior in the context of demands may reflect skill deficits that interfere with following the directions or prompts provided rather than the motivation to escape or avoid the specific tasks. Boelter et al. compared the effects of presenting demands using one-step directions versus three-step directions on the accuracy of task completion and occurrence of challenging behavior for three young boys, aged 3–6 years old, who had developmental disabilities (e.g., attention deficit hyperactivity disorder, developmental delays, autism spectrum disorder) and histories of engaging in challenging behavior. Results showed that each of the participants responded at high levels of accuracy (i.e., 80–100% accuracy) to demands delivered as one-step directions and low levels of accuracy (i.e., 0–40% accuracy) to demands delivered as three-step directions. Although accuracy of responding varied according to the number of task steps presented within each demand for all participants, challenging behavior occurred exclusively during the three-step demand condition for one of the participants. These results show that challenging behavior can be occasioned by how demands are presented rather than to the specific task.

When skill deficits occur as a result of increased difficulty, such as with academic tasks like reading and math, identifying instructional strategies that assist the learner in completing those tasks successfully becomes an important consideration. For example, McComas et al. (2000) evaluated the effects of different instructional strategies on the challenging behavior maintained by escape from academic tasks displayed by three 8-year-old boys with autism spectrum disorder and developmental disabilities. In this study, the researchers developed hypotheses related to the variables establishing escape as a reinforcer for challenging behavior and focused on using instructional strategies to reduce the demand level of the tasks. Based on both their observations of each child and a review of the literature, they next identified which instructional strategies to evaluate for each child, such as manipulatives and a number line for assistance with a difficult math task (Eli), choice of task sequence (Charlie), and inclusion of non-repetitive tasks (Ben). These strategy conditions were compared to a non-strategy condition (e.g., choice of task sequence versus no choice of task sequence) within multielement designs. Each child showed reduced levels of challenging behavior and increased levels of compliance when the identified strategy for that child was included in comparison to the non-strategy condition.

In addition to variables associated with the characteristics of the demands, other variables associated with reinforcement can function as AOs for challenging behavior maintained by negative reinforcement. Some variables that have been evaluated have included noncontingent access to positive reinforcers (e.g., Ingvarsson, Kahng, & Hausman, 2008; Lomas, Fisher, & Kelley, 2010) or negative reinforcers (e.g., Kodak, Miltenberger, & Romaniuk, 2003; Vollmer, Marcus, & Ringdahl, 1995), signaling access to contingent positive reinforcers prior to the demand (e.g., Dowdy, Tincani, Nipe, & Weiss, 2018; Lalli et al., 1999; Schieltz et al., 2017) and providing a choice of positive reinforcers immediately following compliance with the demand (e.g., Kodak, Lerman, Volkert, & Trosclair, 2007). An example of signaling positive reinforcement was presented by Schieltz et al. (2017). These authors evaluated the effects of signaling access to positive reinforcers for compliance prior to the presentation of demands for three typically developing children, aged 2–6 years old, who engaged in challenging behavior maintained by negative reinforcement. In this evaluation, baseline and treatment conditions were compared within a nonconcurrent multiple baseline with reversal design. During the baseline condition, the children were instructed to complete demands. If challenging behavior occurred, escape from the task was provided. The treatment condition was conducted in the same manner as the baseline condition, except that the child was asked to select a leisure activity he/she wanted to play with after completing the work task. When the activity was selected, it was either placed out of reach but within the child's sight or circled on a list that was also within the child's sight. Results showed that challenging behavior decreased for all three children when access to the positive reinforcer was signaled prior to the presentation of demands.

Given that many variables associated with demands can be evaluated to determine the conditions under which challenging behavior is more and less likely to occur, the identification of EOs and AOs, such as those summarized in Table 13.1, can often then be incorporated into a treatment program or perhaps serve as a beginning point for treatment.

Considerations for Treatment Planning Using the results of both consequence and antecedent assessments may be important for individualizing treatment plans for challenging behavior maintained by negative reinforcement. For example, the Richman et al. (2001) study mentioned previously showed that changes in task presentation and response contingencies resulted in changes in target behavior. Treatment, then, might begin with reinforcement for "attempts" (a differential reinforcement of other behavior [DRO] contingency) at the more difficult task level and then gradually be faded to accuracy (a DRA contingency) as skills improve at the difficult task level.

Positive Reinforcement for Tangibles

Challenging behavior maintained by positive reinforcement in the form of access to tangibles is identified in the FA when challenging behavior occurs following the removal or denial of specific stimuli (e.g., toys, leisure activities, food) and then results in the presentation of those stimuli. In DRA programs such as FCT, treatment approaches for challenging behavior maintained by tangibles provide access to the wanted item or activity contingent on appropriate behavior such as a communicative response and withhold those same stimuli for challenging behavior. This approach is often successful, as we noted above, but there are also common problems that occur with treatment. For example, in some cases, after appropriately communicating for an item, the client may not tolerate even a brief delay to obtain the item. Tolerating denials or delays to those items or activities may be needed such as when a favorite dessert is not available or an electronic tablet needs to be recharged. To initiate successful tolerance training, supplemental consequence and antecedent assessments may be useful for identifying the beginning parameters for treatment. For example, identifying how long an individual tolerates a delay before the occurrence of challenging behavior might be beneficial, as beginning treatment with a brief delay may be preferred by the care provider than beginning with no delay. A hierarchical preference assessment might identify other preferred stimuli that the client is willing to engage in during the delay. Similarly, identifying the relationship between how denials are presented and the occurrence of challenging behavior might inform which antecedents to include in treatment. Selected examples of these procedures are provided in Table 13.2 and are briefly described below.

Table 13.2 Summary of selected assessment procedures, rationales, and implications for treatment planning for challenging behavior maintained by positive reinforcement in the form of access to tangibles

Assessment procedure	Procedural steps	Rationale	Implications for treatment planning
Consequence assessments			
Dimensions of reinforcement assessment	1. Evaluate preferences for (a) quality of items and/or (b) magnitude of access to items 2. Evaluate the reinforcing efficacy of lower-quality items	1. Determine the preferred dimension of reinforcement for tangibles 2. Determine if lower-quality items function as reinforcers in the absence of higher-quality items	1. Incorporate the preferred dimensions of reinforcement for tangibles into the treatment plan 2. Use lower-quality items as the alternative reinforcers during delay periods
Delay assessment	Compare levels of challenging behavior during different delay periods using a progressive ratio schedule	Determine the lengths of time that challenging behavior does and does not occur (breakpoint) when tangibles are restricted	Begin the treatment plan at or slightly below the delay breakpoint
Competing reinforcer assessment	Compare levels of challenging behavior during restricted tangibles when alternative reinforcers (e.g., attention, lower-quality tangibles) are (a) present and (b) absent	Determine if differential responding occurs when alternative reinforcers are present during periods of restricted tangibles	Provide access to competing stimuli during periods of restricted tangibles
Antecedent assessments			
Noncontingent reinforcer access assessment	Evaluate the occurrence of challenging behavior when access to preferred stimuli is provided on fixed and/or variable time schedules	Determine if reductions in challenging behavior occur	Scheduled fixed time access may be effective in reducing challenging behavior
Pre-session exposure	Compare levels of challenging behavior during tangible test sessions following (a) pre-session access to tangibles and (b) no pre-session access	Determine if differentiated responding occurs when prior access to the preferred item is provided noncontingently prior to the item being restricted	Provide access to tangibles prior to the removal of tangibles
Presentation of removal assessment	Compare levels of challenging behavior when denial of the preferred item is provided in different ways such as (a) denial with an explanation, (b) denial with an explanation plus alternative activity, and (c) access contingent on completion of a non-preferred task	Determine if differential responding occurs across different methods of denial	The presentation of how preferred items are denied or removed may impact the occurrence of challenging behavior

Consequence Assessments When challenging behavior is maintained by positive reinforcement in the form of access to tangibles, it is presumed that the items and activities that are removed and occasion challenging behavior are preferred. By understanding which items and activities are more preferred (or of a higher quality) over others, treatment plans can be arranged to ensure that those items and activities are available or provided for more appropriate behavior. However, it should be noted that preference for items and activities is relative according to the items and activities available at the time, as well as the motivation to gain or maintain access to those items and activities. Additionally, free access to these items and activities may not always be possible. Therefore, treatment plans may need to identify the components that are needed to decrease challenging behavior during the delay between losing or being denied the preferred item and gaining access to the item. Several options exist for identifying these components, including assessments of (a) the dimensions of reinforcement surrounding the items and activities, (b) stimuli that may compete with access to the items and activities, and (c) the structural and reinforcement parameters of the treatment plan.

To understand the dimensions of reinforcement surrounding tangibles, numerous types of preference assessments are available for identifying these items and activities along a continuum of high to low preferred (DeLeon & Iwata, 1996; Fisher et al., 1992; Pace, Ivancic, Edwards, Iwata, & Page, 1985; Roane, Vollmer, Ringdahl, & Marcus, 1998). Two of the most common procedures are free operant preference assessments (Roane et al., 1998) and paired choice preference assessments (Fisher et al., 1992). Roane et al. (1998) first evaluated the efficacy of a free operant preference assessment, wherein all items were freely available throughout the session and preference was measured as a percentage of item engagement. This method of preference assessment is clinically important because the procedure is very easy and very quick to use. These identified preferred items were then validated using one of two reinforcer assessments. One reinforcer assessment (reinforcer assessment A) included a concurrent choice arrangement, in which allocation to one side of the room resulted in continuous access to the identified preferred item and allocation to the other side of the room resulted in access to nothing. These results showed that the items identified as preferred in the free operant assessment functioned as reinforcers in that the participants allocated their choice of location based on the availability of those items. The other reinforcer assessment (reinforcer assessment B) was conducted in a similar fashion but involved two work stations, one associated with contingent access to the identified preferred stimulus and one associated with contingent access to an identified non-preferred stimulus. The results of the reinforcer B assessment demonstrated that most participants spent more time working on a task that resulted in contingent access to the preferred item. Thus, even as the level of demand increased, the clients continued to allocate to the choice that resulted in the preferred item. Overall, and again important, especially from a clinical standpoint, the results of the free operant preference assessment often matched those of the paired choice assessment.

We highlighted the Roane et al. (1998) study because it describes two procedures for assessing preferences, with the free operant version being quicker and easier to implement and the paired choice version directly showing if preferred items are in fact reinforcing. Selecting which approach to use is based on the purposes of the assessment. If, for example, identifying preferred stimuli to be available during a delay period is important, then the free operant preference assessment is a good option. It is very easy to use and in fact can be conducted during the free play condition of the FA. Recording which toys the client is engaged with during free play provides a hierarchy of engagement across toys. If the challenging behavior then shows a tangible function, one or more of these toys may be inserted into a delay period to increase the client's tolerance for a delay. The paired choice method is more definitive in establishing a preference hierarchy. In the case of Roane et al., the paired choice assessment showed if the preferred stimuli reinforced engagement in a less preferred task. In other examples of paired choice procedures (e.g., Fisher et al., 1992), the results show the actual hierarchy across the stimuli. This hierarchy is identified because every stimulus is paired against every other stimulus, and so the results lead to the exact hierarchy from most to least preferred. This information is more prescriptive than the free operant method but can take quite a bit of time to conduct.

When a FA identifies a tangible function, the client will almost certainly be expected to wait to access the item, either by simply waiting to receive the item or by completing some other activity. In some cases, this is a very straightforward procedure in that the client is willing to wait, the wait times can be increased gradually over time, and the client then (in FCT programs) asks for the item to be returned. In other cases, however, the request to wait, to give up the item, or to complete another task results in challenging behavior. In these cases, further assessment in the form of preference assessments may be needed to identify preferred items and activities. Once identified, these items may serve as competing stimuli that can be offered during the delay period. This may be sufficient to begin treatment, even with items that are not initially highly preferred. For example, Taravella, Lerman, Contrucci, and Roane (2000) identified high and low stimulus items (see Pace et al., 1985, for a description of this procedure). The hierarchy of preference for the "low-preferred" items was then identified using a paired choice preference assessment. The authors showed that these identified items did, in fact, function as reinforcers for task completion. These results show that some items that are low in preference can still function as reinforcers. Similar results were shown by Bowman, Piazza, Fisher, Hagopian, and Kogan (1997) in that items ranked less preferred in a paired choice assessment can still function as reinforcers.

The results of Taravella et al. (2000) and Bowman et al. (1997) show that it is sometimes possible to identify reinforcing stimuli that are not shown to be highly preferred at least initially. This is important for some of our clients who display challenging behavior to obtain one or only a few items or activities. Given the results of a tangible function, and no engagement with any items other than the functional tangible reinforcer, we may decide that further preference assessment is not important. However, further identifying the relative preferences among stimuli, even stimuli that appear less preferred, may improve behavior during delay periods or reinforce task responding. For example, Sumter et al. (2020) showed that the availability of alternative functional reinforcers during the delay period was effective at reducing the challenging behavior displayed by two children, aged 7–8 years old, with autism spectrum disorder. In this study, challenging behavior was shown to be maintained by both access to attention and access to tangibles. Following FCT for each social function, a delay evaluation was conducted within a multielement design across two conditions, a 10-min delay with access to alternative reinforcers and a 10-min delay without access to alternative reinforcers. In the tangible context, the children were offered access to attention following an appropriate communicative response for access to the preferred tangible item. When the delay period ended, access to the tangible item was provided. The same procedures were used for the attention context, except that the tangible item was provided contingent on the communication response for attention and attention was provided contingent on the end of the delay period. Results showed that challenging behavior occurred at zero or near-zero levels during the tangible and attention contexts for one child when the alternative reinforcers were available. For the other child, challenging behavior remained at zero during the attention context with alternative reinforcers but continued to occur in the tangible context with attention as the alternative reinforcer. These results highlight the importance of additional assessments because in some cases alternative reinforcers will be effective, whereas in other cases they will not. And to make matters even more complex, the alternative stimuli may be effective in some contexts but not others for the same client. Again, if the results of the initial treatment are acceptable, then no further assessment is needed. But, if there are problems with beginning treatment, or when the procedures are altered (e.g., via fading), then these additional assessment procedures can be useful in guiding the development of treatment.

The procedures described above are, of course, useful for identifying stimuli that compete with the functional tangible item. We described how items shown to be low preferred can sometimes still function as reinforcers. The reverse can also be true, meaning that preferred stimuli may not function as reinforcers. For example, Roane, Lerman, and Vorndran (2001) evaluated the potency of reinforcers under increasing schedule requirements for four adolescents with developmental disabilities. Following the identification of two equally preferred stimuli that were assessed using a paired choice preference assessment, a reinforcer assessment was conducted using a progressive ratio schedule. During this assessment, each preferred stimulus was presented contingent on the completion of a progressive number of responses such that the response requirement increased after each trial that resulted in reinforcement. Results of this assessment showed that for all participants, only one of the stimuli resulted in continued responding as the schedule requirements increased, suggesting that not all stimuli identified as preferred maintain the same reinforcing value. The results from Roane et al. show that "preferred stimuli" do not always function as reinforcers and that items with similar preference do not always have the same potency as reinforcers. This is why it is important to conduct reinforcer assessments following preference assessments. For treatment planning, we can conduct these reinforcer assessments within the context of treatment by, for example, comparing two preferred items during wait times. A second benefit of this approach is that by conducting these comparisons, we are also identifying the length of wait time, or the tasks the clients will complete, for each of the stimuli being compared. Thus, these assessments do not need to be done prior to initiating treatment, they can be blended directly into treatment.

As summarized in Table 13.2, supplemental consequence assessments may inform treatment planning by identifying (a) which dimensions of reinforcement for tangibles should be programmed for, (b) which relatively lower preferred items effectively function as reinforcers during periods of delay from the wanted item or activity, (c) which conditions highly preferred items function as reinforcers, and (d) how long the initial delay period should be programmed for to ensure success with gaining access to the reinforcers for appropriate behavior.

Antecedent Assessments When challenging behavior is maintained by access to preferred items and activities, the treatment approach often includes increasing the delay to access those items because presumably the individual is required to engage in other activities from time to time. Some antecedent approaches to address challenging behavior maintained by access to preferred items have included providing access to the tangible items on fixed or variable time schedules (Kahng, Iwata, DeLeon, Wallace, & D., 2000; Lalli et al., 1997; Van Camp, Lerman, Kelley, Contrucci, & Vorndran, 2000), providing pre-session access to those items (Rispoli et al., 2011), and modifying the ways in which removal or denial of the items is presented (Mace, Pratt, Prager, & Pritchard, 2011).

Relative to fixed time schedules, Lalli et al. (1997) evaluated the effects of providing three boys, aged 3–9 years old, with developmental disabilities access to their preferred activities on fixed intervals. Each child was informed that he could play with his preferred activity when a timer sounded but needed to play with an alternative activity in the meantime. When the timer sounded, the preferred activities were presented to the children independent of the type (challenging or appropriate) of behavior being displayed. Within multielement (two boys) and multiple baseline across settings (one boy) designs, results showed that challenging behavior decreased and maintained at low levels, even as the fixed time schedule was thinned. These results appeared to have occurred because the children's access to the items at fixed times appeared to abolish the MO for challenging behavior to obtain those items. This, then, is a very practical approach to beginning treatment.

Thus, an often effective option for initiating treatment is to identify the antecedent conditions that alter the MOs for challenging behavior. Vollmer and Iwata (1991) first demonstrated the effects of MOs, in the form of satiation and deprivation of reinforcement for five adult males with profound intellectual disabilities. The experimenters evaluated the effects of deprivation as an EO and satiation as an AO in separate experiments of edible items, music, and social attention as reinforcers for task completion. Using the edible items experiment as an example, preferred edible items were provided on FR schedules contingent on the participant placing blocks in a box during treatment sessions conducted either prior to a meal (i.e., deprivation as the EO) or following a meal (i.e., satiation as the AO). The results of the comparison showed that even though the response-reinforcer contingencies were held constant across the treatment sessions, the target response occurred more frequently during treatment sessions conducted prior to the meal in comparison to the frequency observed during sessions that followed the meal. In this study, when treatment sessions were conducted prior to mealtimes, the absence of food (i.e., deprivation) and potential hunger during these sessions may have increased or established the value of the edible items as reinforcers for the target response, thereby increasing the frequency of the target response. In contrast, when treatment sessions were conducted following mealtimes, consumption of the meal may have decreased or abolished the effectiveness of the edible items as reinforcers, thereby reducing the likelihood of the target response occurring due to satiation for food.

For treatment planning, these results show that the timing of access to the tangible item may be just as important as the access itself. Relative to challenging behavior, Rispoli et al. (2011) tested the effects of providing noncontingent access to preferred tangible items, to the point of satiation, prior to the presentation of classroom instruction with three children, aged 5–6 years old, with autism spectrum disorder who engaged in challenging behavior to access tangible items. Within multielement designs, the participants showed a reduction in challenging behavior and an increase in classroom engagement during sessions preceded by access to the preferred items in comparison to sessions without pre-session exposure to the items.

Despite opportunities to provide access to preferred items throughout the day and the possibility that satiation might not occur with preferred items, there are times that preferred items simply need to be denied. Thus, one consideration for treatment planning may include how the denial is presented. For example, Mace et al. (2011) evaluated the effects of three denial approaches on the challenging behavior displayed by an adolescent male with Waardenburg syndrome and autism spectrum disorder. Conditions included (a) "no" with an explanation, (b) "no" with an explanation plus an alternative preferred activity, and (c) "yes" with a contingency to complete a non-preferred academic task. For conditions with an explanation, the explanation consisted of brief statements of why the preferred item was unavailable. Within a reversal design, results showed that challenging behavior rarely occurred when denial included an explanation plus an alternative preferred activity and when access was given contingent on the completion of a non-preferred task.

Similar to the Schieltz et al. (2017) study described earlier, Suess, Schieltz, Wacker, Detrick, and Podlesnik (2020) provided an additional antecedent approach for use with tangibles because many individuals with tangible functions express concern or frustration relative to what will occur to the functional tangible item when it is removed. For example, some individuals appear to be concerned that the item will not be returned, others express worry that someone else will take the item, and still others just appear to want ongoing visual contact with the item. In these cases, assessment might involve two conditions which alter what happens to the item when it is removed. In the case of Suess et al., a "safespot," which included a piece of paper, was used to signal where preferred activities should be placed during work tasks, whereas Schieltz et al. either placed the preferred item in a bucket or circled it on a written list which were placed out of reach during the work tasks. For the purposes of treatment planning, assessment might evaluate the presence and absence of these signals or "safe spots" for tangibles when they are removed.

Similar to consequence-based assessments and as summarized in Table 13.2, supplemental antecedent assessments might inform treatment plans by demonstrating that (a) fixed time access to preferred items/activities and (b) pre-session access to preferred items/activities are effective at altering the motivation to engage in challenging behavior to gain or maintain access to tangibles when they are denied or removed. Similarly, the "signals" (e.g., instructions, locations for items), such as how denial or removal are presented, may also alter the motivation to engage in challenging behavior for tangibles.

Considerations for Treatment Planning For challenging behavior that is maintained by positive reinforcement in the form of tangibles, both consequence and antecedent assessments, in isolation or combined, may be useful for treatment planning. For example, conducting an assessment of the schedule requirements under a progressive ratio schedule, similar to Roane et al. (2001), may be useful for identifying the starting point for delay tolerance training and may show that different delays can occur with different stimuli. Similarly, conducting an assessment of fixed time access to reinforcers similar to Lalli et al. (1997) may be useful for decreasing the motivation to engage in challenging behavior when preferred items or activities are denied or removed. These may also be used in combination such that the length of the delay is identified as well as reinforcers that can be provided during the delay that effectively compete with challenging behavior. Finally, how items are removed, such as through verbal instructions like Mace et al. (2011) or "safe spots" like Suess et al. (2020), needs to be considered because it may alter the motivation to engage in challenging behavior when preferred tangibles are removed.

Positive Reinforcement for Attention

Challenging behavior maintained by positive reinforcement in the form of access to attention is identified when the contingent presentation of attention is provided following the occurrence of challenging behavior under the diverted or divided attention MOs in the FA. Similar to challenging behavior maintained by access to tangibles, supplemental assessments can facilitate the identification of more prescriptive components of a treatment plan such as the preferred dimensions of attention (e.g., Gardner et al., 2009; Jerome & Sturmey, 2008; Kelly, Roscoe, Hanley, & Schlichenmeyer, 2014; Morris & Vollmer, 2019; Ringdahl & Sellers, 2000; Trosclair-Lasserre, Lerman, Call, Addison, & Kodak, 2008), the current tolerated length of delay without attention (e.g., Kahng, Iwata, Thompson, & Hanley, 2000), and variables that alter the value of engaging in challenging behavior for attention such as pre-session access (e.g., Berg et al., 2000; O'Reilly et al., 2007; Vollmer &

Iwata, 1991) and access to alternative reinforcers (e.g., Austin & Tiger, 2015; Fisher, O'Connor, Kurtz, DeLeon, & Gotjen, 2000; Sumter et al., 2020). The procedures of these selected examples are provided in Table 13.3 and are briefly described below.

Consequence Assessments   One set of procedures for challenging behavior maintained by attention is similar to what we have described previously, in that we are seeking to identify variables that can be used to fade attention or to increase the intervals in which attention is not provided. We do not provide further description of these assessments, in this section, because they are the same as those described for a tangible function (e.g., progressive increases in delays to attention given differential access to distinct preferred tangibles during the delay interval). However, please note that they are often the first set of assessments we conduct if our initial DRA treatment is not effective or if we are attempting to fade the timing or amount of attention that is contingent on more appropriate behavior. Thus, evaluations of (a) access to alternative stimuli during the delay periods (Austin & Tiger, 2015; Sumter et al., 2020) and (b) progressive schedule requirements to determine the reinforcing

Table 13.3 Summary of selected assessment procedures, rationales, and implications for treatment planning for challenging behavior maintained by positive reinforcement in the form of attention

Assessment procedure	Procedural steps	Rationale	Implications for treatment planning
Consequence assessments			
Dimensions of reinforcement	Evaluate preferences for (a) type of attention, (b) quality of attention, (c) person providing the attention, and/or (d) magnitude of attention	Determine the preferred dimensions of reinforcement for attention	Incorporate the preferred dimensions of reinforcement for attention into the treatment plan
Delay assessment	Compare levels of challenging behavior during different delay periods using a progressive ratio schedule	Determine the lengths of time that challenging behavior does and does not occur (breakpoint) when attention is diverted	Begin the treatment plan at or slightly below the delay breakpoint
Antecedent assessments			
Pre-session exposure assessment	Compare levels of challenging behavior during attention test sessions following (a) pre-session access to attention and (b) no pre-session access	Determine if differential responding occurs when exposed to attention prior to its removal	Provide access to attention prior to the removal of attention
Competing stimuli assessment	Compare levels of challenging behavior during restricted attention conditions when competing stimuli are (a) present and (b) absent	Determine if differential responding occurs when competing stimuli are present during periods of restricted attention	Provide access to competing stimuli during periods of restricted attention

value of identified stimuli (Davis, Hodges, Weston, Hogan, & Padilla-Mainor, 2017; DeLeon, Frank, Gregory, & Allman, 2009) may be helpful for further prescribing a treatment for challenging behavior maintained by attention.

Two other approaches to assessment can often be useful in developing treatment plans. First, the effects of attention seem to be highly sensitive to the quality of attention that is received (Gardner et al., 2009). For example, Fewell et al. (2016) showed that the consumption of attention during reinforcement periods varied across participants and appeared to be correlated with the quality of attention being provided by the parent. These results, and those of other investigators (e.g., Gardner et al., 2009; Kelly et al., 2014; Morris & Vollmer, 2019; Trosclair-Lasserre et al., 2008), strongly suggest that for many of our clients, the value of attention can vary substantially by the perceived quality of attention. Thus, identifying an individual's preferences for different types of attention may be a critical component for the over-all success of treatment and may provide a reason for a treatment that appears to work only intermittently. Unfortunately, this also means that the use of attention as a reinforcer may vary greatly and not only across individuals providing and receiving reinforcement but also across sessions with the same individual providing attention to the same client for the same target response. Assessments of the quality of attention are needed to show if clients have preferences for specific types of attention. If so, are these preferences consistent across time, situations, and people delivering attention? To date, studies have shown that responsiveness to attention can be highly individualistic, requiring that functional assessments be conducted to evaluate the potency of different types of attention.

Four sets of assessment procedures have been described in the literature that identify different dimensions or qualities of attention. First, as described by Gardner et al. (2009), high-quality attention can be operationally defined and its effects observed when it is present or absent. In the Gardner et al. study, high-quality attention was either provided or removed during demands, and the results showed that when provided, compliance improved. In this case, an attempt was made to operationalize "high quality" across children because that was the only way it could be evaluated within the confines of a brief outpatient clinic.

A second approach is to assess the effects of attention when it is delivered by different people. For example, Ringdahl and Sellers (2000) showed that the effects of challenging behavior varied substantially dependent on the individual's familiarity with the adult conducting the procedures. In this study, FA procedures were conducted either by the individual's care provider or the clinic therapist. Results showed that the identification of functional reinforcers for challenging behavior varied, not only across functional contexts but across the person who conducted the procedures. These results highlight the importance of considering the impact the person(s) conducting the assessment or treatment procedures may have on challenging behavior.

Third, the specific dimensions or types of attention can be evaluated for each individual. For example, Morris and Vollmer (2019) identified the preferred types of social interactions (e.g., praise, hugs, spins, tickles) for five children, aged 4–11 years old, with autism spectrum disorder. These were then assessed in a subsequent con- current operant assessment, whereby specific responses resulted in access to the corresponding social interaction. Results showed that the majority of children had preferred types of social interactions and that the preferred social interactions func- tioned as reinforcers.

Fourth, once the preferred types of reinforcement have been identified, then fur- ther consequence assessments, such as those described for tangibles, can be con- ducted to determine the point at which treatment might begin. And again, these assessments can be embedded into the treatment program meaning that the results of treatment will identify, for example, how long the wait interval can be for differ- ent types or qualities of attention. For example, based on the results of Roane et al. (2001), we might identify that our client will wait twice as long for the attention from a preferred peer versus a less preferred peer or teacher. Thus, if the results of treatment are less than ideal, if they are variable, or if we are beginning to conduct a fading program, conducting these types of assessments prior to or during treat- ment to provide ongoing prescriptive information should be considered.

As summarized in Table 13.3, there are multiple types of consequence assess- ments that may be useful for treatment planning because they can identify the dimensions of attention that are preferred by the individual. Subsequent assessment can then isolate the conditions under which various types of attention function as a reinforcer and the point at which treatment might begin for increasing tolerance to delays.

Antecedent Assessments   There are two basic antecedent approaches to the assess- ment of antecedents that can be useful for developing or improving treatment. The first approach involves the satiation of attention as a reinforcer (Berg et al., 2000; McGinnis, Houchins-Juarez, McDaniel, & Kennedy, 2010; O'Reilly et al., 2007; O'Reilly, Edrisinha, Sigafoos, Lancioni, & Andrews, 2006; Rispoli et al., 2011; Roantree & Kennedy, 2006). In this approach, the value of attention is reduced or abolished by antecedent manipulations of attention. A second approach is to iden- tify stimuli that compete with attention and can be used to, for example, increase delays to attention (Fisher et al., 2004). For both of these approaches, exposure to a positive reinforcer immediately prior to or during a test condition for challenging behavior maintained by attention is conducted to determine its influence on chal- lenging behavior.

Relative to abolishing the MOs for attention via satiation, several studies (e.g., Berg et al., 2000; Vollmer & Iwata, 1991) have evaluated the effects of providing access to the functional reinforcer on a noncontingent schedule prior to or during the test condition. For example, Berg et al. (2000) used three different functional assessments to demonstrate the effects of pre-session exposure to attention on sub- sequent tests for attention as reinforcement for challenging behavior. The partici- pants were three young children, aged 2–4 years old, with developmental disabilities who had a history of challenging behavior that was maintained by access to atten- tion. Across the different functional assessments used (one functional assessment for each child), each child experienced the presence and absence of noncontingent, positive adult attention during 5-min sessions conducted prior to sessions in which challenging behavior resulted in attention. Similar patterns of responding occurred across each child, such that conditions preceded by adult attention were associated with lower levels of the target behavior. The collective results showed that one way challenging behavior maintained by attention can be reduced is via satiation. Thus, if we know that a child will need to wait or work for a period of time without access to attention, one approach to treatment is to provide noncontingent attention for a period of time before the wait or work period. To improve the effects of this approach, we might also identify if different qualities of attention presented antecedent to wait or demand times result in greater or lesser abolishing effects. Similarly, as described previously for demands and tangibles, a signal might also be associated with waiting (Schieltz et al., 2017). For example, for a child with attention-maintained challenging behavior, the first supplemental assessment might be to conduct an analysis of two different amounts of noncontingent attention prior to a several minute wait period. If one amount of attention results in a greater AO than another, then treatment might begin with that level of attention. To further facilitate the effects of this intervention, a visual symbol (e.g., word card) might show the child that the same amount of attention will be provided (on a DRA or DRO schedule) for successful waiting or task completion. To assess if this symbol is adding to the effects of treatment, some sessions can contain the symbol and others not contain the symbol. In this way, we are assessing both the quantity of attention provided antecedent to the wait or demand session and the effects of the symbol for the same amount (or type) of attention the client will receive following the session.

A second assessment option for treatment planning is to evaluate the effects of competing stimuli on challenging behavior during times of restricted attention. Fisher et al. (2004) compared noncontingent access to competing stimuli and noncontingent access to attention on rates of challenging behavior maintained by access to attention. To identify competing stimuli, caregiver interviews and paired choice preference assessments were conducted to identify stimuli that resulted in item engagement and effectively reduced challenging behavior. These stimuli were then used in a treatment comparison to determine the effects of each treatment approach. Treatment conditions included noncontingent access to competing stimuli and noncontingent access to attention. During the noncontingent competing stimuli condition, the individuals received continuous access to the stimuli along with access to low and moderately preferred toys. Attention was not provided in this condition. During the noncontingent attention condition, the individuals received continuous interactions from another person and had access to the low and moderately preferred toys. Access to the competing stimuli were not available during this condition. Occurrences of challenging behavior were ignored across all conditions. Results of this treatment comparison showed that noncontingent access to competing stimuli resulted in low occurrences of challenging behavior. These results suggest that access to highly preferred tangibles may effectively compete with challenging behavior maintained by access to attention under restricted attention conditions.

As summarized in Table 13.3, antecedent assessments can facilitate treatment planning by demonstrating the conditions under which the value of attention is abolished. This is accomplished in two ways: (a) pre-session exposure to attention as a means for decreasing the value of attention via satiation and (b) access to preferred tangible items during intervals in which the individual must wait for attention. Both of these antecedent approaches are practical and provide a plan for when the individual is going to have to wait or to work without attention.

Considerations for Treatment Planning For challenging behavior that is maintained by positive reinforcement in the form of access to attention, supplemental consequence assessments may inform treatment planning by identifying an individual's preferences for the type and delivery of attention. Supplemental antecedent assessments may identify the conditions under which attention is and is not desired. Both types of information can be used to further enhance the effects of a treatment program and especially when treatment is not resulting in the desired outcomes in a consistent manner. Of particular benefit is that these assessments can be incorporated into ongoing treatment programs such that ongoing assessment is part of ongoing treatment.

Automatic Reinforcement

In applied behavior analysis, one of the early examples of challenging behavior being maintained by automatic reinforcement was provided by Berkson and Mason (1964). This article and many that followed showed that challenging behaviors that occur independent of manipulations to social reinforcers or in the absence of potential social reinforcers (e.g., alone without materials to manipulate or a no interaction condition) appear to be maintained by the behavior itself or potential sensory changes produced by the behavior. These behaviors are described as being maintained by automatic reinforcement because engagement in the behavior provides its own reinforcement; the behavior occurs independent of social consequences and thus occurs when the individual is sometimes ignored or alone, even if other activities are available, or across all conditions.

The identification of an automatic function does not necessarily provide a specific direction on how to treat challenging behavior. Existing successful reinforcement-based treatment approaches typically provide access to stimuli that effectively compete with the occurrence of challenging behavior on both response-independent (e.g., enriched environment; Horner, 1980; Ringdahl, Vollmer, Marcus, & Roane, 1997; Rooker, Bonner, Dillon, & Zarcone, 2018) and response-contingent (e.g., DRO, DRA; Berg et al., 2016; Falcomata, Roane, Hovanetz, Kettering, & Keeney, 2004; Hedquist & Roscoe, 2020) schedules of reinforcement. Reinforcement components of treatment are often combined with other treatment components such as disrupting (e.g., extinction; Rincover, Cook, Peoples, & Packard, 1979; Roscoe, Iwata, & Goh, 1998) or preventing (e.g., response interruption and redirection, blocking, providing protective equipment or restraints; Hagopian, Rooker, & Zarcone, 2015; Roscoe, Iwata, & Zhou, 2013; Spencer & Alkhanji, 2018) the response-reinforcer relationship. However, for the purposes of this chapter, we focus on the reinforcement components.

For challenging behavior maintained by automatic reinforcement, supplemental consequence assessments often focus on schedules of reinforcement, whereas antecedent assessments focus on preferences for stimuli and conditions that alter the motivation to engage in challenging behavior. Selected examples of these procedures are provided in Table 13.4 and are briefly described below.

Table 13.4 Summary of selected assessment procedures, rationales, and implications for treatment planning for challenging behavior maintained by automatic reinforcement

Assessment procedure	Procedural steps	Rationale	Implications for treatment planning
Consequence assessments			
Competing reinforcer assessment	Compare (a) free access to preferred stimuli condition and (b) alone or low stimulation condition	Determine if differentiated responding occurs between the presence and absence of alternative stimuli	Access to competing stimuli may be sufficient to maintain reductions in automatically maintained challenging behavior
Differential reinforcement assessment	Compare (a) access to preferred stimuli contingent on specified alternative behaviors and (b) access to preferred stimuli contingent on the absence of challenging behavior for specified intervals of time	Determine if differentiated responding occurs with contingencies for the occurrence of specified alternative behaviors and/or the absence of challenging behavior	1. Engagement in alternative behaviors suggests DRA might be an appropriate treatment component 2. Reduced occurrences of challenging behavior during specified intervals suggests DRO might be an appropriate treatment component
Antecedent assessments			
Competing stimuli assessment	Compare levels of item engagement and challenging behavior	Determine if stimuli result in higher levels of item engagement and lower levels of challenging behavior	Stimuli with higher levels of item engagement may effectively function as competing reinforcers whether provided noncontingently or contingently
Antecedent analysis	Compare presence and absence of antecedent conditions (e.g., preferred items given to the individual versus placed on a table) that may alter engagement in challenging behavior	Determine if differentiated responding occurs between the presence and absence of the manipulated conditions	Conditions that result in lower levels of challenging behavior may be more effective treatment components to maintain reductions in automatically maintained challenging behavior

Consequence Assessments   The degree to which challenging behavior maintained by automatic reinforcement persists in the presence of alternative stimuli has important implications for the responsiveness of the behavior to specific treatment components for reducing the behavior (Berg et al., 2016; Hagopian, Rooker, Zarcone, Bonner, & Arevalo, 2017). Berg et al. (2016) and Hagopian et al. (2015, 2017) showed that differences in the patterns of responding between a condition with free access to preferred stimuli (e.g., free play) and the alone or low stimulation condition can be informative for selecting treatment components to reduce challenging behavior. A comparison showing minimal to no occurrence of challenging behavior during free play but elevated occurrences during an alone/low-stimulation condition demonstrates a differentiated pattern of responding between the presence versus absence of alternative stimuli. A differentiated pattern of responding between these two assessment conditions suggests that the presence of the stimuli available during the free play condition effectively competes with the automatic reinforcement associated with the challenging behavior. If so, providing access to these alternative stimuli on a continuous or fixed-time schedule may be sufficient to maintain reductions in challenging behavior. This approach to treatment is effective because the stimuli available during the free play condition are relatively more preferred than the reinforcement associated with the challenging behavior, and therefore, responding is allocated toward those alternative reinforcers associated with alternative stimuli. For this treatment to be effective, the types of preference assessments described previously for the tangible function may be sufficient to identify preferred stimuli that effectively compete with challenging behavior. When challenging behavior shows an initial differentiated pattern with few occurrences in the presence of alternative stimuli, a competing stimuli assessment similar to those conducted by Piazza, Adelinis, Hanley, Goh, and Delia (2000) or Ringdahl et al. (1997) may be an effective strategy for identifying alternative stimuli associated with reductions in challenging behavior when provided on a fixed-time or noncontingent schedule (see descriptions of these studies in the antecedent assessment section).

In contrast, when challenging behavior occurs across both a condition with free access to alternative stimuli and a condition without alternative stimuli (e.g., alone with nothing or no interaction conditions), this reflects an undifferentiated pattern of responding (e.g., Berg et al., 2016; Hagopian et al., 2017). In this situation, subsequent assessment will be needed to identify (a) stimuli that are selected to the exclusion of challenging behavior (e.g., via competing stimuli assessments) and (b) the conditions under which responses will be allocated toward gaining the alternative stimuli over automatic reinforcement. By conditions, we are referring to the specific reinforcement contingencies or schedules by which access to the alternative stimuli are provided. Several studies (e.g., Berg et al., 2016; Ringdahl et al., 1997; Shore, Iwata, DeLeon, Kahng, & Smith, 1997) have shown that a change in the contingencies for gaining access to alternative stimuli (e.g., from noncontingent reinforcement [NCR] to DRA or DRA to NCR) may enhance or reduce the value of accessing preferred alternative stimuli in relation to accessing automatic reinforcement. If a change in reinforcement contingencies results in a change in response allocation between alternative stimuli (increased) and the behavior maintained by automatic reinforcement (decreased), treatment can be initiated.

For example, Berg et al. (Berg et al., 2016) showed that for some participants who showed an undifferentiated pattern of responding between the play control condition and the alone condition of the FA, a change in the contingencies for gaining access to alternative stimuli from NCR to a DRA or DRO contingency resulted in increased engagement with the alternative stimuli and reductions in challenging behavior. Berg et al. used a concurrent operant preference assessment with response blocking to identify stimuli that competed with automatic reinforcement when access to the two sources of reinforcement were simultaneously available but mutually exclusive. The experimenters placed masking tape on the floor of the treatment room or used natural barriers (e.g., a sofa) to divide the room in half and placed a set of alternative stimuli on one side and left the other half of the room empty. The participants were placed in the center of the room and shown the choices on either side of the room. If the participant entered the side of the room with alternative stimuli, he or she received continuous access to the stimuli, and attempts at challenging behavior were blocked to prevent access to the automatic reinforcement that maintained the behavior. If the participant entered the empty half of the room, he or she could remain on that side of the room, and challenging behavior was not blocked except to prevent tissue damage. The participants were able to cross back and forth between sides of the room, but they were not allowed to take items from the alternative side to the empty side of the room. Participants who consistently selected at least one set of alternative stimuli during the concurrent operant assessment were then provided a DRA treatment, in which access to the alternative stimuli was contingent on adaptive responding. This successfully reduced the occurrence of challenging behavior.

Both Berg et al. (2016) and Ringdahl et al. (1997) showed that assessment results showing choice allocation to alternative stimuli was predictive of success with DRA treatments. That is, if choice responding showed allocation to preferred stimuli, then a DRA treatment program that required a display of adaptive behavior prior to receiving the alternative stimuli was often successful. In these cases, treatment can involve either NCR access to preferred stimuli or a differential reinforcement schedule to reduce challenging behavior. Unfortunately, these results cannot be assumed for all individuals who display automatically maintained challenging behavior. For example, Shore et al. (1997) showed that three adult participants with profound intellectual disabilities who engaged in challenging behavior maintained by automatic reinforcement allocated their responding to alternative stimuli and away from challenging behavior when the alternative stimuli were freely available. However, when the contingencies for access to the alternative stimuli changed from NCR to DRA, the participants' responding changed to engaging in challenging behavior rather than continuing to engage with the alternative stimuli. Thus, this type of reinforcer assessment is needed prior to or during treatment to make sure that clients respond to alternative stimuli as reinforcers even when the demand to access the stimuli is increased (as occurs when the schedule of reinforcement is changed from NCR to DRA).

Other changes in reinforcement contingencies may result in similar disruptions to the effects of treatment and warrant assessment. For example, Hedquist and Roscoe (2020) evaluated the effectiveness of DRA and DRO treatments in reducing stereotypy maintained by automatic reinforcement for three adolescents with autism spectrum disorder. Within the DRA treatment, the participants received an edible reinforcer contingent on completing a task, and no programmed consequences were provided for stereotypy. During the DRO treatment, the participants received the same edible reinforcer contingent only on the absence of stereotypy for specified intervals of time, and no programmed consequences were provided for task completion. Both treatments were alternated with a baseline condition that included task presentation with no programmed consequences for either task completion or stereotypy. Thus, as described previously, this assessment was conducted as part of an ongoing treatment. The three conditions were compared for their effects on the occurrence of stereotypy, task completion, and item engagement. DRA resulted in greater reductions in stereotypy than observed during DRO for two participants, and similar reductions in stereotypy occurred across the DRA and DRO conditions with the third participant. The DRA condition resulted in more time spent with item engagement and a higher rate of task completion than DRO for every participant. The authors hypothesized that the higher rate of task completion and lower levels of stereotypy within the DRA condition could be attributed to the direct pairing of reinforcement with completion of the task, which may have been incompatible with stereotypy. The DRA condition was also associated with higher rates of reinforcement delivery for each participant, which may have been another reason for why it was relatively more effective than the DRO treatment.

As summarized in Table 13.4, some consequence assessments to consider conducting when developing treatment plans for challenging behavior maintained by automatic reinforcement include competing reinforcer assessments and differential reinforcement assessments. With these types of supplemental assessments, results may indicate that (a) access to competing stimuli is an indicated treatment component because they are sufficient for maintaining reductions in challenging behavior, (b) DRA is an indicated treatment component when the individual engages in alternative behaviors rather than challenging behavior, or (c) DRO is an indicated treatment component when the occurrence of challenging behavior remains low during specified intervals of time.

Antecedent Assessments   For consequence assessments to be effective, preferred stimuli that compete with challenging behavior must first be identified. For example, Ringdahl et al. (1997) used a free operant preference assessment to identify leisure items that competed with self-injurious behavior for three children with developmental disabilities. Within the preference assessment, the investigators compared the time the participants spent engaged in self-injury, a leisure item, or both. Activities that the participants manipulated to the exclusion of self-injury (or nearly to the exclusion) were identified for two participants, and activities that the participant engaged with more often than engaging in self-injury were identified for the third participant. The identified items were freely available to each participant in the context of an enriched environment immediately following the preference assessment. Free access to the leisure items that were selected to the exclusion of self-injury continued to compete effectively with self-injury for two participants as predicted by the assessment results. These same results were demonstrated by other researchers (e.g., Ing, Roane, & Veenstra, 2011; Shore et al., 1997).

Although free access to alternative stimuli can compete effectively with automatically maintained challenging behavior, this condition is not always sufficient as demonstrated by the remaining participant in Ringdahl et al. (1997). This participant engaged with the freely available leisure item but continued to show self-injury. Therefore, the effectiveness of other variables associated with the competing stimuli may need to be assessed. For example, Piazza et al. (2000) identified the preferences for stimuli that were matched and unmatched to the hypothesized sensory consequences being obtained by three individuals with severe intellectual disabilities who engaged in the automatically maintained challenging behavior. Following these results, Piazza et al. compared the effects of providing noncontingent access to the matched and unmatched preferred items that were associated with reductions in challenging behavior during the preference assessment. Results showed that for all individuals, challenging behavior maintained by automatic reinforcement remained lowest when access to preferred stimuli that were matched to the sensory consequences were available noncontingently.

Another example of assessing other variables that might impact engagement with competing stimuli was conducted by Britton, Carr, Landaburu, and Romick (2002). In this study, the researchers conducted a multiple stimulus preference assessment and identified preferred leisure items for three participants. In a subsequent assessment, the investigators provided access to the preferred stimuli on a noncontingent basis and achieved reductions in challenging behavior from baseline levels for every participant. The effectiveness of these stimuli in reducing challenging behavior were then compared when (a) the therapist handed the preferred item to the participant (prompted condition) and (b) when the preferred item was placed on the table in front of the participant (unprompted condition). Each participant showed increased engagement with the preferred item and reductions in challenging behavior during the prompted condition and showed minimal or no engagement with the item, and moderate to high levels of challenging behavior, during the unprompted condition. This study demonstrated that the way stimuli are presented can influence the effectiveness of the item in competing with challenging behavior.

As mentioned above and summarized in Table 13.4, antecedent assessments may focus on identifying the degree to which preferred items are selected to the exclusion of automatically maintained challenging behavior. Results, then, can be used in subsequent consequence assessments to identify the conditions under which the items effectively compete with automatically maintained challenging behavior.

Considerations for Treatment Planning For challenging behavior that is maintained by automatic reinforcement, antecedent assessments may be a critical step prior to any supplemental consequence assessments. This is because preference assessments appear to be needed for identifying preferred stimuli that result in item engagement. This information can then be used when designing the conditions to be assessed during supplemental consequence assessments. Consequence assessments, then, identify stimuli that effectively compete with challenging behavior. Beyond that, the models proposed by Berg et al. (2016) and Hagopian et al. (2015, 2017) provide clear guidance on how to assess and determine which contingencies should be incorporated into the treatment plan.

Summary

The first step in developing a treatment plan for challenging behavior is to conduct a FA because the results indicate the class or classes of reinforcement that are maintaining challenging behavior. These stimuli are referred to as functional reinforcers. Based on these results, traditionally, treatment plans entail the provision of (a) the functional reinforcer for the occurrence of an alternative behavior or the absence of challenging behavior and (b) extinction for the occurrence of challenging behavior. Although these treatment plans can be highly effective at decreasing the occurrence of challenging behavior and increasing the occurrence of desired behaviors, in some cases more information is needed to guide or alter the treatment plans to improve the success of treatment. To gather this information, consequence and/or antecedent assessments can be used to supplement the results of a FA, thereby objectively guiding the inclusion of specific treatment components. Whether used in isolation or combination, these assessments may assist treatment development by identifying (a) relevant reinforcer dimensions, preferences, timing, or contingencies, (b) response requirements with which to begin treatment, and (c) the conditions or stimuli that alter the motivation to engage in challenging behavior.

References

Austin, J. E., & Tiger, J. H. (2015). Providing alternative reinforcers to facilitate tolerance to delayed reinforcement following functional communication training. *Journal of Applied Behavior Analysis, 48*(3), 663–668. https://doi.org/10.1002/jaba.215

Beavers, G. A., Iwata, B. A., & Lerman, D. C. (2013). Thirty years of research on the functional analysis of problem behavior. *Journal of Applied Behavior Analysis, 46*(1), 1–21. https://doi.org/10.1002/jaba.30

Berg, W. K., Peck, S., Wacker, D. P., Harding, J., McComas, J., Richman, D., & Brown, K. (2000). The effects of presession exposure to attention on the results of assessments of attention as a reinforcer. *Journal of Applied Behavior Analysis, 33*(4), 463–477. https://doi.org/10.1901/jaba.2000.33-463

Berg, W. K., Wacker, D. P., Ringdahl, J. E., Stricker, J., Vinquist, K., Dutt, A. S. K., … Mews, J. (2016). An integrated model for guiding the selection of treatment components for problem behavior maintained by automatic reinforcement. *Journal of Applied Behavior Analysis, 49*(3), 617–638. https://doi.org/10.1002/jaba.303

Berkson, G., & Mason, W. A. (1964). Stereotyped movements of mental defectives: IV. The effects of toys and the character of the acts. *American Journal of Mental Deficiency, 68*, 511–524.

Boelter, E. W., Wacker, D. P., Call, N. A., Ringdahl, J. E., Kopelman, T., & Gardner, A. W. (2007). Effects of antecedent variables on disruptive behavior and accurate responding in young children in outpatient settings. *Journal of Applied Behavior Analysis, 40*(2), 321–326. https://doi.org/10.1901/jaba.51-06

Bowman, L. G., Piazza, C. C., Fisher, W. W., Hagopian, L. P., & Kogan, J. S. (1997). Assessment of preference for varied versus constant reinforcers. *Journal of Applied Behavior Analysis, 30*(3), 451–458. https://doi.org/10.1901/jaba.1997.30-451

Britton, L. N., Carr, J. E., Landaburu, H. J., & Romick, K. S. (2002). The efficacy of noncontingent reinforcement as treatment for automatically reinforced stereotypy. *Behavioral Interventions, 17*(2), 93–103. https://doi.org/10.1002/bin.110

Bukala, M., Hu, Y. H., Lee, R., Ward-Horner, J. C., & Fienup, D. M. (2015). The effects of work-reinforcer schedules on performance and preference in students with autism. *Journal of Applied Behavioral Analysis, 48*(1), 215–220. https://doi.org/10.1002/jaba.2015.188

Call, N. A., Wacker, D. P., Ringdahl, J. E., Cooper-Brown, L. J., & Boelter, E. W. (2004). An assessment of antecedent events influencing noncompliance in an outpatient clinic. *Journal of Applied Behavior Analysis, 37*(2), 145–157. https://doi.org/10.1901/jaba.2004.37-145

Carr, E. G., & Durand, V. M. (1985). Reducing behavior problems through functional communication training. *Journal of Applied Behavior Analysis, 18*(2), 111–126. https://doi.org/10.1901/jaba.1985.18-111

Cengher, M., Shamoun, K., Moss, P., Roll, D., Feliciano, G., & Fienup, D. M. (2016). A comparison of the effects of two prompt-fading strategies on skill acquisition in children with autism spectrum disorders. *Behavior Analysis in Practice, 9*(2), 115–125. https://doi.org/10.1007/s40617-015-0096-6

Davis, T. N., Hodges, A., Weston, R., Hogan, E., & Padilla-Mainor, K. (2017). Correspondence between preference assessment outcomes and stimulus reinforcer value for social interactions. *Journal of Behavioral Education, 26*(3), 238–249. https://doi.org/10.1007/s10864-017-9271-x

DeLeon, G. I., Chase, A. J., Frank-Crawford, M. A., Carreau-Webster, B. A., Triggs, M. M., Bullock, E. C., & Jennett, K. H. (2014). Distributed and accumulated reinforcement arrangement: Evaluations of efficacy and preference. *Journal of Applied Behavior Analysis, 47*(2), 293–313. https://doi.org/10.1002/jaba.2014.116

DeLeon, I. G., Frank, M. A., Gregory, M. K., & Allman, M. J. (2009). On the correspondence between preference assessment outcomes and progressive-ratio schedule assessments of stimulus value. *Journal of Applied Behavior Analysis, 42*(3), 729–733. https://doi.org/10.1901/jaba.2009.42-729

DeLeon, I. G., & Iwata, B. A. (1996). Evaluation of a multiple-stimulus presentation format for assessing reinforcer preferences. *Journal of Applied Behavior Analysis, 29*(4), 519–533. https://doi.org/10.1901/jaba.1996.29-519

Dowdy, A., Tincani, M., Nipe, T., & Weiss, M. J. (2018). Effects of reinforcement without extinction in increasing compliance with nail cutting: A systematic replication. *Journal of Applied Behavior Analysis, 51*(4), 924–930. https://doi.org/10.1002/jaba.484

Dunlap, G., DePerczel, M., Clarke, S., Wilson, D., Wright, S., White, R., & Gomez, A. (1994). Choice making to promote adaptive behavior for students with emotional and behavioral challenges. *Journal of Applied Behavior Analysis, 27*(3), 505–518. https://doi.org/10.1901/jaba.1994.27-505

Dunlap, G., Kern-Dunlap, L., Clarke, S., & Robbins, F. R. (1991). Functional assessment, curricular revision, and severe behavior problems. *Journal of Applied Behavior Analysis, 24*(2), 387–397. https://doi.org/10.1901/jaba.1991.24-387

Durand, V. M., & Carr, E. G. (1991). Functional communication training to reduce challenging behavior: Maintenance and application in new settings. *Journal of Applied Behavior Analysis, 24*(2), 251–264. https://doi.org/10.1901/jaba.1991.24-251

Falcomata, T. S., Roane, H. S., Hovanetz, A. N., Kettering, T. L., & Keeney, K. M. (2004). An evaluation of response cost in the treatment of inappropriate vocalizations maintained by automatic reinforcement. *Journal of Applied Behavior Analysis, 37*(1), 83–87. https://doi.org/10.1901/jaba.2004.37-83

Fewell, R. M., Romani, P. W., Wacker, D. P., Lindgern, S. D., Kopelman, T. G., & Waldron, D. B. (2016). Relations between consumption of functional and arbitrary reinforcers during functional communication training. *Journal of Developmental and Physical Disabilities, 28*(2), 237–253. https://doi.org/10.1007/s10882-015-9463-z

Fischer, S. M., Iwata, B. A., & Mazaleski, J. L. (1997). Noncontingent delivery of arbitrary reinforcers as treatment for self-injurious behavior. *Journal of Applied Behavior Analysis, 30*(2), 239–249. https://doi.org/10.1901/jaba.1997.30-239

Fisher, W. W., DeLeon, I. G., Rodriguez-Catter, V., & Keeney, K. M. (2004). Enhancing the effects of extinction on attention-maintained behavior through noncontingent delivery of attention or stimuli identified via a competing stimulus assessment. *Journal of Applied Behavior Analysis, 37*(2), 171–184. https://doi.org/10.1901/jaba.2004.37-171

Fisher, W. W., O'Connor, J. T., Kurtz, P. F., DeLeon, I. G., & Gotjen, D. L. (2000). The effects of noncontingent delivery of high- and low-preference stimuli on attention maintained destructive behavior. *Journal of Applied Behavior Analysis, 33*(1), 79–83. https://doi.org/10.1901/jaba.2000.33-79

Fisher, W., Piazza, C. C., Bowman, L. G., Hagopian, L. P., Owens, J. C., & Slevin, I. (1992). A comparison of two approaches for identifying reinforcers for persons with severe and profound disabilities. *Journal of Applied Behavior Analysis, 25*(2), 491–498. https://doi.org/10.1901/jaba.25-491

Fulton, C. J., Tiger, J. H., Meitzen, H. M., & Effertz, H. M. (2020). A comparison of accumulated and distributed reinforcement periods with children exhibiting escape-maintained problem behavior. *Journal of Applied Behavior Analysis, 53*(2), 782–795. https://doi.org/10.1002/jaba.622

Fuhrman, A. M., Greer, B. D., Zangrillo, A. N., & Fisher, W. W. (2018). Evaluating competing activities to enhance functional communication training during reinforcement schedule thinning. *Journal of Applied Behavior Analysis, 51*(4), 931–942. https://doi.org/10.1002/jaba.486

Gardner, A. W., Wacker, D. P., & Boelter, E. W. (2009). An evaluation of the interaction between quality of attention and negative reinforcement with children who display escape-maintained problem behavior. *Journal of Applied Behavior Analysis, 42*(2), 343–348. https://doi.org/10.1901/jaba.2009.42-343

Golonka, Z., Wacker, D., Berg, W., Derby, K. M., Harding, J., & Peck, S. (2000). Effects of escape to alone versus escape to enriched environments on adaptive and aberrant behavior. *Journal of Applied Behavior Analysis, 33*(2), 243–246. https://doi.org/10.1901/jaba.2000.33-243

Hagopian, L. P., Fisher, W. W., Thibault Sullivan, M., Acquisto, J., & LeBlanc, L. A. (1998). Effectiveness of functional communication training with and without extinction and punishment: A summary of 21 inpatient cases. *Journal of Applied Behavior Analysis, 31*(2), 211–235. https://doi.org/10.1901/jaba.1998.31-211

Hagopian, L. P., Rooker, G. W., & Zarcone, J. R. (2015). Delineating subtypes of self-injurious behavior maintained by automatic reinforcement. *Journal of Applied Behavior Analysis, 48*(3), 523–543. https://doi.org/10.1002/jaba.236

Hagopian, L. P., Rooker, G. W., Zarcone, J. R., Bonner, A. C., & Arevalo, A. R. (2017). Further analysis of subtypes of automatically reinforced SIB: A replication and quantitative analysis of published datasets. *Journal of Applied Behavior Analysis, 50*(1), 48–66. https://doi.org/10.1002/jaba.368

Harding, J. W., Wacker, D. P., Berg, W. K., Lee, J. F., & Dolezal, D. (2009). Conducting functional communication training in home settings: A case study and recommendations for practitioners. *Behavior Analysis in Practice, 2*(1), 21–33. https://doi.org/10.1007/BF03391734

Hedquist, C. B., & Roscoe, E. M. (2020). A comparison of differential reinforcement procedures for treating automatically reinforced behavior. *Journal of Applied Behavior Analysis, 53*(1), 284–295. https://doi.org/10.1002/jaba.561

Horner, R. D. (1980). The effects of an environmental "enrichment" program on the behavior of institutionalized profoundly retarded children. *Journal of Applied Behavior Analysis, 13*(3), 473–491. https://doi.org/10.1901/jaba.1980.130473

Horner, R. H., Day, H. M., Sprague, J. R., O'Brien, M., & Heathfield, L. T. (1991). Interspersed requests: A nonaversive procedure for reducing aggression and self-injury during instruction. *Journal of Applied Behavior Analysis, 24*(2), 265–278. https://doi.org/10.1901/jaba.1991.24-265

Howell, M., Dounavi, K., & Storey, C. (2019). To choose or not to choose?: A systematic literature review considering the effects of antecedent and consequence choice upon on-task and problem behavior. *Review Journal of Autism and Developmental Disorders, 6*(1), 63–84. https://doi.org/10.1007/s40489-018-00154-7

Ing, A. D., Roane, H. S., & Veenstra, R. A. (2011). Functional analysis and treatment of coprophagia. *Journal of Applied Behavior Analysis, 44*(1), 151–155. https://doi.org/10.1901/jaba.2011.44-151

Ingvarsson, E. T., Kahng, S., & Hausman, N. L. (2008). Some effects of noncontingent positive reinforcement on multiply controlled problem behavior and compliance in a demand context. *Journal of Applied Behavior Analysis, 41*(3), 435–440. https://doi.org/10.1901/jaba.2008.41-435

Iwata, B. A., Dorsey, M. F., Slifer, K. J., Bauman, K. E., & Richman, G. S. (1994). Toward a functional analysis of self-injury. Journal of Applied Behavior Analysis, 27(2), 197–209. https://doi.org/10.1901/jaba.1994.27-197. (Reprinted from "Toward a functional analysis of self-injury," 1982, Analysis and Intervention in Developmental Disabilities, 2(1), 3–20, https://doi.org/10.1016/0270-4684(82)90003-9).

Jerome, J., & Sturmey, P. (2008). Reinforcing efficacy of interactions with preferred and nonpreferred staff under progressive-ratio schedules. *Journal of Applied Behavior Analysis, 41*(2), 221–225. https://doi.org/10.1901/jaba.2008.41-221

Kahng, S., Iwata, B. A., DeLeon, I. G., Wallace, M., & D. (2000). A comparison of procedures for programming noncontingent reinforcement schedules. *Journal of Applied Behavior Analysis, 33*(2), 223–231. https://doi.org/10.1901/jaba.2000.33-223

Kahng, S., Iwata, B. A., Thompson, R. H., & Hanley, G. P. (2000). A method for identifying satiation versus extinction effects under noncontingent reinforcement schedules. *Journal of Applied Behavior Analysis, 33*(4), 419–432. https://doi.org/10.1901/jaba.2000.33-419

Kelly, M. A., Roscoe, E. M., Hanley, G. P., & Schlichenmeyer, K. (2014). Evaluation of assessment methods for identifying social reinforcers. *Journal of Applied Behavior Analysis, 47*(1), 113–135. https://doi.org/10.1002/jaba.107

Kettering, T. L., Fisher, W. W., Kelley, M. E., & LaRue, R. H. (2018). Sound attenuation and preferred music in the treatment of problem behavior maintained by escape from noise. *Journal of Applied Behavior Analysis, 51*(3), 687–693. https://doi.org/10.1002/jaba.475

Killu, K., Clare, C. M., & Im, A. (1999). Choice vs. preference: The effects of choice and no choice by preferred and non preferred spelling tasks on the academic behavior of students with disabilities. *Journal of Behavioral Education, 9*(3–4), 239–253. https://doi.org/10.1023/a:1022143716509

Kodak, T., Lerman, D. C., Volkert, V. M., & Trosclair, N. (2007). Further examination of factors that influence preference for positive versus negative reinforcement. *Journal of Applied Behavior Analysis, 40*(1), 25–44. https://doi.org/10.1901/jaba.2007.151-05

Kodak, T., Miltenberger, R. G., & Romaniuk, C. (2003). The effects of differential negative reinforcement of other behavior and noncontingent escape on compliance. *Journal of Applied Behavior Analysis, 36*(3), 379–382. https://doi.org/10.1901/jaba.2003.36-379

Kurtz, P. F., Boelter, E. W., Jarmolowicz, D. P., Chin, M. D., & Hagopian, L. P. (2011). An analysis of functional communication training as an empirically supported treatment for problem behavior displayed by individuals with intellectual disabilities. *Research in Developmental Disabilities, 32*(6), 2935–2942. https://doi.org/10.1016/j.ridd.2011.05.009

Lalli, J. S., Casey, S. D., & Kates, K. (1997). Noncontingent reinforcement as treatment for severe problem behavior: Some procedural variations. *Journal of Applied Behavior Analysis, 30*(1), 127–137. https://doi.org/10.1901/jaba.1997.30-127

Lalli, J. S., Vollmer, T. R., Progar, P. R., Wright, C., Borrero, J., Daniel, D., ... May, W. (1999). Competition between positive and negative reinforcement in the treatment of escape behavior. *Journal of Applied Behavior Analysis, 32*(3), 285–296. https://doi.org/10.1901/jaba.32-285

Laraway, S., Snycerski, S., Michael, J., & Poling, A. (2003). Motivating operations and terms to describe them: Some further refinements. *Journal of Applied Behavior Analysis, 36*(3), 407–414. https://doi.org/10.1901/jaba.2003.36-407

Lerman, D. C. (Ed.). (2013). Special issue on functional analysis: Commemorating thirty years of research and practice [special issue]. Journal of Applied Behavior Analysis 46(1).

Lomas, J. E., Fisher, W. W., & Kelley, M. E. (2010). The effects of variable-time delivery of food items and praise on problem behavior reinforced by escape. *Journal of Applied Behavior Analysis, 43*(3), 425–435. https://doi.org/10.1901/jaba.2010.43-425

Mace, F. C., Hock, M. L., Lalli, J. S., West, B. J., Belfiore, P., Pinter, E., & Brown, D. K. (1988). Behavioral momentum in the treatment of noncompliance. *Journal of Applied Behavior Analysis, 21*(2), 123–141. https://doi.org/10.1901/jaba.1988.21-123

Mace, F. C., Pratt, J. L., Prager, K. L., & Pritchard, D. (2011). An evaluation of three methods of saying "no" to avoid an escalating response class hierarchy. *Journal of Applied Behavior Analysis, 44*(1), 83–94. https://doi.org/10.1901/jaba.2011.44-83

May, M. E. (2019). Effects of differential consequences on choice making in students at risk for academic failure. *Behavior Analysis in Practice, 12*(1), 154–161. https://doi.org/10.1007/s40617-018-0267-3

McComas, J. J., Wacker, D. P., & Cooper, L. J. (1996). Experimental analysis of academic performance in a classroom setting. *Journal of Behavioral Education, 6*(2), 191–201. https://doi.org/10.1007/BF02110232

McComas, J. J., Wacker, D. P., Cooper, L. J., Asmus, J. M., Richman, D., & Stoner, B. (1996). Brief experimental analysis of stimulus prompts for accurate responding on academic tasks in an outpatient clinic. *Journal of Applied Behavior Analysis, 29*(3), 397–401. https://doi.org/10.1901/jaba.1996.29-397

McComas, J. J., Hoch, H., Paone, D., & El-Roy, D. (2000). Escape behavior during academic tasks: A preliminary analysis of idiosyncratic establishing operations. *Journal of Applied Behavior Analysis, 33*(4), 479–493. https://doi.org/10.1901/jaba.2000.33-479

McGinnis, M. A., Houchins-Juarez, N., McDaniel, J. L., & Kennedy, C. H. (2010). Abolishing and establishing operation analyses of social attention as positive reinforcement for problem behavior. *Journal of Applied Behavior Analysis, 43*(1), 119–123. https://doi.org/10.1901/jaba.2010.43-119

Michael, J. (1982). Distinguishing between discriminative and motivational functions of stimuli. *Journal of the Experimental Analysis of Behavior, 37*(1), 149–155. https://doi.org/10.1901/jeab.1982.37-149

Morris, S. L., & Vollmer, T. R. (2019). Assessing preference for types of social interaction. *Journal of Applied Behavior Analysis, 52*(4), 1064–1075. https://doi.org/10.1002/jaba.597

O'Reilly, M. F., Edrisinha, C., Sigafoos, J., Lancioni, G., & Andrews, A. (2006). Isolating the evocative and abative effects of an establishing operation on challenging behavior. *Behavioral Interventions, 21*(3), 195–204. https://doi.org/10.1002/bin.215

O'Reilly, M., Edrisinha, C., Sigafoos, J., Lancioni, G., Machalicek, W., & Antonucci, M. (2007). The effects of presession attention on subsequent attention-extinction and alone conditions. *Journal of Applied Behavior Analysis, 40*(4), 731–735. https://doi.org/10.1901/jaba.2007.731-735

Pace, G. M., Ivancic, M. T., Edwards, G. L., Iwata, B. A., & Page, T. J. (1985). Assessment of stimulus preference and reinforcer value with profoundly retarded individuals. *Journal of Applied Behavior Analysis, 18*(3), 249–255. https://doi.org/10.1901/jaba.1985.18-249

Payne, S. W., & Dozier, C. L. (2013). Positive reinforcement as treatment for problem behavior maintained by negative reinforcement. *Journal of Applied Behavior Analysis, 46*(3), 699–703. https://doi.org/10.1002/jaba.54

Piazza, C. C., Adelinis, J. D., Hanley, G. P., Goh, H.-L., & Delia, M. D. (2000). An evaluation of the effects of matched stimuli on behaviors maintained by automatic reinforcement. *Journal of Applied Behavior Analysis, 33*(1), 13–27. https://doi.org/10.1901/jaba.2000.33-13

Reed, G. K., Ringdahl, J. E., Wacker, D. P., Barretto, A., & Andelman, M. S. (2005). The effects of fixed-time and contingent schedules of negative reinforcement on compliance and aberrant behavior. *Research in Developmental Disabilities, 26*(3), 281–295. https://doi.org/10.1016/j.ridd.2004.01.004

Reichle, J., & Wacker, D. P. (2017). *Functional communication training for problem behavior.* New York, NY: The Guilford Press.

Richman, D. M., Wacker, D. P., Cooper-Brown, L. J., Kayser, K., Crosland, K., Stephens, T. J., & Asmus, J. (2001). Stimulus characteristics within directives: Effects on accuracy of task completion. *Journal of Applied Behavior Analysis, 34*(3), 289–312. https://doi.org/10.1901/jaba.2001.34-289

Rincover, A., Cook, R., Peoples, A., & Packard, D. (1979). Sensory extinction and sensory reinforcement principles for programming multiple adaptive behavior change. *Journal of Applied Behavior Analysis, 12*(2), 221–233. https://doi.org/10.1901/jaba.1979.12-221

Ringdahl, J. E., & Sellers, J. A. (2000). The effects of different adults as therapists during functional analyses. *Journal of Applied Behavior Analysis, 33*(2), 247–250. https://doi.org/10.1901/jaba.2000.33-247

Ringdahl, J. E., Vollmer, T. R., Marcus, B. A., & Roane, H. S. (1997). An analogue evaluation of environmental enrichment: The role of stimulus preference. *Journal of Applied Behavior Analysis, 30*(2), 203–216. https://doi.org/10.1901/jaba.1997.30-203

Rispoli, M. J., O'Reilly, M. F., Sigafoos, J., Lang, R., Kang, S., Lancioni, G., & Parker, R. (2011). Effects of presession satiation on challenging behavior and academic engagement for children with autism during classroom instruction. *Education and Training in Autism and Developmental Disabilities, 46*(4), 607–618.

Roane, H. S., Lerman, D. C., & Vorndran, C. M. (2001). Assessing reinforcers under progressive schedule requirements. *Journal of Applied Behavior Analysis, 34*(2), 145–167. https://doi.org/10.1901/jaba.2001.34-145

Roane, H. S., Vollmer, T. R., Ringdahl, J. E., & Marcus, B. A. (1998). Evaluation of a brief stimulus preference assessment. *Journal of Applied Behavior Analysis, 31*(4), 605–620. https://doi.org/10.1901/jaba.1998.31-605

Roantree, C. F., & Kennedy, C. H. (2006). A paradoxical effect of presession attention on stereotypy: Antecedent attention as an establishing, not an abolishing operation. *Journal of Applied Behavior Analysis, 39*(3), 381–384. https://doi.org/10.1901/jaba.2006.97-05

Romaniuk, C., Miltenberger, R., Conyers, C., Jenner, N., Jurgens, M., & Ringenberg, C. (2002). The influence of activity choice on problem behaviors maintained by escape versus attention. *Journal of Applied Behavior Analysis, 35*(4), 349–362. https://doi.org/10.1901/jaba.2002.35-349

Rooker, G. W., Bonner, A. C., Dillon, C. M., & Zarcone, J. R. (2018). Behavioral treatments of automatically reinforced SIB: 1982-2015. *Journal of Applied Behavior Analysis, 51*(4), 974–997. https://doi.org/10.1002/jaba.492

Roscoe, E. M., Iwata, B. A., & Goh, H. (1998). A comparison of noncontingent reinforcement and sensory extinction as treatments for self-injurious behavior. *Journal of Applied Behavior Analysis, 31*(4), 645–646. https://doi.org/10.1901/jaba.1998.31-635

Roscoe, E. M., Iwata, B. A., & Zhou, L. (2013). Assessment and treatment of chronic hand mouthing. *Journal of Applied Behavior Analysis, 46*(1), 181–198. https://doi.org/10.1002/jaba.14

Roscoe, E. M., Rooker, G. W., Pence, S. T., Longworth, L. J., & Zarcone, J. (2009). Assessing the utility of a demand assessment for functional analysis. *Journal of Applied Behavior Analysis, 42*(4), 819–825. https://doi.org/10.1901/jaba.2009.42-819

Schieltz, K. M., Wacker, D. P., & Romani, P. W. (2017). Effects of signaled positive reinforcement on problem behavior maintained by negative reinforcement. *Journal of Behavioral Education, 26*(2), 137–150. https://doi.org/10.1007/s10864-016-9265-0

Schieltz, K. M., Wacker, D. P., Suess, A. N., Graber, J. E., Lustig, N. H., & Detrick, J. (2020). Evaluating the effects of positive reinforcement, instructional strategies, and negative reinforcement on problem behavior and academic performance: An experimental analysis. *Journal of Developmental and Physical Disabilities, 32*(2), 339–363. https://doi.org/10.1007/s10882-019-09696-y

Schnell, L. K., Vladescu, J. C., Kisamore, A. N., DeBar, R. M., Kahng, S., & Marano, K. (2020). Assessment to identify learner-specific prompt and prompt-fading procedures for children with autism spectrum disorder. *Journal of Applied Behavior Analysis, 53*(2), 1111–1129. https://doi.org/10.1002/jaba.623

Seaver, J. L., & Bourret, J. C. (2014). An evaluation of response prompts for teaching behavior chains. *Journal of Applied Behavior Analysis, 47*(4), 777–792. https://doi.org/10.1002/jaba.159

Shore, B. A., Iwata, B. A., DeLeon, I. G., Kahng, S., & Smith, R. G. (1997). An analysis of reinforcer substitutability using object manipulation and self-injury as competing responses. *Journal of Applied Behavior Analysis, 30*(1), 21–41. https://doi.org/10.1901/jaba.1997.30-21

Smith, R. G., Iwata, B. A., Goh, H.-L., & Shore, B. A. (1995). Analysis of establishing operations for self-injury maintained by escape. *Journal of Applied Behavior Analysis, 28*(4), 515–535. https://doi.org/10.1901/jaba.1995.28-515

Spencer, V. G., & Alkhanji, R. (2018). Response interruption and redirection (RIRD) as a behavioral intervention for vocal stereotypy: A systematic review. *Education and Training in Autism and Developmental Disabilities, 53*(1), 33–43.

Steege, M. W., Wacker, D. P., Cigrand, K. C., Berg, W. K., Novak, C. G., Reimers, T. M., … DeRaad, A. (1990). Use of negative reinforcement in the treatment of self-injurious behavior. *Journal of Applied Behavior Analysis, 23*(4), 459–467. https://doi.org/10.1901/jaba.1990.23-459

Suess, A. N., Schieltz, K. M., Wacker, D. P., Detrick, J., & Podlesnik, C. A. (2020). An evaluation of resurgence following functional communication training conducted in alternative antecedent contexts via telehealth. *Journal of the Experimental Analysis of Behavior, 113*(1), 278–301. https://doi.org/10.1002/jeab.551

Sumter, M. E., Gifford, M. R., Tiger, J. H., Effertz, H. M., & Fulton, C. J. (2020). Providing noncontingent alternative, functional reinforcers during delays following functional communication training. *Journal of Applied Behavior Analysis. Advance online publication.* https://doi.org/10.1002/jaba.708

Taravella, C. C., Lerman, D. C., Contrucci, S. A., & Roane, H. S. (2000). Further evaluation of low-ranked items in stimulus-choice preference assessments. *Journal of Applied Behavior Analysis, 33*(1), 105–108. https://doi.org/10.1901/jaba.2000.33-105

Tiger, J. H., Hanley, G. P., & Bruzek, J. (2008). Functional communication training: A review and practical guide. *Behavior Analysis in Practice, 1*(1), 16–23. https://doi.org/10.1007/BF03391716

Trosclair-Lasserre, N. M., Lerman, D. C., Call, N. A., Addison, L. R., & Kodak, T. (2008). Reinforcement magnitude: An evaluation of preference and reinforcer efficacy. *Journal of Applied Behavior Analysis, 41*(2), 203–220. https://doi.org/10.1901/jaba.2008.41-203

Van Camp, C. M., Lerman, D. C., Kelley, M. E., Contrucci, S. A., & Vorndran, C. M. (2000). Variable-time reinforcement schedules in the treatment of socially maintained problem behavior. *Journal of Applied Behavior Analysis, 33*(4), 545–557. https://doi.org/10.1901/jaba.2000.33-545

Vollmer, T. R., & Iwata, B. A. (1991). Establishing operations and reinforcement effects. *Journal of Applied Behavior Analysis, 24*(2), 279–291. https://doi.org/10.1901/jaba.1991.24-279

Vollmer, T. R., Iwata, B. A., Zarcone, J. R., Smith, R. G., & Mazaleski, J. L. (1993). The role of attention in the treatment of attention-maintained self-injurious behavior: Noncontingent reinforcement and differential reinforcement of other behavior. *Journal of Applied Behavior Analysis, 26*(1), 9–21. https://doi.org/10.1901/jaba.1993.26-9

Vollmer, T. R., Marcus, B. A., & Ringdahl, J. E. (1995). Noncontingent escape as treatment for self-injurious behavior maintained by negative reinforcement. *Journal of Applied Behavior Analysis, 28*(1), 15–26. https://doi.org/10.1901/jaba.1995.28-15

Wacker, D. P., Harding, J. W., Berg, W. K., Lee, J. F., Schieltz, K. M., Padilla, Y. C., … Shahan, T. A. (2011). An evaluation of persistence of treatment effects during long-term treatment of destructive behavior. *Journal of the Experimental Analysis of Behavior, 96*(2), 261–282. https://doi.org/10.1901/jeab.2011.96-261

Wacker, D. P., Lee, J. F., Padilla Dalmau, Y. C., Kopelman, T. G., Lindgren, S. D., Kuhle, J., … Waldron, D. B. (2013). Conducting functional communication training via telehealth to reduce the problem behavior of young children with autism. *Journal of Developmental and Physical Disabilities, 25*(1), 35–48. https://doi.org/10.1007/s10882-012-9314-0

Zarcone, J. R., Fisher, W. W., & Piazza, C. C. (1996). Analysis of free-time contingencies as positive versus negative reinforcement. *Journal of Applied Behavior Analysis, 29*(2), 247–250. https://doi.org/10.1901/jaba.1996.29-247

Chapter 14
Treatments Associated with Mental Health Disorders and Functional Assessment

Joshua J. Montrenes and Johnny L. Matson

Introduction

Mental health conditions are a broadly defined category of psychopathology that may include anxiety disorders (e.g., generalized anxiety disorder; GAD, specific phobia, social anxiety disorder; SAD), depressive disorders (e.g., major depressive disorder; MDD, persistent depressive disorder; PDD), bipolar and related disorders (e.g., bipolar disorder; BPD), and trauma-and-stressor-related disorders (e.g., post-traumatic stress disorder; PTSD) (American Psychological Association; APA, 2013). Among the most prevalent are anxiety disorders (e.g., lifetime prevalence of any anxiety disorder was 31.1% of adults and 31.9% for adolescents in the United States; Harvard Medical School, 2017; Merikangas et al., 2010) and depressive disorders (e.g., lifetime prevalence of major depressive disorder for adults in the United States was 20.6%; Hasin et al., 2018).

Anxiety disorders can be associated with clinically significant emotional distress and physiological symptoms (e.g., increased heart rate) as well as medical conditions including heart attack, asthma, ulcer, and increased risk of suicide (Baxter, Vos, Scott, Ferrari, & Whiteford, 2014; Niles et al., 2015; Sareen et al., 2005). Moreover, in addition to clinically significant symptoms of depressed mood, loss of interest in activities, and feelings of worthlessness (among others), major depressive disorder (MDD) is associated with increased risk for diabetes, stroke, and death by suicide (APA, 2013; Otte et al., 2016).

Given the burden of mental health disorders such as anxiety and depressive disorders, many treatments have been developed to address their negative effects. One

J. J. Montrenes (✉) J. L. Matson
Department of Psychology, Louisiana State University, Baton Rouge, LA, USA
e-mail: jmontr4@lsu.edu

© Springer Nature Switzerland AG 2021   385
J. L. Matson (ed.), *Functional Assessment for Challenging Behaviors and Mental Health Disorders*, Autism and Child Psychopathology Series,
https://doi.org/10.1007/978-3-030-66270-7_14

such method of treatment involves the use of functional assessment. Functional assessment is a tool that can be used in conjunction with treatments for mental health disorders, such as anxiety and depression, to better inform treatment targets (Ferster, 1973; Friman, 2007). Most notably, several of the most widely used treatments for anxiety disorders have been developed through research in classical conditioning (e.g., systematic desensitization; SD; Wolpe, 1954) and behavior analysis (cognitive behavioral therapy; CBT; Beck, 1970; Hazlett-Stevens & Craske, 2002). Treatment targets and progress can be informed through the use of functional assessment. This chapter aims to discuss how functional assessment can supplement behaviorally based treatments for mental health disorders. In order to better inform this discussion, behavioral theories of the development of mental health disorders will be presented, with a specific focus on fear and anxiety, and depression. This will be followed by a discussion of several treatments for mental health disorders from a behavioral perspective. A brief overview of functional assessment, including functional behavioral assessment (FBA) and functional analysis (FA), will follow. Finally, a discussion integrating behavioral theories of mental health disorders, behaviorally based treatments, and use of functional assessment will be presented.

In the following sections, some of this behavioral research will be reviewed followed by examples of these behaviorally based treatments. Finally, functional assessment methods and examples of incorporating these methods into treatment of mental health disorders will be examined.

Behavioral Theories of Psychopathology

Several theories explaining the development of anxiety disorders have been presented historically. Early theories, such as those first developed by Pavlov (1927), Watson and Rayner (1920), and Wolpe (1950), focused on using classical conditioning as a framework to identify the behavioral underpinnings of how fear (and later, anxiety) is acquired. For instance, according to Pavlov (1927), an unconditioned stimulus (UCS) elicits an unconditioned response (UCR) without prior training. He further stated that when a neutral stimulus is repeatedly presented at the same time as the UCS, it elicits the same response as the UCS, thusly becoming a conditioned stimulus (CS). This was demonstrated in Watson and Rayner's (1920) well-known "Little Albert" experiment, where a rat was the neutral stimulus, a loud, aversive noise was the UCS, and crying (emitted by a young boy) was the UCR. Following the conditioning sequence, the rat became the CS with crying as the UCR (Watson & Rayner, 1920). Moreover, this type of conditioning can happen outside of laboratory environments; one may develop fears and maladaptive responses to those fears, such as avoidance (Kaplan, Heinrichs, & Carey, 2011).

Synthesizing this early work, an important addition to theories of conditioned fear was postulated by Mowrer (1939) with his two-stage theory of fear and avoidance. According to Mowrer (1939), fear and anxiety are created as an adverse or painful reaction to an aversive stimulus. Fear itself in this case is considered a powerful motivating tool, and any action that reduces this fear is reinforcing. Thusly, Mowrer concluded that avoidant behaviors become highly reinforcing; avoidance leads to a reduction of fear and becomes further reinforced each time it is enacted. Over time, this theory was found to be insufficient to account for the entirety of human fears, and additional explanations were proposed.

Later theories, such as Rachman's (1976, 1977) neo-conditioning model, proposed that several pathways of fear conditioning may occur; direct contact with feared stimuli was not necessary to develop fear of that stimuli. Processes such as vicarious exposure and vicarious transmission (Rachman, 1977) were also able to produce fears despite the individual never making direct contact with the contingency related to the feared stimulus. For instance, a large part of human learning that influences our emotional responses and overt behavior is due to vicarious, observational learning (Bandura, 1969). In this vein, Rachman (1977) noted that fear and anxiety can be influenced through observing others' fearful experiences which he described as vicarious exposure. In addition to observational learning, humans also learn through information transmitted through language; fears can be transmitted in this manner as well, and individuals do not need direct contact with a feared stimulus to acquire such a fear (Rachman, 1977).

In addition to theories of how fear and anxiety develop, additional theories add insight as to factors that may influence the strength of the fear being conditioned. Asking the question of why not everyone that experiences a traumatic event develops fears or phobias, Mineka and Zinbarg's (2006) work outlined several important factors that can either increase or decrease the strength of fear conditioning. Firstly, they noted that prior experiences can affect the strength of fear conditioning, such that prior, nontraumatic experiences with a CS can reduce the strength of the pairing of the CS and UCS after a traumatic experience. Secondly, Mineka and Zinbarg described that having control or a sense of control during a traumatic event can reduce the strength of the feared stimulus and that the reverse is also true: having less control can increase the strength of the fear conditioning. Lastly, they noted 2 additional processes that can increase the strength of fear conditioning. These include being exposed to an unrelated, traumatic event, which can increase the strength of an unrelated, feared CS. Additionally, information that is acquired verbally or socially can lead to a reevaluation process that strengthens the CS/UCS relationship.

Several behavioral theories of depression have been utilized to explain the development of the disorder. One such theory, Ferster's (1973) behavioral view of depression, indicated that the link between an individual's behavior and the reinforcement for that behavior becomes diminished when they experience depressive symptoms, making reinforcement less successful. Ferster also noted that behaviors affected by these weakening links to reinforcement may be related to several different areas including physiological (e.g., eating) and social (e.g., eating with others). In addition, multiple, observable behaviors of depression exist, which consist of less engagement in pleasurable activities, an escalation of avoidant behaviors, crying and irritable behaviors, and psychomotor retardation (Ferster, 1973).

Further theories of depression include that presented by Lazarus (1968) which described that the development of depression occurs due to either ineffective or a low frequency of reinforcers. Furthermore, the depressed person is suggested to be on an "extinction schedule," such that past, effective reinforcers are discontinued, which sets in motion a state of grief in the individual (Lazarus, 1968). Lazarus also noted that this grief can be combatted by the use of additional reinforcers. However, if none are available, or if the individual is unable to utilize them, then the state of depression may become strengthened.

Lewinsohn and Atwood (1969) and Lewinsohn (1975) stated that depression can be described as a reduced amount of response-contingent positive reinforcement. These authors went on to note that this state serves as an UCS for overt behaviors of depression (e.g., fatigue, dysphoria). Certain contingencies in the social environment serve to positively or negatively reinforce depression (Lewinsohn, 1975; Lewinsohn & Atwood, 1969). For instance, some individuals will provide sympathy and concern to the depressed person, which provides positive reinforcement, while others may avoid the depressed individual, providing negative reinforcement of the depressed behaviors (Lewinsohn, 1975; Lewinsohn & Atwood, 1969). Lewinsohn and Atwood (1969) and Lewinsohn (1975) also described that the positive reinforcement that a person can potentially obtain is dependent on the frequency of events which may be reinforcing, the number of these events which can actually be provided by the environment, and the behaviors of the depressed person that may aid in obtaining reinforcement.

Behavioral Treatments for Mental Health Disorders

Many behaviorally based treatments for mental health disorders are well-known, including systematic desensitization (Wolpe, 1954), CBT (Beck, 1970), and acceptance and commitment therapy (ACT; Hayes, Strosahl, & Wilson, 1999). These are common treatments for mental health disorders such as anxiety, depression, and specific phobia. A select number of these treatments will be described in this section to illustrate the utility of behavior analysis in the development and implementation of interventions for mental health disorders.

An early behavioral treatment for anxiety disorders came in the form of Wolpe's (1954) systematic desensitization. Based on classical conditioning, Wolpe established the use of reciprocal inhibition as a means to counteract anxiety responses, such as avoidance. This was achieved by both repeated exposure to the feared stimulus, as well as by pairing relaxation techniques with the feared stimulus in order to reduce maladaptive behavioral responses (Lazarus & Rachman, 1957; Wolpe, 1954). Wolpe went on to state that this reduction of responses occurs due to the weakening of the link between the feared stimulus and the maladaptive response. To better describe the process of this therapeutic technique, an overview of the procedure is presented.

In order to begin systematic desensitization, first the clinician must gather information concerning what stimuli cause the client's fear or anxiety and construct these items in a list of 5–25 items, which can continually be updated (Lazarus & Rachman, 1957; Wolpe, 1954). Next, as directed by the client, the items on this list are formed into a hierarchy from most to least distressing (Wolpe, 1954). As noted by Wolpe (1954), relaxation techniques are also taught to the client during this time. He then notes that sessions begin by describing to the client which stimulus will be presented and that they may stop the exposure at any time. Following instruction, clients use relaxation techniques followed by visualization of feared stimuli for 5–10 seconds and finally re-engage the use of relaxation techniques. According to Wolpe, it is generally recommended that between 2 and 4 feared stimuli are utilized each session and that clients note reactions to each stimulus to update treatment progress each session. Following a marked reduction in anxiety responses, the next most feared stimulus is presented. Finally, Wolpe noted that this process is then generalized to real-life situations through repeated practice.

Empirical support for the effectiveness of SD most notably exists for the treatment of phobias, including phobic responses to mice (Willis & Edwards, 1969), snake phobia (Lang & Lazovik, 1963), and noise phobia (McGrath, Tsui, Humphries, & Yule, 1990). Although few meta-analyses assessing SD's efficacy exist, one such study reported a large effect size (i.e., 0.91) across outcomes including reduction of anxiety, social relations, and physiological stress (Smith & Glass, 1977).

The work of Reisinger (1972) offered an additional treatment using behavioral techniques. In a 1972 case study, Reisinger proposed the use of response cost in the context of a token economy for treatment of an individual with depression in a psychiatric hospital. Reisinger references Lewinsohn and Atwood's (1969) behavioral theory of depression (which has been previously discussed in this chapter) which considers an individual with depression to have a disruption in positive reinforcement in their environment. With this consideration, Reisinger noted that the structure of this treatment was to reinforce adaptive behavioral responses and response cost maladaptive behaviors in a patient with depression. For example, when the patient exhibited crying, tokens were removed. Conversely, when the patient displayed smiling, they were given a token. Reisinger stated that these tokens were utilized for obtaining rewards such as access to the hospital grounds or time to watch television. The results of the study concluded that a large increase in adaptive behavior (e.g., smiling; 0 instances at baseline to 23 instances during the final week of treatment) and a large decrease in maladaptive behavior (e.g., crying; 30 instances at baseline to 2 instances during the final week of treatment) occurred which was maintained at 14-month follow-up.

Developed by Beck (1970), CBT is a widely used treatment for mental health disorders including anxiety, depression, and PTSD. This therapy is grounded in behavioral theory but also incorporates elements gleaned from cognitive research (Hazlett-Stevens & Craske, 2002). Referencing classical conditioning operant conditioning, learning theory, and cognitive research, Beck (1970) posited that psychological dysfunction was acquired both through learning and information processing. For instance, anxiety may be the result of a combination of factors, including a pairing of an UCS and an aversive stimulus, reinforcement of avoidant behaviors, and cognitive tendencies to attend to threatening information and ignore information that a feared stimulus poses no threat (Hazlett-Stevens & Craske, 2002).

Hazlett-Stevens & Craske (2002) noted that by design, CBT incorporates elements of FA (which will be discussed in-depth later in the chapter) to guide treatment. In this way, the maladaptive behavior of the individual in treatment is considered to be a function of the current, external environment as well as internal, cognitive conditions. Furthermore, Hazlett-Stevens and Craske noted that behavior of the individual can be better understood once its function is identified and that this behavior can then be targeted for treatment. A similar approach is taken to cognitive processes, such that an underlying, core aspect of cognition is assumed to be related to psychological dysfunction which must also be identified and subsequently targeted for treatment.

According to Hazlett-Stevens and Craske (2002), after identifying both behavioral functions and core cognitive processes which are leading to psychological dysfunction, a combination of behavioral and cognitive strategies, including exposure and cognitive restructuring, is utilized during CBT treatment. Thusly, new learning replaces maladaptive processes and behaviors, such that individuals are taught adaptive coping strategies while being exposed to aversive stimuli, and that generalization of these skills occurs, as coping strategies are applied to novel situations. Hazlett-Stevens and Craske also noted that CBT emphasizes continued assessment of the patient's behaviors and cognitive processes so that intervention strategies address relevant maladaptive processes and behaviors as the patient learns new skills.

Regarding efficacy, a comprehensive review of 106 meta-analyses of CBT use across several mental health disorders (e.g., anxiety disorders, depression, and eating disorders) found that there is strong support for its efficacy (i.e., medium to large effect sizes) in treatment of anxiety disorders and modest support for its efficacy (i.e., medium effect sizes) for treatment of depression (Hofmann, Asnaani, Vonk, Sawyer, & Fang, 2012). According to an additional comprehensive review, studies of CBT use across anxiety disorders (vs. waitlist control treatment) found effect sizes ranging from 0.57–1.05 for specific phobia, 0.86 for social anxiety symptoms of social phobia, 1.12 for obsessive-compulsive disorder (OCD), 1.26–1.40 for PTSD, and 0.64–1.15 for GAD (Olatunji, Cisler, & Deacon, 2010). Criticisms of CBT have been raised including mixed findings regarding whether its effects are maintained over time (Olatunji et al., 2010), a need for more empirical evidence across populations (e.g., minority groups) and variable dropout rates (Bados, Balaguer, & Saldaña, 2007). Despite these criticisms, CBT remains an efficacious treatment for anxiety disorders, and its incorporation of functional assessment techniques into its design suggests that functional assessment may, in part, add to this efficacy.

Hayes et al (2006) pioneered an intervention model (i.e., ACT) linked to more recent, contextual theories of behavior, such as relational frame theory (RFT; Hayes, Blackledge, & Barnes-Holmes, 2001). Philosophically, Hayes et al noted that ACT is based in functional contextualism, with the aim to both predict and influence events in the environment (Biglan & Hayes, 1996). Furthermore, this contextual view defined psychological events as the interactions of an organism with their environment in both historical and situational contexts. According to Hayes and colleagues, only events which can be manipulated are the focus of causal analyses, and that through ACT, observable behaviors and contexts are targeted to change thoughts, feelings, and behavior.

Theoretically, Hayes and colleagues (2006) noted that the development of ACT was directed by RFT. According to Hayes et al (2001), RFT posits that the basis of human cognition and language is the acquired ability to relate events (both jointly and in combination) and to manipulate the function of events based on these relations. Considering this theory, psychopathology is thusly related to the way in which language and cognition interact with environmental contingencies and the failure to achieve long-term goals, either by lack of persistence or by the inability to change. Moreover, Hayes et al (2006) noted that a problem underlying psychological dysfunction is psychological inflexibility, which occurs as a result of ineffective contextual control over language processes. An additional theory of psychopathology presented by Hayes and colleagues is cognitive fusion: an instance in which language processes lead to faulty behavioral regulation. To elaborate, when an individual's behavior is not guided by environmental contingencies, but rather by rigid verbal networks, the individual's behavior is inconsistent with relevant contingencies and they are not able to enact value-driven, goal-directed behavior.

ACT consists of 6 core processes which are designed to promote psychological flexibility and help individuals adjust behavior to better meet their goals. Hayes et al (2006) noted that the first core process of ACT is acceptance, which can be described as taking an active approach to experience events (even those that may cause anxiety or discomfort) and not trying to control how these events occur. This method can be described as a means to combat avoidant behaviors and increase values-based behaviors, such as individuals with anxiety being taught to fully experience their anxiety without avoidance.

The next process offered by Hayes et al (2006) is cognitive defusion. This is defined as a process to help transform maladaptive functions of thoughts or other private events, but not to attempt to transform the events themselves. Hayes and colleagues noted that the goal of cognitive defusion is to alter how an individual interfaces with their thoughts by developing contexts in which maladaptive functions are minimized. Put another way, this process helps one reduce the tendency to believe or have a connection to negative thoughts or private events. Several examples of cognitive defusion are presented by Hayes et al, including saying the thought out loud to reduce its literal quality.

Following this, Hayes et al (2006) stated that the next core process of ACT is being present, which is described as a continuous process of connecting to psychological and environmental events in a non-judgmental manner. This process aims to have individuals directly experience events to promote more variable behavior and act in a way that is consistent with their values; this direct experience allows increased contact with effective behaviors and greater behavioral control overall. Hayes and colleagues also emphasized using language as a means to describe and note events rather than to judge or attempt to predict events. Through this process, a sense of self that Hayes described as, "self as process," is able to manifest through defusion, non-judgment, and description (rather than attachment) of thoughts and emotions.

The fourth process presented by Hayes et al (2006) is self as context. This process is based around the notion that an individual can foster awareness of their own continued flow of experiences without developing an attachment to them; this helps to develop acceptance and defusion. According to Hayes et al, an individual can develop self as context by practicing mindfulness, the use of metaphors, and through experiential processes. This concept is derived from deictic frames such as, "I-you," and, "here-there," which indicate a perspective of self as well as a transcendent viewpoint to verbal humans that underlies language functions, including theory of mind and empathy.

Values is the next process put forth by Hayes and colleagues (2006), which is described as qualities of purposeful action which can be enacted in the moment. Several different exercises are used to aid individuals in deciding on how to live purposefully taking important life domains (e.g., career, personal life, spirituality) into account while simultaneously de-emphasizing maladaptive verbal processes which lead to decision making based on social compliance or avoidance, for example. This process also emphasizes that enacting the aforementioned processes (e.g., acceptance, cognitive defusion, being present) incrementally develop the means to live a life consistent with one's values.

Finally, the last process of ACT is committed action (Hayes et al., 2006). Hayes et al (2006) noted that this process promotes development of overarching patterns of effective action which are directly linked to an individual's values. Committed action is enacted through the use of any of a number of appropriate behavioral methods, including shaping methods, exposure, and goal setting. Through committed action, clearly defined goals set by an individual can be achieved through ACT processes, work during therapy sessions, and individual homework assignments which are associated with behavioral change.

As increasing amounts of randomized control trials (RCTs) have emerged in recent years, several meta-analyses have summarized these findings regarding ACT's efficacy (A-Tjak et al., 2015; Öst, 2014; Powers, Zum Vörde Sive Vörding, & Emmelkamp, 2009). Overall, findings have been mixed, with effect sizes ranging from 0.30 to 0.68 when compared to controls and effect sizes ranging from 0.14 to 0.16 when compared to established treatments (i.e., CBT; A-Tjak et al., 2015; Öst, 2014; Powers et al., 2009). Moreover, while A-Tjak et al. (2015) concluded that ACT may be as effective as CBT for treating anxiety orders and depression, Öst (2014) noted that ACT is not currently an established treatment for any disorder and is only possibly efficacious for treating depression and anxiety.

To summarize, Hayes et al (2006) characterized ACT as a behaviorally based intervention linked to recent behavioral theories such as RFT. Psychological inflexibility is a maladaptive style of relational abilities that underlies psychopathology (Hayes et al., 1999). Through the 6 core processes of ACT, the individual is trained to improve their psychological flexibility and to live within the present moment as much as possible (Hayes et al., 2006). Research on the efficacy of ACT is currently mixed, with one meta-analysis suggesting that it is comparable to established treatments for anxiety and depression (A-Tjak et al., 2015) and another meta-analysis suggesting that it is only possibly efficacious for anxiety and depression at this time (Öst, 2014).

An additional, behaviorally based treatment is behavioral activation (BA), which was specifically designed for treatment of depression (Martell, Addis, & Jacobson, 2001). BA was initially a component of cognitive therapy (CT; Beck, 1964) which was found to be as effective as CT when used to address relapsing of depressive symptoms (Gortner, Gollan, Dobson, & Jacobson, 1998). BA aims to identify activities that a depressed individual is avoiding and use these activities in a gradual pattern of exposure to return them to full participation in activities that will present opportunities for them to be positively reinforced (Jacobson, Martell, & Dimidjian, 2001; Veale, 2008). An additional focus is the use of FA to understand and formulate treatment strategies to address maladaptive responding (Jacobson et al., 2001; Veale, 2008). This strategy is, in part, a result of BA's grounding in contextual functionalism; there is emphasis on understanding events and environmental factors that may affect maladaptive responding (Veale, 2008).

At the start of BA, the therapist discusses with the client their current means of coping (e.g., avoidance, other maladaptive strategies) with their depressive symptoms. Next, the therapist and client discuss how these ineffective strategies have been maintaining their depression and only providing short-term relief, rather than addressing the underlying functional variables (Jacobson et al., 2001; Veale, 2008). Over time, clients are taught to perform components of their own FA by recognizing the consequences of their prior, ineffective coping mechanisms (Jacobson et al., 2001). For example, rumination and avoidance may lead to the individual withdrawing from their usual reinforcing activities which exacerbates depressive symptoms (Veale, 2008). Due to the pervasive nature of avoidant behaviors, BA specifically addresses this responding through, "avoidance modification" (Jacobson et al., 2001). Clients are given psychoeducation about avoidant behavioral functions, how to recognize them, and how to choose other, more effective coping mechanisms (Jacobson et al., 2001).

After this discussion, clients are encouraged to develop short-, medium-, and long-term goals with an overarching goal of both returning to a consistent routine and acting in a way that is consistent with their values; this is adapted from ACT's component of goal-directed behavior (Hayes et al., 1999; Jacobson et al., 2001; Veale, 2008). These are called, "graded task assignments," and are tasks of increasing difficulty that help clients gradually move toward full participation in activities that are regular and provide opportunities for positive environmental reinforcement (Jacobson et al., 2001).

A disruption of an individual's regular routine has been found to be an important variable when examining factors that maintain depression (Jacobson et al., 2001). For this reason, BA focuses on re-establishing regular routines that have been disrupted, such as eating, sleeping, and working (Jacobson et al., 2001). Moreover, the therapist will help clients formulate an activity log – this is meant to track the client's engagement (or lack of engagement) in activities (Veale, 2008). These, "focused activities," are meant to be viewed from an FA approach in order to assess how these response patterns affect their mood and to illustrate the effects of adaptive vs. maladaptive responding (Jacobson et al., 2001).

Clients are additionally provided psychoeducation relating to the function of rumination (Jacobson et al., 2001). For instance, negative complaints associated with rumination (e.g., "I hate this," "I don't want to do this anymore") may have served to allow the individual to escape an unpleasant situation (Ferster, 1973). As with other forms of escape, rumination is addressed through exposure (Carr, 1977). BA focuses on activation in this case by designing treatment activities that will maximize an individual's contact with environmental reinforcement and minimize rumination (Jacobson et al., 2001).

To summarize, through the aforementioned strategies of BA, clients are able to identify maladaptive patterns of responding and address them by performing positive actions, such as re-engagement in routine strategies that allow for positive reinforcement (Jacobson et al., 2001). Furthermore, clients enact goal-directed behavior over time, beginning with small steps, to gradually return to a routine of adaptive functioning (Jacobson et al., 2001).

BA has been found to be an efficacious treatment for depression, with large effect sizes ranging from 0.74–0.87 (vs. control conditions) reported by two meta-analytic studies (Cuijpers, van Straten, & Warmderdam, 2007; Mazzucchelli, Kane, & Rees, 2009).

An additional behavioral therapy to briefly mention is functional analytic psychotherapy (FAP; Kohlenberg & Tsai, 1991). Essentially, FAP is characterized by using functional analytic methods within a therapeutic relationship (Hopko, Hopko, & Lejuez, 2007). To elaborate, within a clinical session, therapists identify maladaptive behaviors, purposefully elicit these behavioral responses to aid in modifying them to become more adaptive responses, and provide differential reinforcement for positive behaviors (Hopko et al., 2007).

A final behavioral therapy for mental health disorders to be mentioned here is problem-solving therapy (PST; D'Zurilla, Nezu, & Maydeu-Olivares, 2004; Nezu, 1987). PST was developed from the idea that depressive symptoms are caused and maintained by poor problem-solving strategies (Hopko et al., 2007). According to Nezu (2004), problem-solving skills are thought to moderate the relationship between depression, stressors, and negative attribution. The basic tenants of PST consist of 5 components; these are problem orientation, problem definition and formulation, generation of alternatives, solution implementation, and verification (Hopko et al., 2007). PST asserts the importance of understanding negative contextual events and how maladaptive responses to these events are antecedents of depressive behavior (Hopko et al., 2007).

In this section, several therapies for mental health disorders have been discussed. These involved widely used (e.g., CBT) and lesser used (e.g., FAP) treatments, all of which incorporate, or were developed from, behavioral research methods. Next, a brief overview of functional assessment is offered.

Functional Assessment

Functional assessment refers to both functional analysis (FA), or the process by which one directly tests hypothesis of behavioral functions, and functional behavior assessment (FBA), or broadly defined methods of assessing the function of a given behavior, which include observations, interviews, and conducting FA's (Carr, 1977; Carr, 1994; Jolivette, Scott, & Nelson, 2000). Put another way, functional assessment includes a wide range of strategies which are implemented in order to identify factors controlling a target behavior, including antecedents, consequences, and contextual factors (Carr, 1994; Horner, 1994).

Functional assessment research has identified the importance of identifying behavioral functions as a means to increase the strength of interventions and to decrease or eliminate instances of target behaviors (Carr, 1977; Horner, 1994). As noted by Friman (2007), understanding what consequences are reinforcing a target behavior helps to formulate treatments that allow those consequences to be accessed in adaptive, situationally appropriate ways. Furthermore, FA is recommended to be an additive process, such that it is used to continually adjust interventions over time when they are not as effective as expected, to make changes to elicit desired behavioral responses, and to understand why certain behaviors are occurring in response to treatment (Horner, 1994). For example, if a behavior is maintained by either positive or negative social reinforcement, then the appropriate contingency used to address the target behavior would consist of withholding all forms of social reinforcement (e.g., time-out, extinction; Carr, 1977). However, this method would not be effective for all behavioral functions, such as self-stimulation (Carr, 1977). In addition to allowing early identification of target behaviors, functional assessments can also be used to aid in identifying future behavior problems (Jolivette et al., 2000).

Over time, several common functions occurring across behaviors have been identified, including positive reinforcement (e.g., receiving attention or social praise), negative reinforcement (e.g., escaping demands), self-stimulation (e.g., receiving additional sensory stimulation), physical (e.g., related to physical discomfort or medical conditions), and access to tangibles (e.g., gaining access to an item; Carr, 1994, 1977). It should be noted that multiple functions can underlie a behavior, interact with one another, and strengthen or weaken each other, which may result in ineffective treatment; treatments should not be assumed to work in all cases due to unknown, underlying factors (Carr, 1977; Iwata, Dorsey, Slifer, Bauman, & Richman, 1982).

Other factors that are important to study during functional assessment include contextual influences, or biological and environmental factors occurring both within and outside of an FA which may affect its outcome. (Carr, 1994; Iwata et al., 1982). Contextual influences can include biological events (e.g., lack of sleep, illness, medications) and social events (e.g., being scolded, participating in games, the presence of an unfamiliar person; Carr, 1994). Understanding contextual influences can aid in assessing why an unexpected response occurred or identify environmental factors to manipulate during subsequent treatment (Horner, 1994).

Specific to anxiety disorders and fear, Friman (2007) described 4 functional dimensions of fear and anxiety to investigate during FA. He noted that the first dimension is physiological activity. When an individual experiences an aversive stimulus, they may experience increased physiological arousal in the form of elevated heart rate, shortness of breath, and increased blood flow. Friman also noted that the individual seeks relief from these responses through experiential avoidance, thereby maintaining the anxious behavior. Furthermore, motivating events, including pain, hunger, or fatigue, may also influence these physiological reactions.

Friman (2007) secondly noted cognitive activity as a functional dimension of fear and anxiety. From a behavioral perspective, cognition is examined through verbal behavior of the individual. Friman noted that cognitions of an anxious individual may consist of verbally expressed beliefs that some feared stimulus may bring harm to them that they cannot effectively address on their own. This verbal behavior can consist of short statements but can also include extended, obsessive dialogues. Through these statements, Friman stated that individuals engage in avoidance of language about feared stimuli (e.g., stating, "I can't do this," rather than engaging in dialogue about the feared stimuli directly).

Next, Friman (2007) stated that one should consider behavioral activity as the most important dimension to be assessed during functional assessment of fear and anxiety. He further stated that these behaviors are often the most impairing and are the main referral concern in most cases. Behavioral activity related to fear and anxiety involves overt behavioral responses which are maintained by escape/avoidance. According to Friman, these behaviors can be either exhibited or inhibited. For example, for an individual who has anxiety related to being in a car accident, they may walk instead of riding in a car (i.e., exhibited behavior), or they may refuse to get into a car (i.e., inhibited behavior).

Lastly, Friman (2007) recommended assessing secondary gain, or secondary reinforcers that may be acquired as a result of escape/avoidance or any other behavioral reaction to fear and anxiety. For example, if an individual has anxiety related to school and is engaging in school refusal behavior, they will receive primary, negative reinforcement through avoiding the aversive stimulus (i.e., school). However, staying home may provide secondary, positive reinforcement in the form of leisure activities (e.g., video games, television).

Jolivette et al. (2000) described the process of an FBA to be used to develop and adjust a behavior intervention plan (BIP). They first emphasized using collected data to identify the specific function (or functions) of a target behavior. Next, an equivalent and appropriate replacement behavior should be determined; this new behavior should both serve the same function of the target behavior and be appropriate the social–environmental context. Jolivette and colleagues then stated that the assessor must decide at which point the replacement behavior should be enacted by the client. In order for the new behavior to be maintained, it must occur in a context in which it is properly reinforced. They then stated that a process by which the behavior will be taught to the client should be designed. Following this, Jolivette and colleagues noted that the assessor should manipulate environmental conditions in order to maximize the chances of the new behavior occurring and being reinforced successfully and to minimize the chance that the behavior will fail to occur or fail to be reinforced. Next, the assessor must determine the manner in which the replacement behavior will be reinforced in the environment and which consequences will be implemented when the target behavior occurs. Jolivette and colleagues mentioned that assessors need to keep a clear data collection system in order to understand reductions in target behavior frequency, duration, or intensity. Furthermore, they noted that assessors should create measurable goals that pertain to the occurrence of the replacement behavior.

It should be mentioned that few studies have assessed the efficacy of treatment augmented by functional assessment methods (Gresham, 2003). Three studies were found that examined the efficacy or effectiveness of functionally augmented treatments. Newcomer and Lewis (2004) found that the use of functional assessment to inform a behavioral treatment for problem behavior (e.g., aggression) in a school setting had greater efficacy than behavioral treatment not informed by functional assessment. In a similar study, Ingram, Lewis-Palmer, and Sugai (2005) compared the use of behavioral treatments informed and not informed by a FBA for off-task school behaviors and found that FBA informed treatments have greater effectiveness than those not informed by a FBA. Lastly, Payne, Scott, and Conroy (2007) examined the use of FBA to inform behavioral treatments for off-task behavior in school and found that interventions informed by FBA were more efficacious than those not using FBA. Despite the lack of studies supporting the use of functional assessment methods to inform treatment, these studies suggest some promise for the efficacy of these functionally informed methods.

It should also be noted that the use of functional assessment to inform treatment interventions specific to mental health disorders is not widely studied and thusly lacking in empirical research evidence (Friman, 2007). However, widely used interventions for anxiety disorders use treatment components derived from functionally based treatment research, including exposure and response prevention, which are used to address negatively reinforced functions of escape/avoidance in anxiety treatment (Friman, 2007). Furthermore, certain treatments (i.e., CBT, BA) which were discussed previously in the chapter incorporate elements of functional assessment into their procedures by design and have been found to be efficacious (Cuijpers, van Straten, & Warmerdam, 2007; Hofmann et al., 2012).

Using Functional Assessment to Inform Treatment

This chapter has discussed behavioral theories of mental health disorders, behavioral treatments, and functional assessment. Now, an examination of the literature concerning the use of functional assessment to inform behavioral treatments of mental health disorders will be presented to build upon the previous information that has been discussed in this chapter.

Kearney and Silverman (1999) performed a study examining functionally based treatments for children and adolescents engaging in school refusal behavior that were either prescriptive (i.e., designed to appropriately treat target behaviors based on their functions) or non-prescriptive (i.e., control treatments that were mismatched with the behavioral functions that they were treating). They defined school refusal as either refusing to attend school or difficulty remaining in classes for an entire day. Kearney and Silverman proposed 4 possible functions for this refusal behavior including avoidance (i.e., avoiding school-specific stimuli that provoke negative emotional responses), escape (i.e., escaping aversive situations of evaluation or social interactions), positive social reinforcement (i.e., attention seeking), and positive tangible reinforcement (e.g., access to preferred activities at home; Carr, 1977, 1994). Furthermore, participants who were engaging in school refusal behavior had diagnoses such as specific phobia (SP), generalized anxiety disorder (GAD), major depressive disorder (MDD), separation anxiety (SA), and social anxiety disorder (SAD; Kearney & Silverman, 1999).

It may be recalled that previous discussions of behavioral theories of anxiety disorders proposed several possibilities for the acquisition of fear, such as fear conditioning (Mowrer, 1939; Rachman, 1976, 1977; Watson & Rayner, 1920). Thusly, it could be hypothesized that for some of these individuals, their anxiety related to school developed through the pairing of some aversive stimulus (e.g., getting bullied, getting scolded by teachers) with the neutral stimulus of school attendance (Mowrer, 1939; Watson & Rayner, 1920), or that they simply witnessed others experiencing the consequences of aversive stimuli, or were exposed to repeated verbal modelling related to school aversion, and developed fear and anxiety themselves (Hofmann et al, 2012; Rachman, 1976, 1977). For one participant who was experiencing MDD, this may have developed through a weakening of the expected reinforcers related to the school environment (e.g., social reinforcement: they may have had less positive interactions with peers and poorer grades; Ferster, 1973).

Whatever the origin, the next important step is to identify the functions through functional assessment of these school refusal behaviors in order to implement appropriate treatment strategies. Kearney and Silverman (1999) used the School Refusal Assessment Scale (SRAS; Kearney & Silverman, 1993) which is a 16-item measure used to identify behavioral functions underlying school refusal. It assesses for functions including avoidance, escape, and positive reinforcement (i.e., social, tangible; Carr, 1977, 1994). Across participants, combinations of functions and diagnoses were identified, including escaping from aversive stimuli, GAD, and MDD, attention seeking, SA, and GAD, avoidance of stimuli inducing negative emotional reactivity and SAD (Kearney & Silverman, 1999).

Kearney and Silverman (1999) proposed specific treatment strategies for each individual to align with the identified functions of their target behavior. Treatments included techniques adapted from systematic desensitization (Wolpe, 1954) and CBT (Beck, 1970). For example, for participant 1 who had GAD, MDD, and engaged in school refusal to escape aversive stimuli, his treatment consisted of relaxation training and gradual re-exposure to the school setting. They also proposed for participant 3, who had SA and engaged in school refusal to gain attention, that they use parent training strategies to implement contingencies to provide appropriate consequences to reinforce school attendance and punish school refusal. Other participants initially received non-prescriptive treatments, such as participant 5, who had SA, GAD, and refused school to gain attention, who was administered relaxation training and cognitive therapy.

Overall, Kearney and Silverman (1999) described that participants who had pre-scriptive treatments (including those who switched from non-prescriptive to pre-scriptive treatments in the second half of the study) showed a 94.2% reduction in school absences, 60.7% reduction in daily ratings of anxiety, and 42.0% reductions in ratings of depression. For those receiving non-prescriptive (i.e., mismatched) treatments, participants displayed a 14.6% increase in school absences, 33% increase in daily ratings of anxiety, and a 14.2% increase in depression ratings. The results of this study suggest the importance of properly identifying behavioral func-tions to inform treatments which has been discussed previously in this chapter (Carr, 1977; Horner, 1994).

Another example of functional assessment-informed treatment is described by Jacobson, Martell, and Dimidjian (2001) and their use of behavioral activation (BA) to treat depression. The authors noted that they used FA to assess both underlying functions of depression as well as contextual triggers and their subsequent behav-ioral responses. Frequently, these responses include avoidance of aversive stimuli and disruption of everyday routines. Furthermore, Jacobson and colleagues empha-sized the importance of assessing the client's learning history and how it may have been influenced by insufficient positive reinforcement or aversive control. They noted that they begin FA's with several questions to ask, including what functions underlie the client's depression, what symptoms are they currently experiencing, in what ways are they responding to these symptoms, how might behavioral avoidance be exacerbating symptoms, and what daily routines have been affected? Moreover, understanding the answers to these questions builds an understanding of behavioral functions relevant to the client which helps to create an effective treatment plan. Although, as the authors note, one may not understand whether an FA is accurately identifying behavioral functions until treatment is enacted: an accurate FA should lead to an effective treatment.

To describe the process of using an FA to inform BA treatment for depression, Jacobson and colleagues (2001) presented an example case. They described a client who had recently cheated on his partner with another woman with whom he was now living. This caused him significant emotional distress as well as financial prob-lems. The authors noted several maladaptive patterns of behavior, such that he avoided his ex-partner due to their unpleasant interactions, he avoided spending time with his children, and he avoided speaking with his coworkers. Furthermore, although his work supplied him with positive reinforcement, he often stayed at home and engaged in ruminating behaviors.

Several theoretical explanations of this individual's depression should be consid-ered. For instance, Skinner (1953) would likely highlight that this individual is experiencing an interruption of the previously established behavioral patterns that were once reinforced by the social environment. Previously established behavioral patterns may have included this individual's previous routine of working and spend-ing time with his family, which are currently disrupted. Moreover, the current environment may not be providing enough reinforcement to this individual (Lazarus, 1968; Lewinsohn, 1975) who may, in turn, engage in less frequent acts of behavior that have the potential to be positively reinforced, such as spending time with his children (Ferster, 1965, 1966).

Considering the patterns of behavior that this individual displayed as described by Jacobson and colleagues (2001), a FA may reveal the function of these to be negatively reinforced through escape or avoidance of negative stimuli (e.g., unpleasant interactions with an ex-wife; Carr, 1977). Furthermore, the function of rumination would likely be categorized as negative reinforcement through escape or avoidance as well; Ferster (1973) noted that individuals have likely terminated unpleasant situations with this behavior in the past and may continue to do so even when there is no direct benefit. Relatedly, as discussed earlier, Friman (2007) noted that engagement in verbal behavior expressing an inability to confront an aversive stimulus may allow escape/avoidance of verbal behavior directly relating to the feared stimulus.

After identifying these behavioral functions, Jacobson and colleagues (2001) noted that treatment should begin by addressing several contextual variables, including improving financial security, promoting relationship stability with the client's new partner, promoting focus on being more involved with parenting, and promoting a healthy relationship with their ex-wife to reduce conflict. As discussed in the overall description of BA earlier in this chapter, these would be accomplished through BA strategies, including graded task assignments (e.g., providing tasks on an increasing gradient of difficulty to build up to being fully involved in activities) and avoidance modification (e.g., facilitating understanding of the negative effects of avoidance and offering alternative coping strategies) and routine regulation to re-establish a routine of life activities that increase mood and the potential for positive environmental reinforcement. For example, addressing rumination could be accomplished through re-establishing a regular working routine on a task gradient (e.g., begin working 1 day a week, move up to 2 days, and so on; Jacobson et al., 2001). Addressing avoidance of the client's ex-wife may require avoidance modification and work to understand that avoidance serves to maintain the client's depression, but a long-term goal of reducing stressful interactions will require the client to interact with their ex-wife over time (Jacobson et al., 2001).

An additional example case given by Jacobson and colleagues (2001) includes a woman who had depressive symptoms related to a work environment that was causing her significant distress. Her initial means of coping was to stay home from work, stay in bed, and avoid engaging in social interactions with others. An FA would likely reveal that the function of this individual's behavior was negative reinforcement (i.e., escape/avoidance) in this case (Carr, 1977). Given this finding, strategies of avoidance modification as well as graded tasks to re-establish a regular work routine would be used to address functional (i.e., escape/avoidance) and contextual (e.g., negative work environment) variables maintaining depressive symptoms (Jacobson et al., 2001).

Friman (2007) additionally described several, brief case studies involving the usage of functional assessment-informed treatment. First, Friman and Lucas (1996) described a case study of a 14 -year-old boy with social phobia who exhibited adverse reactions to corrective feedback (e.g., verbal outbursts, behavioral problems). Following a functional assessment, the outbursts were determined to serve a function of negatively reinforced escape/avoidance and an important contextual factor (i.e., being reprimanded in public) was found to maintain this behavior due to the individual's social phobia. Treatment involved sustaining a regular schedule of reprimands, and these were given in a private space away from peers. Following treatment, the frequency of outbursts was reduced to nearly zero and was maintained at long-term follow-up.

An additional example presented by Friman (2007) involved a case study by Swearer, Jones, and Friman (1997) of treatment of a 15 -year-old boy with social anxiety. The presenting problem consisted of the client biting the inside of their cheeks during social interactions until his mouth bled. A functional assessment revealed that the cheek biting provided the function of self-stimulation through physiological arousal and negative reinforcement through escape/avoidance from social engagement. Treatment in this case consisted of training the client in relaxation exercises to reduce aversive physiological arousal and to chew gum during aversive social situations to provide an equivalent consequence to the cheek biting behavior. After treatment, the frequency of biting behavior dropped to nearly zero and was maintained at long-term follow-up.

A final case study from Hopko et al (2007) is offered. The client in this case study was reportedly exhibiting depressive symptoms (e.g., depressed mood, loss of appetite, anhedonia), anxiety symptoms (e.g., uncontrollable worry regarding her career, finances, family), and physiological symptoms (e.g., shortness of breath, nausea). The client additionally reported psychosomatic symptoms (e.g., muscle tension, insomnia) and cognitive symptoms (e.g., feelings of failure regarding her work and home life). According to Hopko and colleagues, several overt behavioral symptoms were noted by the client, including substance use, gambling, anger, and social withdrawal.

Following an initial psychological assessment, Hopko et al (2007) noted that the client was given a diagnosis of MDD and GAD. Following this, she began recording her daily activities as a part of a shortened BA protocol (brief behavioral activation treatment for depression; BATD; Lejuez, Hopko, & Hopko, 2001). According to Hopko and colleagues, the client's activities related to her career and household responsibilities as well as gambling and binge drinking.

Using the values process of ACT (Hayes et al., 1999), the client identified main values and goals. Hopko et al (2007) noted that the client's values and goals consisted of family and other close relationships, education and career, recreational activities, and spirituality, among others.

Following this, Hopko et al (2007) noted that a FA was performed to identify relevant contextual factors which may be maintaining depressive and anxious symptoms. The FA found that these symptoms were frequently maintained by negative reinforcement. The client overexerted herself at her job, which was negatively reinforced by avoidance of feelings of inadequacy. Furthermore, this overexertion led to failures in the client's home life (e.g., rarely had time to spend with her spouse and children). Hopko and colleagues described that these failures led to the client's binge drinking and gambling behaviors, which were negatively reinforced by the avoidance of experiencing feelings of failure related to her home life.

Hopko et al (2007) stated that an initial treatment goal was to increase the client's engagement in behaviors related to her values in order to maximize positive reinforcement. Using BATD techniques, the client created a list of graded tasks, including spending time with family, exercising, connecting to spirituality, and engaging in muscle relaxation (Lejuez et al., 2001). The client attempted to engage in a number of these tasks each week, which was discussed with the therapist to assess whether the client was successful or had problems with an activity.

According to Hopko et al (2007), the client was also instructed to engage in cognitive defusion exercises (Hayes et al., 1999). The client was taught to approach negative feelings (e.g., sadness) and cognitions (e.g., fear of failure) with acceptance. Moreover, the client's feelings of inadequacy were shown to be a function of negative life experiences (e.g., the client experienced harsh treatment by her father as a child), and this understanding allowed the client to re-evaluate negative thoughts as passing cognitive experiences that were not necessarily true.

Over the course of treatment, the client made marked improvements in quality of life, with a reduction in anxious and depressive symptoms as well as gambling and binge drinking (Hopko et al., 2007).

Conclusion

Within this chapter, factors related to the functional assessment of mental health disorders have been discussed. Early behavioral research such as classical conditioning (Pavlov, 1927; Watson & Rayner, 1920) led to the development of behavioral theories of fear and anxiety as well as models of treatment such as systematic desensitization (Wolpe, 1954). Later behavioral analytic and contextual research led to more robust theories of fear, anxiety (Rachman, 1977), depression (Ferster, 1973), and psychological distress (Hayes et al., 1999) as well as behaviorally based treatments, including CBT (Beck, 1970) and ACT (Hayes et al., 1999).

These behavioral theories and interventions allowed for a behavioral conceptualization of treatment where functional assessment can inform treatment targets based on relevant functions of behavior. Although there is a need for greater empirical evidence, the widespread use of treatments which incorporate functional assessment methods (e.g., CBT) suggests that identifying behavioral functions to develop treatment targets may be useful when treating mental health disorders (Friman, 2007; Hazlett-Stevens & Craske, 2002).

References

American Psychiatric Association, & American Psychiatric Association. (2013). *Diagnostic and statistical manual of mental disorders: DSM-5* (5th ed.). Arlington, VA: American Psychiatric Association.

A-Tjak, J. G. L., Davis, M. L., Morina, N., Powers, M. B., Smits, J. A. J., & Emmelkamp, P. M. G. (2015). A meta-analysis of the efficacy of acceptance and commitment therapy for clinically relevant mental and physical health problems. *Psychotherapy and Psychosomatics, 84*(1), 30–36. https://doi.org/10.1159/000365764

Bados, A., Balaguer, G., & Saldaña, C. (2007). The efficacy of cognitive–behavioral therapy and the problem of drop-out. *Journal of Clinical Psychology, 63*(6), 585–592. https://doi.org/10.1002/jclp.20368

Bandura, A. (1969). Social learning of moral judgments. *Journal of Personality and Social Psychology, 11*(3), 275–279. https://doi.org/10.1037/h0026998

Baxter, A. J., Vos, T., Scott, K. M., Ferrari, A. J., & Whiteford, H. A. (2014). The global burden of anxiety disorders in 2010. *Psychological Medicine, 44*(11), 2363–2374. https://doi.org/10.1017/S0033291713003243

Beck, A. T. (1964). Thinking and depression: II. Theory and therapy. *Archives of General Psychiatry, 10*(6), 561–571.

Beck, A. T. (1970). Cognitive therapy: Nature and relation to behavior therapy. *Behavior Therapy, 1*(2), 184–200. https://doi.org/10.1016/S0005-7894(70)80030-2

Biglan, A., & Hayes, S. C. (1996). Should the behavioral sciences become more pragmatic? The case for functional contextualism in research on human behavior. *Applied and Preventive Psychology, 5*(1), 47–57. https://doi.org/10.1016/S0962-1849(96)80026-6

Carr, E. G. (1977). The motivation of self-injurious behavior: a review of some hypotheses. Psychological bulletin, 84(4), 800.

Carr, E. G. (1994). Emerging themes in the functional analysis of problem behavior. *Journal of Applied Behavior Analysis, 27*(2), 393–399.

Cuijpers, P., van Straten, A., & Warmerdam, L. (2007). Behavioral activation treatments of depression: A meta-analysis. *Clinical Psychology Review, 27*(3), 318–326. https://doi.org/10.1016/j.cpr.2006.11.001

D'Zurilla, T. J., Nezu, A. M., & Maydeu-Olivares, A. (2004). *Social problem solving: Theory and assessment*. Washington, DC: American Psychological Association.

Ferster, C. B. (1965). Classification of behavioral pathology. *Research in behavior modification*, 6–26.

Ferster, C. B. (1966). Animal behavior and mental illness. *The Psychological Record, 16*(3), 345–356.

Ferster, C. B. (1973). A functional analysis of depression. *American Psychologist, 28*(10), 857–870. https://doi.org/10.1037/h0035605

Friman, C. P. (2007). The fear factor: A functional perspective on anxiety. In P. Sturmey (Ed.), *Functional analysis in clinical treatment* (pp. 335–356). New York, NY: Academic Press.

Friman, P. C., & Lucas, C. P. (1996). Social phobia obscured by disruptive behavior disorder: A case study. *Clinical Child Psychology and Psychiatry, 1*(3), 399–407.

Gortner, E. T., Gollan, J. K., Dobson, K. S., & Jacobson, N. S. (1998). Cognitive–behavioral treatment for depression: Relapse prevention. *Journal of Consulting and Clinical Psychology, 66*(2), 377.

Gresham, F. M. (2003). Establishing the technical adequacy of functional behavioral assessment: Conceptual and measurement challenges. *Behavioral Disorders, 28*(3), 282–298. https://doi.org/10.1177/019874290302800305

Harvard Medical School, 2007. National Comorbidity Survey (NCS). (2017, August 21). Retrieved from https://www.hcp.med.harvard.edu/ncs/index.php. Data Table 1: Lifetime prevalence DSM-IV/WMH-CIDI disorders by sex and cohort.

Hasin, D. S., Sarvet, A. L., Meyers, J. L., Saha, T. D., Ruan, W. J., Stohl, M., & Grant, B. F. (2018). Epidemiology of adult *DSM-5* major depressive disorder and its specifiers in the United States. *JAMA Psychiatry, 75*(4), 336. https://doi.org/10.1001/jamapsychiatry.2017.4602

Hayes, S. C., Blackledge, J., & Barnes-Holmes, T. (2001). Language and cognition: Constructing an alternative approach within the behavioral tradition. In *Relational frame theory. A post-Skinnerian account of human language and cognition* (pp. 3–20). New York, NY: Plenum.

Hayes, S. C., Luoma, J. B., Bond, F. W., Masuda, A., & Lillis, J. (2006). Acceptance and commitment therapy: Model, processes and outcomes. *Behaviour Research and Therapy, 44*(1), 1–25. https://doi.org/10.1016/j.brat.2005.06.006

Hayes, S. C., Strosahl, K., & Wilson, K. G. (1999). *Acceptance and commitment therapy: Understanding and treating human suffering*. New York, NY: Guilford.

Hazlett-Stevens, H., & Craske, M. G. (2002). Brief cognitive-behavioral therapy: Definition and scientific foundations. In F. W. Bond & W. Dryden (Eds.), *Handbook of brief cognitive behaviour therapy* (pp. 1–20). Chichester, UK: John Wiley & Sons Ltd. https://doi.org/10.1002/9780470713020.ch1

Hofmann, S. G., Asnaani, A., Vonk, I. J. J., Sawyer, A. T., & Fang, A. (2012). The efficacy of cognitive behavioral therapy: A review of meta-analyses. *Cognitive Therapy and Research, 36*(5), 427–440. https://doi.org/10.1007/s10608-012-9476-1

Hopko, D. R., Hopko, S. D., & Lejuez, C. W. (2007). Mood disorders. In P. Sturmey (Ed.), *Functional analysis in clinical treatment* (pp. 307–334). New York, NY: Academic Press.

Horner, R. H. (1994). Functional assessment: Contributions and future directions. *Journal of Applied Behavior Analysis, 27*(2), 401–404.

Ingram, K., Lewis-Palmer, T., & Sugai, G. (2005). Function-based intervention planning: Comparing the effectiveness of FBA function-based and non—function-based intervention plans. *Journal of Positive Behavior Interventions, 7*(4), 224–236. https://doi.org/10.1177/10983007050070040401

Iwata, B. A., Dorsey, M. F., Slifer, K. J., Bauman, K. E., & Richman, G. S. (1982). Toward a functional analysis of self-injury. Analysis and intervention in developmental disabilities, 2(1), 3-20.

Jacobson, N. S., Martell, C. R., & Dimidjian, S. (2001). Behavioral activation treatment for depression: Returning to contextual roots. *Clinical Psychology: Science and Practice, 8*(3), 255–270. https://doi.org/10.1093/clipsy.8.3.255

Jolivette, K., Scott, T. M., & Nelson, C. M. (2000). The link between functional behavioral assessments (FBAs) and behavioral intervention plans (BIPs). ERIC Digest E592.

Kaplan, G. B., Heinrichs, S. C., & Carey, R. J. (2011). Treatment of addiction and anxiety using extinction approaches: Neural mechanisms and their treatment implications. *Pharmacology Biochemistry and Behavior, 97*(3), 619–625. https://doi.org/10.1016/j.pbb.2010.08.004

Kearney, C. A., & Silverman, W. K. (1993). Measuring the function of school refusal behavior: The School Refusal Assessment Scale. *Journal of Clinical Child Psychology, 22*(1), 85–96.

Kearney, C. A., & Silverman, W. K. (1999). Functionally based prescriptive and nonprescriptive treatment for children and adolescents with school refusal behavior. *Behavior Therapy, 30*(4), 673–695. https://doi.org/10.1016/S0005-7894(99)80032-X

Kohlenberg, R. J., & Tsai, M. (1991). *Functional analytic psychotherapy: Creating intense and curative therapeutic relationships*. New York, NY: Plenum Press. https://doi.org/10.1007/978-0-387-70855-3

Lang, P. J., & Lazovik, A. D. (1963). Experimental desensitization of phobia. *The Journal of Abnormal and Social Psychology, 66*(6), 519.

Lazarus, A. A., & Rachman, S. (1957). The use of systematic desensitization in psychotherapy. South African Medical Journal, 31(11), 934-937.

Lazarus, A. A. (1968). Learning theory and the treatment of depression. *Behaviour Research and Therapy, 6*(1), 83–89.

Lejuez, C. W., Hopko, D. R., & Hopko, S. D. (2001). A brief behavioral activation treatment for depression: Treatment manual. *Behavior Modification, 25*, 255–286.

Lewinsohn, P. M. (1975). The behavioral study and treatment of depression. In Progress in behavior modification (Vol. 1, pp. 19–64). Elsevier. https://doi.org/10.1016/B978-0-12-535601-5.50009-3.

Lewinsohn, P. M., & Atwood, G. E. (1969). Depression: A clinical-research approach. *Psychotherapy: Theory, Research & Practice, 6*(3), 166.

Martell, C. R., Addis, M. E., & Jacobson, N. S. (2001). *Depression in context: Strategies for guided action.* New York, NY: WW Norton & Co..

Mazzucchelli, T., Kane, R., & Rees, C. (2009). Behavioral activation treatments for depression in adults: A meta-analysis and review. *Clinical Psychology: Science and Practice, 16*(4), 383–411. https://doi.org/10.1111/j.1468-2850.2009.01178.x

McGrath, T., Tsui, E., Humphries, S., & Yule, W. (1990). Successful treatment of a noise phobia in a nine-year-old girl with systematic desensitisation in vivo. *Educational Psychology, 10*(1), 79–83. https://doi.org/10.1080/0144341900100107

Merikangas, K. R., He, J., Burstein, M., Swanson, S. A., Avenevoli, S., Cui, L., ... Swendsen, J. (2010). Lifetime prevalence of mental disorders in U.S. adolescents: Results from the National Comorbidity Survey Replication– Adolescent Supplement (NCS-A). *Adolescent Psychiatry, 49*(10), 10.

Mineka, S., & Zinbarg, R. (2006). A contemporary learning theory perspective on the etiology of anxiety disorders: It's not what you thought it was. *American Psychologist, 61*(1), 10–26. https://doi.org/10.1037/0003-066X.61.1.10

Mowrer, O. H. (1939). A stimulus-response analysis of anxiety and its role as a reinforcing agent. *Psychological Review, 46*(6), 553.

Newcomer, L. L., & Lewis, T. J. (2004). Functional behavioral assessment: An investigation of assessment reliability and effectiveness of function-based interventions. Journal of Emotional and Behavioral Disorders, 12(3), 168-181.

Nezu, A. M. (1987). A problem-solving formulation of depression: A literature review and proposal of a pluralistic model. *Clinical Psychology Review, 7*(2), 121–144.

Nezu, A. M. (2004). Problem solving and behavior therapy revisited. *Behavior Therapy, 35*(1), 1–33.

Niles, A. N., Dour, H. J., Stanton, A. L., Roy-Byrne, P. P., Stein, M. B., Sullivan, G., ... Craske, M. G. (2015). Anxiety and depressive symptoms and medical illness among adults with anxiety disorders. *Journal of Psychosomatic Research, 78*(2), 109–115. https://doi.org/10.1016/j.jpsychores.2014.11.018

Olatunji, B. O., Cisler, J. M., & Deacon, B. J. (2010). Efficacy of cognitive behavioral therapy for anxiety disorders: A review of meta-analytic findings. *Psychiatric Clinics of North America, 33*(3), 557–577. https://doi.org/10.1016/j.psc.2010.04.002

Öst, L.-G. (2014). The efficacy of acceptance and commitment therapy: An updated systematic review and meta-analysis. *Behaviour Research and Therapy, 61*, 105–121. https://doi.org/10.1016/j.brat.2014.07.018

Otte, C., Gold, S. M., Penninx, B. W., Pariante, C. M., Etkin, A., Fava, M., ... Schatzberg, A. F. (2016). Major depressive disorder. *Nature Reviews. Disease Primers, 2*(1), 16065. https://doi.org/10.1038/nrdp.2016.65

Pavlov, I. P. (1927). Conditioned reflexes: an investigation of the physiological activity of the cerebral cortex. Oxford Univ. Press.

Payne, L. D., Scott, T. M., & Conroy, M. (2007). A school-based examination of the efficacy of function-based intervention. *Behavioral Disorders, 32*(3), 158–174. https://doi.org/10.1177/019874290703200302

Powers, M. B., Zum Vörde Sive Vörding, M. B., & Emmelkamp, P. M. G. (2009). Acceptance and commitment therapy: A meta-analytic review. *Psychotherapy and Psychosomatics, 78*(2), 73–80. https://doi.org/10.1159/000190790

Rachman, S. (1976). The passing of the two-stage theory of fear and avoidance: Fresh possibilities. *Behaviour Research and Therapy, 14*(2), 125–131. https://doi.org/10.1016/0005-7967(76)90066-8

Rachman, S. (1977). The conditioning theory of fear acquisition: A critical examination. *Behaviour Research and Therapy, 15*(5), 375–387. https://doi.org/10.1016/0005-7967(77)90041-9

Reisinger, J. J. (1972). The treatment of "anxiety-depression" via positive reinforcement and response cost. *Journal of Applied Behavior Analysis, 5*(2), 125–130.

Sareen, J., et al. (2005). Anxiety disorders and risk for suicidal ideation and suicide attempts: a population-based longitudinal study of adults. *Archives of General Psychiatry, 62,* 9.

Skinner, B. F. (1953). Science and human behavior. New York: Macmillan.

Smith, M. L., & Glass, G. V. (1977). Meta-analysis of psychotherapy outcome studies. *American Psychologist, 32*(9), 752.

Swearer, S. M., Jones, K. M., & Friman, P. C. (1997). Relax and try this instead: Abbreviated habit reversal for oral self-biting. *Journal of Applied Behavior Analysis, 30,* 697–700.

Veale, D. (2008). Behavioural activation for depression. *Advances in Psychiatric Treatment, 14*(1), 29–36. https://doi.org/10.1192/apt.bp.107.004051

Watson, J. B., & Rayner, R. (1920). Conditioned emotional reactions. *Journal of Experimental Psychology, 3*(1), 1.

Willis, R. W., & Edwards, J. A. (1969). A study of the comparative effectiveness of systematic desensitization and implosive therapy. *Behaviour Research and Therapy, 7*(4), 387–395

Wolpe, J. (1950). The genesis of neurosis, an objective account. *South African Medical Journal/ Suid-Afrikaanse Tydskrif Vir Geneeskunde, 24*(30), 613–616.

Wolpe, J. (1954). Reciprocal inhibition as the main basis of psychotherapeutic effects. *AMA Archives of Neurology & Psychiatry, 72*(2), 205–226.

Chapter 15
Ethical Issues in Functional Assessment

Renee O. Hawkins, Tai A. Collins, Kamontá Heidelburg, and James A. Hawkins

Functional behavioral assessment (FBA) is an umbrella term incorporating a variety of behavioral assessment strategies used to identify environmental variables that contribute to problem behavior (Peterson & Neef, 2020; Steege, Pratt, Wickerd, Guare, & Watson, 2019). As described throughout this chapter, the goal of FBA is to identify the stimuli, events, and activities that present just prior to and after the occurrence of challenging behavior and to use this information to develop effective intervention plans. Both antecedents, which precede problem behavior, and the consequences that follow affect the probability that problem behavior will occur. Antecedents can set the stage for problem behavior to occur or, alternatively, can decrease the likelihood that a specific behavior will present. Following the occurrence of problem behavior, consequences affect how likely that same behavior is to occur in the future. By carefully examining the relationships between antecedent, problem behavior, and consequences, functional hypotheses are generated as to why the behavior is occurring. Intervention plans are then developed to manipulate the environment in ways to decrease inappropriate behavior and increase appropriate behavior.

The literature describes three types of FBA, including indirect assessment, descriptive assessment, and functional (experimental) analysis (FA) (Peterson & Neef, 2020; Steege et al., 2019). These three types of FBA represent increasing intensity of assessment in terms of time, effort, and expertise to complete as well as increasing confidence in the results, with FA requiring the most resources but often yielding the strongest data (Peterson & Neef, 2020). Indirect FBA includes the use of interviews, questionnaires, checklists, and rating scales to gather information

R. O. Hawkins (✉)
University of Cincinnati, Cincinnati, OH, USA

School of Human Services, University of Cincinnati, Cincinnati, OH, USA
e-mail: renee.hawkins@uc.edu

T. A. Collins · K. Heidelburg · J. A. Hawkins
University of Cincinnati, Cincinnati, OH, USA

© Springer Nature Switzerland AG 2021
J. L. Matson (ed.), *Functional Assessment for Challenging Behaviors and Mental Health Disorders*, Autism and Child Psychopathology Series,
https://doi.org/10.1007/978-3-030-66270-7_15

regarding the context for problem behavior from individuals who are familiar with the individual and have observed the problem behavior. As reflected in its name, this approach relies on indirect sources of information and does not include direct observation of the behavior. In contrast, direct observation is at the core of descriptive FBA. Through ABC (antecedent-behavior-consequence) narrative recording, scatterplot assessment, or systematic direct observation methods, the problem behavior is observed in the natural context in which it occurs, without any manipulation of the environment. In descriptive FBA, direct observation data are used in combination with data collected through indirect methods to help generate functional hypotheses. Both indirect and descriptive FBA lead to the identification of functional hypotheses regarding environmental variables contributing to problem behavior; however, these approaches do not verify these hypotheses. FA is used to test functional hypotheses by systematically manipulating antecedent and consequences linked to the problem behavior in order to isolate their effects. FA is often conducted in analog settings but can also be carried out in the natural environment in which the behavior occurs.

There is a great deal of research supporting FBA as a valid method for assessing problem behavior (Hanley, Iwata, & McCord, 2003). Concerns have been raised regarding the use of indirect FBA alone due to the reliance on secondary reports that are often unreliable (Steege et al., 2019) and use of interviews and questionnaires lacking sufficient technical support (Dufrene, Kazmerski, & Labrot, 2017; Hanley, 2012). Research has also called into question the validity of relying solely on descriptive FBA to determine function, which often results in false-positives for attention serving as the function (Thompson & Iwata, 2007). However, indirect and descriptive FBA can be critical for developing function-based intervention methods and the use of FBA is well supported by research (Ervin, Radford, Bertsch, & Piper, 2001; Goh & Bambara, 2012). In addition, these less-intense FBA methods can help inform FA procedures, which have the most extensive research base supporting its use and are considered by many as the "gold standard" of behavioral assessment (Hanley et al., 2003; Peterson & Neef, 2020). Given that FBA is a research-based approach to assess client behavior, professionals engaging in FBA should be aware of and adhere to relevant ethical guidelines. Guidelines for assessment are included in the ethical codes of the American Psychological Association (APA), Behavior Analyst Certification Board (BACB), and the National Association of School Psychologists (NASP). APA's *Ethical Principles of Psychologists and Code of Conduct* (2017), the BACB's *Professional and Ethical Compliance Code for Behavior Analysts* (2014), and the NASP *Principles for Professional Ethics* each refer to the use of reliable and valid assessment methods that are based on current research as ethical behavior. Further, the BACB code explicitly states that "When behavior analysts are developing a behavior-reduction program, they must first conduct a functional assessment." Behavior analysts, psychologists, and other professionals engaging in FBA must keep in mind a number of considerations to ensure that their assessment practice is aligned with the ethical guidelines of professional organizations.

Informed Consent

The APA, BACB, and NASP ethics codes all require professionals to obtain and document informed consent for assessment services. Exceptions for consent in the APA Code include "when conducting such activities without consent is mandated by law or governmental regulation or as otherwise provided in the Ethics Code" (APA, 2017). The NASP ethics code provides some exceptions for seeking informed consent with the following: "Parent consent is not ethically required for a school-based school psychologist to review a student's educational records, conduct classroom observation, assist in within-classroom interventions and progress monitoring, or to participate in educational screening conducted as part of a regular program of instruction." Nor is parental consent required in urgent situations or for a few initial meeting following student self-referral. However, the NASP code also makes it clear that consent is required when consultation for a student is likely "to be extensive and ongoing," as would typically be the case when there is a need for FBA. Given that FBA is individualized and goes beyond the scope of instruction and assessment provided to all students, school psychologists should seek informed consent consistent with the ethical guidelines of the profession.

Key to informed consent is that the individual providing consent understands exactly what will be involved. Section 3.03 of the BACB Code indicates "(a) Prior to conducting an assessment, behavior analysts must explain to the client the procedure(s) to be used, who will participate, and how the resulting information will be used." The APA Code states that when conducting research or providing psychological services, including assessment, psychologists "obtain the informed consent of the individual or individuals using language that is reasonably understandable to that person or persons..." (Section 3.10). NASP further states that the explanation of services "...taking into account language and cultural differences, cognitive capabilities, developmental level, age, and other relevant factors so that it may be understood by the person providing consent" (Standard I.1.3). In regard to the use of FBA, in many cases the individual who is the focus of assessment is a minor and/ or may have intellectual disabilities that interfere with their capacity to provide consent. Under these circumstances, professionals must ensure that the person responsible for providing consent (parent, legal guardian) clearly understands the process and procedures. In addition, whether or not an individual has the authority to consent or not, they should be provided a clear explanation of the assessment procedures and be given the opportunity to provide assent whenever possible. A key principle reflected in the APA, BACB, and NASP ethics codes is a respect for the dignity, rights, and worth of all individuals, and consistent with this principle are efforts to include individuals in their treatment planning and allow them to participate in decisions affecting their well-being to the greatest extent possible.

Competence

For FBA to be useful in informing treatment planning, appropriately qualified individuals must conduct the assessment to increase the accuracy of the results. All of the ethical codes indicate that professionals must not practice outside their areas of competence (APA, 2017; BACB, 2014; NASP, 2010). Staff must have the appropriate educational training and professional experience to competently conduct an FBA, as well as the appropriate credentials, which may include the Board Certified Behavior Analyst (BCBA) credential or licensure from a state board of psychology or state department of education. With regard to coursework, academic preparation would include basics of learning theory, single case design, ethics, behavioral interventions, behavior analytic assessment, and behavior recording procedures (Steege et al., 2019). It is also necessary for individuals conducting FBAs to obtain the necessary supervised experience from supervisors who are competent in FBA methodology (BACB, 2014; Steege et al., 2019). If necessary, practitioners should refer the work to others if they have not acquired the appropriate skills to conduct an FBA (APA, 2017). This is particularly important in schools and community agencies, as limitations in staffing may be problematic with regard to staff training. In these settings, it is crucial that staff are well qualified to conduct FBA procedures or they seek out colleagues with the appropriate training and supervision.

Do No Harm

The concept of do no harm is a key ethical principle of all of the ethics codes guiding behavior analytic practice (APA, 2017; BACB, 2014; NASP, 2010). Practitioners must ensure that their service delivery confers a benefit to clients and does not introduce or exacerbate harm for clients and families. With regard to FBA, one of the first things to consider is the length of the assessment process. The FBA process must be thorough enough to ensure a valid assessment of the antecedents, behaviors, and consequences associated with clients' behaviors; however, it must not be so long that the clients' behaviors continue without intervention for an inordinately long amount of time. Research indicates that a traditional FA may involve 30 or more sessions, with sessions lasting up to 30 min each (Nortup et al., 1991; Steege et al., 2019). It is estimated that, on average, a traditional FA requires six and a half hours to administer (Iwata, Dorsey, Slifer, Bauman, & Richman, 1994; Tincani, Castrogiavanni, & Axelrod, 1999). As such, practitioners must balance the need for a strong FBA with the need to intervene in a timely manner, especially for dangerous behaviors. It is also important to remember that FBA is an ongoing process that can be informed by intervention efforts, allowing practitioners some flexibility in determining when intervention is necessary to reduce or eliminate harm.

Functional analysis is particularly relevant to the concept of do no harm. As the goal of an FA is to test functional hypotheses by systematically altering antecedents and consequences, it is typically necessary that problem behaviors are allowed to occur during the FA. As such, the fact that Fas' occasion problem behaviors pose some ethical challenges, especially when the problem behaviors are severe and/or dangerous (Heath & Smith, 2019). Although they found that injuries occurred infrequently, Kahng et al. (2015) indicated that injuries resulting from self-injurious behavior were 8.5 times more likely to occur during an FA than outside of an FA when controlling for time. When conducting FAs, it is imperative that safeguards are put into place to protect clients and staff. For example, the original Iwata et al. (1982/1994) studies included safeguards such as medical examinations and clear termination criteria. Other important safeguards include the use of protective equipment (although this may alter the results of the FA), utilizing an appropriate number of well-trained staff, and consistent documentation of injuries (Kahng et al., 2015). Researchers have developed briefer versions of FAs (e.g., Northup et al., 1991) discussed later in this chapter, as well as methods of analyzing less severe or dangerous precursor behaviors within FA (e.g., Heath & Smith, 2019), allowing for greater flexibility in choosing the appropriate FA to minimize the risk of harm to clients and staff.

Right to Effective Treatment

Behavior analysts must advocate for "scientifically supported, most-effective treatment procedures" and for the "appropriate amount and level of service provision and oversight required to meet the defined behavior-change program goals", as explicitly outlined in section 2.09 of the BACB Code (2014). Conducting an FBA can be critical to treatment planning because results can lead to the identification of effective intervention plans (Napolitano, Knapp, Speares, & McAdam, 2012). However, an FBA, particularly a traditional FA, may not always be needed to develop an effective treatment plan (Poling, Austin, Peterson, & Mahoney, 2012). Research exists suggesting that the use of FBA results in more effective intervention plans and better outcomes than developing intervention without FBA data (Crone & Horner, 2000; Gage, Lewis, & Stichter, 2012; Vollmer & Northup, 1996). However, research also exists suggesting that interventions based on FBA results do not result in more improved outcomes as compared to interventions developed without a preceding FBA (Gresham et al., 2004). Further, as previously discussed, with any FBA, particularly an FA, there is a potential ethical issue related to delay in treatment due to the time required to complete the assessment. Professionals considering whether or not to carry out at FBA should conduct a cost–benefit analysis to make decisions about the assessment plan based on available resources and feasibility (BACB, 2014). In some instances, it may be more appropriate to design and evaluate an evidence-based intervention without a clear functional hypothesis rather than collect extensive FA data before allowing the client to access potentially effective treatment.

Once a FBA is conducted, it is important and dictated by ethical codes that the results of the assessment be presented in a way that can be readily understood by those being served, as outlined in sections 3.01b and 3.04 of the BACB Code (2014), 9.10 of the APA Code (2017), and Standard II.3.8 of the NASP Code (2010). Moreover, the results must be presented in a way that can be clearly understood by all of the members on the treatment planning team to effectively develop an evidence-based plan. When interpreting FBA results, behavior analysts and psychologists must consider the various factors and unique characteristics of the individual being assessed (i.e., situational, linguistic, environmental conditions, and cultural differences), all of which could affect the accuracy of the interpretations and the treatment plan (APA, 2017; NASP, 2010).

Functional Analysis Alternatives and Ethics

In order to address ethical issues related to the extended delay of treatment that may be associated with conducting a full FA, alternative FA procedures can be used. Described in more detail in Chap. 11, brief FA, trial-based FA, and Interview-Informed Synthesized Contingency Analysis (IISCA) reduce the time required to conduct an FA. Brief FA includes the same conditions and procedures included in traditional FA but reduces the number and duration of sessions (Northup et al., 1991). As compared to the average six and a half hours required to complete an FA, a brief FA takes just 90 min on average (Asmus, Ringdahl, Sellers, Call, Andelman, & Wacker, 2004). Trial-based FA embeds trial-based assessment of contingency conditions (attention, escape, tangible, automatic) within the individual's daily activities (Sigafoos & Saggers, 1995). The maximum trial duration is just 60s and 10–20 trials are delivered for each condition, significantly reducing the time needed to conduct the FA (Sigafoos & Saggers, 1995). IISCA also reduces the number and duration of assessment sessions included in the FA, including just one test and one control condition (Jessel, Hanley, & Ghaemmagami, 2016). Reported estimates of the time to complete IISCA range from 15 to 75 min, requiring far less time than a traditional FA (Hanley, Jin, Vanselow, & Hanratty, 2014; Jessel et al., 2016).

In addition to reducing the time to complete an FA, latency-based FA can reduce the number of times the problem behavior has to occur in order to complete the FA, which is important when the problem behavior is severe and/or presents risk of harm (Lambert et al., 2017; Thomason-Sassi, Iwata, Neidert, & Roscoe, 2011). In latency-based FA, an establishing operation is present and remains until the problem behavior occurs (or until a predetermined time limit), at which time the session ends. The latency from the presentation of the establishing operation to the occurrence of the problem behavior is analyzed across conditions, with one session per condition.

As another alternative to conducting a full, traditional FA, a FA of precursors can be a preferred option when evoking the problem behavior even once may represent a significant risk of harm to the individual or others in the environment (Heath &

Smith, 2019). Rather than evoking and analyzing the problem behavior, behaviors that predictably precede the problem behavior can be the target of a FA. Results from precursor FA have been used to develop effective intervention plans for the severe behavior (Heath & Smith, 2019). As FA procedures are developed, these alternatives should be considered when there are ethical concerns regarding delays in treatment and evoking dangerous behavior.

FBA in Schools

The Individuals with Disabilities Improvement Act (2004) mandates the use of FBA for students with disabilities who engaged in problem behavior. The law requires that an FBA be conducted when there is a change in a student's educational placement as a disciplinary action because of the student's misconduct and the misconduct is due to either the student's disability or the school's failure to adhere to the Individualized Education Program (IEP). Further, IDEA also suggests that schools conduct an FBA whenever a student's behavior interferes with their learning and/or the learning of others. Given the extensive research supporting FBA methods, it is not surprising that it is explicitly included in school law (Gresham, Watson, & Skinner, 2001; Steege et al., 2019). However, with these mandates, schools must ensure that they have capacity to conduct FBAs, including having appropriately trained and credentialed staff who have the professional knowledge and skills to competently conduct an FBA. Available staff within schools may include school psychologists with behavior analytic training. In addition, increasing numbers of educational professionals are seeking and obtaining the BCBA credential and may be employed in schools as school psychologists, intervention specialists, or special education teachers. It is the responsibility of schools to ensure that they have qualified personnel and to fairly evaluate the competence of school professionals to complete FBAs well in order to adhere to IDEA mandates. To support the development of qualified staff, researchers have identified successful methods for training staff to effectively conduct FBA in schools (Loman & Horner, 2014; Strickland-Cohen & Horner, 2015; Strickland-Cohen, Kennedy, Berg, Bateman, & Horner, 2016).

Although the law requires a FBA in certain circumstances, it does not provide specific requirements as to what is involved in the procedures of the FBA. That is, it is up to schools to decide what methods (i.e., indirect FBA, descriptive FBA, FA) may be used to meet this legal requirement. Some states provide more guidance in their state laws, which can help school teams make decision on how to proceed (Collins & Zirkel, 2017). FA is the most supported FBA approach described in the research (Peterson & Neef, 2020; Steege et al., 2019); however, conducting a full FA may not always be feasible due to the often limited resources in schools (Lewis, Mitchell, Harvey, Green, & McKenzie, 2015). Further, a FA may not be necessary in order to develop an effective intervention. Lewis et al. (2015) found that many of the functional hypotheses generated by school personnel based on indirect and descriptive FBA methods matched those from FA. The researchers noted that the results were in contrast to previous studies finding inconsistencies across functional hypotheses derived from FA versus indirect and descriptive FBA (e.g., Payne, Scott, & Conroy, 2007). The authors suggest that improvement in the training of school personnel and more widely available technical support for FBA in schools may be leading to overall better accuracy in FBA data collection and subsequent hypotheses generation (Lewis et al., 2015).

Factors including the severity of the problem behavior, the consistency of data collected through indirect and descriptive FBA methods leading to hypothesized functions, and the capacity of school personnel to implement a FA well should all be considered when deciding which FBA methods will be used. For example, for low-intensity problem behavior that is readily observed in the classroom, with antecedents and consequences consistently described across staff and observed, an FA may be unnecessary and represent a waste of resources. However, for challenging behavior that is high intensity or lacking a discernable pattern based on environmental stimuli, an FA may be critical for effective intervention planning. Regardless which FBA methods are used, it is important that school teams collect data on the effects of the function-based intervention plans developed on student behavior. Problem-solving is a cyclical process and teams should continuously evaluate plans and make changes as necessary when interventions are not having the desired effect. FBA is an ongoing process teams should continue to think functionally about the problem behavior as interventions are implemented and evaluated (Dunlap & Kern, 2018).

Conclusion

Behavior analysts and psychologists are held accountable to the professional behaviors described in relevant ethical codes, including those of the BACB, APA, and NASP. A professional conducting a FBA is engaging in assessment, which is explicitly discussed in these codes. Professionals must consider issues related to the client's right to effective treatment and risk of harm when planning a FBA, especially those involving FA. Several alternatives to traditional FA procedures have been developed to address some of these issues. Further, it is important that informed consent is obtained is documented and that the results of FBA are presented in such a way that the individual being assessed and others involved in treatment planning can understand them to help develop effective intervention plans.

References

American Psychological Association. (2017). *Ethical principles of psychologists and code of conduct*. Washington, D.C.: Author.

Asmus, J. M., Ringdahl, J. E., Sellers, J. A., Call, N. A., Andelman, M. S., & Wacker, D. P. (2004). Use of a short-term impatient model to evaluate aberrant behavior outcome data summaries from 1996-2001. *Journal of Applied Behavior Analysis, 37*, 283–304.

Behavior Analyst Certification Board. (2014). *Professional and ethical compliance code for behavior analysts*. Littleton, CO: Author.

Collins, L. W., & Zirkel, P. A. (2017). Functional behavior assessments and behavior intervention plans: Legal requirements and professional recommendations. *Journal of Positive Behavior Interventions, 19*(3), 180–190.

Crone, D. A., & Horner, R. H. (2000). Contextual, conceptual, and empirical foundations of functional behavioral assessment in schools. *Exceptionality, 8*, 161–172.

Dufrene, B. A., Kazmerski, J. A., & Labrot, Z. (2017). The current status of indirect functional assessment instruments. *Psychology in the Schools, 54*, 331–350.

Dunlap, G., & Kern, L. (2018). Perspectives on functional (behavioral) assessment. *Behavioral Disorders, 43*(2), 316–321.

Ervin, R. A., Radford, P. M., Bertsch, K., & Piper, A. L. (2001). A descriptive analysis and critique of the empirical literature on school-based functional assessment. *School Psychology Review, 30*, 193–210.

Gage, N. A., Lewis, T. J., & Stichter, J. P. (2012). Functional behavioral assessment-based interventions for students with or at-risk for emotional and/or behavioral disorders in school: A hierarchical linear modeling meta-analysis. *Behavioral Disorders, 37*, 55–77.

Goh, A. E., & Bambara, L. M. (2012). Individualized positive behavior support in school settings: A meta-analysis. *Remedial and Special Education, 33*, 271–286.

Gresham, F. M., McIntyre, L. L., Olson-Tinker, H., Dolstra, L., McLaughlin, V., & Van, M. (2004). Relevance of functional behavioral assessment research for school-based interventions and positive behavioral support. *Research in Developmental Disabilities, 25*, 19–37.

Gresham, F., Watson, T. S., & Skinner, C. H. (2001). Functional behavioral assessment: Principles, procedures, and future directions. *School Psychology Review, 30*, 156–172.

Hanley, G. P. (2012). Functional assessment of problem behavior: Dispelling myths, overcoming implementation obstacles, and developing new lore. *Behavior Analysis in Practice, 5*(1), 54–72.

Hanley, G. P., Iwata, B. A., & McCord, B. E. (2003). Functional analysis of problem behavior: A review. *Journal of Applied Behavior Analysis, 36*, 147–185.

Hanley, G. P., Jin, C. S., Vanselow, N. R., & Hanratty, L. A. (2014). Producing meaningful improvements in problem behavior of children with autism via synthesized analyses and treatments. *Journal of Applied Behavior Analysis, 47*, 16–13.

Heath, H., & Smith, R. G. (2019). Precursor behavior and functional analysis: A brief review. *Journal of Applied Behavior Analysis, 52*, 804–810.

Individuals with Disabilities Education Improvement Act of 2004, P.L. 108-446, 20 U.S.C. § 1400 et seq.

Iwata, B., Dorsey, M., Slifer, K., Bauman, K., & Richman, G. (1994). Toward a functional analysis of self-injury. *Journal of Applied Behavior Analysis, 27*, 197–209. (Reprinted from *Analysis and Intervention in Developmental Disabilities, 2*, 3–20, 1982).

Jessel, J., Hanley, G. P., & Ghaemmaghami, M. (2016). Interview-informed synthesized contingency analyses: Thirty replications and reanalysis. *Journal of Applied Behavior Analysis, 49*, 576–595.

Kahng, S., Hausman, N. L., Fisher, A. B., Donaldson, J. M., Cox, J. R., Logo, M., & Wiskow, K. M. (2015). The safety of functional analysis of self-injurious behavior. *Journal of Applied Behavior Analysis, 48*, 107–114. https://doi.org/10.1002/jaba.168

Lambert, J. M., Staubitz, J. E., Roane, J. T., Houchins-Juarez, N. J., Juarez, A. P., Sanders, K. S., & Warren, Z. E. (2017). Outcome summaries of latency-based functional analyses conducted in hospital inpatient units. *Journal of Applied Behavior Analysis, 50*, 487–494.

Lewis, T. J., Mitchell, B. S., Harvey, K., Green, A., & McKenzie, J. (2015). A comparison of functional behavioral assessment and functional analysis methodology among students with mild disabilities. *Behavioral Disorders, 41*(1), 5–20.

Loman, S. L. L., & Horner, R. H. (2014). Examining the efficacy of a basic functional behavioral assessment training package for school personnel. *Journal of Positive Behavior Interventions, 16*, 18–30.

Napolitano, D. A., Knapp, V. M., Speares, E., & McAdam, D. B. (2012). The role of functional assessment in treatment planning. In J. L. Matson (Ed.), *Functional assessment for challenging behaviors* (pp. 213–233). https://doi.org/10.1007/978-1-4614-3037-7

National Association of School Psychologists. (2010). *Principles for professional ethics*. Bethesda, MD: Author.

Northup, J., Wacker, D., Sasso, G., Steege, M., Cigrand, K., Cook, J., & DeRaad, A. (1991). A brief functional analysis of aggression and alternative behavior in an outclinic setting. *Journal of Applied Behavior Analysis, 24*(3), 509–522.

Payne, L. D., Scott, T. M., & Conroy, M. (2007). A school-based examination of the efficacy of function-based intervention. *Behavioral Disorders, 32*, 158–174.

Peterson, S. M., & Neef, N. A. (2020). Functional behavior assessment. In J. O. Cooper, T. E. Heron, & W. L. Heward (Eds.), *Applied behavior analysis* (3rd ed., pp. 628–653). Hoboken, NJ: Pearson.

Poling, A., Austin, J. L., Peterson, S. M., & Mahoney, A. (2012). Ethical issues and considerations. In J. L. Matson (Ed.), *Functional assessment for challenging behaviors* (pp. 213–233). https://doi.org/10.1007/978-1-4614-3037-7

Sigafoos, J., & Saggers, E. (1995). A discrete-trial approach to the functional analysis of aggressive behaviour in two boys with autism. *Journal of Developmental Disabilities, 20*, 287–297.

Steege, M. W., Pratt, J. L., Wickerd, G., Guare, R., & Watson, T. S. (2019). *Conducting school-based functional behavioral assessments: A practitioner's guide* (3rd ed.). New York: Guilford Press.

Strickland-Cohen, M. K., & Horner, R. H. (2015). Typical school personnel developing and implementing basic behavior support plans. *Journal of Positive Behavior Interventions, 17*, 83–94.

Strickland-Cohen, M. K., Kennedy, P. C., Berg, T. A., Bateman, L. J., & Horner, R. H. (2016). Building school district capacity to conduct functional behavioral assessment. *Journal of Emotional and Behavioral Disorders, 24*(4), 235–246.

Thomason-Sassi, J. L., Iwata, B. A., Neidert, P. L., & Roscoe, E. M. (2011). Response latency as an index of response strength during functional analyses of problem behavior. *Journal of Applied Behavior Analysis, 44*, 51–67. https://doi.org/10.1901/jaba.2011.44-51

Thompson, R. H., & Iwata, B. A. (2007). A comparison of outcomes from descriptive and functional analyses of problem behavior. *Journal of Applied Behavior Analysis, 40*, 333–338.

Tincani, M. J., Castrogiavanni, A., & Axelrod, S. (1999). A comparison of the effectiveness of brief versus traditional functional analyses. *Research in Developmental Disabilities, 20*, 327–338. https://doi.org/10.1016/S0891-4222(99)00014-1.

Vollmer, T. R., & Northup, J. (1996). Some implications of functional analysis research. *Research in Developmental Disabilities, 17*, 229–249.

Index

© Springer Nature Switzerland AG 2021
J. L. Matson (ed.), *Functional Assessment for Challenging Behaviors and
Mental Health Disorders*, Autism and Child Psychopathology Series,
https://doi.org/10.1007/978-3-030-66270-7